W9-CFV-242

Psychotic Symptoms in Children and Adolescents

Psychotic Symptoms in Children and Adolescents

Assessment, Differential Diagnosis, and Treatment

Claudio Cepeda

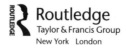
Routledge
Taylor & Francis Group
New York   London

Routledge is an imprint of the
Taylor & Francis Group, an informa business

Routledge
Taylor & Francis Group
270 Madison Avenue
New York, NY 10016

Routledge
Taylor & Francis Group
2 Park Square
Milton Park, Abingdon
Oxon OX14 4RN

© 2007 by Taylor & Francis Group, LLC
Routledge is an imprint of Taylor & Francis Group, an Informa business

Printed in the United States of America on acid-free paper
10 9 8 7 6 5 4 3 2 1

International Standard Book Number-10: 0-415-95364-2 (Hardcover)
International Standard Book Number-13: 978-0-415-95364-1 (Hardcover)

No part of this book may be reprinted, reproduced, transmitted, or utilized in any form by any electronic, mechanical, or other means, now known or hereafter invented, including photocopying, microfilming, and recording, or in any information storage or retrieval system, without written permission from the publishers.

Trademark Notice: Product or corporate names may be trademarks or registered trademarks, and are used only for identification and explanation without intent to infringe.

Visit the Taylor & Francis Web site at
http://www.taylorandfrancis.com

and the Routledge Web site at
http://www.routledgementalhealth.com

Table of Contents

The author has received consultation fees from Lilly, AstraZeneca, Bristol-Myers Squibb, and Pfizer Pharmaceuticals, but does not have any financial affiliation to any of these companies or to any other pharmaceutical manufacturer.

Preface

Psychosis in childhood is not rare. Actually, psychosis is a rather common phenomenon in severe psychiatric conditions. Although psychotic features may go unrecognized for a long time, quite often these features are influential if not determinative of maladaptive behaviors. Psychotic symptoms may be reliably identified with simple questions. Identifying psychotic features is rather simple. Deliberate engagement and systematic and nonleading questioning are the main diagnostic skills that examiners should apply in this area.

Psychiatric examination places a great deal of attention on the nature of the clinical communication and on the detailed analysis of issues related to the presenting symptoms.

The author has extensive experience in dealing with moderate to severe child and adolescent psychopathology, and has developed a simple and systematic method of inquiry to explore these symptoms.

On one occasion, the author made a presentation on psychotic disorders in children and adolescents. One member of the audience objected to the presenter's recommendation for a methodic and systematic exploration of perceptual disorders and delusional symptoms. The objecting psychiatrist asserted that exploring psychotic symptoms in the manner recommended by the author would be very time consuming. To this, the author retorted that to not explore psychotic features in a systematic fashion was a risky practice psychiatrists could not afford. The author reminded the audience that a comprehensive and systematic examination is the most cost-effective intervention that a physician can offer to his or her patients.

Some physicians and some child and adolescent clinicians feel mystified by the process of evaluating psychotic behavior. It should not be so. Children give reliable responses to an interviewer's questions about subjective experiences. Rarely, parents know about the child's psychotic experiences, and usually they are skeptical about the existence of psychotic features in their children. For this reason, in very small children, the author conducts the evaluation of psychotic experiences in the parents' presence and, as indicated in the text, the author engages parents in the diagnostic enquiry.

All the cited cases were seen by the author at the Southwest Mental Health Center (SMHC).[1]

This book is preeminently a clinical text, mostly descriptive. It will be useful to child psychiatrists and child psychologists, to adolescent and general psychiatrists, and to the great variety of mental health professionals (nurses, clinical social workers, special education specialists, and other clinicians) who specialize in the child and adolescent field.

The author agrees with experts who maintain that psychosis in childhood is consequential. Psychotic experiences can certainly submerge, leaving no trace. On the other hand, a significant number of psychotic experiences endure, and they either become organizing psychopathological cores, or they aggravate other comorbid psychiatric conditions.

Chapters 1, 2, 3, 4, 6, 7, and 9 are readily accessible to nonmedical readers; the rest of the book is rather technical and requires some medical or biological background. No matter what the reader's background may be, the chapters on the use of medication with children (chapters 10, 11, 12), and the ones that overview medication side effects (chapter 13) and the treatment of medication side effects (chapter 14), will benefit any reader involved in the process of assessing and treating children and adolescents.

In contemporary psychiatry, biochemical issues at the subcellular levels are the order of the day. The author overviews the most relevant aspects of biological psychiatry that he considers fundamental in clinical practice. It is hoped that the technical aspects of the book do not become too overbearing to nonmedical readers.

The author is sympathetic with international readers who may want to pursue some of the cited references. About 15% of the bibliography relates to Continuing Medical Education (CME) literature that may be inaccessible in foreign countries. In the same vein, another 15% of references are found in new clinical publications that have limited international distribution. The CME presentations were chosen among other things for the relevance of the topics, the clarity of the expositions, the didactic aspects of the programs, the reputation of the faculty, and/or the visual aspects of the programs including graphs and tables.

Acknowledgments

The late Otto Will, M.D., a superb Sullivanian psychotherapist of schizophrenia in the 1970s, used to say that his best teachers were his patients. I do agree with him; we owe a great deal to the people we serve. Each child and each family leave teachings and memories that contribute to our expertise and personal growth. I want to express my gratitude to the multiple children and parents I have had the privilege to treat.

I was invited to organize a conference on Psychosis in Childhood at the Annual Meeting of the Puerto Rico Academy of Psychiatry in 2001. The idea for this book germinated during the preparation for that conference. I am grateful to Jose Manuel Pou, M.D., for such an invitation.

If the best gift of love is the provision of time, I want to express my immense gratitude to so many persons who in one way or another contributed to the culmination of this book. I appreciate and recognize that without the collaboration of so many persons this book might not have reached a successful conclusion. It is likely that my recollection would betray me in remembering many persons who to greater or lesser degree have contributed to making this endeavor a success. That risk notwithstanding, I take such a risk and give public recognition to a number of persons who assisted me in a significant way in the preparation, content, and readability of the text. Nonetheless, I take sole and complete responsibility for the quality of the content.

If being lucky is to have a good wife and a good boss, I am very lucky indeed. I am particularly grateful to my "boss," Graham Rogeness, M.D., for the moral, logistic, and intellectual support of this project. As Medical Director of the Southwest Mental Health Center (SMHC) and President of the Southwest Psychiatric Physicians (SPP), to which I belong, he allowed our busy secretarial staff to assist me in many practical aspects of the preparation of the manuscript. In the same vein, I am very grateful to Fred Hines, CEO of SMHC at San Antonio, for his support of this effort, and for the staff and logistic support provided during the last four years.

Special gratitude is due to Sheila Ortiz, Director of Operations, for the interest she demonstrated in this project, and for the time she spent proofreading a number of chapters. I want to express many thanks to the SPP secretarial staff, and to Diana Gonzales, in particular, for her ongoing assistance throughout the evolution and completion of the book.

As was the case with my first book, *The Concise Guide to the Psychiatric Interview of Children and Adolescents* (APA, 2000), I am immensely indebted to Marie Beyer, LPC, for the enthusiasm that she demonstrated for the new book and for her generosity in spending uncountable time reading and correcting drafts and making suggestions regarding the clarity and readability of the text.

I am very thankful to my SPP colleagues for their professional support and for sharing and discussing a number of vignettes presented in the text. Geoff Gentry, Ph.D., Vice President of Clinical Services and Rick Edwards, LPC, Director of Inpatient Services, at the SMHC, gave helpful suggestions to improve the quality of chapter 9.

Cynthia Mascarenas, PharmD, MS, BCPP, Clinical Assistant Professor, University of Texas College of Pharmacy at Austin and University of Texas Health Science Center at San Antonio, provided input in the psychopharmacological book chapters.

Upon acquaintance with preliminary drafts of the book, Herb Reich, Senior Editor, gave strong support to me, and strove to carry the draft to publication. I am most grateful to him for his editorial assistance and for ironing out the publication contract; his ongoing support for this book is greatly appreciated.

David Booth and Quint Taylor, Director of Information Technology and Network Administrator, respectively, at the SMHC, offered ongoing computer expertise. On more than one occasion, David and Quint helped me to get off a "computer jam." David assisted in the technical aspects of digitizing the drawings and algorithms, and both Dave and Quint were always available and offered assistance on a variety of computer and information processing issues. I want to express my special gratitude to both of them.

Early in the development of the book, Lisa Gustafson, LMSW, former Director of Admission SMHC, read drafts of the first two chapters and gave valuable suggestions.

I disrupted the retirement of my good friend, Gonzalo Mesa, by asking him to assist me in the correlation and completeness of the bibliography, a tedious job. I thank Dr. Mesa for his meticulous job.

Many Child Fellows and General Psychiatric Residents from the Department of Psychiatry, University of Texas Training Program at San Antonio, assisted me with multiple bibliographic searches. Former General Psychiatric Residents Ricardo Salazar, M.D. and Ashley Chen, M.D., as well as former Fellows in Child and Adolescent Psychiatry Jennifer Herron, M.D., Annita Mikita, M.D., Soad Michelsen, M.D. (now a member of SPP), James Brown, M.D., Henry Polk, M.D., and Melissa Watson, M.D., assisted me in this endeavor. In the same vein I am thankful to Juan Zavala, M.D., Tracy Schillerstrom, M.D., Ilianai Torres-Roca, and Lucille Gotanco, M.D., Fellows in Child and

Adolescent Psychiatry at the University of Texas Health Science Center at San Antonio (UTHSCSA) for assisting me in the same area. Dr. Schillerstrom also gave a number of suggestions regarding the clarity of chapters 5 and 6. Special thanks to Peta Clarckson, M.D., former Child Fellow, for her interest, eagerness, and diligence in procuring bibliographic references. Many senior medical students who elected to rotate at the SMHC also assisted me in obtaining bibliographic references. Equally, I express gratitude to Jody Gonzalez, Ph.D., a faculty member at UTHSCSA, for her contribution with important bibliographic references.

My deepest appreciation goes to the staff of EvS Communications for the meticulous job done with the correction of the manuscript and for the enhancement they provided to the readibility of the text.

I am most thankful to David Guadarrama, R.Ph., John Gaston, Chris Rios and Bryan E. Vacek, Alex Camacho and Ana Pechenik, and Bill Simmons, pharmaceutical representatives from Lilly, Jenssen, Astro-Zeneca, Bristol-Myers/Otsuka Pharmaceuticals, and Pfizer, respectively. They provided me with scientific information when requested and facilitated contact with the regional scientific representatives. I want to express my deepest appreciation to each one of them.

Last but not least, I am grateful to my wife Rosalba's unswerving support for the new book; her support is laudable considering her state of ill health. In spite of her delicate health and decreasing energies, she has been excited about this endeavor no matter how much time it has taken away from family and marital life.

CHAPTER 1

Overview of Psychotic Symptoms in Childhood

This chapter will review the following propositions:

- Psychotic symptoms are rather common in clinical practice.
- Psychotic symptoms are common in severe psychiatric disturbances.
- Most of the psychotic features in children and adolescents are associated with affective disorders.
- The great majority of psychotic symptoms of children and adolescents respond to appropriate treatment.
- There are a number of barriers that examiners need to overcome to objectify psychotic disorders.
- Psychotic symptoms in childhood may represent incipient signs of serious psychiatric disorders or may foreshadow serious future psychopathology.
- Oftentimes, psychotic symptoms are not apparent; clinicians need to explore their presence systematically in all patients.
- Serious psychotic disorders may continue into adulthood.
- Psychotic symptoms are seldom trivial. They need close monitoring

THE CONCEPT OF PSYCHOSIS

The concept of psychosis has different levels of explanation. As a symptom, psychosis has traditionally referred to the presence of hallucinations and delusions; as a disorder, and applying the DSM-IV-TR (APA, 2000) definition of mental disorder, the term *psychotic disorder* refers to a significant clinical behavioral and psychological pattern or syndrome that occurs in an individual and that is associated with distress and disability (impairment in one or more important areas of functioning, or developmental progression), or with a significant increased risk of death (suicide), suffering pain (due to distressing symptoms), disability, or an important loss of freedom due to fear or misinterpretation of reality, secondary to abnormal perception, paranoia, or thought disorder,

1

among others (DSM-IV-TR, 2000, p. xxxi). The *Dorland's Illustrated Medical Dictionary* (1994) gives a very succinct definition of illness: "a condition marked by pronounced deviation from the normal healthy state." The subheading of "Mental Illness" refers the reader to the concept of *disorder* (p. 819), and the term is defined as a "derangement or abnormality of function; a morbid physical or mental state" (p. 492). This short definition of illness agrees with the explanatory definition of disorder obtained from the DSM-IV-TR described above. The concept of psychiatric disorder is customarily used to describe what is informally designated as mental illness.

Psychotic symptoms may emerge in isolation from other disturbances, be coterminous with other disturbances (frequently affective disturbances), or be a substantial component of a major psychotic disorder. Isolated psychotic symptoms, not associated with other psychiatric symptoms, are of no clinical concern because they do not interfere with adaptive functioning. Psychotic symptoms may be secondary to substance abuse or may be associated with other psychiatric disorders, such as mood disorders, anxiety disorders, and others. The DSM-IV-TR established that psychotic symptoms represent an element of severity of the mood or anxiety syndromes, but they become indispensable, prominent, and incapacitating symptoms in patients with severe primary psychotic disorders (so-called "functional" psychotic disorders).

Thought disorder and negative symptoms are also cardinal associated symptoms of severe psychotic disorders (schizophrenic spectrum disorders). Bipolar disorder, in its moderate and severe presentations, may be associated with significant psychotic features. At times, it is difficult to differentiate one category of disorder from the other. Formerly, there was a rigid separation between the so-called thought disorders (schizophrenic disorders) and the mood disorders (unipolar and bipolar disorders), the belief being that certain forms of thought disorder were exclusive of the schizophrenias. Although, this belief is now considered inaccurate, the distinction between thought disorders and mood disorders is still maintained. However, the boundaries of these disorders are not as distinct and specific as was previously postulated (see chapter 8).

In recent years, a number of accompanying deficits such as disorganized behavior, cognitive deficits, and a variety of neuropsychological deficits have been recognized, and added to the definition of severe psychotic disorders.

In the study of psychosis in childhood and adolescence, the dimension of development needs to be considered. A severe psychosis in childhood causes developmental deviations, impairs the acquisition of adaptive skills, and handicaps the child in a multiplicity of adaptive domains: neuromotor, cognitive, learning, interpersonal, social–adaptive, and subjective functioning.

There is a growing consensus regarding the progression and continuity of the symptomatology (illness/disorder) from childhood to adulthood for a number of psychotic disorders. There is also an increasing recognition that severe, chronic, and progressive psychotic disorders have a neurobiological substrate, and that genetic, neurodevelopmental, neurodegenerative, and neurochemical factors, as well as adverse environmental conditions, contribute to the expression (onset and maintenance) of the disorder. Most of these issues will be discussed in chapter 8.

RISKS FACTORS FOR PSYCHOTIC DISORDERS

Multiple risks factors have been considered in the development of psychotic disorders. These include: changes in mental status, such as depression or anxiety; subjective complaints, impaired cognitive, emotional, motor, and automatic functioning; changes in bodily sensations and in external perception; low tolerance for normal stress; drug and alcohol usage; neurocognitive impairment; obstetric complications; and delays in milestones achievement. Possible trait markers include neurological abnormalities and poor premorbid adjustment (Phillips et al., 2002, p. 261). Patients at risk for psychotic disorders have some positive neurological findings; however, the nature of the neurological abnormalities is unclear. Curiously, patients with larger (though still within the normal range) left hippocampal volumes at intake were more likely to develop a psychotic episode in the subsequent 12-month period. Furthermore, comparison of the MRIs of patients who underwent a psychotic episode with MRIs at intake revealed neurological structural changes in the left insula cortex and in the left posteriomedial temporal structures, including the hippocampus and posterior hippocampus gyrus during the transition to psychosis (Phillips et al., 2002).

PREVALENCE OF PSYCHOTIC SYMPTOMS

Psychotic symptoms are not uncommon experiences in the lives of children; they are not uncommon findings in clinical practice, either. Psychotic features occur more frequently in children than originally thought. Severe psychotic disorders are uncommon in childhood. This proposition is supported by Reimherr and McClellan (2004), who asserted that "Although, psychotic illnesses are relatively rare in youths, especially younger children, these disorders are not uncommon in clinical settings and must be considered in the evaluation of every individual patient" (p. 10). Although psychotic symptoms are rather common in clinical practice, this is not so in regard to the frequency or prevalence of psychotic disorders.

In clinical populations, the prevalence of psychotic symptoms in children and adolescents has been reported as 4 and 8%, respectively. Psychosis becomes more prevalent with increasing age (Birmaher, 2003, p. 257).

In community samples, prevalence of psychosis (psychotic symptoms) in children and adolescents has been estimated to be about 1%. Auditory hallucinations (about 8%) are the most frequent psychotic symptoms. Delusional beliefs in children are less complex than those in adolescents, and their frequency is estimated at about 4% (Ulloa et al., 2000).

In epidemiological studies in adults, 3 to 5% of the subjects report psychotic symptoms before age 21. In a cohort of 2,031 children aged 5 to 21, evaluated at a mood and anxiety disorder clinic, 4.5% of the evaluated children had a definite psychosis (defined as having the presence of a definite hallucination and a definite delusion), and 4.7% had probable psychosis (defined as having the presence of a suspected or likely hallucination, or a suspected or likely delusion). For patients with definite psychotic symptoms, 41% had a major depressive disorder; 24% were diagnosed with bipolar disorder; and 21% were diagnosed as depressive disorder not fulfilling criteria for major depressive disorder. In 14% of the cases, patients received a schizophreniform spectrum disorder diagnosis: four patients had schizophrenia, and nine patients had schizoaffective disorder. Patients with anxiety and disruptive disorders who presented with definite psychotic symptoms always had a comorbid mood disorder (Ulloa et al., 2000, p. 339).

Mood disorders were the most frequent conditions associated with psychosis. These observations are in line with prevalence community studies in general populations; for instance, in a representative sample of 7,076 subjects (aged 18 to 64 years), psychoticlike symptoms were strongly associated with psychotic disorders (van Os, Hanssen, Bijl, & Volleberg, 2001, p. 667).

Among the psychotic symptoms, hallucinations were the most prevalent symptoms in 80% of patients (73.6% endorsed auditory command hallucinations), followed by delusions (22%) and thought disorder (3.3%). Thought disorder was only present (or perhaps only recognized) in adolescents. Hallucinations perceived as coming from outside of the head were more common in adolescents than in children. The frequency of other perceptual disturbances in psychotic children was as follows: 38.5% visual hallucinations, 26.2% olfactory hallucinations, and 9.9% tactile hallucinations. Delusions of reference were the most common type of delusions: delusions that people "could read my mind," "could know my own thoughts," or that other people "could hear my thoughts" were less common (Van Os et al., 2001). Usually, these delusional symptoms are rare and only present in severe psychotic disorders, and when present, they are more common in middle to late adolescence and beyond.

REASONS PSYCHOSIS IS UNDERDIAGNOSED IN CHILDREN AND ADOLESCENTS

Clinicians have hesitated to explore perceptual abnormalities or delusional thinking in childhood. Some clinicians feel mystified when they explore psychosis in children. This contributes to the high rate of misdiagnosis and underdiagnosis of psychotic disorders in childhood.

Problems with misdiagnosis probably reflect clinicians' reluctance to consider this diagnosis, a lack of familiarity with clinical presentations of psychosis in childhood, or idiosyncratic practices; it is also true that many cases are difficult to characterize until enough time has passed for the disturbing process to provide a clear pattern of the unfolding illness. The use of standardized diagnostic practices, adherence to diagnostic criteria, and systematic symptom exploration improve accuracy.

Children typically do not share their disordered perceptual experiences or delusional beliefs with parents or other trusted adults. For children, psychotic features belong to the realm of private or secret experiences that are seldom divulged to significant others. Frequently, parents only become aware of the presence of psychotic symptoms when the child starts displaying abnormal behaviors.

Older children and adolescents who develop a psychotic illness often have some recognition that something is wrong with their thinking, perception, or behavior; they feel frightened due to a feeling of confusion in their sense of reality. Perceptual disturbances and paranoid feelings further limit a patient's willingness to discuss symptoms with caretakers or providers because the individual has a penumbra of awareness of his or her abnormal experiences.

Some parents normalize psychotic experiences or expect that "children will grow out" of them. This idea may be reinforced by professionals; sometimes pediatricians and even mental health professionals support these naïve expectations and give parents false reassurances. Parents are often told that these unusual experiences are trivial and temporary. Sadly, this contributes to delays in identification and treatment of early presentations of psychotic symptoms. Even psychiatrists may miss the symptoms underlying psychosis as they focus on presenting behavioral manifestations such as aggression or suicide (Semper & McClellan, 2003, p. 682).

As an example of how parents are misguided or falsely reassured, Schaffer and Ross (2002) describe initial experiences of parents of schizophrenic children with professionals:

> Once the psychotic symptoms began, the common predominant theme was frustration with the lack of a clear and finite diagnosis at an earlier stage of development. Consistently, they reported telling pediatricians and school psychologists that something was "seriously wrong." Of those [parents] who recognized psychotic symptoms early, three (out of 17) were explicitly told by a medical professional that "schizophrenia does not exist in children." Eight families (out of 17) specifically stated that they questioned schizophrenia as a possible cause of the child's symptoms but were told by more than one mental health or medical professional that psychotic symptoms in childhood are not necessarily schizophrenia, and, since the diagnosis could not be made, antipsychotic medications were not indicated.

One mother quoted a psychologist as having told her: "Let's make friends with the voices." This confusion over the meaning of psychotic symptoms was associated with a mean two-year delay in diagnosis, and the trial and failure of alternative treatment plans. Specifically, many trials of mood stabilizers occurred during this period, as did trials of alternative treatments. In all cases, once the diagnosis of schizophrenia was determined and antipsychotic medications were used, a significant change was seen in baseline symptoms. (p. 543)

Psychotic symptoms are baffling for children and parents. Children with psychotic symptoms experience a lack of understanding and support from significant others when they reveal disturbing perceptions or beliefs; as a consequence, they learn to keep abnormal experiences to themselves, increasing, then, their fear and sense of alienation. It is not uncommon to hear from disturbed children that they have suffered from psychotic experiences for a long time, even years, or that the psychotic experiences began in early childhood. It is when the child no longer feels able to control the psychotic influence that the psychosis becomes manifested in unmistakably abnormal or bizarre behaviors.

Some parents become defensive when they become aware that their children are experiencing psychotic symptoms. Others attribute an ominous connotation to psychotic symptoms, not knowing that most of the psychotic symptoms are amenable to appropriate interventions.

Psychotic symptoms in their offspring often confront parents with their own disturbed sense of reality. Not infrequently, psychotic symptoms in children trigger in the parents painful memories of their own developmental experiences: these symptoms remind parents of their own unusual experiences, of psychotic parents or relatives, or of other disturbing events in their past. It is not unusual, when a child endorses psychotic features, that other family members may endorse psychotic symptoms as well.

Psychotic symptoms should be taken seriously and clinicians need to alert parents to take appropriate steps to prevent the disturbed child from acting out his or her psychotic beliefs. When dealing with psychotic symptoms, the first priority for parents should be to guarantee the safety of the child and that of siblings and caretakers. This is particularly true when the child experiences auditory command hallucinations telling the child to either kill others or to kill himself. A child misguided by distorted beliefs may also pose a serious risk to others when he believes that he needs to defend himself against a falsely perceived persecutor or external danger.

Psychotic symptoms do not occur in isolation; therefore, psychotic symptoms in the context of an otherwise normal mental status examination warrant skepticism (Reimherr & McClelland, 2004, p. 6). Relevant psychotic symptoms impair the child's adaptive capacity in a variety of areas.

TABLE 1.1 Risk factors of psychotic disorders

- Homicidal behavior
- Suicidal behavior
- Terroristic behavior
- Impulsive/self-defeating behaviors
- Alcohol and drug abuse
- Gang participation/antisocial behavior
- Unwanted pregnancies/STDs
- Poor compliance and relapse risk
- School difficulties
- Social and vocational problems
- Self-neglect
- Victimization

RISKS ASSOCIATED WITH PSYCHOTIC SYMPTOMS

Psychotic patients, especially those who are paranoid, have an increased potential for violent and homicidal behaviors. These risks need to be explored and monitored systematically.

Homicidal Behavior

The risk is higher if the patient has history of aggressive/violent behaviors, or if he or she has already planned or has taken steps to do personal harm. The Tarasoff decision places a burden of disclosure and creates confidentiality challenges for clinicians and physicians; the specific rules of disclosure vary from state to state. The physician needs to be familiar with the obligations to warn potential victims in the state where he or she practices.

Here is an example of a psychotic adolescent with strong homicidal feelings:

Crissy, a 15-year-old white teenager, was evaluated because she threatened to hurt herself and the family. She had never received a psychiatric evaluation before, in spite of extensive behavioral difficulties and ongoing psychological distress.

The patient reported feeling suicidal for at least a couple of years and endorsed a history of multiple suicidal attempts. She disclosed strong and enduring homicidal thoughts against her stepfather. She had been close to stabbing him with a butcher knife and harbored the plan of "cutting his balls during his sleep." She said she would put the "balls" in his mouth for him to choke. She claimed that he had sexually abused her for a number of years, subjecting her to a variety of sexual acts except vaginal intercourse. Crissy stated that she had told her mother about this but her mother had not done anything about it. She reported that she was aware that her stepfather was abusive to her mother, and that the family had been in a shelter for battered women the year before.

Crissy stated that she was not attending school, that she was being home-schooled. Actually, she informed the examiner that her mother was not following the prescribed curriculum and that she was "way behind the learning she was supposed to have."

Crissy also reported that her mother needed her and felt very strongly that, without her around, her mother would fall apart. Crissy claimed that, instead of studying, she was expected to clean the house and help her mother with the younger sisters, 8 and 4 years old. Crissy stated that although her mother said she loved her, she did not feel it nor believe it. She said she had substituted her mother's love for that of one of her friends. At the time of the psychiatric evaluation, Crissy was dating a 23-year-old illegal immigrant of whom her family strongly disapproved. She was sexually involved with him.

Crissy stated that the only time she did not feel sad or bored was when she was with her friends. She said she had been depressed for years. She denied any drug use or any legal trouble but acknowledged that she had run away a number of times, the longest for four days. She asserted that she wanted to leave home and join her friends, some of whom were homeless. She forcefully affirmed that she did not want to return home.

The mental status examination revealed the presence of a rather attractive, though mildly overweight adolescent, who appeared to be her stated age. Long strands of her hair covered most of her face; she made only limited eye contact, and frequently became downcast. She was guarded, distant, and disdainful, but was very articulate. Her mood appeared depressed; she displayed marked constriction of affect. At times, she displayed an inappropriate smile and represented a veiled grandiosity. She endorsed suicidal and homicidal ideation and, as indicated, she harbored a homicidal plan toward her stepfather.

She endorsed command hallucination and visual hallucinations; voices told her to kill her stepfather and other people. Voices told her to kill herself, too. She indicated she could not control the voices but had learned to manage them by writing poetry, drawing, and listening to music. She also endorsed florid para-noid ideation. Crissy seemed very intelligent; she demonstrated good abstracting capacity and used very sophisticated language.

Because Crissy had expressed intentions to hurt herself and to kill her step-father, and since she stated she did not want to return home, she was referred to an acute psychiatric program. Child Protective Services (CPS) was contacted.

In the following vignette the child's psychotic perception put her younger brother in clear danger.

Rosa was an eight-year-old Hispanic female who was admitted to a preadolescent inpatient psychiatric program after she attempted to stab her four-year old brother with a knife. Her mother reported that, for a long time, Rosa had attempted to hurt her brother. She was very physically abusive and mean to him. Rosa had suffered prolonged sexual abuse by her stepfather, the father of her brother. The abuse entailed intercourse for many months. The abuse finally stopped when Rosa revealed the abuse to one of her teachers.

When the examiner attempted to understand the reasons for Rosa's ongoing homicidal ideation toward his half-brother, she said that her brother looked pretty much like his abusive stepfather, whom she felt extremely angry about. Her mother confirmed that there was a striking resemblance between the brother and his father. Rosa's identification of her hateful step-father with her half-brother was to a great extent the explanation of her homicidal behavior.

Suicidal Behavior

Suicidal behavior is common in psychotic children and adolescents. At times, children and adolescents feel helpless when experiencing auditory command hallucinations telling them to kill themselves, and often, give in to the self-destructive commands. Other times, suicidal behavior arises from a deep sense of hopelessness and despair, from an overwhelming sense of internal damage, or from a sense of having a hopelessly deranged mind. Stressors at home, school, and in interpersonal relationships also contribute, as do alcohol and drug abuse. Lack of compliance with psychotropic medications increases suicide risk. If the patient is on psychotropics, compliance helps reduce the risk of self-harm. Attending to the child's depression and to negative environmental imput (expressed emotion, see chapter 9) also lessens the risk. Above all, improving the psychotic state ameliorates the child's subjective state and helps to restore the patient's trust in him- or herself and the feeling that it is good to be alive.

Terroristic Behavior

Paranoid children who feel ostracized by peers, and those who harbor grievances against teachers or other school authority figures or authority in general, may develop plans or actually attempt to implement destructive and homicidal schemes to avenge wrongs and other perceived injustices. These adolescents' hatred is frequently extended against symbols of authority or of government representatives. Any child or adolescent who makes even a veiled terroristic threat should receive a comprehensive psychiatric evaluation. Assessment of these children is discussed in chapter 3.

Currently, every time a child makes a veiled or overt terroristic threat in the school setting, he is referred for an emergency psychiatric evaluation. The stereotypic picture is the one of an adolescent male (14–16 years old), depressed and paranoid, who feels isolated and ostracized by peers. This individual carries intense resentments against the authorities at school, or authorities in general, and feels the need to avenge the slights or rejections he experiences from peers or persons in power. Universally, this type of adolescent feels misunderstood, and complains that nobody, including his parents, listens or pays any attention to him. Commonly, the family is unaware of the child's feeling or of the severity of the adolescent's anger and potential destructiveness. Such children often endorse suicidal and homicidal ideation, and feel paranoid and hopeless.

Recent reports of massacres in schools are tragic and sad; it is tempting to think that some of these catastrophes could have been averted with early detection and timely intervention for the youths at risk.

Impulsive/Self-Defeating Behaviors

Psychosis increases suicide risk and the risk for self-abusive behaviors.

> A 12-year-old white boy was referred for a psychiatric evaluation after he attempted to break a glass display containing firearms. He was arrested and charged. This child was very psychotic and harbored active homicidal ideation. He stated that procuring a gun would allow him to actualize his delusional beliefs of being Superman.

In this example, the psychotic and impulsive child came into conflict with the law. Had he accomplished his goal, the consequences would have been disastrous.

At other times, psychotic children go on "joy rides" and wreck cars, putting their own and other people's safety at risk. Delusional, grandiose adolescents falsify checks, develop schemes for making "lots of easy money," and are driven by unrealistic expectations: they want be in the hall of fame or to become football or basketball superstars. In a more grandiose delusional vein, they believe they are superheroes capable of extraordinary actions. These children commit antisocial acts due to their poor judgment and their marginal sense of reality.

Alcohol and Drug Abuse

Abuse of and addiction to illegal substances is a common complication of psychotic illness. Frequently, patients attempt to self-medicate by using mind-altering substances. Substance abuse needs to be explored systematically in the diagnostic assessment and in the follow-up with psychotic patients. Some patients attempt to cope with feelings of alienation or with the terror of a mental breakdown by using drugs that alter their sense of reality or their dysphoric emotional state. Alcohol and drugs make children and adolescents "forget" their disturbing worries or ameliorate psychotic anxieties at the cost of impairing judgment, motivation, and adaptive coping.

Children and adolescents with psychotic and drug abuse problems are designated as dual diagnoses cases. The presence of substance abuse in a psychotic child demands concomitant treatment of the alcohol or chemical dependency problem.

The lifetime prevalence of alcohol and drug abuse disorders in persons with schizophrenia is 58.5% and 47% respectively (Brunette, Noordsy, & Green, 2005, p. 29).

Gang Participation and Antisocial Behaviors

Paranoia is rampant in gang members; a delusion shared by the entire group may provide coherence and a sense of identity to its members. Grandiose and paranoid leaders do not appreciate the potential danger by which they are surrounded.

> Al, an 18-year-old Latino male, with long history of conduct disorder and many years of bipolar illness with broad paranoid features, revealed to his psychiatrist in a follow-up session that he was "the president of a gang." He was very proud of his role in the group. A few weeks later, he was assaulted by rival gang members and was badly beaten with brass knuckles. He sustained multiple fractures of the facial bones and suffered severe injuries of the soft facial tissues necessitating extensive facial reconstructive surgery. He had barely recovered from the assault when he organized a party. Al got into a conflict with an uninvited guest and asked that individual to leave. This fellow became irate and left. Al and some friends, believing that the conflict had been resolved, left the apartment and continued conversing in the street. Unexpectedly, the uninvited individual drove his truck into the group. Al was not able to evade the oncoming speeding truck. The truck ran over him, causing a severe brain injury. Al was comatose for more than a month. Surprisingly, he came out of the coma and began to recover from a massive right hemispheric injury.

This is but one example among the innumerable media accounts of murders, assaults, drive-by shootings, and other criminal incidents associated with gang activity.

Unwanted Pregnancies/STDs

Psychotic females run a high risk of being sexually victimized; sexual assaults have the associated risks of sexually transmitted diseases and unwanted pregnancies. Psychotic females are inconsistent in attending to appropriate birth control or protective methods. If the pregnancies are maintained, they are often complicated by poor nutrition and limited medical care, as well as exposure of the embryo/fetus to alcohol or illegal substances, which contribute to severe neurodevelopmental problems in children thus conceived. Mothers with a poor sense of reality provide erratic mothering at best, and are at a higher risk of neglecting and abusing their children than nonpsychotic mothers.

Poor Compliance and Relapse Risk

A report has indicated that psychiatrists underestimate the problems of medication compliance and treatment adherence. In one study clinicians only detected one case in 21 as having compliance difficulties. In reality, 13 of 21 cases displayed adherence problems when electronic monitoring and other more objective measures were used (see chapter 10). Oftentimes, compliance issues are related to medication side effects such as dysphoria, affect flattening, sexual side effects, or poor therapeutic effects. Such side effects or lack of response need to be identified. Weight is an important cause of noncompliance. Weight gain has become a major obstacle for consistent mood stabilizers and antipsychotic adherence because most of these medications promote weight gain. The weight increase may be considerable; some antipsychotics promote it more that others. These complications will be addressed in the discussion of mood stabilizers' side effects (see chapter 13) and atypical medications side effects in general, and in the discussion of each atypical medication in particular (see chapter 12).

Occasionally, patients do not want to give up a symptom's secondary gain and stop medication to reactivate the psychosis, which gives them a sense of power and a unique identity.

> A 13-year-old African American girl was evaluated for violent behavior and issues associated with her sexual identity. The mental status examination evidenced strong delusional beliefs: she thought she was born on Mars. She also reported that she hated to be a girl and that she hated to dress like one. This patient was placed on neuroleptics and by all external appearances she had a very positive response to the medication. The family was pleased with the change in her mood and demeanor, especially with the decrease of her hostility. She was more pleasant and began behaving in a more feminine manner.
>
> After a number of weeks, this adolescent surprised her psychiatrist by complaining about the changes she was experiencing. She asserted that the medications had taken her anger away and she did not like that; she also protested that the medications were making her act more like a girl and she hated that, as well.

The next example illustrates why some adolescents adhere to psychotic features:

> About the time that Crissy's psychiatric evaluation (cited above) was ending, the examiner asked Crissy how he could help. She said that she didn't feel the examiner could help. The examiner confronted her with her depression and she

responded by saying that she was used to it; the examiner confronted her with the suicidal ideation, and she replied that she did not care to get rid of those feelings. She certainly stressed she did not want to get rid of the homicidal feelings toward her stepfather. When the examiner confronted her with the voices, she said she did not want to get rid of the voices because they gave her company when she felt lonely.

The need to reactivate the symptom(s) may be suspected in patients who do well for a while and then stop adhering to the medication regime.

School Difficulties

Psychotic children and adolescents have difficulties applying themselves to academic tasks. Although poor motivation is a major factor, other problems, such as difficulty with sustained attention and information processing difficulties, memory difficulties, and other neuropsychological problems, may also play a role. For many psychotic children, going to school is a major effort in itself. Parents struggle on a daily basis to send chronically psychotic children to school. Schoolwork and assignments require an inordinate amount of prompting and encouragement. Children with chronic psychosis, regardless of the degree of their intelligence or the intactness of their neuropsychological functioning, lag behind the scholastic achievement levels of their nonpsychotic peers.

Social and Vocational Problems

Persons with chronic psychosis seldom attain independent living status. Many children and adolescents (and young adults) with psychotic disorders suffer from chronic social, vocational, and adaptive handicaps. The most successful patients are able to continue their college education, go into technical careers, or enter more specific vocational training programs. Others with more severe problems need support from social agencies and live in semi-independent, supervised, or sheltered environments, at best. The most impaired may require intermittent or chronic institutionalization. The vast majority of chronically psychotic individuals are supported by a variety of government programs on a permanent basis.

In one study, early onset schizophrenia (nonaffective) spectrum disorders showed a chronic course with a poor outcome in 79% of the patients, while 74% of early onset affective psychosis patients showed a good to intermediate outcome. The poor outcome of 26% of the patients with affective psychosis was related to mental retardation in 7% of the patients, and to a progression to schizoaffective disorder in 12% of the patients. The worst outcome was seen in schizophrenia spectrum patients with a family history of nonaffective psychosis (Jarbin, Ott, & von Knorring, 2003, p. 176; see chapter 7 and table 7-3).

Self-Neglect

Chronically psychotic children and adolescents are usually careless in matters of hygiene and self-care. Some become malnourished because they do not eat on a regular basis. Others become obese because of poor nutritional habits and the influence of antipsychotic medications. Because of a lack of attention to their bodies, many psychotic children and adolescents have chronic untreated medical conditions including infections, STDs, hepatitis, diabetes, TB, HIV, or skin conditions (tineas, skin infections, etc.). Dental health is usually poor.

> Chris, a 14-year-old Latino, was evaluated for severe depression and suicidal ideation necessitating acute care hospitalization. He had a long history of difficulties relating to others and had a number of prior psychiatric treatments.
>
> During the psychiatric assessment, he displayed prominent negative symptoms and inappropriate smiling. He also endorsed positive symptoms. During the physical examination, the psychiatrist noticed poor hygiene. Upon inspecting his feet, he noticed extensive fungal infection on both feet ("athlete's foot"). Actually, the patient displayed the longest, most unsightly toenails the psychiatrist had ever seen. The examiner jokingly wondered if the patient was planning on participating in the *Guinness Book of Records*. The psychiatrist ordered a clipping of the toenails and ordered antimichotic medication. A couple of days later, the physician wanted to check the progress of treatment of the patient's feet; the patient became paranoid and objected to removing his shoes and socks. He feared that people were going to look at his feet, and became very secretive when the physician inspected his feet because he had refused the clipping of his toenails.

Victimization

For psychotic children and adolescents, by and large, the most common and hurtful victimization occurs in the school setting. Psychotic children are frequently teased and ostracized. These children's peers play embarrassing pranks on them, and abuse them verbally or physically. Some psychotic, vulnerable children fall prey to manipulation and machinations by their brighter and more adept class- and schoolmates. The author recalls a white teenager, who was psychotic and had Asperger's and wanted to have friends. Some schoolmates devised conditions for their "friendship," such as, telling her she would have to eat pebbles, or even more disgustingly, she would have to eat feces. Sadly, she complied.

Chronically psychotic adolescents are frequently victims of crimes and exploitation. Since they are not adept in social situations, their social judgment is faulty. Mentally ill adolescents are frequently taken advantage of by adults, more so if they are females. Victimization is common in runaway psychotic adolescents who do not have any place to stay or anything to eat. Rape is not rare in chronically psychotic female adolescents.

IS THE CHILD PSYCHOTIC OR IS HE IMAGINING THINGS?

The age when children are able to discriminate reality from make-believe, when normal children are able to differentiate reality from fantasy, is relevant for the assessment of psychosis. Pilowsky quotes Despert (1948) who asserted that a normal child of average intelligence is fully able to distinguish between fantasy and reality by the age of 3 years (Pilowsky, 1998, p. 3). The present writer concurs with Despert.

A case of a psychotic 4½-year-old child is described (Cepeda, 2000). Briefly, this 4½-years-old Hispanic child would take a knife to his room to defend himself and his family against the "jingle," which was coming to kill them (pp. 112–113). Another 4½-year-old white boy was unable to sleep because the "scable" was coming to kill him and his family. The following vignette reports an even younger preschooler example. Notice that in both examples there was a neologistic creation.

Blond was 3 years and 1 month old when he was brought in for a psychiatric evaluation due to marked aggressiveness and hyperactive behaviors. According to his biological mother, Blond was very aggressive toward her and toward his 2-month-old baby brother. With precocious language, Blond had threatened to kill his mother and had made frequent threats to kill other people; he even reported that he would like to kill and eat people, "to roll up people in a taco and eat it." Blond's mother reported that he had tried to hit his baby brother with a bat. The child had difficulties sleeping at night. As an example of how mean Blond was, mother reported that, a number of times, he had gone to people who were sleeping and had hit them in the face; she also said that he also had tried to choke a kitten. A number of times, he had gone to a neighbor's home and been openly aggressive to unfamiliar children.

Blond's mother said that the child started to display behavioral problems by the second year of life and that it appeared his behavior had worsened when it became apparent that his mother was pregnant. He hit mother in the stomach many times while she was pregnant.

His mother reported that Blond was an out-of-wedlock child. He was a full-term baby who was delivered by C-section. He was described as a cuddly and affectionate baby. His mother reported no delays in developmental milestones (crawling, walking, or speaking); he had poor social skills, however. He had been unsuccessful in making and keeping friends. Blond could indicate that he needed to go to the bathroom but had not acquired complete toilet training by the time of the evaluation.

Blond's 5-year-old brother had an extensive psychiatric hospital history for related behaviors, and had been hospitalized for violent and destructive behaviors. CPS had been involved with the family in connection to the older brother, but that agency had not received any complaints regarding Blond. Apparently, Blond's biological father had been abusive to his biological mother in front of the children in the past. Blond's father also had a history of drug use and possibly had been incarcerated in the past.

Blond's mother reported suffering from depression and claimed that she had been on medications related to a "postpartum depression." She also claimed that her live-in boyfriend had problems with bipolar disorder and that, at times, he had problems controlling himself.

Blond was a very small and handsome, blue-eyed child; he moved around the evaluation room displaying no regard for the adults around him. He showed no gross motor difficulties. He used his hands, demonstrating good coordination and satisfactory fine motors skills. Although he maintained good eye contact with the interviewer, he did not utter a single word during most the evaluation.

The mother had brought in the child's baby brother, in a baby carriage, to the evaluation room; during the examination Blond moved around the baby in a careless and impulsive manner. Blond would not respond to his mother's verbal redirections and very soon it became apparent that Blond was very testy and quite defiant. It also became apparent that mother addressed the child in an irritated tone.

When the interviewer attempted to explore some facts related to mother's background she became defensive. The examiner had to reassure her that he was trying to help her with the child, and that the more he knew about her, the better he would be able to assist her. She seemed to accept this proposition.

Although the examiner attempted some verbal engagement, the child remained electively mute. When the examiner brought a pail of large Legos of multiple colors, the child increased the interaction with the examiner at a non-verbal level. The child showed the examiner a tall tower he constructed with the Legos. The examiner praised the child and assisted him in building supports for the tower. During these playful interactions the examiner explored whether the child could tell the Legos' colors, and other basic vocabulary and cognitive probings. In a short time, the child was offering Legos to the examiner; however, the child was not talking yet.

Blond's mood was euthymic, but at times he appeared to be a bit reserved; his demeanor was serious until he became nonverbally engaged with the examiner. When the examiner questioned if the child was ever scared, the mother reported that at times Blond seemed to be scared at night. When the examiner asked if Blond was scared of monsters, the mother readily indicated that, as a matter of fact, Blond had been saying that monsters bothered him. The examiner invited Blond to talk about the monsters. Blond said this time, that the monsters hid in the closet. When the examiner wondered what the monsters did, Blond stated the monsters tried to "poke" him, and when the examiner asked Blond what he wanted the psychiatrist to do with the monsters, the child responded that he would like the doctor "to take the monsters away from the closet, away from the home." He said that he "did not like to see the monsters." Her mother stated that the child had told her that the monsters said scary things to Blond. The content was unclear. When the examiner asked Blond what he would like to do to the monsters, Blond replied, "I'd like to step on them."

This is the youngest child with clear psychotic features the author has encountered. It is clear that the psychotic symptoms were dystonic, and that he wanted the monsters to go away. The undeniable family dysfunction had an important bearing on the child's maladaptive functioning and on the child's reality testing difficulties.

Pilowsky (1998) warns that,

> At times a child may deliberately withhold information about his or her hallucinations as a result of very specific situational anxieties, such as the fear of being hospitalized and thus separated from the parents or the fear of admitting to "bad thoughts" when the content of the hallucinations is of an aggressive or sexual nature.

We should also consider that the child's fear that they "are going insane" or "crazy" may contribute to him or her withholding information about hallucinations, or to the denial of delusional beliefs. Adults do not credit children with the capacity to distinguish fantasy from reality (reality testing function), even though intelligent children as young as 3 to 4 years of age are able to differentiate reality from fantasy. Children as early as 5 to 6 years of age (and probably younger), can accurately state whether a reported experience is "pretend or real."

Parents often dismiss their children's idiosyncratic experiences by attributing them to imagination, as creations of the infantile mind, or as byproducts of the influence of movies or TV. In more religious or superstitious milieus, psychotic symptoms are attributed to the influence of the devil or to other malignant or supernatural sources.

Often, significant others express skepticism about the child's endorsement of psychotic features. In order to ascertain if the child's productions are the result of a vivid imagination or psychosis, the psychiatrist needs to challenge the child's account; if the child persists in his distorted perceptions or beliefs, a gentle confrontation adds a sense of conviction to the attribution of psychosis. Thus, after the child says, for instance, that he is hearing voices, the examiner may challenge her or his assertion: Could it be that your imagination is playing a trick on you? Are you imagining this? Or, in stronger terms, is this real? Are you putting me on? Psychotic children stick to their claims and persevere in the factuality of their complaints.

A 7-year-old white boy, with a history of some neurodevelopmental delays (delays in the milestones, delays in speech development), and with an extensive history of aggressive and violent behaviors, was convinced he was Superman. In spite of the psychiatrist's challenges to his beliefs he persisted in asserting he was "the man of steel." When the psychiatrist demanded proof, the child said he had special powers in his eyes, he could burn things with "the lava that comes from my eyes." This child had also attempted to fly on many occasions. Other times, he attempted to demostrate his superstrength by attempting to lift tables or to move the walls.

The diagnosis of psychosis is not always definitive:

At one end of the spectrum are instances of vivid imagination, such as eidetic imagery, imaginary companions, and so forth. At the other end there are clear-cut hallucinations. Between these extremes is a gray area that includes those cases where it cannot be determined with a reasonable degree of certainty whether the child is hallucinating. I postulate that looking at other areas of the child's functioning is the key to evaluating these children (Pilowsky, 1998, pp. 2–3). The same can be said about delusional symptoms.

The consideration for the actuality of psychotic symptoms is strengthened when the child gives overt evidence of the presence of abnormal internal perceptions or of the disturbing paranoid ideation. Thus, if the child holds his/her head, or shakes it, expressing despair and a feeling of helplessness against his distressing experiences, it is more likely that phenomenology described by the child is "real" and beyond the child's control. Skeptical parents promptly change their minds about the child's psychotic revelations when they see the child's terror or his/her efforts to keep the unusual experiences under control. The psychotic child feels frightened and unsafe and seeks continuous protection and reassurance. The psychotic child also show other signs of adaptive impairment, that is regressive behaviors, when he/she avoids going to the room at night, needs company to go to the bathroom, or expresses persistent preoccupation for the safety of the family, responding to paranoid fears. Major concerns are raised when the child's takes active steps to deal with perceived persecutors, and attempts to cope with feelings of danger and persecution by procuring weapons or other means to deal with the anticipated dangers.

PSYCHOTIC SYMPTOMS AS PREMONITORY SYMPTOMS OF SEVERE PSYCHOTIC DISORDERS

A number of German studies have described various subjective phenomena that antecede the full-blown picture of a major psychotic syndrome (schizophrenia). The basic deficiencies (*Basis Symtomes*) are premonitory, unstable neuropsychological deficiencies; these include impaired attention, hyperacusis, perceptual distortions, misattribution of meaning, and feelings of conviction.

Coenesthetic phenomena relate to fluctuating sensations of the body, often unpleasant and painful, probably related to third ventricle enlargement. The term *Trema* relates to an ominous increase in general affective responsivity. Subdelusional or predelusional state (*Wahnstimmung*) refers to a general affective state of suspiciousness before forming distinct delusions. By paying close attention to the patients' subjective experience these states could be identified (Oepen, 2002, p. 108). Premonitory symptoms are not described in the standard psychiatric texts, and often, patients have difficulties verbalizing those peculiar experiences. Identification of these distressing states assists in the creation of a therapeutic alliance (Oepen, 2002, p. 109).

Some cautionary statements about prodromal research are in order. Even if reliable indicators were elucidated, there is no reason to believe that the identification of these markers will provide any clue to relevant treatment. It is likely that many risk factors for severe psychotic disorders will not be directly causally related to psychosis. Such factors need to be eliminated since treatments aimed at such noncausal risk factors are spurious (Knowles & Sharma, 2004, p. 601).

A number of studies have demonstrated, rather consistently, that preceding the psychotic outbreak, patients with a serious proclivity for psychosis evidenced neuropsychological deficits. Thus, Schubert and McNeil (2005) report that offspring with a genetically heightened risk for schizophrenia showed significant impairment of verbal memory, selective attention, and grammatical reasoning compared with normal-risk offspring. The authors assert that, "These repeated findings support the hypothesis of a genetically mediated disturbance in the neurodevelopmental maturation in a subgroup of individuals at presumed risk for schizophrenia" (p. 764).

Retrospective and prospective observations of children, who later develop bipolar disorder, confirm early manifestations of mood dysregulation and anger dyscontrol. These children have pervasive difficulties in the social–relational areas, display low tolerance for frustration, and are prone to explosiveness and affective storms. Children who later develop bipolar disorders or other mood disorders are a challenge to parents due to the high levels of irritability, the lack of response to soothing parenting behaviors, and the pervasive alteration of the biorhythms. Difficulties with separations, problems with babysitters, difficulties in day care, and early evidence of interpersonal aggression, among others, are common in the developmental background of these children.

CONTINUITY OF PSYCHOTIC SYMPTOMS

Accumulating data support the notion of continuity of psychotic diathesis into adulthood. However, there is also controversy regarding the significance of psychotic features in childhood and adolescence. Some authors believe that these symptoms are innocuous. Other authors believe that psychotic features in childhood herald important psychopathology in adulthood.

In the first camp are authors like Garralda and Schreier. Garralda (1984a, 1984b) distinguishes nonpsychotic children who hallucinate from psychotic children: the nonpsychotic children "are not delusional, they do not exhibit disturbances in the production of language; they do not evidence decreased motor activity or signs of incongruous mood; and they do not present with bizarre behavior or social withdrawal." Schreier (1999) asserts that long-term follow-up of hallucinations has little prognostic significance. In Schreier's view, "[H]allucinations of critical voices or those demanding that the patient do horrific acts to the self or to others do not predict severity nor necessitate a poor prognosis. The presence of a single voice seems to indicate a good prognosis. The presence of internal versus external voices do not have any predictive value." Hallucinations may persist for several years without a major role in the child's functioning. Schreier has found an association between migraines and nonpsychotic hallucinations (p. 624).

In the other camp, are authors like Poulton, Del Beccaro, Fenning, and others who espouse a more serious view of the presence of hallucinations in childhood. In a study conducted by Poulton et al. (2000), a cohort of 761 children who, at age 11, endorsed hallucinations and delusional beliefs, were reinterviewed 15 years later, at age 26. Self-reported psychotic symptoms at age 11 predicted a very high risk of schizophreniform diagnosis at age 26; 42% of the schizophreniform cases at age 26 had endorsed one or more psychotic symptoms at age 11. Psychotic symptoms at age 11 did not predict mania or depression at age 26. The authors propose a continuity of psychotic symptoms from childhood to adulthood (p. 1053).

Del Beccaro, Burke, and McCauley (1988) reported that children who hallucinate continue to exhibit behavioral disturbances and that 50% of the children continue to report hallucinations at follow-up. The authors felt that the latter number could be an underestimation (p. 465).

Fennig et al. (1997) also found that 5.3% of adult psychotics (N = 341) endorsed previous hallucinatory experiences in childhood. Most of these respondents had not revealed the hallucinations to their parents or caregivers. Only 2 of 18 subjects had received treatment in a mental health center while experiencing isolated childhood hallucinations. Seven of the 18 subjects (38.9%) received the diagnosis of schizophrenia. The authors concluded that, "although the majority of children with such isolated childhood hallucinations may not develop psychotic disorders, these hallucinations appear to confer an increased risk for these disorders" (p. 115).

Adolescents who report auditory hallucinations are at an increased risk for general psychiatic impairment as young adults. In a Dutch longitudinal study conducted by Dhossche et al. (2002) of 914 adolescents aged 11 to18 years, 5% reported auditory hallucinations; these patients also had higher scores of externalizing symptoms (35 vs. 9% of controls) and internalizing symptoms (44 vs. 8% of controls). When assessed eight years later, 17.8% of 783 young adults from the original group met diagnostic criteria for at least one psychiatric disorder: 7.4% specific phobias; 5.1% depressive disorder; 4.2% substance abuse; 2.2% PTSD, and 1.5% social phobia. Fewer than 1% had psychotic bipolar disorders, and none had schizophrenia, schizoaffective disorder, or delusional disorder (p. 622). The adolescents who experienced auditory hallucinations had a fourfold risk of developing psychiatric disorders as adults. Adolescents who had experienced visual hallucinations did not have any added risk for psychiatric pathology in adulthood (p. 624).

Robinson, Woerner, McMeniman, Mendelowitz, and Bilder (2004) conducted a study on 118 first-episode young adult schizophrenic or schizoaffective disorder patients (70% of the subjects were diagnosed as schizophrenics, 30% as schizoaffective). Patients were assessed at baseline and treated according to an established algorithm (fluphenazine, haloperidol, haloperidol plus lithium, either molindone or loxapine, and clozapine). Full recovery was defined as a remission of positive and negative symptoms and evidence of adequate social/vocational functioning. After five years, 47% of the subjects achieved symptom remission, and 25.5% displayed adequate social functioning for two years or more. Only 13.7% of the patients met full recovery criteria for two years or more. Better cognitive functioning and stabilization were associated with full recovery, adequate social/vocational functioning, and symptom remission.

In the presence of psychotic features at a very early age, the psychiatrist needs to give neither a prematurely hopeless prognostication nor a false sense of reassurance; the psychiatrist may indicate to the family that the great majority of these children grow up without any significant impairment; however, it is impossible to tell which children will suffer an enduring effect. It is difficult to tell what the meaning and implications of the symptoms are when they are first identified. Regular monitoring and longitudinal observations, in the context of other variables, will clarify the unfolding clinical picture.

DIAGNOSTIC STABILITY

How stable is the diagnosis of a psychotic disorder? Schwartz et al. (2000) reevaluated a cohort of 547 subjects 6 to 24 months after they received an initial psychotic disorder diagnosis: 72% of the initial diagnosis was congruent with current status. The most temporally consistent diagnoses at six months were: schizophrenia (92%), bipolar disorder (83%), and major depression (74%); the least stable diagnoses were psychosis NOS (44%), schizoaffective disorder (36%), and brief psychosis (27%). The most frequent shift in diagnosis at 24 months occurred in schizophrenia spectrum disorders (45 subjects).

In a 10-year follow-up study of affective and schizophrenia spectrum disorders in an original adolescent sample of 88 patients, there was a 5% (N = 39) shift from schizophrenia spectrum disorders to affective disorder, and 16% (N = 49) shift from nonschizophrenia to schizophrenia spectrum disorders (Jarbin, Ott, & von Knorring, 2003, p. 181).

When psychotic disorder NOS patients were reevaluated in follow-up (2–8 years later), 50% (13 patients) met the following Axis I mood related diagnoses: 3, schizoaffective disorder; 4, bipolar disorder; and 6, major depressive disorder. The other 13 patients met criteria for psychotic disorder NOS, and the majority were in remission; but disruptive behaviors were exceedingly common in follow-up (Nicolson, Lenane, Brookner, et al., 2001). For additional follow-up related studies, see the studies by Del Beccaro et al. (1988); Dhossche et al. (2002); Fennig et al. (1997) Poulton et al. (2000), and those quoted in the previous section.

RECOVERY FROM PSYCHOTIC DISORDERS

Benign and transitory psychoses are by their nature time-limited. There are many psychoses that resolve on their own, leaving no trace of their prior existence and creating no adaptational consequences. The psychosis associated with neurodevelopmental disorders, such as Asperger's syndrome, autism, and others tend to be episodic and stress-related; the same could be said for psychosis associated with borderline, multidimensional impairment, and personality disorders. Psychosis symptoms associated with medical conditions, in general, improve when the medical conditions are appropriately treated.

In general, the psychoses associated with mood disorders (major depressive episodes and bipolar disorders) are state-related; that is, the psychotic features tend to resurface when the mood disorder is destabilized. Frequently, this is an indicator of noncompliance or of a major adaptational stressor. On the other hand, psychoses associated with schizophrenic spectrum disorders tend to be chronic and are usually severe and incapacitating. Even with the psychopharmacological advances in the field of psychosis, schizophrenia spectrum disorders still carry a guarded prognosis. This is more so for very early onset schizophrenia (VEOS) and early onset schizophrenia (EOS), since the early emergence of these disorders disrupts and deviates psychosocial development and disturbs the optimal adaptation to school and the social milieu.

There is limited data in the child and adolescent literature regarding the rate of recovery from schizophrenia spectrum disorders. There is an accepted view of continuity of the clinical course from childhood to adulthood, and there is a growing unification of etiology, course, and treatment of childhood and adult schizophrenic disorders.

A sample of adult onset schizophrenic patients was compared with a sample of patients whose schizophrenia had started before age 18. All the patients belonged to the same catchment area and the same clinic. Those patients with earlier onset had greater social disability on a number of variables. This could be accounted for by the greater number of patients with insidious onset schizophrenia (correlated with poor outcome), the probability that schizophrenia greatly impedes normal development with greater ensuing disability, or it may indicate that an earlier onset represents a more virulent disease process. Whatever the cause, final social disability appears greater in the early onset than in adult onset psychosis (Merry & Werry, 2001, p. 284).

Merry and Werry (2001) commented on the difficulties in assessing outcomes both in the adults and child studies: there are no commonly agreed-upon definitions of outcome, and there is the common use of the term *improved*, with different criteria used to judge improvement. Defining adjustment is not an easy task. The two main components of adjustment are psychopathological symptoms and social function. Symptoms and functions are correlated but the correlation is not close and the two domains can behave independently of one another. Furthermore, both in adult and in child literature, the studies are retrospective. Most of the studies are often short-term (1–2 years) and the point at which outcome is reported may not be truly the end-state in the disease process (pp. 283–283).

A shorter duration of psychosis before the study predicted both full recovery and symptom remission. More cerebral asymmetry was associated with full recovery and adequate social/vocational functioning; a schizoaffective disorder predicted symptom remission. Full recovery is associated with longer term social and vocational functioning. The authors mentioned that although early course determines long-term outcome, there is a small subgroup of patients that improves after a number of years of severe illness. In general more negative symptoms at baseline predict a poorer outcome.

Since there have been studies comparing first-generation antipsychotics (FGAs) with atypical antipsychotics' effectiveness, it is unlikely that the findings would be substantially different if the algorithm had included only second-generation antipsychotics (SGAs), see CATIE studies 2005, 2006 in text. The authors rightly conclude that, "[P]atients with first-episode schizophrenia or schizoaffective disorder can recover. However, the low rate of recovery during the early years of the illness highlights the need for continued efforts to develop better treatments to promote recovery for patients with schizophrenia" (p. 478).

In Robinson et al. (2004) a low full recovery percentage, mentioned above, is in line with a number of studies reviewed by Merry and Werry (2001, pp. 283–284).

It is likely that no more that one in eight (12.5–15%) of VEOS/EOS patients obtain a full recovery in long-term follow-up (more than 5 years). The recovery rates for children with affective psychosis are probably better, around 20 to 25%; the rates for recovery from Psychosis NOS are around 30 to 40%.

CHAPTER 2

Psychiatric Assessment

This chapter deals with the psychiatric examination of psychotic symptoms in children, preadolescents, and adolescents. Because of the strong association of psychosis with affective disorders, assessment of mood will be covered in a separate chapter. The examiner will attempt to approach the nature and severity of psychotic symptoms with sensitive and systematic exploration. As with any other internalizing symptom, the child will be the most important reporter of the disturbing symptoms. The child provides confirmatory evidence of the presence of psychotic features or of a psychotic syndrome.

The following propositions represent a summary of the issues covered in the chapter:

- The diagnosis of psychotic disorders in children and adolescents is a preeminent clinical enterprise.
- Examiners need to develop a diagnostic and therapeutic alliance with children and their families to obtain effective diagnostic and therapeutic data.
- The psychiatrist needs to be deliberate and systematic in the exploration of psychotic symptoms in children and adolescents.
- Developmental history, family history, comprehensive exploration of the presenting problem, keen observations during the examination, coupled with a systematic examination of multisensory perceptual disturbances, and paranoid perceptions, provide the diagnostician with solid leads in the diagnostic process.
- Diagnosis in children and adolescents is a dynamic process. Many heterogeneous disturbances begin with common manifestations in early childhood; as the child grows and develops, features that differentiate one disorder from another begin to emerge. To achieve categorical diagnoses in children and adolescents, longitudinal observations are necessary in the majority of clinical presentations.
- It is advisable to keep an open mind in the diagnostic process; parents should not be discouraged with prognostications of hopelessness, nor should they be falsely reassured in the face of serious maladaptive symptoms. "Time will tell" is a dictum with immense wisdom.

- Difficulty in diagnosing psychosis in children and adolescents does not mean that interventions should be postponed until a precise categorical diagnosis is achieved. Dimensions of behavior that are maladaptive need to be addressed as soon as they are detected.

INFORMATION GATHERING

Despite major advances in the child psychiatric field, the diagnosis of the major psychotic disorders (schizophrenic spectrum disorders and psychotic features associated with mood disorders; that is, major depressive disorders and bipolar disorders) in children and adolescents still relies preeminently on clinical skills.

Symptom checklists and rating scales complement but do not supplant the clinical interview. The validity of some of the assessment tools for children and adolescents has not been conclusively demonstrated. On the other hand, the use of structured diagnostic interviews in psychotic children improves diagnostic accuracy (Reimherr & McClellan, 2004, p. 10).

A complete history and physical examination are essential elements for the initial assessment of psychotic children and youth. Careful and systematic history taking is the most valuable tool in the understanding of the clinical presentation of the child. History should be gathered from all the available sources, including the child or adolescent, family members, teachers, other treatment providers, and supportive community staff. The psychiatric history should focus on the presenting symptomatology and the timelines and evolution of the symptoms and associated features (behavioral problems, school problems, sleep disorder, substance abuse, etc.). It is important to address the longitudinal presentation of the illness rather than simply to develop a cross-sectional checklist of symptoms (Semper & McClelland, 2003, p. 682).

No psychiatric examination is complete without a thorough review of the family history, which should be scrutinized for psychiatric illnesses in the patient's generation and in at least the two prior generations. Developmental history, history of physical/sexual abuse, history of sexual behavior, history of alcohol or drug abuse, history of legal problems, school performance, and medical, surgical, or traumatic history, among others, are all relevant. In addition, previous responses to prior psychiatric treatment interventions should be explored.

EXAMINATION OF PSYCHOTIC SYMPTOMS

The field of psychosis is expanding in scope. Initially, attention to positive symptoms was emphasized. This was followed by the progressive attention given to negative symptoms. There is an increasing interest in the affective, social, vocational, and neurocognitive functioning disturbances in schizophrenia and mood spectrum disorders.

Since psychotic functioning impairs the patient's adaptive functioning in multiple domains, it is important to demonstrate objective evidence of the impact of psychosis in multiple areas. A child who simply reports experiences that sound psychotic, and for which there is no functional significance or corroborating evidence in the mental status examination, or in the adaptive level of functioning, is likely not to be truly psychotic. Conversely, a child who denies hallucinations or delusions, but who has a marked deterioration in functioning and associated bizarre behavior and thinking, is likely to have a psychotic condition (Semper & McClellan, 2003, pp. 682–683).

Issues of Validity

Children may misunderstand questions during the psychiatric interview. In a study examining the validity of structured interviews, questions regarding rare or unusual phenomena, including psychotic symptoms, had the highest rate of false positives. Therefore, simply because children respond affirmatively to a question regarding hallucinations or delusions, that does not automatically mean they are psychotic (Reimherr & McClellan, 2004, p. 7). In order to obtain valid data from the child, the examiner needs to use language (vocabulary) that is understandable by the child; that is, the examiner's language and vocabulary should be developmentally fitted to the child. Furthermore, the examiner needs to be redundant in the exploration to eliminate the possibility that the patient assents to leading questions, agrees to questions without understanding the content, consents to questions to please the examiner, or that the child may be responding to leading questions if feeling pressured or cornered to agree to the suggestive inquiry. The latter should be avoided at all times.

In ascertaining the presence of hallucinations in a child, Caplan (1994b) expresses a cautionary note:

> First, has the child comprehended the clinician's question about hallucinations? Second, did the child confirm having a hallucination simply to please the interviewer or to get attention? Third, does the child realize that the hallucinatory experience was unusual and was not experienced by others? Fourth, would the child act on the basis of the hallucinatory percept? Fifth, is the hallucinatory experience associated with an affective response of fear, dread, or elation? (p. 17).

Caplan's cautions and reservations are valid; however, if we were to apply the same criteria for hallucinations in adults, many valid hallucinations would not withstand Caplan's reservations. Nevertheless, ascertaining the understanding of the nature of the questions is fundamental to give credibility to the patient's responses. These cautions are also pertinent to the understanding of questions related to delusional beliefs.

Caplan asserts that the validity of psychotic symptoms should be questioned when:

> 1. The reports are inconsistent and there is no other documented evidence of a psychotic process.
> 2. The qualitative nature of the reports is not typical of psychotic symptoms; that is, greatly detailed descriptions or reports more suggestive of fantasy or imagination.
> 3. The reported symptoms occur only at specific times or are clearly reinforced by environmental circumstances, for example, hearing voices only after an aggressive outburst. (1994b, p. 17)

EVALUATION OF POSITIVE OR PRODUCTIVE SYMPTOMS

Frequently, overt psychotic symptoms in preadolescence and adolescence only come to light when the psychiatrist explores and inquires about these symptoms directly and specifically. The clinical task is obvious and the transition into the realm of the exploration of psychosis is smooth when the child discloses from the very beginning of the psychiatric evaluation that a psychotic feature is present. In this situation a comprehensive and systematic symptom exploration, should ensue.

Examination of Psychotic Symptoms When They Are Revealed During the Exploration of the Presenting Problem

The term *hallucination* comes from the Latin word *alucinari*, "to wander in mind;" Esquirol introduced it to the psychiatric literature in 1837 (Boza, http://www.priory.com/halluc.htm). When the child reveals the presence of psychotic symptoms from the beginning of the interview, the examiner needs to determine the extent and the degree of influence of these symptoms. It could be stated that psychotic symptoms are clinically relevant when:

1. The child endorses perceptual experiences or individual beliefs that do not receive consensual validation by the family or child's cultural milieu.
2. The child attributes an influence (that is, the child believes that these experiences are somehow determinative) on the child's behavior.
3. The child feels that he does not have control over these experiences.
4. The child, as a result of these experiences, takes actions to endanger his own safety or that of others, puts the surrounding environment at risk, or,

based on the perceived dangers, takes obvious measures to defend him- or herself.

5. The psychotic symptoms disrupt the child's attention and motivation.
6. The psychotic symptoms disrupt sleep and other aspects of the child's daily life, and above all,
7. The psychotic symptoms torment children with an unrelenting sense of fear and dread.[1]

According to the above criteria, if a child says that she hears an angel telling her to behave or that an angel is around her most of the time, we would not conclude that these experiences are psychotic unless the child is demonstrating adaptational difficulties at school or at home, for instance.

PERTINENT ISSUES RELATED TO THE EXAMINATION OF PSYCHOTIC SYMPTOMS

If the child endorses positive symptoms, the clinician will attempt to elucidate relevant components of the psychotic symptoms; they are listed in Table 2.1.

Because auditory hallucinations are very complex and have a multitude of clinical perspectives, they will be taken as the prototype for the discussion that follows. The discussion is also applicable to other types of hallucinations and to delusional beliefs to a greater or lesser extent. If, during the process of a psychiatric evaluation, the child states that he has heard or is hearing voices, for instance, the examination begins with the exploration of the following psychotic components (see table 2.2).

TABLE 2.1 Basic Elements in the Exploration of Hallucinations

1. Auditory hallucinations
   Do you hear any "creepy" sounds? Do you hear any noises?
   Do you hear voices talking to you when nobody is around?
   Does your brain talk to you?
2. Visual hallucinations
   Do you see things that are not real? Do you see monsters? Ghosts? Shadows? People?
3. Olfactory hallucinations
   Do you smell thing that are not real? Do you feel any smells that are weird?
4. Other hallucinations
   Haptic hallucinations
      Do you feel someone touching you when there is nobody around?
   Gustatory hallucinations
      Do you have any strange taste in your mouth?
   Autoscopic hallucinations
      Have you ever seen yourself other than seeing yourself in a mirror?

TABLE 2.2 Exploration of Auditory Hallucinations and Other Positive Symptoms

1. Content
2. Control
3. Frequency
4. Familiarity
5. Source
6. Understandibility
7. Duration
8. Syntonicity
9. Communication
10. Sensorium disturbance
11. Nonverbal behavior
12. Affective display
13. Unusual experiences
14. Conviction
15. Response to previous treatments
16. Association of psychosis with abuse of illegal substances
17. Association of psychosis with physical and/or sexual abuse
18. Association of psychosis with complex partial seizures
19. Psychotic symptoms are suggested during the clinical evaluation but are denied by the child

Content

The nature and subject matter of the hallucinations should be assessed. What are you hearing? What is the voice or the voices telling you? Is the voice (voices) telling you to do things? What things? Do you recognize the voice? Here, the examiner needs to explore the presence of command hallucinations: What are the voices telling you to do? Are the voices telling you to harm yourself? How? Are the voices telling you to kill yourself? How? This exploration should be extended to an inquiry into command hallucinations that tell the patient to harm or kill other people; the examiner should ask then: Are the voices telling you to harm people? How? Are the voices telling you to kill people? How? Have you shared your thoughts or plans with anyone? The examiner should inquire if the patient has made any plans to carry out the hallucinatory commands: How close have you been to obeying these commands?

Volkmar (1996) advises clinicians to attend to safety issues: "If psychosis is suspected, consideration for the patient's safety—and, as appropriate, that of others—should be the initial consideration" (p. 848). It is not uncommon for children to hear voices telling them to hurt the family; some children attempt to carry this out while family members sleep. It is not rare for some psychotic children to reveal that they have entered the parents' room in the middle of the night armed with knives with the intention of killing the parents or significant others. More often than not, parents or significant others are unaware of these risks. Thus the clinician should ask, have you ever tried to hurt your family while they sleep? What about when they nap?

The exploration of psychotic symptoms should continue into other perceptual domains and into the area of delusional beliefs: Do you see things that are not real? Do you see monsters, ghosts, shadows, or people? Do you smell things that are not real? When you smell weird things, does something else happen to your body? What? Do you feel confused? Have you passed out? Do you have any unusual taste in your mouth? Please describe. Do you feel somebody is touching you when nobody is around?

The assessment of hallucinations is not always clear-cut: there is a gray area that includes cases where it cannot be decided unequivocally if the child is hallucinating or not (Pilowsky & Chambers, 1986, p. 2). Frequently, the answers to the above questions transition the examination into the exploration of delusional beliefs; many patients respond, spontaneously, that they feel somebody is behind them or that somebody follows them.

For children, reactions to being alone in their rooms at nighttime have particular psychological and emotional relevance. When children are asked to retire to their rooms some fears emerge: fears about a number of places in the bedroom, bathroom, and other areas in the house (see table 2.3).

Questions such as the following allow the exploration of delusional preoccupations or beliefs: Do you feel people talk about you? What do they say? Do you feel people watch you? Do you feel people spy on you? Do you feel watched when you are alone? Do you feel somebody is behind your back? Do you feel somebody is in your room? Are you afraid of closets? What about the windows in your room? Of what might be under your bed? Do you feel that people follow you? Please explain. When you walk, do you have to turn to check if somebody is behind you, following you? Do you feel people are out to get you? Do you feel somebody is after you? Whom? Why? Do you have or have you ever experienced any other weird and unusual experience? Complaints that cameras are taking pictures of children wherever they go are not infrequent in middle and late latency children.

Classical delusional symptoms should also be explored. Do you ever feel the television or the radio is talking to you or sending messages to you? These and related questions of thought intrusion or thought broadcasting, the so-called Schneiderian symptoms, are likely to be endorsed by severely psychotic adolescents and young adults. Occasionally, young children endorse feelings of being controlled by external sources (i.e., a robot, or other powers).

TABLE 2.3 Focus of Delusional Beliefs in Preadolescents

1. Child's room
2. Bathroom
3. Closets
4. Windows
5. Under the bed
6. Ceilings and vents
7. Darkness

Control

The examiner needs to ascertain what control the child has over the psychotic symptoms by asking, for example: Tell me what do you do when you hear the voices? Can you ignore the voices? If the answer is negative, the examiner needs to examine the degree to which the patient follows or is about to follow the psychotic commands. Can you control the voices? Can you make the voices go away? How close have you been to doing what the voices tell you to do? Have you already tried to do what the voices have told you to do? Please explain.

The examiner needs to explore the risk the patient poses to her- or himself, to others, or the external environment. If the patient endorses command hallucinations, the psychiatrist should ascertain the degree of control the patient has over these experiences and to determine how compelled he or she is to act on this ideation or belief. If the psychiatrist concludes that the child does not have control over the psychotic ideation he or she will take action to insure the patient and others' safety.

Children who experience command hallucinations during the day, frequently report that they continue, "hearing the voices at night," while they attempt to sleep. Some children report distressing auditory hallucinations during sleep. These experiences need to be monitored; the psychotic process will not be considered resolved until these experiences vanish, or become sufficiently decreased.

> Liz, an 11-year-old white child, was severely sexually abused by her stepfather for more than a year when she was 8 years old. She complained of disturbing auditory and visual hallucinations, as well as paranoid ideation, during both the day and night. A recurrent experience that promoted suicidal ideation occurred "during sleep." She claimed that, while she was sleeping, she heard "the voices" on a regular basis; the voices tormented her by putting her down, by stating she was worthless and hopeless, and by telling her that she should kill herself. She also reported that during sleep and with the same regularity, every night, she saw a little girl who made fun of her and who carried an ax in her hand advancing toward Liz with the intention of killing her.
>
> It is difficult to understand Liz's reports of a suicidal response upon hearing the voices "during sleep." Was she really sleeping? Was she in an altered state? It seemed that there was a continuity of self-awareness and cognitive processing from the wakening to the dreaming state; during the night, she reported experiencing perceptual disturbances.

There are times when the voices tell the child not to talk to the psychiatrist and even threaten the child if he or she does so. The psychiatrist needs to be aware of this probability and explore it.

Frequency

The clinician should determine how often and at what times the hallucinations or delusions occur. How often do you hear the voices? When do hear them? Do you hear the voices during the day? Do you hear the voices in the classroom? Do you hear the voices at night? Often, patients reveal that they hear voices at night, this being the reason they cannot sleep. It is also at night when patients may feel a stronger pressure to carry out the hallucinatory commands.

Familiarity

Children with trauma-related psychosis frequently recognize the identity of the disturbing voice; commonly, that voice belongs to the perpetrator threatening the child with new injuries or abuse, or with punishments, by announcing that new abuse for the child and the family is coming. At times, the perpetrator's perceived voice continues to intimidate the child and persists in threatening the child if he or she discloses events related to the abuse to psychiatrists, therapists, and others.

The voice identity is also clear in children and adolescents who hear voices from deceased loved ones, inviting them to join them "in the other life." In other situations, children are unable to identify who the voice or voices belong to. Younger children inculpate members of the immediate family as the disturbing source (mother, father, siblings, etc.), whereas older adolescents inculpate extrafamilial persons as the tormenting source. Pertinent questions include: Do you recognize the voice? Voices? Do the voices tell you not to talk to me? Why don't the voices want you to say it? Do the voices want you to get help?

Source

In general, older preschoolers and early preadolescents indicate that the voices come from their heads; as children grow older, they externalize the source of the perceptual disturbance. By late adolescence, auditory hallucinations associated with serious psychosis are identified as coming from outside. Small children complain that their brains talk to them; this may be the initial step in the process of depersonalization, splitting, and projection characteristic of the psychotic process. For some children, scary characters from recent TV series or movies such as Michael Meyers, Freddie Kruger, the Scream, Chucky, and others become the feared persecutors of childhood.

Understandability

Some psychotic children state that they hear the auditory hallucinations clearly; others indicate that they hear mumbling or whispering, and that they cannot make sense of what the voice (voices) say or what the voices intend to say. The clearer the voices are heard, the more influential the voice is perceived. Some children identify a single voice; others mention a number of voices. At times, the voices talk to the patient, but at other times, the voices talk among themselves. In the presence of multiple voices the examiner should consider the possibility of alter phenomena related to complex dissociative syndromes (like dissociative identity disorder). Some patients report that the voices have long conversations, and that voices talk in long and elaborate sentences; others report that they hear short phrases or even single intimidating or scary words.

Duration

The clinician should determine how long the patient has experienced hallucinations or delusions, how long the episodes last, and whether they have changed or progressed in any way. How long have you been hearing the voices? When did you start hearing them? Did you tell anyone? Since you started hearing the voices, has there been any time you have not heard them? How have the voices changed since they started? Are they the same? Are they better? How? Are they worse? How? Some adolescents and even adult psychotics report that they have experienced psychotic features since early childhood.

Syntonicity

This exploration focuses on the subjective response to the psychotic experiences. More specifically, the psychiatrist ascertains if the psychotic symptoms are ego syntonic or ego dystonic. In the former case, the symptoms are accepted, tolerated, or recognized as part of the self. Occasionally, symptoms may even get overvalued. The term *ego dystonic* refers to symptoms that are experienced as alien and not part of the self. It is accepted that when the symptoms are ego dystonic it is easier to build a working or therapeutic alliance against them. There is limited therapeutic success when the psychotic features are ego syntonic. Most children dislike experiencing auditory hallucinations, or other psychotic experiences; commonly, they report that they feel scared, that hearing voices, for instance, makes them feel crazy, angry, or depressed. The same is true for the experience of delusional beliefs (being watched, or followed, or feeling somebody is after them). So a patient may be asked, What do you do when you hear the voices?

Frequently, children try to fight the voices; some know how to distract the voices by getting busy, by occupying themselves with something, by increasing the volume of the radio, by playing a game, or by listening to music.

Sometimes, patients like or seem to enjoy experiencing psychotic features; it is understandable that a child might want to enjoy having the belief that she is Superwoman, and that she has special powers. It is more difficult to understand why a child would assert that she likes to hear a frightening or commanding voice. However, some children do. Some children state that, "the voices" provide them with company.

Communication

The clinician should explore whether the child has reported the symptoms or kept them secret. Have you told any body about the voices? What happened? How come you have not told anybody about what you are going through? Some patients are secretive about the content of the hallucinations and delusions. The child may say, for example, "The voices do not want me to tell you this." The clinician needs to explore why "the voices" do not want someone or the examiner to know what they are saying or what they are planning to do. Efforts will be made to assist the child to articulate the "voices' fears or concerns."

Sensorium Disturbance

Delirium is frequently associated with psychotic features. The examiner will suspect the presence of delirium when the psychotic patient demonstrates disturbances of the sensorium or when there is evidence of confusion or autonomic dysregulation. These findings should alert the physician to etiological causes that require immediate medical or neurological attention (see "Delirium," chapter 6, pp. 124–125).

Nonverbal Behavior

The examiner will observe the quality of the patient's relatedness and will notice if the patient is open, reserved, or suspicious. The clinician will also closely observe the quality of the child's eye contact, the nature of the gazing, or the presence of staring. The examiner will notice if there are overt indications that the patient is responding to internal perceptions. The examiner will observe if the patient is subvocalizing, indicating the presence of ongoing auditory hallucinations. The examiner will also ascertain the presence of negative emotions: fear, anxiety, perplexity, confusion, or anger, as well as feelings of helplessness, hopelessness, or despair.

Affective Display

From the very beginning of the examination the examiner will pay close attention to the child's emotional reactions, to the flow of emotional expression, to the associations, and to the appropriateness of the affective display. Every time the examiner observes a discrepancy between the child's thought content and the affective display, efforts will be made to elucidate the reasons for the incongruity.

Unusual Experiences

Somatic sensations, derealization, depersonalization, déjà vu phenomena, and others, are perceptual disturbances frequently heard in clinical practice; they have important diagnostic implications. Autoscopic phenomena, occurring when the patient sees him- or herself, may be associated with seizure activity. Probably this symptom is not as rare as has been previously proposed. Hypochondriacal preoccupations, depersonalization and derealization may the first indicators of a major psychotic disorder (i.e., schizophrenia).

Morbid fantasies and magical thinking present a diagnostic challenge for two reasons: First, they occur in children without underlying psychiatric disorders. Second, they might be developmental precursors of delusions. Similar to delusions, magical thinking and morbid fantasies can impair the child's functioning if they become pervasive and if the child acts on these thoughts without understanding their imaginary quality (Caplan, 1994b, p. 18).

Conviction

The examiner will attempt to determine if the reported unusual experiences correspond to perceptual disturbances (or delusional thinking) or to a more benign category. The examiner may query the child as to whether his or her imagination is playing a trick on the patient, or in stronger terms, and expressing disbelief, the examiner may wonder if what the child is reporting is real or not. A child who experiences true perceptual disturbances asserts, even with vehemence, that what he or she reports is real, that it is not made up. When the child is convinced of his or her perceptual distortions and the examiner challenges the patient's assertions ("Is that real? Is it your imagination . . . ?"), it is common for the child to respond with anger and even indignation because the child perceives that the examiner is doubting the veracity of what has been disclosed; challenged children may expressed frustration, if not despair, that the examiner, like the family or others, disbelieves him or her. The examiner needs to know, then, that challenging the validity of a hallucination or of a delusion is not without its perils, and that the therapeutic alliance may be compromised.

Response to Previous Treatments

It is important to determine what has been the response to previous treatments, which symptoms have responded and which ones have not. The examiner needs to inquire about compliance and adherence to prior treatments. If there have been lapses of compliance or no compliance at all, the examiner will attempt to understand reasons why the patient (and the family) was not able to follow through with the psychiatric and other treatment recommendations. When the patient discontinues antipsychotic medication, the examiner will inquire as to reasons underlying such a decision; exploration regarding the nature of potential medication side effects should be thoroughly pursued because this is a common cause of medication discontinuation. Has the child ever been in therapy? Has she revealed these psychotic experiences to the therapist? Why not? Has the patient ever used alcohol or drugs to attempt to cope with the psychosis?

Association of Psychosis with Abuse of Illegal Substances

Substance abuse must be considered a causative factor of psychosis in children and adolescents. It is also a common complication of chronic psychosis. The psychiatrist needs to explore this issue in every psychotic child.

Association of Psychosis with Physical or Sexual Abuse

Sexual and physical abuse and its associated posttraumatic stress disorder are common causes of a multiplicity of psychotic features in children and adolescents (see chapter 7, "Traumatic Psychosis").

Association of Psychosis with Complex Partial Seizures

Complex partial seizures are the grand simulators of psychiatric symptomatology. Seizure disorders need to be considered regularly in the differential diagnosis of psychosis in childhood.

PSYCHOTIC SYMPTOMS ARE SUGGESTED DURING THE CLINICAL EXAMINATION BUT ARE DENIED BY THE PATIENT

Seriously disturbed children do not have an observing ego and are not attuned to the happenings of their internal world. If they do not endorse psychotic symptoms but display significant adaptive impairments or developmental deviations, serious consideration will be given to the possibility of a psychotic disorder, even when children deny the presence of positive symptoms. The overall weight of dysfunction and symptomatology as indicated by negative symptoms, behavioral disorganization, regressive behaviors, and adaptive failures may be converging factors of a serious psychotic disorder.

Not infrequently, children report that the "voices" tell them not to say anything to anybody, including the examiner. Children also report that the "voices" threaten them with retaliation (doing something bad to the family or to them) if they break this command. In the presence of a very defensive and guarded child, the examiner may opt to make an inquiry about these symptoms in the past. By accepting the patient's illusion that the symptoms are no longer present, the child might be more forthcoming with the disclosure. When was the last time that you heard voices? What did the voices tell you to do, then? When was the last time you saw things?.

NATURE AND EVALUATION OF NEGATIVE SYMPTOMS

Nasrallah and Smeltzer (2002) list the most common and clinically relevant negative symptoms: affective flattening or blunting; alogia (poverty of speech, poverty of content of speech, blocking, prolonged response latency); anhedonia (inability to experience joy or pleasure); asociality (lack of social relatedness, no interest in relating to people); avolition (apathy, lack of spontaneity, lack of initiative); and inattentiveness (p. 57). Odd and hebephrenic behaviors may also be considered as negative symptoms.

Marin (2005) affirms that decreased motivation is found in apathy, abulia, and akinetic mutism, and that these conditions share a common pathogenesis, a dysfunction of the anterior cingulate-basal ganglia-thalamic circuit. Symptoms of diminished motivation include anergy, and lack of interest, initiative, and drive. Other disorders of diminished motivation include the Kluver-Bucy syndrome, negative symptoms of schizophrenia, and emotional indifference associated with right hemispheric dysfunction. Anergy plays a role in diminished motivation. People with conditions such as chronic fatigue syndrome, Lyme disease, and testosterone deficiency often experience a lack of energy, resulting in decreased motivation (p. 15).

Clinicians Distinguish Primary Negative Symptoms (Deficit Symptoms) from Secondary Negative Symptoms

Primary negative symptoms are considered an inherent component of schizophrenia and related illnesses. Secondary negative symptoms result from other factors, such as poorly controlled positive symptoms, antipsychotic-induced extrapyramidal side effects (EPS), depression (demoralization), institutionalization, or a lack of environmental stimulation (Nasrallah & Smeltzer, 2002, p. 56).

The term *affective flattening* or *blunting* refers to the quality of affect that indicates a neutral or negative affective tone, a lack of oscillation of affect, poor affective reactivity, or the incapacity to resonate with the interlocutor's affective valence. Children with affective blunting are hard to engage and they do not disclose; the verbal exchanges are perfunctory and they neither smile nor cry. In spite of the examiner's efforts to make emotional connection to the patient, the examiner feels that he or she has not been able to make any emotional contact with the child nor that a working or therapeutic alliance has been built. A common countertransference response to this effort of engagement is the feeling of tiredness or exhaustion.

Poverty of speech content relates to the child incapacity to keep an interactive level of verbal communication with the examiner; the verbal and nonverbal patient's exchanges disrupt the interpersonal communication and interrupt the creation of emotional rapport. Language is either monosyllabic or overtly concrete for the child's age. Each verbal exchange produces blocking in interpersonal exchange rather than adding information to keep the communication going. As a result of this communication failure, the examiner is left with a feeling of detachment, if not of boredom. In these circumstances, it is difficult for the examiner to keep a productive level of alertness, and as a result he or she may experience drowsiness. Other patients have overt thought disorders that interfere with interpersonal resonance and the transmission of meaning.

Children with anhedonia are not able to experience fun anymore. They do not feel happy and withdraw from activities that were pleasurable before: games, sports, going out, or being with friends. They do not seem to care; the lack of caring frequently overlaps with a sense of hopelessness. Children in this emotionless or detached state have stopped caring and trying. Anhedonic children feel that life is a big frustration, that nothing is worthwhile or exciting, and that nothing pans out, that nothing will happen. In other words nothing matters, it is futile! Why try?

Amotivation relates to the lack of an inner drive, to the loss of personal goals and ambitions, and to the progressive immersion in detachment, withdrawal, and passivity; this results in an increased dependency on significant others. Amotivational children have given up the drive for progressive autonomy. Deep inside, these adolescents feel unable to cope, to take care of themselves, and seldom entertain thoughts of leaving home. A related concept is the one of avolition that refers to the lack of will or purpose, to the lack of planning or personal goals.

Issues with inattentiveness often relate to executive functioning deficits. Attention is a fundamental function for the resolution of most internal and external adaptation demands. It is proposed that in premorbid phases (pre-schizophrenia) impaired attention may be causally associated with social deficits that emerge in later stages (Knowles & Sharma, 2004, p. 599).

Negative symptoms have important diagnostic, prognostic, and therapeutic implications. Regarding adults, "The negative symptoms factor was the best predictor of both diagnosis and outcome. Negative symptoms are hallmark characteristics of schizophrenia and often have profound effects on social and occupational functioning" (McClellan, McCurry, Speltz, & Jones, 2002, p. 797). The same could be considered for negative symptoms in childhood.

School interest, school attendance, and school performance suffer significantly when motivation falters; children or adolescents with an amotivational syndrome do not seem to care, and see no purpose in trying. Children with amotivation report no goals in life, and do not have a sense of future. Typically, when these children are asked, what do you want to do in life? They respond, "I don't know." The same response is heard when they are asked, what do you want to do in the future? What kind of jobs would you like to have?

In children, negative symptoms are a major hindrance for socialization and for family closeness and intimacy. Negative symptoms separate atypical children from their normal counterparts due to their unusual demeanor and their awkward relatedness. In the same manner, children and adolescents with negative symptoms have serious problems transitioning from home to the larger social sphere.

Children with negative symptoms also display difficulties achieving a satisfactory quality of life. Psychotic children with negative symptoms have problems fitting into social milieus and are frequently ostracized by their peers. Deficits in relating (i.e., difficulties making friends) interfere with social bonding and meaningful adaptation. Problems in social relating often interfere with the development of independent functioning.

According to Caplan (1994a), loose associations and illogical thinking reflect two different cognitive deficits in schizophrenic children. Loose associations reflect distractibility and are considered a positive sign of childhood-onset schizophrenia. Problems with logical reasoning are hypothesized to reflect a deficit in the ability to perform controlled processing. The latter deficit is considered a negative symptom of childhood-onset schizophrenia (p. 610).

Children with seizure disorders, especially those with lower IQ, earlier seizures, and poor seizure control, have an increased prevalence of formal thought disorder (illogical thinking) even in the absence of schizophrenic symptoms; these children do not evidence loose associations, however. In one study, despite the presence of interictal schizophrenialike symptoms in one fifth of the children with complex partial seizures, none of those children had loose associations (Caplan, 1994a, p. 608). Whether the psychoticlike symptoms represent underlying neuropathology that produces seizures or represent a secondary effect of seizures, remains unclear (King, 1994, p. 6; see the phenomenon of forced normalization, chapter 6).

Galderisi et al. (2002) consider that negative symptoms represent enduring deficits in a subgroup of schizophrenics. Patients with these symptoms have poorer premorbid adjustment (probably indicating an early onset of the illness), a greater genetic loading for schizophrenia, and a more insidious illness. These patients also display resistance to antipsychotic treatment and a worse long-term outcome (p. 983).

Schizophrenic patients without such a deficit state have a better premorbid adjustment and have a better long-term prognosis. Schizophrenics with a deficit syndrome exhibit more neurological and neuropsychological impairment than patients without this deficit. In particular, patients with deficits demonstrate problems of sequencing of complex motor tasks and difficulties in the domain of focused and sustained attention reflecting fronto-parietal dysfunction. However, patients without these deficits show a greater impairment in executive functions likely related to a lower IQ (Galderisi et al., 2002, p. 988).

Gheorghe, Baloescu, and Grigorescu (2004) reported that conscripts who later developed schizophrenia, and who had a higher risk for that illness, scored lower in the Raven's Progressive Matrices tests than normal controls. Schizophrenic patients also scored worse in the subscales of "neuroticism" and "psychosis" than controls; 8% of the patients had a seriously mentally ill parent compared to 1.5% in the control group. Equally, parental death or separation was reported in 23.6% of the patients versus 10.7% of the controls (p. 606).

The presence of negative symptoms has obvious implications for social success and overall adaptational outcome. In schizophrenics, affective symptoms are often difficult to distinguish from schizophrenic dysphoria; frequently, they are a prodrome of the illness.

Negative symptoms by themselves do not make the diagnosis of schizophrenic illness. Many if not most of the children with primary negative symptoms do not grow up to develop schizophrenia. In order to qualify for this diagnosis, children need to demonstrate, in addition to negative symptoms, the presence of active positive psychotic symptoms, formal thought disorder, and a progressive deterioration in adaptive functioning.

Enduring negative symptoms are present in a variety of psychiatric conditions and neurological disorders. Schizoid disorders, Asperger's syndrome, mood and psychotic disorders, developmental disorders (global and specific), and even seizure disorders and other neurological conditions (cerebral palsy, muscle diseases, and others): all these conditions must be considered in the differential diagnosis.

Tandom, quoted by Bowes (2002), states that although positive symptoms are the most obvious features in schizophrenia, what is frequently more important is the patient's functioning or quality of life that is considerably affected by negative and cognitive symptoms (p. 57).

The assessment of negative symptoms is based on data gathering from a number of sources: developmental history, history of the presenting problem, past history (including affectivity and social relations), family history, observations during the psychiatric examination, and systematic inquiry.

Developmental History

Cepeda (2000) suggested some general guidelines for the exploration of psychotic symptoms in the section, "Evaluation of Psychotic Symptoms." Some components of the suggested inquiry have particular relevance for the assessment of negative symptoms. Thus, regarding developmental history,

> The following questions are pertinent. . . . How was the pregnancy? Were there any problems during labor and delivery? Were there any neonatal complications? Was the baby responsive to the mother (or primary caregiver)? Did the child cuddle? Did he or she mold into the mother's arms? At what point did the major milestones occur? In particular, when did the social smiling and stranger anxiety first occur? How was the child's socialization progress? What progress has the child made in the process of separation-individuation? Relevant questions regarding the child's psychosocial development include the following: Does the child play with other children or does he prefer to be alone? Is the child able to share? How easy is it for the child to make friends? Is the child able to keep the friends that he or she makes? Is the child invited to birthday or slumber parties? Does the child behave or play in a gender-appropriate manner? Does the child demonstrate empathy or concern for others? (pp. 150–151). Other considerations include, Is the child able to play interactively with other children, or is he/she only capable of parallel play? Is the child caring or sensitive to his or her pets?

It is important for the examiner to ascertain the timelines of motor and speech development and the acquisition and progress in social relatedness. For preschoolers, the quality of the child's play and the use and care of toys is relevant; of equal importance is the child's behavior toward pets. Is there any history of cruelty to animals? Questions related to child's social development include: Has the preschooler been able to form social links with persons other than the immediate family? Does she demonstrate interest in being with people, in being around people? Does the child show initiative to be with other children? With other persons? Does the child display appropriate social pragmatics around other children? Does the child display appropriate pragmatics around grown-ups? Does the child initiate contact with unfamiliar persons? Does he befriend strangers?

HISTORY OF THE PRESENTING PROBLEM

When the child displays negative symptoms, the psychiatrist will attempt to track down the epigenesis of those symptoms. Are the negative symptoms new? Do these symptoms represent a change? How? Was the child like this before he received psychotropics? The elucidation of the history of negative symptoms has fundamental diagnostic and prognostic significance.

Past History

As indicated above, background inquiry regarding social development is of cardinal importance. When the child is around other children of the same age, does he or she attempt to join the group or make attempts to participate in other children's play and activities? Is the child able to make friends? Is the child able to keep the friends that he or she makes? Does the child display age-appropriate social and communication pragmatics?

Family History

It is common to discover a family history of major psychoses, manic–depressive illness, major depression, or substance abuse in the families of children afflicted with childhood psychoses, more so if the disorders are severe. When making the inquiry about family psychiatric history it is easy to skip the parents' generation and "jump" into questioning whether the child's grandparent or great-grandparents had a history of mental illness or had committed suicide. The line of inquiry ought to start with the parents themselves. The examiner will attempt to ascertain the presence of psychiatric illness in either parent, history of psychiatric hospitalizations, history of substance abuse, or suicidal history.

OBSERVATIONS DURING THE PSYCHIATRIC EVALUATION

The psychiatrist makes significant diagnostic impressions as she first meets the patient and before any word is spoken during the interviewing process. Prior to any verbal engagement, the examiner observes the child's demeanor and other nonverbal behaviors, and makes assumptions regarding the child's presence of mind, her sense of social propriety, and reality orientation. This initial gestalt influences rapport and the technical management of the diagnostic interview.

Important observations during the psychiatric examination focus on the child's overall demeanor, the degree and appropriateness of the child's relation to the family and to the examiner, the propriety of the child's social behavior, the child's sense of boundaries, the capacity for engagement with the examiner, his or her spontaneity or degree of warmth.

First impressions are fundamental; they relate to how the child and the family come across: Are they likable? Are they engaging? Do they elicit warmth and interest? Do they evoke compassion? Do they elicit concern and apprehension? Is there open hostility or disregard? Does the child demonstrate regard for acceptable social behavior? Does the child show social pragmatics? Here is an example of significant negative symptoms in a preadolescent girl.

> During the first psychiatric contact, Katie, an 8-year-old, intelligent girl, displayed poor self-care: her hair was in disarray and clumps of hair covered her face, but she did not seem to care; it appeared her hygiene was lacking. She sat with open legs, revealing her panties. She showed no regard for her sitting or for her regressed posture and social deamenor. Katie got involved with a number of rocks she had brought to the office. Mother reported that she was obsessesed with her rocks, and that she would even wake up in the middle of the night to play with them. At the psychiatrist's office, she turned her back to the examiner and mother, and got absorbed in smashing some of the rocks. Her mother indicated that Katie was looking for crystals. The child was oblivious to whatever was going on around her and disregarded her mother's concerns with the "mess" she was creating when pulverizing the rocks. Katie went on breaking some more rocks in spite of her mother pointing out to her what she was doing to the office carpet.

SYSTEMATIC INQUIRY

During the psychiatric interview of a child or adolescent it is important to gauge the level of cognitive development, as well as the level of speech and language skills (Labellarte & Riddle, 2002, p. 3). The examiner should ask open-ended questions and attempt to avoid leading and suggestive questions. Open-ended questions will allow the examiner to observe the quality of the patient's narrative, the nature of the child's thought process, and the emotional associations to it. The examiner will observe how the patient presents and elaborates his answers, and will also pay attention to the patient's cognitive resources and the state of the patient's sensorium.

Pertinent inquiry will focus mostly on the quality of social relationships. The examination of negative symptoms should be systematic in each psychiatric evaluation. A systematic inquiry into the quality of the child's social relatedness includes: Do you have friends? Tell me about them. Who is your best friend? Why do you say that Jim/Jane is your best friend? What kind of things do you do with your friend? A question that is very telling about the child's emotional bonds and the quality of his or her affective bonds is: Tell me who is the most important person for you? A child who feels loved and cared for by the parents universally mentions the parents first. When this does not happen, the examiner will attempt to clarify. If the answer is a parent, for instance, it is helpful to ask: Who is important after your mom, dad, etc.?

In summary, the evaluation of negative symptoms is based on history, observations during the psychiatric evaluation, deductions obtained from the child's capacity to engage with the interviewer, and the child's emotional affective display.

EXAMINATION OF PSYCHOSIS WHEN THERE ARE NO INDICATIONS OF ITS PRESENCE DURING THE EXPLORATION OF THE PRESENTING PROBLEM

When there is not a hint of psychosis during the initial exploration, the exclusion of psychotic features is carried out by exploring relevant issues related to the presenting problem and during the completion of the mental status examination. The more unusual the symptom, especially if the initial presentation is bizarre, the greater the suspicion that a psychosis may be present. The clinician will strive to clarify the nature of the unusual symptoms and to make sense of the patient's bizarre behavior, disturbed speech, peculiarities of the patient's narrative, abnormalities of thought processes, or affective display, as well as the unusual quality of the patient's relatedness, or the patient's odd demeanor.

Schneiderian symptoms, such as the fear or belief that people could read the patient's mind, or that, on the contrary, the patient could read other people's minds, are rarely endorsed before middle adolescence (see the case of Jimmy, chapter 8). The more florid the multiperceptual disturbance and the broader the paranoid ideation is, the higher the chances the patient may endorse Schneiderian symptoms.

The examiner may notice from the very beginning of the interview abnormalities in the way the patient presents her- or himself (bizarre clothing or makeup), disturbances in eye contact, abnormalities of speech, or in thought processes: blocking, loose associations, non sequitur responses, neologisms, or inappropriateness in the display of affect (ranging from bluntness to overt inappropriateness of affect). The examiner also will strive to ascertain the patient's capacity for interpersonal relatedness, the patient's empathic abilities, and his or her sense of interpersonal boundaries.

Nighttime is a very sensitive and vulnerable time for the emergence of psychotic symptoms. The separation from the support of significant others and the relaxation of adaptive defenses bring forward a degradation of reality testing. Literally, at bedtime, children have to face their own fears and their own demons. Sleep behavior and sleep disturbances are common and persistent problems in some preadolescents and adolescents; exploration of problems in this area allows an easy transition to exploring psychosis in childhood.

The examiner may begin by asking the child: How do you sleep at night? If the child indicates the he has difficulties settling or falling asleep, the examiner may ask, What sort of things keeps you up? Are there any scary things that don't let you fall asleep? If the child endorses this, the examiner proceeds: What kinds of fears do not let you fall asleep? Do weird things happen at night? Do you hear any creepy noises? Do you hear any voices? If the child endorses any of these symptoms, the evaluation of psychosis proceeds as indicated before. For preadolescents and early adolescents, the child's bedroom is a frequent focus of fears and wariness. Other venues that are frequent targets of projection and fear are the closets, the space under the bed, and the windows. Are you afraid of the closets..., windows..., under the bed?

If the patient gives evidence of psychosis, the examiner will continue the exploration of other perceptual disturbances, and will strive to complete the exploration of paranoid fears as suggested above. Fears are also a sensitive area for initiating the exploration of the presence of psychotic features.

Sometimes, preadolescents and even adolescents do not endorse "hearing voices," but readily acknowledge that their brains "talk" to them. In these cases, the exploration needs to ascertain if the patient can control the brain talking to them, for how long has the brain talked to them, or if the brain tells the child to do things. The presence of psychosis is strongly suggested by circumstances listed in table 2.4.

If a child does not endorse psychotic features, that does not mean that the child is not psychotic. Many psychotic children hide their psychosis tenaciously and are able to maintain secrecy over this abnormal ideation and associated behaviors. Children may fear actualizing the psychotic ideation by the mere fact of talking about it and, at a more realistic level, they fear hospitalization and being separated from the family; these children may also be afraid of being

TABLE 2.4 Factors that Raise the Index of Suspicion of the Presence of Psychosis in Children and Adolescents

Persistent suicidal behavior
Homicidal behavior
Loss of significant adaptive capacity
Regressive behavior
Unusual and bizarre behaviors
Presence of inappropriate affect
Presence of multiple developmental delays
Prior history of psychosis
Labile and unstable mood
History of alcohol/substance abuse
History of physical/sexual abuse

labeled "crazy" if they reveal their peculiar experiences. As has been mentioned before, some psychotic children are proscribed to reveal their psychosis by their own psychotic influences: there are "voices" telling the child not to reveal anything; otherwise, dreadful consequences may ensue.

There are times when the child is an unreliable historian, and therefore, the answers to the mental status examination questions are much skewed. The patient may be aware that disclosing certain symptoms may send him or her to the hospital. When the patient appears unreliable or the patient's history is unclear, due to the patient's level of adaptive behavior, collateral information and the observations of the examiner clinician during the psychiatric evaluation are of definitive importance.

> Rupert, a 15-year-old male, was referred for an emergency psychiatric evaluation following a violent episode in which he threw a fan at his parents. At the time of the psychiatric assessment the parents were not available, but referral information indicated that Rupert had been diagnosed with Paranoid Schizophrenia in the past.
>
> During the diagnostic interview, Rupert reported three previous extensive psychiatric hospitalizations and acknowledged that he had been psychotic in the past; however, he did not endorse the presence of perceptual disorders or paranoid thinking when a thorough exploration of psychosis was performed. The examiner was not satisfied; he maintained a high index of suspicion.
>
> When the patient was taken to the examination room for a physical examination his paranoia became florid; he became suspicious of the stethoscope, he thought the neurological hammer was a knife, and he feared that the physician was going to stab him.
>
> The stepmother arrived, a short time after these observations. She was terrified of Rupert because he had shaken his baby brother and had taken aggressive stances against his parents.

If the examiner suspects psychosis, he or she needs to be persistent and comprehensive in the exploration of those symptoms and attentive to observations that may indicate the presence of psychotic behavior. Also, if the examiner suspects psychosis, he or she needs to pay attention to countertransference, to clinical sense and experience, and be persistent in the exploration of indicators of psychosis. The clinician will be rewarded when the patient's trust is gained.

Pato's example is a case in point.

> Pato, a 12-year-old Hispanic boy with a background of severe developmental difficulties, was admitted for the third time to an acute preadolescent program for bizarre behavior including wanting to skin himself. He had carved a 2-inch square area off his left arm. He stated that he wanted "to taste [his] own flesh, put salt on [his] body, and to eat [his] skin." He had a history of autistic features in the preschool years and he was described as aloof, and having no friends. He wished

he was an armadillo, "to burrow a hole and to stay away from people." When Pato was asked what would happen if another armadillo would come to his hole, he immediately replied, "I would bite him."

Pato had a prominent frown most of the time (omega sign). In previous admissions he had denied auditory, visual, olfactory, or haptic hallucinations. He had also denied paranoid ideation in spite of the fact that a therapist overheard him asking if there were any cameras in the bathroom taking pictures of him when he masturbated. During the latest admission, Pato denied he heard noises or voices, and repeated his denials regarding experiencing paranoid ideation.

Pato displayed a very unusual and disturbing smile. On one occasion, while he was smiling inappropriately, the examiner inquired if he was hearing his brain talking to him. Pato acknowledged that for more than a year he has been hearing his brain talking to him. He claimed the brain was telling him to cut himself. He stated that he could not control his brain.

The examiner suspected that Pato experienced other perceptual difficulties and that he suffered from broad and prominent paranoid ideation. Upon pursuing this issue, he found that Pato's bizarre ideation centered on eating people. He asserted that, "We should eat dead people, not the ones with maggots and worms, but freshly dead people." When discussing his mother making barbecue, he immediately associated this with the idea that, "the insides of dead people could be barbecued." He actually suggested, "grilling the bowels and stuffing the human heart with eggs." He felt so strongly about his ideas of eating flesh that he suggested writing to the president to make eating freshly dead people a rule.

During the evaluation, the examiner was struck with Pato's negative symptoms: lack of relatedness, his poverty of thought, the concreteness of his thinking, and the bluntness of his affect. Pato's blunt affective display only broke down when the examiner explored his inappropriate smiling. The examiner also noticed that Pato got very involved in and excited by his bizarre ideations.

One and a half years later, Pato was readmitted to an acute psychiatric program because he continued injuring himself. He had been anorexic and insomniac, and he had refused to take his medications. The physical examination revealed a fresh 2-inch square lesion on the right arm; previous lesions had left the skin without epidermis. There were scars of similar nature and dimensions in the left arm and in the right upper thigh; those were areas from which he had removed the epidermis before. When a nurse was attending to his most recent wound, Pato remarked, "I did not cut deep enough!" During this admission he was more withdrawn and appeared more depressed. He got very irritated when he was queried regarding perceptual or delusional beliefs. Pato, then, 13½ years old, was more asocial and his eating had been limited; he had lost about 25 pounds since the previous admission (it is tempting to think that his anorexia was a defense against his cannibalistic tendencies).

Although Pato denied psychotic features, his preoccupation with death was evident. When the examiner discussed the patient's problems with insomnia, he compared lying in bed with the position of a corpse; he acknowledged that sometimes he felt like a dead person.

To reiterate, when the patient reveals psychotic symptoms, it is the clinician's responsibility to ascertain their strength, their intensity, and the patient's efforts to deal with them. As has been highlighted, it is of particular relevance to determine if the patient is hearing command hallucinations or to ascertain if the patient's behavior is being activated by paranoid distortions.

If paranoid ideation activates the patent's abnormal behavior and motivates the child to act out his or her distorted beliefs, the examiner should explore the source of the paranoid distortion, in order to provide reality testing and alternative explanations to the patient's irrational beliefs. If the examiner concludes that the psychosis is activating behavior that puts the patient's life or that of others at risk, he or she will take steps to avert that.

A bigger clinical challenge occurs when the patient is not forthcoming with the symptoms. The clinician needs to be attentive to windows of opportunity, to "openings" in the patient's narrative, to explore circumstances that are frequently associated with psychotic behavior.

Because the rate of misdiagnosis at the time of initial assessment of psychosis is high, longitudinal monitoring and reassessment are necessary to achieve diagnostic accuracy (Semper & McClellan, 2003, p. 684).

CHAPTER 3

Examination of Other Psychotic Symptoms

This chapter will cover the following areas:

- Examination of thought disorder, disorganized behavior, and grandiosity.
- Other pertinent explorations in preadolescents and adolescents with psychosis.
- Examination of psychosis in preschoolers and early preadolescents.
- Completing the mental status examination.
- Psychosis in nonverbal patients, in patients with mental retardation, and issues related to violence associated to psychosis.

EXAMINATION OF THE THOUGHT PROCESSES

It is important to distinguish between developmental thought disorder slippage and clinically significant thought disorder. It is also important to recognize that young children may have difficulties describing their symptoms and experiences; in part this help to explain that younger normal children have higher thought disorder index scores than older children. It is doubtful that a thought disorder could be reliably diagnosed before 7 years of age (Asarnow, Tompson, & McGrath, 2004, p. 181). Because of this, and due to other diagnostic objectives, the present writer has advocated the involvement of significant others (the mother, in particular) in the interviewing assessment of early latency children and preschoolers (see below).

The term *psychosis* refers to problems with reality testing and the presence of hallucinations or delusions. The term *thought disorder* refers to problems with the process of thought production, thought concatenation, and thought organization (Cepeda, 2000, p. 109).

The thought examination section of the Appearance, Mood, Sensorium, Intelligence, and Thought (AMSIT) as it pertains to children and adolescents,

TABLE 3.1 Relevant Issues in the Examination of Thought Processes

Issues related to logic
Issues related to goal directedness
    Circumstantiality
    Tangentiality
Issues related to associations
    Quality of thought transitions
    Loose associations
    Flight of ideas
    Word salad
    Blocking
Other disturbances of thought processes
    Non sequiturs
    Thought slippage/reality disruption
Pressure of speech

contains 12 elements: coherence, logic, metaphoric thinking, goal directedness, reality testing, associations, perceptions, delusions, content of thought, judgment, abstracting ability, and insight. The presence of severe language disorders makes the identification of a thought disorder difficult. Developmental and academic histories are helpful in assisting in this differentiation (Cepeda, 2000, p. 108).

It will be repeated a number of times that there are no pathognomonic signs of schizophrenia or bipolar disorders; although thought disorder is commonly present in schizophrenia, thought disorder by itself is not sufficient to establish the diagnosis of schizophrenia. First rank psychotic symptoms (the Schneiderian criteria) have been demonstrated in mood disorders with psychotic features. Clinically, relevant elements of thought disorder include those listed below in table 3.1.

Issues Regarding Thought Coherence

Attention should be paid to the logical flow and convergence of reasoning in the patient's thinking. Are the child's thoughts "threaded" together to express the intended idea? Does the narrative make sense? Is the exposition clear? Are the topics or themes connected to one another? Can the child's train of thought be followed?

Issues Related To Logic

Does the child the child discourse respect the laws of reasoning? Does the child discourse respect the laws of time and space? Does the child narrative respect the laws of the contradictory nature of opposites? Do the child's conclusions derive from established premises? Are cause–effect relationships respected in the child's arguments?

Issues Related to Goal Directedness

Does the child include details in the narrative that are relevant to the understanding of the idea he or she intends to communicate? Does the child branch off into unimportant details? Does the child deviate from the point he or she initially intended to make?

The most common disturbances in goal directedness are tangentiality and circumstantiality. In circumstantiality, the child's train of thought branches into irrelevant details, but the child eventually gets back to the main idea. In tangentiality, the main idea is lost, and the child goes off into extraneous content or unrelated ideas.

Issues Related to Associations

The term *associations* refers to the manner in which the child's thoughts are connected among themselves. The examiner observes the flow of the child's thoughts. Do they flow smoothly? The examiner also notices the quality of thought transition. Does the child return to the original thought after elaborating or digressing into other topics? *Affective prosody* relates to the emotional coherence of the thought content. *Ideoaffective dissociation* relates to a noticeable incongruence between the expressed thoughts and associated emotions.

The main disturbances of associations are blocking, loose associations, flight of ideas, and word salad. *Blocking* refers to the interruption of the train of thought. The child stops presenting the main idea and either becomes silent, or after a pause goes off onto another thought that is not connected to the unfinished thought. *Loose associations* relate to ideas that are weakly connected to one another. In *flight of ideas*, the chain of thought is presented as an apposition of ideas that are not connected among themselves. In extreme cases, the ideas are so disconnected to one another, so jumbled together, that the condition is described as *word salad*. Other thought process disturbances include slippage of thought, non sequiturs, and neologisms.

Slippage of thought or reality disruption refers to the insertion of irrational, illogical, fantasy-based, nonreality-based content into the logical, actual, reality-based discourse. Technically, this thought disturbance is a form of confabulation. Two examples illustrate this disturbance:

> Meg, a 7-year-old child with about five years of psychiatric disturbance, had a day pass from an acute psychiatric program. She carried the diagnosis of very early

onset schizophrenia (VEOS). Meg's parents terminated the pass early because Meg displayed an aggressive and explosive flare-up. When she was debriefed the following day, Meg indicated that there had been three incidents during the pass. She mentioned that she had problems with her sister (a 4-year-old), with her dog (he had fallen), and also mentioned that she had a problem with her mom. She got in trouble with her sister because Meg did not want to share toys with her. Meg explained that she had taken her dog "high up" and that the dog had fallen. When Meg began to talk about the problem with her mom, she said she wanted to kill her mother. As Meg proceeded, her account became confusing and difficult to follow. She mentioned that her father had dropped his gun and that he had said to her mother, "I am sorry." Since Meg mentioned a gun, the examiner sought clarification.

Meg repeated the same story when she was interviewed again. To corroborate Meg's narrative, the examiner asked her to draw all the described events. She proceeded to draw the falling of the dog and then she drew the gun incident. She drew her sad mom hastily, blackening her body with dark and fast markings. She also drew her father with a gun, which looked like a pistol.

The psychiatrist became concerned with the content of her disclosure and with the drawing content. He called an emergency family meeting. The parents indicated that Meg had been doing ok during the pass at home till the mother set limits on Meg's wearing some clothing items from the closet. Meg contravened this limit and put on items she was not supposed to wear. When her mother realized this, she reprimanded Meg. Meg became angry and told her father to bring his gun to kill her mother. The tantrum continued and Meg made further threats to kill her mother and sister, and to strangle them both. Since Meg did not calm down and had become progressively more aggressive and unyielding, her parents terminated the pass.

The parents were alarmed at Meg's distortion of events. The drawings assisted the father into realizing how disturbed his daughter was. He had a tendency to doubt the seriousness of Meg's difficulties. He realized then that Meg had problems with her sense of reality, and that "a story," like the one she had made up, could jeopardize his career.

Although the content and narrative regarding the events with her sister and the dog were factual, the narrative and portrayal of the problems with her mother and the alleged gun incident, were not. Meg narrated and depicted the fantasized events related to the gun as if they had been factual.

Meg continued demonstrating slippage of reality testing six months later. At that time, she needed hospitalization again after she assaulted the school bus driver's aide. On that same day, she attempted to kill her mother with a steak knife. Actually, she cut her mother's arm in three places. When the examiner wondered why she was back in the hospital, Meg replied that she had killed her mother with a knife and that her mother was in heaven.

Here is another example of a similar thought disorder:

Joe, a 7-year-old white boy, with a diagnosis of VEOS, was in a seclusion room following a major explosive event. The examiner evaluated the child in the seclusion room after the child made attempts to remove one of his own teeth. The following day, the examiner interviewed the child.

When the child was debriefed, he stated that he had been placed in the seclusion room because he had hit a child, because he had hit staff, and because he had kicked chairs. The examiner asked the child to talk about what he had attempted to do in the seclusion room the day before. The examiner reminded Joe that he had tried to harm himself while in the seclusion room; to this Joe stated that, "I tried to kill myself, I tried to stab myself with a knife."

Joe certainly had hit a peer and had also attacked staff and overturned chairs the day before, but it was not true that he had tried to kill himself with a knife. Joe had a long history of neurodevelopmental problems. His most prominent delays centered on poor frustration tolerance, poor anger control, severe and profound regressive tendencies, and extreme difficulties in forming and maintaining friends. He was frequently self-absorbed. Joe did not interact with other children. He often had a vacant look, and when he was talked to, he appeared inwardly preoccupied. Joe was a very good-looking child and at times he was endearing. When faced with minor difficulties, he would become utterly helpless; he would cry and appeared as if he did not know what to do. At these moments, he would act like a helpless child and expected that others would take care of him, refusing to do even the most basic of his self-care activities. Joe was perpetually preoccupied with plants and insects: while his peers enjoyed the playground and the basketball court, Joe would go around the hospital campus looking for insects and worms. He collected seeds and would put them in pots, watering them attentively. He spent a great amount of time drawing plants and flowers.

Joe had a history of multiple psychiatric hospital admissions for aggressive behavior at home and at school. The last hospital admission occurred after Joe cut his younger sister's lip with a knife.

Non sequiturs are defined (Shorter Oxford English Dictionary, 2002) as, "(2), an inference or conclusion that does not follow from the premises; a response, remark, etc., that does not follow from what has gone before" (p. 1939). A non sequitur changes the referent of the communication because the dislocated statement is not connected to the nature of previous exchange. Usually, a non sequitur creates a sense of bafflement in the listener. A common reaction to a non sequitur is a subjective pondering: Where did he come up with this? The non sequitur disrupts the communication and interrupts the listener's train of thought. Here is a telling example:

> During the daily rounds at a local psychiatric hospital, the author asked a 17-year-old schizophrenic male if anything had changed since he had come to the hospital (he had been in the acute care program for a week). His response was concrete and a non sequitur: "Yes, now I can move my bowels better." He had been admitted for violent behavior toward his family and for inappropriate and disorganized behaviors.

Neologisms refer to created, "made up" words that are not in ordinary language or in the local parlance; nor are they colloquialisms. A neologism frequently makes reference to meanings that are sui generis or dereistic. Interestingly, when aphasics and schizophrenics were compared regarding communication difficulties, the aphasics made up more neologisms than schizophrenics (Cummings & Mega, 2003, pp. 90–92).

The presence of thought disorder is commonly observed in schizophrenic children; thought disorder by itself does not make a child schizophrenic. Here is an example of a nonschizophrenic adolescent's trend of thought reflecting a prominent thought disorder.

> On one occasion, as the psychiatrist escorted an adolescent to the office, the adolescent noticed some ongoing construction and started saying, in a loud and rather dysprosodic tone: "I am good at building...I and other friends could complete the project faster...we don't charge anything. My father makes me work for nothing....How did you get the hair cactus you have in your office?"
>
> In the office, after he was asked to sit down, he said then, "I feel funny today." When the examiner asked him to explain, he said, "I am not talking too much today...when I got up this a.m. and I looked at the light, I had a headache between my temples...that indicated to me that the lithium is low.... I need my lithium back....I might burst at any time....I'll leave the 22nd (he had been told that he would be discharged by that day)....I might have to come back....I'm able to speak better without lithium." The examiner redirected him to the statement that he was "feeling funny today." He stated, "My blood pressure was 140 over something, it is not good, guanfacine controls my blood pressure...I miss my little brother." He continued, "I am working on a fish (an occupational art project) for him....I don't want my aunt Joanna to have it; she is very overprotective of me."
>
> On another occasion when his father went to sea (he was a seafarer), the patient said, "I'm worried about my dad, he could get hurt in the storms (this was the hurricane season), I'm worried about the white sharks.... There is a war going on (the Iraq war)....My father has to go by Mexico and Guatemala...."
>
> This 13-year-old white adolescent had been transferred from an emergency room and had been committed to an acute psychiatric program after he attempted to slash his stepmother's neck. In the emergency room, he claimed that he was enacting a dream. He stated that his stepmother "was an alien who had sent [him] to slavery. I fought and killed the slavery officers." He reported that he "was dropped from a helicopter and that [he] installed a bomb on it and blew it in four pieces." He said that he "went to the living room and saw that the alien had turned into [his] stepmother. The alien (stepmother) lay in the chair;" he claimed that he "heard voices telling [me] to hurt my stepmother." In the emergency room he said that he "woke up when voices in [my] brain were telling me to harm my stepmother." He said he loved his stepmother and that he did not want to listen to those voices. He stated that his "heart told [him] not to harm her, but I could not control these urges." He claimed he felt bad about his behavior.
>
> The patient had lived with his father, stepmother, and a 20-month-old half-sister for the previous two years. The stepmother described this child as "kind-hearted"; he was gentle to his 20-month-old sister and to animals. He had not been hospitalized before, but had a long history of psychiatric difficulties; he

had seen psychiatrists for over five years and had received treatment with lithium and guanfacine before.

The family had received family therapy for the previous two years, "to learn ways to handle the child." There had been behavioral deterioration, and emergence of regression since his half-sister's birth.

After the alarming incident, in which he attempted to cut his stepmother's throat, the family indicated that, "It was not him; he has never been aggressive with family or others." He had been more argumentative but he had displayed no physical aggression before.

The patient had been born 2½ months premature; he had been exposed to drugs and alcohol in utero and was in the neonatal ICU for 110 days. He had a history of developmental delays, including walking and talking late; he had received speech therapy and had been in special education. He also had a history of asthma and ear infections, and had some hearing loss (left ear more than right).

The patient had been unable to make friends. He was aware that peers complained that he talked too much and that he was "annoying." The biological mother was said to have bipolar and substance abuse disorders; the maternal grandmother had been diagnosed with bipolar disorder and also had problems with substance abuse. The grandmother had a history of suicide attempts. The grandfather had a history of aggressive behavior and poor impulse control. Two of the patient's biological brothers (14 and 8 years of age) had problems with impulsivity and ODD. One of the brothers had been diagnosed with bipolar disorder as well.

This adolescent had spent his early childhood with his biological mother and grandmother. Apparently, he suffered a great deal of physical abuse (and possible sexual abuse) at that time. He hated his biological mother intensely, and harbored a great deal of resentment toward her. He said his natural mother "was a jerk, an idiot, and a bastard." He expressed that he wanted to tell this to his mother all his life. He said his biological mother would beat him and did not feed him. "She didn't know what she was doing; she could not take care of us, me, my brother, and my sister." He also complained about his maternal grandmother saying that, "She was not fair . . . she was a bastard, she didn't think right and she also abused us." He claimed that his 20-month-old baby brother had drowned in a toilet when the patient was 2 years old and that he had witnessed that (apparently, this was a factual event). He felt responsible for it. He claimed that someone had put a letter on his desk asking, "Why did you kill your brother?"

At age 7, the patient apparently suffered a stroke; it was reported that the patient had a "toxic shock syndrome" as a result of a chronic sinus infection. He was in a coma for several weeks. His motor assessment at 7 years of age revealed a marked delay in gross motor development; the motor skills were at the 30-month level, with scattered skills at the 48-month level with a broad based and a waddling gait pattern. He also evidenced hypotonia and bilateral coordination difficulties. The patient had visuomotor and fine motor deficits, difficulties with spatial relationships, and problems with manual dexterity (he held the pencil with thumb-wrap grasp indicating an intrinsic weakness of the hand musculature).

The physical examination revealed the presence of a child who was small for his age with obvious dysmorphic features: he had close-set eyes and flat zygomatic processes.

The mental status examination revealed that he was hypertalkative, loose, and overinclusive. He displayed somewhat pressured speech. He was distractible and required frequent redirection regarding the content of his verbalizations; he was markedly tangential. He responded well to redirection and during the interviews he made an ongoing effort to be polite and to respect social conventions. He never uttered any expletives. When he had to refer to obscenities, he would spell them out. There was a strong overanxious quality about him and he expressed multiple worries about himself and his family. During the initial examination, he stated that he had had a dream about being a slave and getting beat up by the slave owner. He said he knew he had to kill the slave owner, and that when he got the knife to cut his stepmother's neck, he was still having a dream. When he was asked about the voices, he said these were the voices of his dream.

On another occasion he came to the interviewing room making growling and other strange noises; he explained that those were dinosaur noises, and added that, "I think a lot about dinosaurs; this is most the important thing for me in the whole world."

The vignette illustrates clear evidence of looseness of association, tangentiality, and incoherence. Also the background and developemental history overlap with the histories of children diagnosed as child onset schizophrenia (COS) or VEOS. The child's narrative was difficult to follow and he needed redirection to focus his trend of thought. He was overinclusive and markedly anxious. The content of his thinking was heavily bound to environmental events. Because the breaks in this child's reality testing were not persistent, and since he demonstrated persistent misperceptions of reality, ongoing faulty judgment, and a frequent change in the content of the hallucinations and delusions, strong consideration was given to an "organic etiology" to his psychosis. The history of drug exposure in utero, as well as the history of coma and probable stroke, made an "organic" etiology likely.

It is proposed that the disordered thought of schizophrenic patients is due to an activated and disinhibited associative network (Kuperberg & Caplan, 2003, p. 455). In some schizophrenic patients the degree of atrophy of the left temporal lobe is correlated with the severity of the thought disorder (p. 457).

In summary, thought disturbance usually indicates the presence of a severe psychiatric disturbance; however, thought disturbance is not a specific sign of schizophrenia. Thought disturbance may be manifestation of delirium, substance abuse, or of a medical or neurological condition that demands timely identification and treatment. Thought disturbance may also be present in a number of personality disorders, and in neurodevelopmental and pervasive developmental disorders (PDDs).

EXAMINATION OF DISORGANIZED BEHAVIOR

Parents and other informants (teachers, relatives, friends, etc.), as well as the examiner's observations, are the best sources of information for the assessment of the child's problems related to *behavior organization*, a term that refers to the degree to which the patient's behavior is self-structured. It indicates the capacity to generate adaptive activities independent of surrounding circumstances (Cepeda, 2000, p. 97). Behavioral organization is an executive function that assumes initiative, goal setting, motivation, planning, sequencing, focused attention, problem solving, and other functions.

Two main disturbances are observed in the area of behavioral organization:

1. The child appears aimless or seems lost, "He or she does not seem to know what to do in a given moment or circumstance." It is as if the child had a "psychic apraxia." He or she knows what to do, but is unable to activate the steps of a behavioral program, to carry out the task that the child needs to perform to meet the current circumstances or what he or she intends to do. When facing a task or demand, the child appears mindless, helpless, without a presence of mind, and expects somebody to do the tasks for him or her (see Joe's example above). Becoming angry or having a tantrum is a common response to dealing with the frustration of being unable to cope with the immediate task. Since the child is unable to solve problems in an organized and consistent way, he or she displays regular difficulties with frustration tolerance. This pattern of disturbance increases the child's dependence on significant others.

2. The child is driven, hyperactive, and has no apparent behavioral objective. Instead of the mind guiding the child, the motor activity seems to be propelling the child into a purposeless hyperactivity. Some children appear to be in a frenzy, moving aimlessly day and night, unable to settle and to have a respite; these children seldom get tired and are unable to sleep. Due to impulsivity and extreme lack of judgment, they require intense supervision to stop them from harming themselves or to prevent them from damaging the surrounding environment. Akathisia, mania, excited catatonia, and a seizure disorder need to be considered in the differential diagnosis.

Some patients undergoing an acute psychotic episode (see chapter 6, "Primary Psychosis") appear confused and displayed significant disorganization of behavior. They appear aimless or lost; they wander, stare, seem self-absorbed, and behave as if they are disregarding the surrounding environment or the people around them. They may also posture, display unusual gestures, or stereotypical movement. The most conspicuous and unusual presentation of behavioral disorganization is catatonia. This condition is discussed in chapter 7.

Helpful questions in exploring behavioral organization, that should be asked of parents, are: Is there any time when your child seems to be at a loss and does not know what to do? Give me examples of that. Have you observed your child being unable to do the things he knows how to do, appearing as if he is confused and helpless, and unable to carry out a mental plan? The caveat is that patients with agnosias and apraxias secondary to progressive neurological illnesses may report similar problems. Tell me, what activities your child is able to do. Is the child able to take care of his basic needs? Is he or she so "mindless" that you have to remind the child to eat or go to the bathroom?

Have you ever noticed any unusual movement in your child? Does he or she stare, pace, posture? Does the child become immobile? Does he or she display robotlike movements? Does the child respond when being addressed? When the child responds, is the response coherent? Does the child make sense when he or she speaks?

Since the driven behavior puts these children at risk to themselves, to others, or to the external environment, these risks need to be immediately attended to. Problems with behavioral organization may indicate unfolding brain pathology; the examiner needs to explore for other symptoms indicative of a medical or neurological disorder.

EXPLORATION OF GRANDIOSITY

Abnormal grandiose ideation is out of context with the situation and the developmental level of the child. The child may become hypersexual and inappropriately touch dolls, peers, or adults in an attempt to engage them in "sex." Adolescents may display promiscuous sexual behavior or engage in binge drinking, drug use, or shopping.

Hypersexuality is present in about half of youth with bipolar disorder, and in less than 1% in children with backgrounds of abuse (DelBello & Grcevich, 2004, pp. 13–14). These statistics may be true for outpatients but not for inpatients; in the latter population, the prevalence of sexual abuse is very high (30–80%).

Grandiose children describe in colorful ways how they are special; these children describe being powerful and having the ability to do things other children cannot do. Some manic children describe feelings of inexhaustible energy, such as, "I feel I have six engines running my body," "I can be faster than the wind," "I have billions of energy," "I feel I can walk around the earth many times." One manic adolescent tightened his muscles and showed the examiner how strong he felt. He revealed that he was so strong he could lift anything he wanted.

Exploration of grandiosity is mandatory when the patient shows elated mood or when the psychiatric evaluation elicits the presence of manic symptoms. The examiner will also suspect grandiosity when the patient displays condescension, or when the child shows devaluing behaviors toward the examiner or toward significant others (i.e., parents, teachers, friends, etc.). Relevant questions include: Do you feel you can do things other children can't do? Tell me about it. Do you feel you are better than other children? How? Do you feel you have special powers? Which ones? Do you feel that you are a superhero? Superman? A Power-Ranger? Superwoman? Have you ever tried to fly? Clinicians may be surprised at the frequency with which children endorse these questions. Here is an illustrative example:

Kelly, a 9-year-old white girl, had been followed by a pediatric neurologist with the diagnoses of frontal lobe dysfunction and episodic dyscontrol. She was brought in by her parents for a psychiatric evaluation for "out of control" behavior at school. Kelly had been in the behavior modification classroom on the day of the evaluation and had been told she could not go outside for recess. Upon hearing this, she began rearranging all the desks in the classroom. She then stood on top of the desks and started to scream. This continued for approximately two hours. Her parents were called, and when they arrived, Kelly ran from them. When she was caught she held her hand up to her head as if it were a gun and pretended to shoot herself in the head.

Kelly's parents reported that she has always been hyperactive, impulsive, and frequently irritable. These symptoms had been notably worse over the previous 1½ weeks since her medications were last adjusted. She had been on Trileptal, Seroquel, and Zoloft for quite some time. She had side effects with Trileptal and the plan had been to taper off her meds and to try a new regimen. When the Trileptal was decreased, 1½ weeks previously, Kelly's mood became significantly more irritable. Her parents felt they had to "walk on eggshells" around her. She was increasingly aggressive with peers at school. Her mood would quickly change throughout the day from extreme silliness to rageful behavior. She frequently talked about not "wanting to live anymore" or wanting to kill herself. These statements were usually made at times when she was angry or getting into trouble. One month before, Kelly grabbed a knife and superficially cut the skin at her wrist. Her mother described daily outbursts that could last for several hours; after these episodes Kelly would seem fine, as if nothing had happened. With Seroquel she slept through the night. However, prior to the initiation of Seroquel, Kelly would have difficulty staying asleep. She would regularly stay awake and active from midnight to 3 or 4 a.m.

Kelly agreed that, recently, she had been more easily angered. She endorsed racing thoughts, stating, "It's like a whole city is in my head and I can't stop it or slow them down." She called her racing thoughts "jumping thoughts." To dramatize this, she tapped her fingers rapidly against the table to show how the thoughts jumped quickly from subject to subject.

She felt she had special powers and described feeling like she was "all the superheroes mixed together." She felt she could, "Fly like Superman and run like

Flash Gordon;" she could also "shoot lasers from my eyes," and felt she had "claws like a wolverine." She stated she knew she didn't really have these powers but she often felt like she did. She had climbed onto roofs and jumped from trees on occasions when she had these feelings.

Kelly felt that people talked about her. She heard a voice telling her to "kill." Sometimes this meant to kill her brother and other times it meant to kill herself. She stated that "usually" she could ignore the voice.

Kelly's Mental Status Examination: Appearance: The patient appeared to be her stated age of 9 years old. She was dressed casually and exhibited increased psychomotor activity, changing positions in the room frequently, wrapping a blanket around her like a cape; she needed redirection for frequent interruptions. She alternated between sitting in a chair and lying on the couch. She cooperated with the interview, but was easily frustrated. Her speech was pressured and increased in volume. Her eye contact was fair. *Mood*: Her mood was moderately elated with an expansive affect. Lability was noted as she quickly became irritable or tearful and quickly returned to moderate elation. *Sensorium*: She was oriented to person, place, time, and situation. Her concentration was impaired as evidenced by her inability to spell the word *world* backward. She was able to recall 3/3 objects immediately and at 5 minutes. Her response to similarities was abstract. *Intellectual function*: Her intelligence was considered high average based on vocabulary and complexity of concepts. *Thought*: Her thoughts were coherent but illogical. She denied ongoing auditory or visual hallucinations. She exhibited flight of ideas and positive grandiose delusions believing that she had superhero powers. She endorsed florid paranoid ideation: she felt that people talked about her, felt that people watched and spied on her, felt that people followed her, and that somebody was after her. Her judgment was impaired and her insight was fair as she was able to recognize that she had difficulty controlling herself. Her reality testing was variable: She recognized that she did not truly have superhero powers, but at other times she believed she had those powers.

The clinical presentation was compatible with a bipolar disorder, mixed, with psychotic features; she also displayed features of the so-called affective storms.

In the following example, grandiosity reaches new heights. The vignette also illustrates the vicissitudes of grandiosity.

God was a 15-year-old male Hispanic, who had a psychiatric follow-up for more than 10 years. His two older brothers (22 and 19 years old) had been treated for bipolar disorder for the same length of time. The oldest brother was on SSI for psychiatric disability. The second oldest brother was very unstable and was prone to depressive episodes and to suicidal behavior. That brother was very impulsive and aggressive. Both brothers have significant histories of drug use and of participation in gangs. The second brother had already fathered a child.

The children's biological father was alcoholic and mother had suffered from severe depression, but she was an exemplary mother. The children had been exposed to the marital violence that their father episodically inflicted on their mother. God was first seen for sleeping difficulties, paranoid fears at night, and dysphoric erections. Over time a bipolar disorder condition began to unfold with florid manifestations.

Seven months before, mother began to notice clear mood fluctuations. God began to voice that he was in control of the school and that everybody looked up to him. He felt he was a priest, but at the same time he felt like a vigilante, a gang leader. Obviously, God felt more important than his teachers. Because he didn't like to see people being abused, he felt compelled to rescue and to save people. He indicated he was hearing a girl talking to him and that he could not rid her from his mind. He felt invincible and felt very energetic and felt like hurting (killing) everybody.

Three months before, he began to feel he was God and that people were following him. He felt higher and bigger than anybody. He felt he had special powers and that he had the power of psychokinesis. He also began to feel paranoid: he felt persecuted by his enemies. The manic episode abated following treatment with mood stabilizers and atypicals, but was followed by a significant depression; he began to feel like "Jell-O" and "watery," as if, "there was no bone." He complained of bad memories and started worrying about bad things happening to him. He disclosed strong homicidal ideation. He feared that he could hurt all the people that hurt him. God had nightmares of being killed, having his head chopped off, and had started seeing dead people.

As depression worsened he felt like he wanted to die. However, he denied suicidal ideation saying, "I am already dead." These feelings of despair were mixed with feelings of grandiosity. Hallucinations (auditory and visual) continued. He felt there was nothing to live for and felt paranoid. He experienced command hallucinations telling him to kill people.

Six months later, God's grandiosity had resolved. He was no longer feeling as if he were God or as if he had special powers. However, he still felt he could control people. Depressive feelings remained strong. He did not want to go to school. Although he still felt paranoid, he no longer complained of command hallucinations.

For this patient, family history, developmental history, course of illness, and phenomenology converged into a classical manic–depressive illness (bipolar disorder I, with psychotic features).

Roxanne, an 11-year-old female with history of neurodevelopmental problems, revealed other unusual forms of grandiosity. She believed that she could make rain and knew what other people were thinking. She stated that she understood what cats, dogs and snakes were thinking. Her family which, lived in a farm, reported with a great of concern that in one occasion Roxanna had attempted to grab a poisonous snake to communicate with her. Roxanna had also tried to fly and believed she was a superheroine.

It is not unusual during the process of an evaluation to observe preadolescents enacting efforts to lift the tables or enacting feelings they can move the walls. Here is a clinical vignette of a preschooler:

A 4½-year-old white boy was brought for an emergency evaluation after he put his 1¾-year-old brother in a drier. The family had noticed a rather drastic change in his overall demeanor for the previous two weeks. He had been laughing inappropriately, had been mean to the kitten, and had threatened to kill it and eat it; he also had threatened to kill his father and brother, to cut them with a knife and to eat them too. The child had become more hyperactive and impulsive and had ventured outside of the house a number of times. He could not sleep. This child had verbalized to mother that he heard people talking by his window, and a number of times he had asked mother to answer the door believing somebody was at the door. Mother also reported that the child was scared at night, he avoided or even refused to go to his room and had developed the habit of coming to sleep with his parents. The child had voiced that his father was trying to kill him. Mother reported that on one occasion the child had made an inappropriate remark to her, "You have nice boobs." On another occasion when the mother entered the child's room she found him in bed with a large Barbie covered with a sheet. The child did not want mother to check under the sheet.

The examiner faced a very handsome, intelligent, well-groomed, high spirited, verbal, and elated preschooler. He was markedly overfriendly and displayed a broad and continuous smile. The child was distractible and needed redirection. The child was given paper and a pencil for him to draw whatever he wanted. As he got involved in the process of drawing he kept on "puffing himself up" expanding his chest with a clear air of arrogance, while at the same time voicing he was a giant. At some point the child became attentive to the examiner and started drawing the doctor; to depict him he drew a rather small sketch. When the examiner asked the child to draw himself he filled the whole page stating he was a giant. All along he kept an elated mood. The examiner made the diagnosis of psychotic mania in a preschooler.

Now, an example of an early school age child. A white, male, manic 6-year-old, who had severe difficulties at home and school, had voiced defiantly that he did not have to go to school, that he wanted to go to college. He said he wanted to go to South America to hunt whales, and wanted to go to Africa on a safari to chase tigers! The author observed this child when a significant other was giving him redirection for his impulsive and bullish behavior; following this and without any restraint, the child began to mock the adult female, to imitate and ridicule her without any sense of boundaries and with blatant disrespect.

The case of Gus is an excellent illustration because he was able to articulate many subjective experiences related to unmistakable manic behavior:

Gus was a 9½-year-old-adopted Hispanic boy with an extensive psychiatric history. He had been in psychiatric treatment for years and had needed acute psychiatric hospitalization many times before. Prior to his adoption at age 4 he had been a victim of physical and sexual abuse. The latest psychiatric evaluation had occurred a couple of weeks following an acute inpatient treatment. Significant medication changes had been implemented by the outpatient psychiatrist that apparently were unhelpful. The psychiatrist had discontinued the atypical (risperidone 3 mg/day), and had added carbamazepine instead.

During the latest crisis, the child became violent toward his mom, held a knife to her, hit her, and threw a coat hanger at her. He also threw his maternal grandfather's glasses away. His mother reported that the child became totally disinhibited: repeatedly tried to grab her breasts and attempted to "suck" them, he took all his clothes off, and masturbated openly. All along, the child was laughing inappropriately and would not respond to redirection. Gus became more unruly and unrestrained. He also had difficulties falling sleep and would stay up until "it became bright," at dawn.

When Gus was interviewed, he was elated and lucid. He could not stop laughing. He was interested in explaining "the reason why I could not control myself was that lots of things were flashing in my mind, that my thoughts were going quick, and I can't control them." He added that, "things would pop-up in [his] mind." He revealed that during this time he felt special, "like a king; a king can do whatever he wants to do and nobody can say no to the king . . . a king can spit at people, can kill people, can kill a policeman with a chain saw, can break a window . . . ." Gus was laughing without restraint when narrating his sexually inappropriate behavior. He said that, "sexual feeling popped into [his] mind," and stated that he felt that "hot girls" were looking at him. He also endorsed believing that the police were after him and that he was afraid that somebody was going to "rape" him. Significantly, Gus explained that he felt he had lot of energy, that he felt he had superpowers, superstrength; he gestured saying, "I can lift a car and throw it to the police . . . I can lift a chair up over my head with only one hand . . . ."

In adults, according to Lake and Hurwitz (2006), paranoia and fear often hide grandiosity that is diagnostic of bipolar disorders (p. 57). These considerations are be applicable to related symptoms in children and adolescents.

Other delusional ideas center on feelings that the child can read other people's minds, or that the child has telekinetic abilities; these latter beliefs are not uncommon. Some of the pertinent questions include: How strong do you believe you are? Do you have special powers? Are there things you can do better that anyone else? Can you do things nobody else can?

It is difficult to interpret early precocious and unusual behaviors, and how these behaviors might be related to unfolding primary psychotic disorders. Some preschoolers appear to be fearless, bold, and unrestrained. They do not show apprehension about strangers. Some children even attack strangers, or inappropriately believe they can confront adults or a person in power. A 4-year-old female child boldly asserted that, "I can fight the police." Some of the behaviors in question may be explained by the presence of ADHD, deprivation, abuse, or inappropriate parenting. The author observed a 5-year-old boy's father teaching the child to fight, "to be a man and to be strong." Bullish behavior has been proposed as a precursor or equivalent of grandiosity in preadolescents and adolescents. Other times these maladaptive behaviors do not seem to have an exogenous explanation. A bright 8-year-old girl managed to misuse her grandmother's credit card, so she went on the Internet and requested a credit card in her own name; to her grandmother's dismay, the child got the card.

When the psychiatrist suggested to grandmother that she should destroy the card, the child threw a big tantrum.

The clinician will pay attention to the presence of condescending behavior, to airs of superiority, or to devaluating attitudes toward others. The latter contributes to these children's inability to make and to keep friends. They alienate peers with their arrogant and condescending attitude. A child may give evidence of grandiosity during the psychiatric evaluation when he announces that he knows more than his teachers or anybody else, or when the child reports arguing about subjects of expertise with teachers or doctors.

> A known weather newscaster visited an acute adolescent psychiatric program. After a short presentation about issues with weather, patients were given an opportunity to ask the weatherman some questions. A grandiose adolescent argued with the weather expert, claiming that the weatherman was not right, that he was not telling the truth, that he did not have the facts straight. The patient claimed that he knew more about the weather than the expert!

Some grandiose children are secretive. For example, an 11-year-old boy reported that he had special abilities but refused to discuss them for fear he could lose his special powers. Another psychotic, paranoid, and grandiose child claimed to have "some patents," but did not want to discuss them fearing the examiner "could steal his secrets."

EVALUATION OF PSYCHOTIC SYMPTOMS IN PRESCHOOLERS AND EARLY LATENCY AGE CHILDREN

Parents are frequently unaware of their children's psychotic symptoms. Often, the revelation of psychotic experiences causes a sense of shock or disbelief in the parents. This reaction is stronger when the child is a preadolescent or even a preschooler. In the case of preschoolers, it is a good technique to ask parents to become assistants to the examiner; the parent is instructed to ask the child a series of probing questions. This technique lessens the parent's resistance and disbelief when the child reveals psychotic symptoms. In general, parents are able to use appropriate and developmentally attuned language when phrasing the questions. The clinician can take advantage of the parent–child interaction to observe the parent's style of communication with the child, the degree of empathy for the child, the sense of caring, and other parenting behaviors.

When the interview is conducted by the parent, and he or she elicits psychotic symptoms, the parent's tendency to minimize or to deny the presence of psychosis is decreased. When children incorporate recent movie figures or themes into their psychotic thinking, parents become skeptical about the factuality of psychotic features. In truth, children *do* use recent figures/events, or contemporary experiences to concretize their fears and abnormal turmoil. Children *do* get afraid of such creations as Chucky, Michael Meyers, the Shining, or Kill Joy. In the same vein, some children incorporate recent political and world events into their psychotic thinking. For example, a 7-year-old believed that Bin Laden was after him, that Bin Laden was going to end the world. In general, latency stage and older children are frequently cooperative and reliable in their response to the exploration of psychotic symptoms.

EXPLORATION OF PSYCHOTIC SYMPTOMS IN LATE LATENCY AND PREADOLESCENCE

For preadolescents, sensitive situations that become organizers of paranoid ideation and other psychotic features are elements of the child's immediate familiar environment. Table 3.2 lists common situations that become paranoid organizers for preadolescents.

A number of preadolescents are afraid of going to their rooms at night; others are afraid of going to the bathroom. In exploring this, children reveal they are scared that someone might be in the bedroom or bathroom. Closets are "filled" with "monsters and ghosts;" these are the hiding places for "bad people" at night. "Bad people and persecutors come through the windows"; "the monsters hide under the bed" to terrify preadolescents at night. Preadolescents who are afraid of going into the bathroom may leave the door open and carry on an oral communication with significant others while they sit on the toilet.

> An 8-year-old white boy stated that the monsters would come from under his bed at night and that they would "exchange his blood for green liquid." The child asked his father to board up the underneath of his bed to stop the monsters from bothering him at night.

> Another child, a 6-year-old Hispanic boy with a history of Marfan syndrome, asked his maternal grandmother to buy him a flashlight. At night, he would use the flashlight to search under his bed for "a scary hand that was coming from underneath, to grab me in the middle of the night."

TABLE 3.2 Organizers of Paranoid Ideation in Preadolescence

- Darkness
- Own room at night
- Room windows
- Bathroom
- Closet
- Under the bed

TABLE 3.3 Other Features Suggestive of Psychosis in Preadolescents

- Children are unable to sleep by themselves; they always need to sleep with an adult or prefer to sleep in the living room. They fear something may happen to them or that somebody may harm them if they sleep alone.
- Children put things in their ears, to block auditory hallucinations. Some children raise the volume of the radio or TV to counteract the distressing voices.
- Children bring knives or other "weapons" to their rooms to defend themselves against perceived persecutors.

Some psychotic children are frightened of the windows at night: they fear somebody might get through the window(s); somebody might scare them or might watch them.

An 8-year-old white boy stated that he could not sleep at night. He said he heard scary noises and voices by the window. He would get up and go to check the window to see where the noises and conversations came from.

Other indicators of psychosis in childhood and preadolescence are listed in table 3.3.

- The child is unable to sleep in his or her own room, and needs to sleep with a parent because of fears at night. When the child insists on sleeping with a parent, the possibility of psychosis needs to be explored.
- The child consistently increases the volume of the radio or TV: Some children increase the volume to counteract the hallucinatory voices or noises disturbing them.
- The child displays unusual behaviors such as putting things in his ears with the objective of blocking disturbing auditory hallucinations.
- The child keeps knives or other kind of "weapons" in his room with the goal of defending himself if somebody "intrudes into my room and attempts to hurt me."
- Children's behavior toward teddy bears, pets, or their toys is a sensitive indicator of psychosis in preschoolers or early school-age children. If a child removes the teddy bear's eyes or if he dismembers dolls on a regular basis, psychosis should be suspected. For example: A 7-year-old boy removed his teddy bear's eyes because "he was looking at me funny."
- Persistent aggressive and injurious behavior of a child toward his or her newborn sibling is sometimes mistakenly attributed to benign sibling rivalry. Persistent injurious behavior toward a younger sibling may represent an early manifestation of a psychotic disorder. Experts in preschool and latency age are familiar with experiences of children who have tried to smother younger siblings by putting pillows over their heads, poked their eyes, pushed them, or, at a more serious level, pushed siblings down

the stairs or off sidewalks, or of children who have attempted to stab their younger siblings with knives, screwdrivers, and the like.

Sleep time is a vulnerable time for children with psychotic tendencies. The issue of sleep offers the examiner an excellent subject with which to start the exploration of psychotic symptoms. When the patient reveals that he or she cannot sleep, the clinician could explore this problem further by asking: Is there something in your mind that keeps you awake? Do you have any thoughts or ideas you can't get rid off? Are there any fears that do not leave you alone? At this time the examiner may become more direct in the exploration of psychotic symptoms: I wonder if you hear noises at night. Do you hear any sounds? Any creepy sounds? Do you hear voices at night? Do you see any things that are not real? Do you see any monsters, ghosts, or shadows? If the patient endorses any of those questions, the examination will proceed to determine the extent to which the psychotic symptoms are related to the child's behavior, or the degree to which psychosis influences or contributes to the child's maladaptive functioning, as has been described above.

It is not uncommon for early latency children to disclose the presence of both "good" and "bad" voices. The "good" voices are associated with God, a guardian angel, the conscience, or supportive relatives who give them good advice or reassurance, or provide them with needed support. Children very clearly distinguish those supportive voices from the "bad" or "mean" ones. Often, a child will report internal struggles among the voices vying for supremacy in the child's mind. In consequence, if a child reports hearing "good voices," the examiner will explore if he also hears "bad or evil voices." Some children report a transformation of the good voices into bad ones or vice versa.

As previously discussed, some children do not endorse hearing voices, but acknowledge that "their brain talks" to them; this experience needs to be explored when the child denies hearing voices and the examiner has reasons to believe that the child is responding to internal stimuli. Even adolescents, may deny hearing voices but endorse hearing their brains talking to them.

Most children are open to discussing psychotic symptoms in their parents' presence. Actually, it is a good practice to conduct this part of the psychiatric interview in the parents' presence. Children rarely object to this. Adolescents avoid talking to the parents about sexual behavior, drug use, or delinquent behavior. However, they rarely object to discussing psychotic features in front of their parents. Tables 3.2 and 3.3 lists factors which raise the index of suspicion about the presence of psychosis in children and adolescents.

COMPLETING THE MENTAL STATUS EXAMINATION

To complete the mental status examination in a way that will allow the discovery of psychotic symptoms and help to differentiate psychosis from other conditions, the following questions need to be asked of all patients on a routine basis: Does your mind ever play tricks on you? How? Many children request clarification of this question. When this occurs, the examiner could ask: When you are alone, do your hear noises? Do you hear creepy or scary noises? Do you hear voices talking to you when there is no one around you? If the patient endorses this, the exploration proceeds as outlined previously. Otherwise, the clinician moves on to explore other psychotic features as indicated above, followed by the systematic exploration of delusional thinking and other unusual experiences. For example, Do you see things that no one else can see? Do you see monsters, ghosts, or shadows of people? What do they do? Do you smell things that are not real? Do you smell anything you cannot account for?

Children with a history of abuse report smelling the perpetrator's cologne or alcoholic breath. Disgusting smells (olfactory hallucinations), at times associated with a bad taste in the mouth (gustatory hallucinations), may be associated with complex partial seizures or other active intracranial pathology; when that is the case, a prompt neurological consultation should be demanded.

Do you ever feel somebody is touching you when nobody is around? Abused children often report that they feel they are being touched. This is a sensory memory related to experiences of abuse and is distressing to the victims. Formications (feelings that insects are crawling in the patient's skin) are common in children and adolescents who are delirious, and in those who abuse stimulants, cocaine, and other illegal substances.

Seizure disorder is an important condition in the differential diagnosis of psychosis. Complex partial seizures need to be considered in the differential diagnosis of psychosis in children and adolescents. This topic is covered in chapter 6, "Differential Diagnosis of Psychotic Disorders."

Other pertinent questions to explore when complex partial seizures are suspected include: Do you ever feel confused? Have you ever had times when the world around you feels unfamiliar and strange (derealization experiences)? Have you ever felt strange and unfamiliar with yourself (depersonalization experiences)? Have you ever gone to places you never visited before and you felt that you had been there already (déjà vu experience)? Have you ever been in places familiar to you and felt that you had never been there before (*jamais vu* experience)? Have you had the feeling that you can foretell the future? Have you ever found yourself in a place and you did not know how you got there? All of these unusual experiences are common in complex partial epilepsy.

Complementary questions in this regard are: Have you ever had any seizures? Have you ever fainted, blacked out, or fallen? Have you ever had any "accidents"? Have you ever urinated in your pants? Have you ever lost control of your bowel? When you wake up in the morning, have you ever found blood on your pillow? Have ever you bitten your tongue? Complex partial seizures represent a neuropsychiatry condition that must be considered in the differential diagnosis of perceptual disturbances and other psychotic disorders (see Ruby's case).

After exploring the perceptual disturbances discussed above, the examiner completes the assessment of perceptual disturbances by exploring other sensory disturbances, and other less frequently occurring perceptual disturbances by asking, for example: Do you ever feel any other unusual feeling in your body? What about other unusual feelings? Do you have any other feelings about yourself or around you?

In preschoolers or young latency children, paranoid ideation may have a subtler presentation: Children complain that nobody likes them, that nobody wants to be their friend, or that nobody loves them.

EXAMINATION OF DELUSIONAL BELIEFS

Paranoia in children has subtler coloring than parallel manifestations in adults. Feelings that "peers do not like me" or that "nobody likes me" are common manifestations of paranoia in early latency.

In children and adolescents, the paranoid feelings frequently center on the immediate family. This is even true for some preadolescents and adolescents. The case of Jess illustrates a case of severe paranoia toward a family member.

Jess, an 11½-year-old white preadolescent girl, consulted for the first time for suicidal ideation. She had become irritable, had started to display temper outbursts, and had twice attempted to run away. She felt unloved and stated that she did not want to go home at all. She had tried to stab herself with a nail file, but was stopped by her stepfather, who was the focus of her hostility and paranoia.

For Jess, her stepfather represented everything that was wrong in her life; he was the cause of all her problems. The stepfather was Jess's target of systematic paranoia. Jess had no friends and expressed difficulties relating to peers. She had been diagnosed with ADHD at age 4 or 5 years. She had walked at 15 months and had been enuretic until the age of 8.

TABLE 3.4 Exploring Delusional Thinking

---

1. Do you feel people talk about you?
2. Do you feel people watch you? Do feel people spy on you?
   When you are alone, do you feel somebody is watching you?
   Do you feel there are cameras taking pictures of you?
3. Do you feel people follow you?
   When you walk, do you have to turn to check if somebody is following you?
4. Do you feel somebody is after you?
   Do you feel somebody wants to hurt you? Why?

The mental status examination revealed an attractive preadolescent girl who displayed limited eye contact and blunted affect. She was guarded, evasive, and suspicious. At times she was circumstantial. She indicated that sometimes she heard her "loud thoughts" and that "I can't remember what I think." Jess believed that she could tell the future, that she had premonitions, and that she could move objects with her mind. She was not sure if she wanted to be alive and was not able to contract for safety.

On one occasion, after an argument with her stepfather, Jess cut her wrists, blamed her mother for it, and called 911. When she was interviewed, shortly after this incident, she reported hearing a scary voice. She was secretive about the content of this hallucination. Jess's strong denials about having any emotional or behavioral problems were remarkable.

Jess was extremely guarded and very evasive. She was also very constricted, if not blunted, in her affective display. It was quite striking how paranoid she was about her stepfather. Jess remained distant and uninvolved throughout the ensuing follow-up appointments and continued to have no insight. She received the provisional diagnosis of VEOS.

One year later, Jesse remained markedly aloof and emotionally blunted. She was not spontaneous or engaging and her eye contact was poor. With intense family therapy and tutorial support, she advanced to the next grade. Her family had to put forth lots of energy to motivate her to do her schoolwork. When she was queried about the presence of hallucinations, she denied them; she also denied paranoid ideation. However, from time to time, she uttered "off the wall" statements, that were totally inappropriate and often disconnected from whatever was being discussed (non sequiturs). These unusual comments had a sexual and inappropriate content. The clinical picture did not change during the following three years. Her prognosis remained guarded. At age sixteen, Jess received the diagnosis of paranoid schizophrenia following a new aggressive and paranoid crisis with her family. This time, the biological mother was the target of Jess' hostility and paranoia. Jess stated repeatedly that she did not want to go back home, that she would rather go to live with her boyfriend's family. She was convinced she could move in with that family and that the boyfriend was marrying her. During the mental status examination, Jess evidenced a thought disorder and bizarre thinking; she revealed that she was continuously in a dream-like state, and that she was, "coming in and out of reality." She affirmed that she could control his reality drift.

The more bizarre the delusion the greater the likelihood the patient belongs to the schizophrenia spectrum disorder category. This is not absolute, though. All along, the clinician will pay special attention to the mood, to the affect (range and appropriateness), and to the flow and organization of the thought processes (for exploration of mood, refer to chapter 4). These observations and discriminations will be fundamental in the differential diagnosis.

In clinical practice, the exploration of psychosis may be followed by questions related to symptoms of obsessive–compulsive disorder. Are there any thoughts or feelings you cannot put out of your mind? Are there any thoughts that keep on coming to your mind, even though you don't want them in your mind? Are there any thoughts or feelings that get stuck in your mind? Do you have any urges you can't control? Do you have any habits you can't stop? Do you need to check things over and over? And so forth. Paranoid preoccupation often assumes an obssesional quality; this may create diagnostic confusion. Depending on the circumstances, further exploration of psychotic symptomatology may be indicated.

Referential ideation such as "feelings that people talk about me" and "feelings that people watch me" are the most common paranoid feelings in children and adolescents. Feelings that people "follow me," and persecutory ideation, the feeling that, "people are out to get me" follow these, on a scale of severity. The feeling that "people talk about me" is so common in clinical populations that its presence, without other paranoid or psychotic features, is of minor clinical significance. However, there are some insidious delusions that cause an enduring negative impact. The following vignette exemplifies an enduring delusion and its negative impact throughout this child's life.

> Lucy, a white 16-year-old, received an emergency psychiatric evaluation following a new episode of self-abusive behavior the night before. Lucy claimed that she was thinking about her dead mother (the biological mother had died in a car crash five years before when Lucy was 11) and that she still missed her biological mother a great deal. Along with the self-abusive behavior, she felt like ending her life. She had cut her left arm and forearm with a knife; shortly after, Lucy went to her family (father and stepmother) and told them what she had done. Her parents got upset with Lucy's action and apparently voiced the concern that "It will not be covered by the insurance." This aggravated Lucy even more; she took off from the house before midnight. Her stepmother attempted to bring her back. One of her brothers persuaded her to go back home. The police had been called; they found and mandated her to an emergency evaluation under an order of protective custody.
>
> Lucy had an extensive history of psychiatric disturbance, mostly centered on a continuous depressive mood and repeated suicidal behavior. She had tried to kill herself multiple times. Lucy had a protracted history of self-abusive behavior. She had been "raped" by one of her aunt's friends when she was 5. Lucy claimed that she seldom remembered the incident and that "nothing had happened to the perpetrator." She had done well at school.
>
> The mental status examination revealed the presence of an unattractive female adolescent who appeared to be her stated age. She appeared disheveled and unkempt. She looked moderately to severely depressed and displayed markedly constricted affect. She endorsed ongoing suicidal ideation but voiced no plan. She denied homicidal ideation.
>
> Lucy's thought processes were intact; she denied auditory, visual, olfactory, or haptic hallucinations. She endorsed no paranoid ideation. However, when the examiner asked Lucy what did she see when she looked at herself in the mirror, she replied she saw an ugly person who did not deserve to live. She added that the reason why she thought about suicide so frequently was that she did not feel she

deserved to live. When the examiner asked Lucy how long she had felt like that, she replied that she had felt like that since she was 5 years old.

This delusion was hidden, but it seemed that it had actively contributed to the patient's unremitting depression and to her ongoing suicidal behavior. In adolescents, body-centered delusions, so called dysmorphophobias, may represent early forerunners of schizophrenia. The case of Van Gogh is illustrative:

Van, a white 18-year-old, was referred for a psychiatric consultation related to self-mutilation. He had presented to a psychiatric emergency room some time before after he cut the tip of his nose following an argument with his mother.

Convinced that his nose and other facial features were ugly, Van had contemplated plastic surgery for many years but claimed that the evaluations for the surgery "were always postponed." A year prior to this consultation, Van cut his earlobes; because of this bizarre behavior he was committed to the local state hospital. At the state hospital, he displayed ideas of reference and reported bizarre delusions such as feeling that a dog knew his thoughts and that he was speaking with birds when they were not around. Van felt helpless and frustrated because of the surgery delays, but he also indicated that he felt somewhat pleased and relieved by the results of the mutilation he had made on himself. He denied auditory hallucinations and asserted that, on a prior occasion, the previous examiners "tricked him" into saying he was hearing voices telling him to cut himself. He denied suicidal and homicidal ideation.

Although Van displayed depressed mood, he denied loss of interest, problems with concentration, or other disthymic features. He did acknowledge, however, that he suffered from excessive sleepiness and poor appetite. He denied visual hallucinations, but displayed overt paranoia. He believed that the postponed plastic surgeries could be a part of a grand plot to prevent him from reducing his ugliness. Van denied mind reading, thought projection, or other beliefs; however, he was fixated on what he perceived as his misshaped and grotesque facial features. These perceptions clearly had delusional qualities. Van denied any current ethanol or drug use, but he admitted that he had experimented with cocaine and cannabis some months prior to the evaluation. Van stated that while he was at home, he did not think about his nose, but when in public, he was constantly vigilant and concerned as to how others perceived him.

Van's parents had divorced when he was a baby; his mother remarried when he was 2 years old. Apparently, his stepfather began to abuse Van when he was 10. Van also witnessed his stepfather being physically abusive to his mother. Van's mother divorced for the second time when Van was 12. Van's biological father had killed his own girl friend and had committed suicide when Van was 12 years old.

His mother and stepfather raised Van until their divorce; there was also a 13-year-old brother whom the patient described as a "pretty boy." Van reported that since puberty he had been made fun off by his peers for having a nose that drooped at the end and was wide at the bridge. Allegedly, Van was able to function well prior to age 16 and also had friends prior to that age. It was also stated that he had done well academically. At age 16, however, he had begun to feel depressed and to have constant concerns about his appearance. He had developed an extreme preoccupation about his perceived ugliness. He quit high school and stayed at home doing little and sleeping most of the time. He let his appearance go. Van claimed that prior to dropping out of high school he had made good grades and had been in honors classes. After age 16, Van started gaining weight. He reported depressive symptoms over the two previous years, increased sleep, decreased interest, and decreased appetite during the previous year. He also reported an increased sense of helplessness, hopelessness, and worthlessness. Van had not sought any kind of employment and remained idle. He had become socially withdrawn.

Van was suspicious, moderately depressed, and markedly constricted (blunted affect). His affect was decreased in range and intensity. He perseverated on his need for surgery, believing that it would change his entire life. He displayed poor eye contact, decreased rate and volume of speech, and decreased psychomotor activity. His thought processes were unclear and illogical; he was delusional about his nose. The sensorium was intact.

The clinical course and the progressive loss of adaptive capacity justified the diagnosis of a schizophrenic spectrum disorder (Van carried the diagnosis of paranoid schizophrenia). Van's depressive syndrome could be a source of diagnostic difficulties; however, a depressive syndrome is not uncommon as a prodromal manifestation of schizophrenic illness.

Somatic-centered delusions may begin in preadolescence.

A very handsome and intelligent 10-year-old boy, had a prior history of psychiatric hospitalization for unrelenting suicidal ideation with prominent psychotic features, which included command hallucinations telling him to kill himself. He also reported seeing blood and dead people hanging from the ceilings and the walls. This boy had a great deal of difficulty distinguishing reality from unreality. On one occasion, after the psychotic features had been stabilized and his mood disorder was better, he asked his mother to leave the office because he needed to discuss some private thing with his doctor. After the mother left, the child asked the doctor to reassure him that his mother would not be made aware of his concerns. The child confided in his doctor that he felt that his penis was very small and that his behind was too big.

The need for a systematic inquiry cannot be emphasized enough. The following example shows how a thorough and systematic exploration provided diagnostic material, which was fundamental for a pertinent therapeutic decision.

Lee, a sixteen-year old Asian-American male, came for an outpatient consultation following his family relocation into the USA southwest area. Lee's family had been living in Japan, on a temporary military assignment. While in Japan, six month before the psychiatric consultation, Lee had a psychotic episode. He had been an outstanding and outgoing student before. At the time of the psychotic break, Lee had become very withdrawn, and started experiencing derealization and depersonalization symptoms; he also complained that the radio was talking to him, etc. About six months prior to the psychotic break, Lee's motivation and school performance had begun to falter and some personality changes were evident: he became withdrawn and at times, he became immobile for longer periods of time (catatonia?).

Since the military did not have facilities nor expertise locally, to deal with this psychiatric crisis, Lee was transferred to a psychiatric hospital in Hawaii where he received treatment for six weeks. The child had been discharged from the Hawaii psychiatric hospital 4 weeks prior to the consultation.

At the time of the consultation, the family had the strong impression that the child had recovered substantially. Basically, the family came to ask if the child still needed the medication (ziprasidone, 60 mg/evening), or at least they hoped the consultant psychiatrist would recommend a dose decrease.

During the Mental Status Examination, the adolescent was quiet, mildly withdrawn, non spontaneous but cooperative. His affect was very constricted but appropriate. Lee denied suicidal or homicidal ideation. The child did not show any evidence of thought disorder. Lee did not endorse auditory, visual, olfactory or haptic hallucinations. On the other hand he endorsed feelings that people talked about him, that people watched him and that people follow him. Moreover, when the examiner explored Lee's difficulties with falling sleep, he stated that he could not fall sleep because his feared that the devil would come to kill him.

The parents, who were present during the mental status examination, readily understood that their child was far from being asymptomatic and that he needed to continue on antipsychotics. Actually, the consultant psychiatrist indicated that Lee actually needed a medication increase.

OTHER PERTINENT EXPLORATIONS IN PREADOLESCENTS AND ADOLESCENTS WITH PSYCHOTIC SYMPTOMS

Alcohol and substance abuse issues, along with other health-related issues are of major significance.

Exploration of Alcohol and Substance Abuse

Brunette, Noordsy, and Green (2005) indicate that the prevalence of alcohol and drug abuse disorders in patients with schizophrenia is surprisingly high, with a lifetime prevalence estimated in 58.5% for alcohol and 47% for substance abuse (p. 29). Alcohol and substance abuse complicate the treatment of schizophrenia in a number of ways (see table 3.5).

TABLE 3.5 Complications of Treatment of Chronic Psychosis
Caused by Alcohol and Substance Abuse

1. Treatment nonadherence
2. Increased risk of relapse
3. Suicidality
4. Hospitalization
5. Homelessness
6. Victimization
7. Violence
8. Increased risk for HIV, hepatitis B, and hepatitis C
9. Lower adaptive capacity

Source: Modified from Brunette, Noordsy, & Green (2005, p. 29).

Exploration of Health Related Issues

Patients with severe psychosis have a higher prevalence of medical disorders (i.e., diabetes mellitus, visual problems, and others); on the other hand, patients who receive antipsychotic medication treatment carry a higher risk of medical complications like obesity, diabetes mellitus, metabolic syndrome, cardiovascular complications, and others. It is mandatory then, that the treating psychiatrist makes a systematic review of systems of the cardiovascular background (prior history heart disease, history of long-QTc syndrome, history of fainting, dizziness, and others); endocrinological background (history of obesity, history of polycystic ovarian disease, history of menstrual abnormalities, history of hyperprolactinemia, and others); history of cholesterol and other blood lipid levels abnormalities, history of sexual dysfunction, and visual abnormalities.

PSYCHOSIS IN NONVERBAL PATIENTS WITH DEVELOPMENTAL DISABILITIES

Patients with developmental disabilities may exhibit some unusual behaviors indicative of psychosis, yet are actually almost never reflective of psychosis (Ryan, 2001, p. 51). The examiner should be cautious in diagnosing psychosis in such circumstances (see table 3.6).

The following symptoms are never indicative of psychosis:

Volitional self-talk, vocal tics—consider Tourette's syndrome.
Phenomena that are modeled directly from other people.
Phenomena that the person can start and stop at will.
Phenomena thought to be the result of circumstances or programming
Displays of aggression, agitation, shouting, or self-injury (Ryan, 2001, p. 51).

TABLE 3.6 Indication of Psychosis in Developmentally Impaired Children and Adolescents

- Patients stare to the side, nod and gesture as though listening to a conversation others do not hear.
- Patients seem to be shadow boxing with unseen others.
- Patients brush unseen material off themselves.
- Patients wear multiple layers of clothing unrelated to weather.
- Patients cover their eyes and ears as though shutting out stimuli.
- Patients place unusual wrappings (e.g., feminine hygiene products) around their ankles, sleeve ends, ears, or collars.
- Patients glare at others out of context, and display an angry or intensely fearful expression at strangers or previously liked persons.
- Patients wrap bandannas or extra scarves around the head or ears when this is not congruent with the weather or the rest of the person's clothing.
- Patients wear costumes that are associated with a false role (e.g., wearing full firefighting gear when the patient is not a firefighter)
- Patients inspect food and beverages with new and out of context intensity.
- Patients grimace or wince as though smelling or tasting something foul.

Source: Ryan (2001, p. 51).

In persons with developmental disabilities, referred for psychiatric consultation, between 70 and 85% of them, have one or more untreated, undertreated, or undiagnosed medical problems influencing their behavior (Ryan, 2001, p. 51). Many of these conditions may produce delirium, which may include psychosis. Between 60 and 100% (depending on the sample) of individuals with developmental disabilities have experienced trauma, usually repeated incidents of abuse.

PTSD and other trauma sequelae need to be considered. Mood disorders with psychotic features are more common in people with developmental disabilities than are conditions in the schizophrenic spectrum (Ryan, 2001, p. 51).

ASSESSEMENT OF VIOLENCE RISK IN PSYCHOTIC CHILDREN

Violence may be associated with both command hallucinations and other psychotic symptoms. According to the Epidemiological Catchment Area survey, approximately 13% of schizophrenic patients engage in violent behavior (Basil, Mathews, Sudak, & Adetunji, 2005, p. 60).

Violence is even more likely if delusions are present. Delusions plus an aggressive cognitive style, characterized by external hostile attributions, make violence likely. Violent behavior by psychotic patients results from a complex array of neurobiological, psychological, interpersonal, contextual, and socioeconomic factors (McNeil, Eisner, & Binder, 2001, p. 386). Of equal or even greater importance, is the psychotic child's compulsion to carry out a major act of revenge against a teacher or peers in the school environment, paralleling celebrated mass killings in unfortunate schools. Thus, the question regarding the presence of psychosis is often raised by school authorities when making decisions regarding potentially dangerous students.

Any child who makes even a veiled terrorist threat merits a comprehensive psychiatric and psychosocial asessment. According to Twemlow, Fonagy, Sacco, O'Toole, and Vernberg (2002), the levels of risk that should be considered in the evaluation of youth with homicidal violence include,

> High level risk: this includes children with behaviors that pose direct, specific threats that are plausible when concrete plans and steps have been taken.
>
> Medium level risk: this includes children whose threats may be concrete and detailed, but no plans or action has been taken.
>
> Low level risk: this includes threats that are often indirect. Details are inconsistent and nonplausible.

In assessing risk, these authors advise examiners to pay attention to a number of factors: previous warning communications; ambiguous messages; grievances: (these are most often communicated to peers); threats of suicide, and a history of depression and despair; the presence of cluster A and B personality disorders; and adolescents with paranoid, narcissistic, or passive–aggressive traits (pp. 475–476). Factors that need to be considered in the evaluation of potential for violence in children and adolescents are listed in table 3.7.

Children who shot their classmates and teachers felt disconnected from their peers and adults. They had been bullied at school and had experienced humiliation. Many shooters had suffered significant losses, had symptoms of depression, and had thought about suicide a great deal (Brown, Kennedy, & Pollack, 2005, p. 14). Similar concerns relate to hate crimes. Youth who perpetrate hate crimes demonstrate impulse control problems, thrill seeking behaviors, bullying, conduct or aggressive problems, a drive to be competent (to be noticed and recognized), or a need to deal with feelings of betrayal and

TABLE 3.7 Factors that Need to be Considered When Evaluating Potential for Violence in Children and Adolescents

- Availability of guns and knowledge of how to use them
- History of victimization by social groups or individuals
- Previous concerns expressed by adults or peers
- Mimicry of media figures: copying a movie plot, a novel, or recent events (i.e., following a previous massacre school scheme)
- History of change in emotions and interests
- Offspring of families low in emotional closeness and knowledge of adolescent life
- Over-involvement in fantasy or behavior with aggressive and violent behavior

Source: Modified from Twemlow, Fonagy, Sacco, O'Toole, & Vernberg (2002, pp. 475–476).

underlying hurt. It has been reported that similarities exist between those violent youth with rigidity of thinking, and those diagnosed with depression or paranoia. Both of these types of youth feel that they have been betrayed, they believe that someone is responsible for the betrayal, and they also believe that the person or the group needs to be punished for the betrayal (Steinberg, Brooks, & Remtulla, 2003, p. 984).

An aggressive cognitive style, characterized by external hostile attributions, represents a unifying construct that could explain the associations of command hallucinations and violence in the context of psychotic symptoms (such as some types of delusions) that are also correlated with violence (McNeil et al., 2001, p. 386).[1,2] These considerations for adults need corroboration in the field of child and adolescent psychiatry. It is true that many psychotic children hear command hallucinations and that only a few of them follow the voices' commands. The following case illustrates a case of severe risk of homicidal behavior toward the family:

Leo, a 15-year-old Hispanic male, with no prior psychiatric history, was taken by the local police to an acute psychiatric center, on an emergency detention order, due to homicidal ideation toward his father. According to the police, the patient told his school counselor that he had stabbed his father in the leg the night before, adding that he wished he had "finished off the job." He then stated that he still had thoughts of killing his father.

Leo's mother stated that on the night prior to admission they discovered that he had been tattooed on his neck without their permission. He and his father argued about this, at which point Leo grabbed a knife and cut his father's thigh (actually he punctured his father's left gluteal area). His parents had left him alone for the remainder of the night.

Leo's mother reported no prior problems with Leo until his last academic year when he switched to his current charter school and began associating with gang members. Since that time he became more oppositional. His mood became more irritable and he had been quicker to lose his temper. She worried that Leo was a "follower" and that he was acting up because of his new friends. She also worried about Leo using drugs because she knew his friends did. The day following the initial contact, mother found a small stash of marijuana in the child's room.

Leo stated he had problems with depressed feelings, primarily in the wintertime. Over the previous few months he felt that his depression had been converted into a feeling of rage. He asserted that he liked the feeling of rage because it made him feel "powerful." He felt rage most days. He stated that when he did not feel the rage he felt weak. The rage was mostly directed at his father; Leo justified his anger by saying that his father was too strict and that he also resented that father did not understand him.

Leo had revealed another plan to kill a peer at school stating, "I know it will happen, I just don't know when." Upon further questioning he admitted that he often had thoughts of killing people when angered. He denied having thoughts of wanting to kill himself, but stated he "was not afraid to die." He got angry at the suggestion that he was a follower, stating that people followed his lead and that he felt rather proud that he had always been a troublemaker. He denied that he belonged to a gang but said he had plans to join one soon.

Leo had been smoking marijuana for over a year. He claimed that "a dime bag lasted [him] approximately 3 weeks." Marijuana took away the rage and made him feel "calm." He felt this was the main reason he continued smoking it. He denied other drug use with the exception of drinking "approximately three beers per month."

Leo often felt that people were talking about him or out to get him. He often had to check behind him while walking. He occasionally heard footsteps at night and saw shadows. These feelings had been present even when he was not smoking marijuana. He had some difficulty falling asleep at night because he feared somebody was in the room; he also worried about what his future would bring. He denied any changes in his energy level, interest, appetite, or ability to concentrate. He denied any decreased need for sleep or racing thoughts. However, he felt hopeless about the future and wondered if he was going to end up in jail or if somebody was going to kill him.

The mental status examination revealed the presence of a dark complected Hispanic youth who appeared to be his stated age of 15. He was dressed all in black with baggy pants. He had a tattoo of "Guadalupe" on the left side of his neck and one of three black dots on his left forearm. His hair was greased and arranged in numerous slick clumps. He sat slouched in the chair and stared at the floor, making intermittent eye contact with the examiner. His speech was mumbled at times but understandable. His answers were brief and he needed encouragement to elaborate his answers.

His mood was depressed and he frequently leaned his head over his forearms avoiding eye contact; he also displayed mild irritability. Leo's affect was congruous with thought content, although he became cocky if not arrogant when discussing his homicidal ideation. No affective lability was noted.

The sensorium was intact: Leo was oriented to person place, date, and situation. His concentration was intact: he was able to spell the word *world* backwards. He recalled 3/3 objects immediately and 2/3 at 5 minutes. His responses to similarities were concrete. Intellectual functioning was considered average based on his fund of knowledge and complexity of concepts.

Leo's thoughts were coherent, logical, and goal directed. There were no loose associations, flight of ideas, or obsessive thoughts. He initially denied hearing voices, but when he was asked again if his brain talked to him, he disclosed that "for a while" he had been hearing his mind talking to him. His mind told him to do things, including killing his dad. Leo said that his mind had told him "to go ahead and stab your father." He also heard his mind telling him to kill his peer. At night, his mind told him that somebody was behind him, that he needed to check the room. He said he could shut the voices off but not always. He added that some times he liked to hear the voices, that sometimes "the voices cracked jokes." He exhibited florid paranoia in that he felt that people talked about him, watched him, and followed him. He also felt that people were out to get him. He denied ongoing suicidal ideation but endorsed homicidal ideation toward his father. His judgment was poor based on the disregard for his behavior toward his father. His insight was poor in that he did not seem to think that there was anything wrong with the way he felt toward his father.

It is obvious that this adolescent was a very high homicidal risk. Treatment of this adolescent was fraught with difficulties because his anger and even some of his psychotic features were ego syntonic.

MENTAL RETARDATION AND PSYCHOSIS

It is difficult to ascertain the diagnosis of schizophrenia in children with mental retardation; linguistic and cognitive obstacles demand integration of information from a wide range of relevant sources. This information needs to be standardized and reliable; symptoms such as thought disorder are particularly difficult to identify reliably in persons with mental retardation, indicating the need for caution when making the diagnosis. Using the term *diagnostic hypothesis* rather than *diagnosis* opens the possibility of change in the light of subsequent assessments (Lee, Moss, Friedlander, Donnelly, & Honer, 2003, p. 167). The diagnostic imprecision of incongruous affect highlights a crucial issue in relation to the diagnosis of schizophrenia in mentally retarded people. Negative symptoms have the potential for being confused with behaviors that may occur in people with mental retardation who are not mentally ill (Lee et al., 2003, p. 166). When interviewing children with cognitive deficits, the examiner's language should be simple, concrete, and redundant. Findings need to be corroborated from a variety of clinical angles.

It is possible to make the diagnosis of early onset schizophrenia in adolescents with mental retardation, provided the assessment is carefully structured and attention is paid to all the important sources of information (Lee et al., 2003, p. 168).

CHAPTER 4

Examination of Mood and Affect

The examination of mood is one of the fundamental components of the mental status examination; the other components of the exam include, the description of general appearance and demeanor, the examination of the sensorium and thought processes, and the determination of intellectual functioning.

The propositions to be reviewed in this chapter include:

- The examiner needs to explore mood related disorders in every case of psychosis in children and adolescents.
- The mental status examination or the observations gathered during the psychiatric evaluation are not enough to rule out a mood disorder. Background information, developmental history, family history, and other clinical and testing information are important auxiliaries in the diagnostic process.
- Children's and adolescents' mood and affect change significantly from moment to moment, creating diagnostic confusion. At times, although the child looks euthymic, significant others report that the child is isolative, that the child has cut communications with friends and the family, that the child is unmotivated, or that he or she is preoccupied with death or with suicide.
- Even when the phenotype is ostensibly schizophreniform, the examiner needs to be open to schizophreniform phenocopic presentations of mood disorders. It has been stated a number of times before that mood disorders may have an acute presentation that is indistinguishable from schizophrenia.

In the assessment of psychotic disorders in childhood, the evaluation of mood and affect is of preeminent importance because the great majority of psychoses in children and adolescents are associated with mood disturbances. As in the evaluation of negative symptoms (see chapter 2), discussion of the assessment of mood will include: exploration of the presenting problem, past history including developmental history, observations during the psychiatric assessment, and a systematic inquiry during the mental status examination.

DATA GATHERING

The examiner will gather systematic information regarding the child's presenting problem, past history, developmental background, and history of ongoing stresses. Family history is fundamental in the diagnosis of mood disorders of children, adolescents, and adults. The same is true of the exploration of medical and neurological history, use of drugs, intake of prescribed medications, and over-the-counter products. Of equal importance is to obtain a full overview of the child's adaptive capacity in the major milieus: school, family, friends, play, and other areas of interest to the child. Progress in the development of autonomy and individuation, and the child's capacity for behavioral organization are important. Last, but not least, the examiner will gather information regarding past treatments, with emphasis on medication history, detailing what medications have been tried, doses, compliance, responses, and side effects.

Major depressive episode (MDE) will be discussed as a prototypical mood disorder. This disorder is a common affliction of children and adolescents,

---

TABLE 4.1 Criteria for Major Depressive Episode

A. Five or more of the following symptoms, representing change from previous level of functioning, should be present for at least two weeks. Either (1) depressive mood or (2) loss of interest or pleasure must be present. Symptoms should not be obviously related to a general medical condition, or mood incongruent psychotic features
   1. Depressed mood, most of the day, nearly daily. Children and adolescents may display irritable mood.
   2. Diminished interest or pleasure in almost all activities, most of the day, nearly daily.
   3. Weight loss when not dieting or weight gain, or decrease or increase of appetite. In children there might be a failure to make expected weight gain.
   4. Insomnia or hypersomnia nearly daily.
   5. Psychomotor retardation or agitation nearly daily.
   6. Fatigue or loss of energy nearly daily.
   7. Feelings of worthlessness or inappropriate guilt nearly daily.
   8. Diminished ability to think or concentrate, or indecisiveness nearly daily.
   9. Recurrent thoughts of death, or recurrent suicidal thoughts, or a suicidal attempt or a specific suicidal plan.
B. Symptoms do not meet criteria for a mixed episode
C. Symptoms cause clinically significant distress or impairment in social, occupational or other important areas of functioning.
D. Symptoms are not related to effects of a substance (alcohol, drugs, medications), or a general medical condition.
E. Symptoms are not better accounted for by bereavement.

Source: American Psychiatric Association. (2000). *Diagnostic and statistical manual of mental disorders. Text revision* (p. 356, 4th ed. rev.).Washington, D.C.

and is frequently associated with psychotic features. Table 4.1 summarizes the DSM-IV-TR criteria for MDE (APA, 2000).

In florid cases of MDE, the child or adolescent will experience sadness, usually accompanied by crying. Sudden and unexplained spells of crying are not uncommon, and often, the child cannot verbalize the reason for the crying. Parents report emotional withdrawal from the family, and growing isolation from friends. Commonly, the child loses interest in activities he or she had previously been invested in, such as sports, outings, avocations, or other extracurricular activities. The most telling indicator of a mood disorder (depression) is the deterioration of academic performance or the loss of interest in school. Academic decay is due to a number of factors associated with depression: concentration difficulties, motivational problems, boredom, anhedonia, hopelessness, and others.

Serious evidence of depression includes suicidal ideation and behaviors (to be discussed below), irritability and anger control difficulties, anhedonia, anergy and tiredness, sleep abnormalities, and loss of weight. It is not uncommon for depressed patients to activate other comorbid conditions such as anxiety related features, psychosis (both hallucinations, and delusions), drug abuse, eating disorders, and others.

In serious depressions during adolescence patients frequently report, "being depressed" all their lives. A pertinent inquiry in the exploration of severe depression would include questions such as the following: How long have you been depressed? Since you started feeling depressed, have you had any times when you are not depressed? How long did these periods last? Is there anything you can do to make yourself feel better? What is the worst your depression has been? What sort of things have you tried to get rid of the depressive feelings? Have you used any drugs?

Children and adolescents with severe mood disorders report that they wake up in a bad mood. A revealing question is, how do you feel when you wake in the mornings? Patients endorse irritability or a "grouchy or cranky" mood when they wake up. They also endorse lack of energy, tiredness, or lack of restorative sleep. Clinician will ascertain if the child suffers from initial, middle, or terminal insomnia.

Initial insomnia gives plenty of opportunities to explore psychotic features as indicated in chapter 2. What keeps you away from sleeping? Any worries? Any fears? Does your mind play tricks with you at night? The examiner also needs to enquire for the presence of reverse neurovegetative symptoms: How much do you sleep? Do you sleep during the day? How much do you eat? Do you eat more than you need? These questions are of limited relevance if the patient is receiving atypical antipsychotics (see below).

Adolescents are quite vulnerable to interpersonal rejection, more so if it comes from a close friend, or from a boyfriend or girl friend. Emotional breakups throw adolescents into hopelessness and despair. Suicidal potential is high in these circumstances. A recent death of a loved one is an event that

TABLE 4.2 Risk Factors That May Predict Suicide in Youths

- Pubertal age
- Male gender
- Depression and feeling of hopelessness
- History or evidence of mania
- Mixed mood states
- Psychosis
- Victim of physical or sexual abuse
- Co-occurring disruptive disorders
- Comorbid substance abuse
- Impulsivity
- Easy access to means, such as firearms, lethal toxins, or medications
- Lack of family support, family dysfuction
- Acute stressors (i.e., a romantic breakup, death of a close one, peer teasing, and peer rejection)
- Family history of suicide
- History of suicidal behavior

Source: Modified from Fuller & Fuller (2005, p. 89).

frequently elicits depression and suicidality. The suicide of a close friend or a peer is another negative stimulant for depression and suicide. Suicides within the family are major triggers of self-destructive behavior. Table 4.2 highlights risk factors associated with suicide in children and adolescents.

The major clinical challenge in the field of adult and child psychiatry, in the process of mood assessment, is the differentiation of major depressive episodes and unipolar depressions (MDD) from bipolar depressions. Table 4.3 indicates the DSM-IV-TR criteria for the diagnosis of bipolar I disorder, most recent episode depressed.

TABLE 4.3 Diagnostic Criteria for Bipolar Disorder, Most Recent Episode Depressed

Current or most recent evidence of a major depressive episode
Previous history of at least one manic episode or a mixed episode
Mood episodes of criteria A and B cannot be explained by the presence of schizoaffective disorder, delusional disorder or psychotic disorder NOS

Specifiers:

Mild, moderate, severe without psychotic features or severe with psychotic feature.
Chronic
    With catatonic features, with melancholic features, with atypical features, with postpartum onset

In partial remission, in full remission
Chronic
With catatonic features, with melancholic features, with atypical features, with postpartum onset

With or without interepisode recovery
With seasonal pattern
With rapid cycling

Source: American Psychiatric Association. (2000). *Diagnostic and statistical manual of mental disorders* (p. 391).

According to the National Institute of Mental Health, about 2% of children between 6 and 12 years of age suffer from major depression at any one time. At puberty, the rate increases to 4%. In adolescence, girls have a higher rate of depression than boys and this difference is lifelong. While depression before school age (i.e., 2–5 years of age) is rare, it definitely exists. By the time they become adults, about 20% of these youths will have suffered from one or more episodes of major depression. Of those who have adolescent depression, approximately 40% will have recurring depression, with some experiencing lifelong illness, if not treated (Sussman, 2005, p. 11). MDD is a common psychiatric ailment, with an estimated lifetime prevalence of 15% for adolescents 15 to 18 years of age (Gabbay, Silva, Castellanos, Rabinovitz, & Gonen, 2005, p. 52).

The distinction between MDD and bipolar depression has important treatment implications; if the diagnosis is incorrect and the psychiatrist orders antidepressants alone, there is a risk of precipitating mania. In the presence of chronic and severe preadolescent or adolescent depressions, the clinician will strive to ascertain the presence of a history of hypomanic or manic episodes, presence of family history of affective disorders (in three previous generations), history of pharmacological mania or hypomania, history of preadolescent psychotic depression, or history of early depression associated with alcohol or substance abuse, among others. In chronic depressions, it is important to explore the presence of hypomanic features; that is, experiences of elation or euphoria, feelings of having too much energy and not needing sleep, "feelings of being on top of the world," racing thoughts, beliefs in having special powers, and other grandiose traits, hypersexuality, affective storms, or suicidality. Perlis, Brown, Baker, and Nierenberg (2006) state that in bipolar disorders there is a greater prevalence of atypical depressive features or reversed neurovegetative symptoms: hypersomnia, hyperphagia; also, irritability, anger, subthreshold mixed symptoms (overactivity), and psychosis are more common in bipolar depression. One prospective study suggests a high specificity with a combination of clinical predictors, such as early onset symptoms, bipolar family history, and hypersomnia or psychomotor slowing as high as 98% (p. 225). Moreover, tension/edginess and fearfulness are more severe in patients with bipolar depression than in patients with unipolar major depressive disorders. On the contrary, anxiety and somatic complaints (muscular, respiratory, genitourinary), are more common in the unipolar group (Perlis, Brown, et al., 2006, p. 229).

If the data are complex and inconclusive, it is sound practice to consider the diagnosis and treatment of a bipolar depression and implement treatment of mood stabilizers rather than using antidepressants alone. In acute or relapsing clinical situations, parents become aware of symptoms of mood disturbances earlier than symptoms of thought disorders. In general, parents have more access to information and observations related to affective disturbances than to symptoms related to psychotic disorders. Parents inform examiners of the reappearance of sadness, interpersonal withdrawal, and appetite or sleep problems. More pertinent for the consideration of a severe mood disorder are parents' reports of moodiness, increasing irritability, if not explosiveness and escalation of oppositional behavior; these demeanors may contrast to the child's previous behavior or represent a worsening of previous behavioral and emotional baseline.

With severe mood disorders, behavior and performance difficulties at school are omnipresent. The decrement in school performance parallels parents' observations regarding a lack of motivation for schoolwork and family life, disinterest in friends or in activities that used to draw the child's interest and attention. For anhedonic children, not even the Internet, TV, friends, partying, or other fun activities have any appeal anymore. Difficulties getting out of bed, lack of school interest, or problems with elementary hygiene are sources of serious concern. Even personal care or taking regular meals become recurrent difficulties for many seriously disturbed mood-disordered children.

There are a number of recurrent clinical situations that stimulate the search for a mood disorder and of an increased suicidal risk:

1. The child loses considerable weight or his or her physical condition becomes a matter of concern.
2. The child conveys that he or she does not care anymore, and overtly loses interest in areas where the child was previously involved. Somehow, the child reaches the conclusion that no matter how much he or she tries, nothing will change, that any effort is useless, that life is hopeless.
3. The child begins to display self-abusive behavior, or makes veiled or overt declarations that he or she wants to die. Adolescents frequently express in writing or otherwise that they want to die, or that they are thinking about or contemplating suicide. If they write poetry, they express interest in and preoccupation with morbid topics; the content of their poetry, notes, or essays is gloomy and depressing, filled with anger and resentment, disillusionment and despair. Without exception, these children indicate that nobody understands them, and that they feel lonely and unloved. These adolescents have lost hope that parents can help or soothe them, and seek emotional support somewhere else, often, in a community of friends. Psychologically and emotionally, these other individuals become as important as or even more important than the parental figures. To the question, who is the most important person in your life? A parent or parents is not the first person that the adolescent mentions. The examiner needs to clarify the reason for such a choice.
4. The child feels overwhelmed with ongoing stressors, feeling that interpersonal injuries are catastrophic. This is the case when adolescents break up with a boyfriend or girl friend, when parents divorce or separate, when a close friend dies, or when a perceived failure feels beyond repair.
5. Suicide of a parent or of a close friend, or even of a peer increases the potential for suicide.

6. The child cannot cope with family stresses. If there is overt discord between the parents, including violence, or a history of sexual abuse, the child or adolescent feels unsafe and unprotected; in these circumstances, the adolescent fears further traumatization while at the same time he or she longs for a parental source of emotional support. Moreover, between 20 and 50% of depressed children and adolescents have a family history of depression (Sussman, 2005, p. 11).

7. The adolescent feels that he or she cannot live up to the expectations or standards of a demanding family.

8. The child feels ostracized in the school environment due to overweight/ obesity, presence of a handicap, physical peculiarities, or for possessing intellectual or learning limitations. A counterpart to this is the child who feels bullied and intimidated, if not abused, by dissocial or antisocial peers, and feels helpless in confronting ongoing threats. Similar risk is present in adolescents with conflictive sexual identity, or when the adolescents' sexual preferences are revealed and disapproved of by the family.

9. The adolescent suffers from a medical condition, such as asthma, juvenile diabetes, seizures, arthritis, renal failure, cancer or others that encumber the individual's self-image and imposes limitations on physical and social activities.

10. The child or adolescent suffers from body image disturbances that become the focus of acceptability in the social milieu, as well as the explanation for everything the individual feels is wrong in his or her life.

11. The child displays a personality transformation, behaving in ways that are alien to previous deportment: The child begins to sneak out of the house, becomes promiscuous, or worse, begins to display antisocial behavior; the adolescent gets involved in behavior that leads to legal problems, associates with the "wrong crowd," or demonstrates involvement with drugs or alcohol.

12. The child displays demeanors that are uncharacteristic: although formerly restrained, maybe inhibited, he or she now becomes impulsive, unrestrained, and disinhibited. The child who formerly respected rules and authority becomes unruly and enamored with anarchy, detesting rules and disapproving of social norms.

13. Girls and boys who previously demonstrated modesty or controlled sexual behavior become overtly sexually preoccupied. It is not unusual for adolescent females to allow male companions into their rooms, or "to sleep around" with multiple boys. Unprotected sex is the norm.

14. Female and even male adolescents reveal despair and hopelessness when unwanted pregnancies are confirmed, anticipating rejection or even ejection from the home environment.

15. Dramatic changes in mood and demeanor are common sources of parental concern and confusion. Sudden mood changes, aggressive storms,

outbursts of violence and destructiveness, among others, may be early manifestations of bipolar disorders and of increased suicidal risk.

16. The adolescent stops taking medications that have demonstrated a benefit, and refuses to attend psychiatric and psychotherapeutic appointments. Frequently, these behaviors are part of an overall pattern of denial, of disregard for rules and expectations, and of open defiance and rebelliousness. These behaviors may represent a lack of medication compliance indicating hopelessness and despair.

17. Because of lack of response to discipline or consequences, the adolescent gets into "heated" confrontations with parents who feel progressively helpless, disrespected, and without effective authority. These situations increase the risks of parental dyscontrol, of the development of physical abuse, creating further alienation of the child from the family.

18. It is important to abide by the new FDA recommendations when prescribing antidepressants to youth: close monitoring of suicidal ideation and behavior at the beginning of antidepressant induction is mandatory.

Sometimes, children and adolescents do not conceive of the thought of killing themselves but entertain the idea of provoking others to cause their demise. For instance, adolescents may commit some minor misdemeanor when they know there are police officers around, and run or flee the scene, hoping police will shoot them down; other times, when there are sources of violence in the neighborhood, children conceive the idea of provoking one or more gang members, expecting a lethal retaliation. These provoked deaths are known as suicide by proxy.

Theme variations of the recurrent clinical situations, described above, are the rule. These situations, among many, are sources of concern, conflict, and developmental problems. They pose a significant challenge to the children, adolescents, and their families' adaptation and sense of well-being. Attentive parents notice disturbing changes at once and take appropriate action immediately. In families where there is parental discord or family disorganization, or in environments where the children's welfare is not a priority, response and solutions to ongoing problems are delayed if not denied. Certainly, in abusive environments, families do not have the children's best interests at heart. In families where the parents have suffered from mood disorders, their norms of normality and propriety are lax and "are not in sync" with the social milieu or the school environment. These families postpone professional intervention until external pressures move them to take action.

In clinical situations such as those cited above, it is assumed that for some children, mood and psychotic disorders are discontinuous or episodic, or that once the condition recedes, the child will return to his or her baseline, "normal" condition. It is also frequently assumed that the child started out with integrity of the genome and the CNS; that pregnancy, delivery, and perinatal life were uneventful; that development proceeded according to normative schemes; and that the family environment has been caring and supportive, among other things.

Unfortunately, for a significant proportion of children afflicted with mood and psychotic disorders, these assumptions are invalid. These children, to a greater or lesser degree, carry the negative results of genetic, congenital, developmental, or environmental adversities that contribute to the severity and chronicity of the disorders. For many children, prior to the identification or diagnosis of a mood or psychotic disorder, their background has already been compromised. Often, after psychiatric and psychotherapeutic interventions the disorders are not thoroughly resolved and their psychiatric conditions may become chronic, creating an added impediment for the child's progression in multiple developmental domains: self-regulation, self-soothing, self-concept, emotional regulation (anger control), social relations, language, cognitive development, and others.

Children and adolescents with chronic mood disorders display significant comorbidities such as ADHD, conduct disorder, substance abuse, anxiety disorders, and others that complicate the primary disorder or that make treatment more difficult; comorbidities also complicate the psychiatric rehabilitation process.

PRESENTING PROBLEM

When the initial presentation is depression, for instance, the examiner will explore the what, how, when, where of the depressive symptoms, and finally the examiner will attempt to understand the why of the depressive features. The clinician will inquire into the presence of melancholic symptoms: lack of energy, anhedonia, amotivation, loss of appetite, and sleep disturbances. Each symptom needs to be explored and elaborated independently. Relevant consequences of melancholia in children, such as loss of school days, physical complaints and visits to pediatricians, school deterioration, loss of motivation, weight loss, and concentration difficulties, need to be substantiated.

Above anything else, suicide risk needs to be explored thoroughly and in depth. Among all the psychiatric conditions, mood disorders and psychotic-spectrum disorders carry the highest level of lethality. In the United States, about 500,000 suicide attempts and 2,000 completed suicides occur on a yearly basis in adolescents. Suicide is the fourth leading cause of death among children and adolescents 10 to 14 years of age, and the third leading cause of death for adolescents 15 to 19 years of age (Silva, Gabbay, Minami, Munoz-Silva, & Alonso, 2005, p. 43). The risk of suicide in affective disorder is high; suicidal risk in bipolar disorders is estimated to be around 15%. Lewinsohn, Seeley, and Klein (2003) reported that a history of suicidal attempts was significantly elevated in adolescents with bipolar disorder (44.4%); in comparison to adolescents with a subsyndromal picture, major depressive disorder, and controls. For subsyndromal bipolar disorder the incidence of suicide was 17.6%, in the major depressive disorder group it was 21.8%, and in the group without a mood disorder the incidence was 1.2%. The bipolar disorder group also had a higher frequency of suicidal ideation than the subsyndromal and control groups, but was similar in this regard to the major depressive group. Also, the bipolar disorder group had an earlier history of attempts and of multiple attempts when compared to the other mood disordered groups. Furthermore, the bipolar disorder group displayed a higher level of lethality in their suicidal attempts (p. 12). Thus, the risk of suicide is higher for bipolar than for unipolar children and adolescents.

The suicide risk for schizophrenic disorders is approximately the same as for bipolar disorders. Each one of the recurrent clinical situations, listed above, has an increased suicide potential. This potential needs to be explored.

Suicidal children and adolescents are also at a heightened risk to hurt others, including the immediate family. Homicidal tendencies need to be explored in depth. According to the Epidemiological Catchment Area survey, about 13% of schizophrenic patients engage in violent behavior and mentally ill patients who come from violent backgrounds are often violent themselves. Violence is more common during acute psychotic episodes. In acute psychiatric settings lack of insight is a highly predictive factor for violence potential (Basil et al., 2005, p. 60).

Relevant for the diagnosis and psychopharmacological treatment and even genetic counseling, is the elucidation of genetic factors or family pathology in the immediate family, as well as the presence of mood disorders or a history of suicide in the two previous generations. At the same level of relevance is the elucidation of manic, hypomanic, or cyclothymic behaviors, as well as the rate or frequency of mood changes, including seasonal mood variations in extended family and prior generations.

Most recent observations indicate that a number of disorders antecede the presentation of bipolar disorder in adolescence or early adulthood. Antecedent conditions are, first and foremost, depressive disorders; the earlier the onset and the more melancholic the picture, the greater the chance that a bipolar disorder may develop in the future. Also important in this regard, is the presence of ADHD (considered a prodrome in children with a family history of bipolar disorders), anxiety disorders (separation anxiety, social phobia, panic disorders—considered a marker for genetic heterogeneity—and obsessive–compulsive disorders). At the root of panic disorder/bipolar disorder comorbidity, behavioral inhibition is proposed as the common diathesis for both disorders (Papolos, 2003, pp. 89–90). Substance abuse and bipolar disorder are considered to exist on a bipolar disorder spectrum (Camacho, 2004, p. 44).

CHAPTER 5

Aids in the Diagnostic Process

The chapter will elaborate on the following propositions:

- The psychiatrist needs to attend to multiple indicators of the presence of a psychotic disorder.
- There are a number of clinical techniques that the clinican can use to ascertain the presence of psychosis in childhood.
- A number of reliable diagnostic scales can be used to ascertain the presence and extent of psychosis.
- Psychological testing is a helpful aid in the diagnosis of psychosis.
- The psychiatrist may seek a neurological consultation or may request neuroimaging or other related studies.
- So far, there are no definitive studies that corroborate the presence of a serious psychotic disorder.
- The identification and diagnosis of childhood psychosis is still preeminently a clinical exercise.
- Significant progress is being made in many fields (genetics, electrophysiology, biochemistry, imaging, and others) to identify diagnostic underpinnings of chronic psychosis.

A number of techniques and tests are used to advance the diagnosis and to assist in the differential diagnosis of psychoses of childhood, including play, drawings, the use of diagnostic protocols, and rating scales (WASH-U-K-SADS, K-SADS, BPRS, PANNS, YMRS, and other diagnostic scales; see below), physical and neurological examination, neurologic consultation, neuroimaging studies, psychological and neuropsychological testing, and others.

The DSM-IV-TR and the ICD-10 are the most universally used indexes of the classification of psychiatric illnesses. The DSM sytem establishes criteria for categorical diagnosis of psychiatric disorders, and each diagnostic category has inclusionary and exclusionary criteria. The DSM and ICD systems are the accepted diagnostic manuals for the provision and administration of mental health services around the world. The DSM system is a necessary resource for the diagnosis of psychiatric disorders and for consideration of differential diagnosis.

DRAWINGS

Drawings give a good indication of the child's level of intelligence and of the child's creative and artistic talents; they may also hint at the presence of possible neuropsychological deficits. The quality of the child's pencil grasp, how the child approaches this task, the nature, content, and quality of the drawings themselves, and other related observations, give the examiner opportunities to further the diagnostic assessment.

Psychotic children often give indications of their psychotic preoccupation in their drawings, and their drawings frequently reflect their disturbed psychotic thinking or their abnormal thought processes. Frequently, there is evidence of intrusive ideation during the task, and drawings commonly show unusual or bizarre preoccupations.

It is recommended that four or five drawings, in a prestablished order, be obtained from the patient during the examination. The order that the author commonly recommends is the following: (1) a spontaneous drawing; (2) drawing a person; (3) drawing a person of the opposite sex; (4) the family kinetic drawing ("draw your family doing something together"); and (5) the drawing of a tree (Goudenough test). Asking the child to draw any reported hallucination(s) is helpful to add credence to the presence of psychotic symptoms; this visual evidence helps to change the mind set of skeptical parents.

A 10-year-old Hispanic boy was evaluated for suicidal and homicidal behaviors. The child had a borderline IQ. His mother reported that over the previous month, the child had been progressively aggressive toward the family and had even threatened to kill her. Over the previous month or so, he had also started hearing voices; he disclosed to his mother that the voice had told him that, "[it] was coming to get him, that [it] would get a knife and cut his heart out." This child also claimed that he had seen the bad voice, and that, "It looked like the devil." A few days prior to the evaluation, the child started to hear a toy talking to him; that particular toy had been a "survivor" of a house fire the year before. Apparently, the toy told him that the fire "was [his] fault." The child had received no prior psychiatric treatment.

The child had a history of delayed milestones: he sat by six months and crawled by the eighth month. Although, he could stand by one year, he had only started walking by age 5. He also had speech delays. He repeated second grade and had been receiving special education for academic difficulties. Allegedly, he had no friends at school because he was frequently involved in fights.

Much more consequential in this child's life were the family's frequent moves and the birth of a baby sister two months prior to the examination. The child had changed schools four times during the previous year. The family denied any physical or sexual abuse history. However, this child had attempted to touch his biological father's girl friend's breasts a year before. The child's biological father had been in prison for child molestation.

The mental status examination revealed the presence of an overweight boy who displayed significant separation anxiety when he was interviewed without his parents. The child was very concrete and his vocabulary was limited. He revealed that the devil was in the room and that the devil was telling him not to cooperate with the examiner. The child became progressively anxious without the parents around and began to say that there was nothing wrong with him. At this time, the examiner invited the child to do some drawings. The drawings were very revealing of the child's psychotic functioning, as described below:

First Drawing: Spontaneous drawing. The drawing represented his heart stabbed with a knife by the devil. Blood was pouring from the stabbed heart.

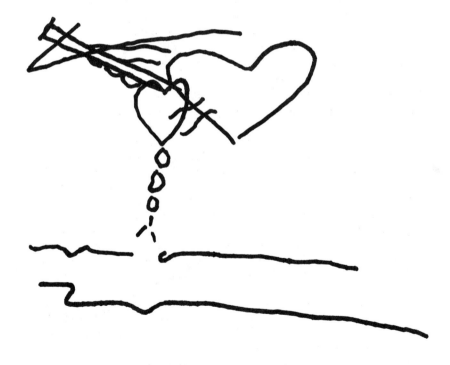

Second Drawing: Draw a person. The child drew a boy whose heart had been removed by the devil. He elaborated that the devil had entered into the child's body and that "he" looked ugly (dark face).

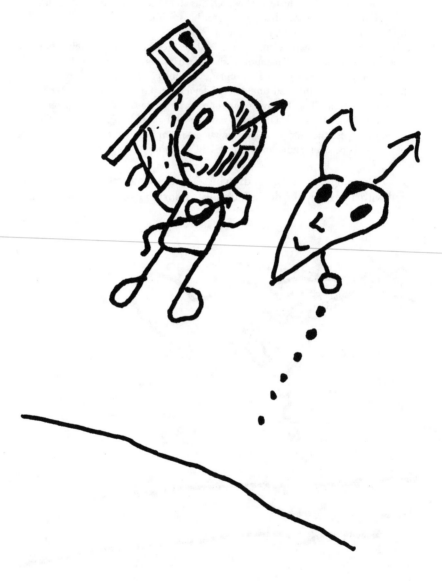

Third Drawing: Draw a girl. He drew a girl who had been chopped up by the devil.

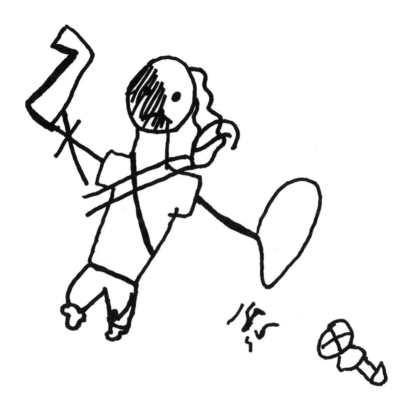

Fourth Drawing: Draw your family doing something together. He drew his scared mother and two younger siblings running away, fleeing from the persecuting devil.

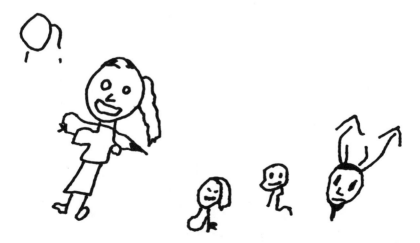

The parents began to waver in their resolve to seek treatment when they saw the child's separation anxiety and his desperate assertions that there was nothing wrong with him. When the parents were presented with the child's drawings, they regained their resolve and were able to agree to an intensive intervention for the child. In this case, the drawings were instrumental in corroborating the presence of psychois and in assisting the parents in understanding the severity of their child's condition. Contrary to the child's denials, the drawings showed a morbid preoccupation with aggression and a persistent paranoid ideation about the devil.

Another example of the usefulness of drawings can be seen in the case of Louis (chapter 7, pp. 174–176). Louis suffered from very early onset schizophrenia (VEOS). In the first drawing, Louis, a 10-year-old, drew himself. The body parts are disconnected and there are no limbs. When he was asked to explain the drawing, he mentioned that the top part was "a cap, a hat," and that below the head was a "bone, the body." He stated that the lower part was "a penis." At the right side of this drawing, there is an intrusion of peculiar ideation or preoccupation; he displayed this disturbance throughout the process when doing other drawings.

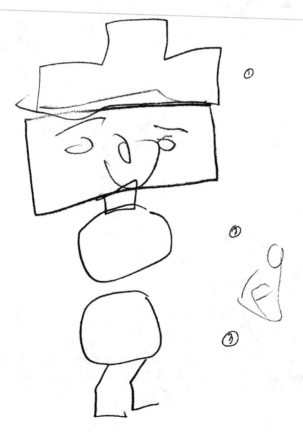

Notice that in the second drawing, in the section of the drawing corresponding to the head, he wrote the word *mom.*

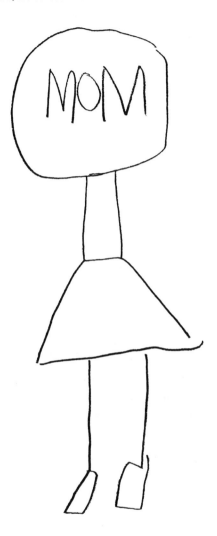

In the third drawing, the name of the person (J.F.) represented the image of that person. This person was supposed to be sweeping (for confidentiality purposes the name of this person has been blurred out).

These drawings are dramatic examples of a profound thought disorder. Louis's drawings show an extraordinary confusion of images and words. Images and words are transposed and interchanged without the patient's awareness of

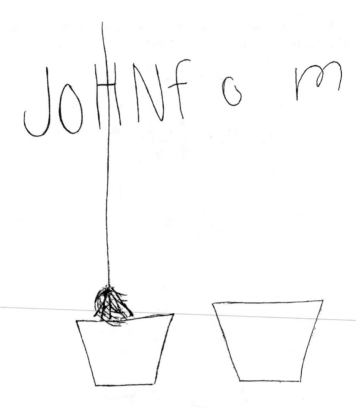

the categorical violation. Louis seemed completely unaware to his trangressions of communicational conventions. Louis's drawings also hint at his severe body image disturbance and ongoing intruding peculiar ideation. How common are these imagery and language confusions in psychotic children? We speculate that this disturbance is probably present in other severely psychotic children. It is not difficult to imagine how difficult and confusing Louis's thinking processes would be.

PLAY

For preschoolers and early latency children, play offers the opportunity to observe a number of psychological and emotional functions that assist clinicians in the clarification of important diagnostic questions. The clinician observes the child's quality of relatedness, and the child's capacity or willingness to communicate with the examiner, or to involve the examiner in the child's play. Examiners observe the themes of the play (the content) and attempt to understand the plot (narrative or drama) of the play. Examiners will also notice the process of the play and how the child changes the play content or action from one moment to the next. These observations and explorations allow diagnosticians to observe the nature of child's reality testing and the quality of the child's thought processes. Diagnosticians should also give special attention to the process of the affective display (flow of affect) and the relationship of the affect to the content of the play. During play observations, the examiner may observe bizarre content or paranoid trends, magical or illogical thinking or other features of inappropriateness of affect or thought disturbance.

DREAMS

Occasionally, psychotic children become uncommunicative or secretive, and it is impossible to fathom what is going on in their minds. When the examiner approaches these children, she receives monosyllabic replies, or noncommittal responses. To questions, such as, "How are you feeling?" "What are you thinking?" The clinician hears, "I am OK," "I'm fine," or the like. Any further attempts to elicit disclosures regarding the patient's internal world are usually frustrating.

Dreams may offer a window of insight into this private world; frequently, children and adolescents are more revealing and straightforward when reporting their dreams. Since dreams are commonly cryptic, if not puzzling, children are less inclined to withhold disclosing the content of their oneiric experiences. The dream content could provide the examiner with important clues as to the nature of the child's psychotic world. Here is an example of how dreams may illuminate the patient's split-off internal world.

> Jess, an almost 16-year-old female, whose case is described as an illustration of preschizophrenic symptoms and behavior, came in to an outpatient appointment accompanied by her mother. As in previous follow-up contacts, she displayed prominent negative symptoms including blunt affect, poor eye contact, secretive behavior, and a strong paranoid attitude; evidence of a thought disorder was commonly observed. When the examiner attempted to engage Jess in an overview of what had been accomplished during the previous three years, she stated she was not feeling suicidal anymore. When the psychiatrist inquired, "How is your mood?" she replied she was feeling ok. The examiner asked the patient to share the last dream she had. She reported a dream she had the previous week. She said that in the dream she was ok, but she was dead. Actually she was dead and people were ripping at her flesh. She had been impaled with a metal bar. Vampires came in to suck her blood. At this point the patient woke up.

The patient reported the dream in a matter of fact manner, contrary to the emotional reaction of her listening mother who was horrified. The patient manifested a prominent disavowal of her persecutory paranoid internal world.

The dream was very morbid and its content reflected problems with self-image and strong paranoid and persecutory ideation. When the patient reported the dream, she evidenced thought disorder; that is, incoherence and illogical thinking.

Papolos and Papolos (2002) report that many children with bipolar disorders suffer from night terrors. Sometimes patients do not wake up, remaining in a semiconscious state, and continuing to experience the frightening events. Papolos and Papolos point out that whereas the nonbipolar child wakes up just before he or she is injured, the bipolar child does not. The authors stated that bipolar children's dreams are often filled with blood and gore. Papolos and Papolos quote Charles Popper's 1990 article "On Diagnostic Gore in Child's Nightmares": "Bipolar children explicitly report the appearance of blood in their dreams, (visualized blood), and make description of mutilations of bodies, dismembering, and the insides of body parts. Their dreams are more affectively intense than regular nightmares" (quoted in Papolos & Papolos, 2002). Popper thinks that the unconscious sensors of painful affects are not working effectively even in bipolar patients' dreams. Papolos and Papolos conclude that bipolar children deal with horrifying imagery of bodily threat, dismemberment, and death (pp. 10–11). The case of Jess described above has some parallel features to the ones Papolos and Papolos describe in bipolar children, but differs substantially from them in Jess's lack of intense affect when she narrated the dream.

DIAGNOSTIC SCALES FOR MOOD AND PSYCHOTIC SYMPTOMS

The PANSS, K-SADS, the WASH-U-KSADS, the Hamilton, and Other Scales

The Positive and Negative Syndrome Scale (PANSS) and the Positive and Negative subscales are the research measurement tools most frequently used in psychotic disorders research. The scales are impractical for regular clinical practice, but may be used for comprehensive overviews, and to assess periodic longitudinal progress. It needs to be stated that the use of the PANNS (Positive and Negative Scales) in children and adolescent needs further studies in areas of validity, reliability and developmental sensitivity.

The PANSS positive scale measures: (1) delusions, (2) conceptual disorganization, (3) hallucinatory behavior, (4) excitement, (5) grandiosity, (6) suspiciousness or persecution, and (7) hostility. The PANSS negative scale measures are:(1) blunted affect; (2) emotional withdrawal; (3) poor rapport; (4) passive/apathetic or social withdrawal behaviors; (5) difficulties with abstract thinking; (6) lack of spontaneity and flow of conversation; and (7) stereotyped thinking. To a large extent, the PANSS negative scale attempts to measure relatedness, mood, and quality of thinking. Both scales are rated from 1 to 6 according to severity. Few serious studies on psychosis are done without the use of these scales.

The Schedule for Affective Disorders and Schizophrenia for School Age Children (K-SADS) has a number of versions: K-SADS-E (epidemiological), K-SADS-P/L (present and lifetime), K-SADS-P (present state), and the Washington University K-SADS-P (expands the definitions of mania) (McClellan, 2004, p. 143). The Schedule for Affective Disorders and Schizophrenia (SADS) for school age children, affectionately known as K-SADS-P (KIDDIE-SADS Present Episode) is frequently used as a research assessment protocol. It is an extensive and comprehensive diagnostic protocol that requires a high level of training and expertise for its administration and diagnostic determinations; in addition, it is time consuming. What makes this examination survey different, is that it has explicit definitions (criteria of inclusion and exclusion), and guides the examiner in the process of data gathering; it specifically suggests examples of probing questions that could be asked when exploring any given issue.

The WASH-U-KSADS is currently, the most widely used diagnostic assessment instrument for pediatric bipolar disorder. This protocol expands on symptoms that differentiate ADHD from preadolescent mania, highlighting symptoms of a restricted phenotype of preadolescent mania: grandiosity, reduced need for sleep, pressured speech, elation/euphoria, hypersexuality, daredevil acts, silliness, and others (DelBello, Axelson, & Geller, 2003, p. 4). Tillman and Geller (2005) developed a brief screening protocol for the identification of the prepubertal and early adolescent disorder phenotype using the Conner's Abbreviated Parental Questionnaire, a 10-item scale. Items 7 (demands must be met immediately/easily frustrated), 8 (cries often and easily), 9 (mood changes quickly and drastically), and 10 (temper outbursts, explosive and unpredictable behavior) were all significantly higher in the prepuberal and early adolescent bipolar disorder phenotype than in the ADHD group. The abbreviated questionnaire performs as well as the Mood Disorder Questionnaire, a screening tool used in adult outpatients (pp. 1215–1216).

Among the most commonly used scales for the assessement of mood, the Hamilton Rating Scale for Depression is one of the best known. The Montgomery-Asberg Depression Rating Scale (MADRS) is frequently used in affective disorders research.[1]

Besides the K-SADS, there are a number of interviewing protocols that provide coverage for schizophrenic symptoms in childhood: National Institute of Mental Heath Diagnostic Interview Schedule for Children (NMIH DISC; 2000), Child and Adolescent Psychiatric Assessment (CAPA; 1995) and the Interview for Children's Disorders and Schizophrenia, 1989 (ICDS; Asarnow, Tompson, & McGrath, 2004, pp. 180–181). The Brief Psychiatric Rating Scale for Children (BPRS) is another measurement tool that is widely used in psychosis research. It consists of 21 individual items that deal with differents aspects of psychopathology. Three of the 21 items deal specifically with psychotic features: Item 7, Peculiar Fantasies—recurrent, odd, unusual, or autistic ideation; Item 8, Delusions—Ideas of reference, persecutory or grandiose delusions; and Item 9, Hallucinations—visual, auditory, or other hallucinatory experiences or perceptions. These items are rated from 0 (not present) to 6 (extremely severe). Neither the PANSS nor the BPRS gives any guidance about how to gather pertinent psychiatric data.

PHYSICAL AND NEUROLOGICAL EXAMINATION

Prior to the physical and neurological examination the psychiatrist will conduct a comprehensive review of systems; previous and ongoing medical problems need to be identified. The patient's prenatal, perinatal, and developmental histories are relevant. History of seizures, head trauma, fractures, and prior surgeries will be noted. In females, menarche, menstrual cycle, and any pregnancy history are pertinent. History of alcohol or drug abuse is also of particular importance. For both sexes, history of sexual behavior, contraception, and STDs is relevant. Any history of physical or sexual abuse must be obtained.

The psychiatric assessment is enriched when the psychiatrist conducts the physical and neurological examinations. The examiner will seek evidence of dysmorphic features compatible with 22q11 syndrome. It is advisable to have a parental figure accompanying the child or adolescent during the examination, especially if the child is a female. Rectal and genital examinations are deferred to the primary care physician or to specialists when indicated. When there are indications of sexual abuse or of rape, the child will be referred for a forensic examination. Rape crisis evaluations, specially designated for this objective, provide developmentally sensitive examinations for small children. These diagnostic and treatment centers are available in designated medical–surgical hospitals across the nation.

For most female patients, and for children in general, the performance of the physical and neurological examination (even when is done by the psychiatrist) is an uneventful experience without any detrimental side effects. These examinations pose no significant risks for the building of a therapeutic alliance with the psychiatrist (Cepeda, 2000, p. 57).

When the psychiatrist performs the physical examination, he or she will pay attention to the child's relatedness and the degree of the child's participation during the examination. The presence of dysmorphic features or of facial features suggestive of identifiable syndromes should be noted (i.e., facial features suggestive of chromosome 22q11 delesion syndrome, or velocardiofacial syndrome (VCFS) may clarify the clinical presentation; see chapter 8, pp. 207–208).

Minor physical anomalies (MPAs) and dermatoglyphic abnormalities are associated with risks for schizophrenia. A Danish study found that children

(11–13 years of age) with MPAs were more likely to go on to develop schizophrenia spectrum disorders in adulthood. MPAs are more frequent in children with early onset schizophrenia (EOS). For a subset of these patients who underwent MRI examaination, the MPA scores were positively correlated with ventricular enlargement (Buckley, Mahadik, Evans, et al., 2003, p. 44).

Reassurance and a greater sensitivity should be exercised during the physical evaluation of a psychotic child. Explaining to the child what the examination entails and describing to the patient what the physician is about to do is helpful in lessening anxieties and dispelling apprehensions. During the examination, the physician will have the opportunity to notice the degree of the patient's cooperation and orientation to reality. The physician should pay attention to other valuable observations such as the degree and appropriateness of the child's relatedness, evidence of suspiciousness or paranoia, disturbances of reality testing, signs of anxiety, or evidence of drug abuse. The physician will observe the degree of the child's neglect to his body (poor oral and body hygiene, untreated skin infections, unclipped finger or toenails, ingrown toenails, and others).

The patient's complexion, baseline weight, and vital signs will be registered. Regularity of the pulse will be noted. Any evidence of injury needs to be investigated. Signs of self-abusive behavior should be noted and addressed in further interviewing, as should evidence of substance abuse, obesity, or cachexia. The physician will assess the thyroid size, its firmness and its regularity.

Acanthosis nigricans and other cutaneous and neurocutaneous findings should be pursued with further inquiry, testing, or consultation referrals. The evaluation of the cardiorespiratory systems is particularly pertinent. When the patient has a history of fainting or blacking out, a history of shortness of breath or exercise dyspnea, further investigation is mandatory. The presence of rhythm dificulties, murmurs, or any other cardiovascular finding will be noted; these require further testing and consultation. It is prudent to assume that every obese child has cardiomegaly requiring a pediatric cardiologic consultation. Any ongoing illness or medical–surgical condition will be appropriately attended to.

In the neurological examination, the physician will make observations on the patient's degree of alertness, orientation to time and place, and his or her sense of boundaries. Attention should be given to the quality of language and melody of speech (prosody), as well as the child's affective display. Fundoscopy should be performed on every child; the physician will identify the presence of cranial nerve signs, deficits in the gross or fine motor movements, abnormal reflexes, or difficulties with praxis or coordination. Problems with right to left differentiation, finger sequencing difficulties, or difficulties with bimanual behavior may also shed some light in the child's neurodevelopmental problems; such is the case of language deficits, learning disorders, and cognitive deficits.

In addition to the above observations, testing may reveal neurological abnormalities, apparently specific to schizophrenia, that indicate neurological compromise in the left heteromodal association cortex and cerebellum. Motor abnormalities are common in schizoprenia and in nonschizoprenic psychosis, and correlate with cerebellum and straital abormalities, but with limited involvement of the heteromodal area (Keshevan et al., 2003, p. 1302). A bedside neurological evaluation derived from the Neurological Evaluation scale may assist in the differential diagnosis (p. 1299). Items that particularly correlate with a decrease in heteromodal association cortex and cerebellum volume in schizophrenia are:

- NES, item 7, Audiovisual Integration. The patient is asked to match a set of tapping sounds with one of the three sets of dots presented on a 5 × 7-inch card.
- NES, item 13, Memory. The patient is told four words and he is asked to repeat the words immediately after they are presented. The subject is asked to recall the words again 5 and 10 minutes later.
- NES, item 18, Extinction (Face–Hand test): the subject, with his eyes closed, is simultaneouly touched in the following order: right cheek-left hand, left cheek-right hand, right cheek-right hand, and left cheek-left hand. The patient needs to identify where he was touched. For a complete review of the NES testing items and their scoring, see Buchanan and Heinrichs (1989, pp. 345–350).

Deficits in the examination of items are common in schizophrenia and nonschizophrenic psychosis: Item 10—Fist-Ring test; Item 11—Fist-Edge Palm test; Item 12—Alternating Fist-Palm (Ozereski Test); and Item 15—Rapid Alternating Movements (Keshevan et al., 2003, p. 1302).

It is interesting that adult offspring of mothers with schizophrenia had significantly more abnormalities than either the offspring of mothers with affective disorders or offspring of healthy mothers. Also these neurological abnormalities at age 6, but not in infancy, correlated with neurological abnormalities in adulthood (see Schubert & McNeil, 2004).

Soft neurological signs, frequently found in chronic psychotic patients, are not stable findings; they change with the state of the illness. Soft neurological signs decreased in first-episode adult schizophrenic patients at a follow-up period of 14 monthss. This effect was related to better outcome. Despite the improvement, soft signs remained elevated in schizophrenic patients relative to heathy controls. Findings are in harmony with the concept that neurological soft signs range among the most consistent neurobiological characteristics of schizophrenia. Patients with decreasing soft signs scores experienced further stabilization of psychiatric symptoms, whereas patients with stable scores foreshadowed a chronic course (Bachmann, Bottmer, & Schroder, 2005, p. 2340).

Related issues of the presence of neurological signs in psychotic children have been known for a long time. Goldfarb (1974) stated many years ago that,

> Evidence for central nervous system impairment in a proportion of diagnosed schizophrenic children, however, is quite convincingly derived from many sources. Many studies have demonstrated a higher incidence of prenatal and perinatal complications.... In addition to deviations in neurological history, a proportion of schizophrenic children tend to give observable, though soft, evidence of neurological dysfunction in physical examination, including deviations in gait, posture, balance, motor coordination, muscle tone, and integration of multiple simultaneous stimuli. In one clinical sample, neurological examination diagnosed neurological dysfunction in 65% of a group of schizophrenic children. (pp. 97–98)

Even though the diagnosis of schizophrenia has gained precision over the years, Goldfarb's assertions still stand today. Interestingly, an increasing number of neurological, morphologic, physiologoical, and neuropsychological deficits are being described in pediatric bipolar disorder children, too.

Disturbances of visual attention and smooth pursuit eye movement are common in schizophrenic patients (more than 30% and more than 40%, respectively), and are frequently found in schizophrenics' relatives who suffer from schizophrenia spectrum disorders or personality disorders (30 and 35%, respectively). Antisaccade performance and verbal working memory disturbances follow similar trends (Tamminga, 2003, p. 1578).

Of particular relevance for the treatment and follow-up of psychotic children is the identification and documentation of involuntary movements. The examiner will document the presence of tremor, choreathetosis, cogwheeling, and other oro-bucco-lingual or facial movements.

NEUROLOGICAL CONSULTATION

A neurological consultation in children and adolescents with a psychotic disorder is indicated in a number of clinical circumstances (see table 5.1).

TABLE 5.1 Indications for a Neurological Consultation

- The history suggests "organicity" or neurological compromise.
- There are demonstrable positive findings in the neurological examination.
- There is a history of neurodevelopmental difficulties, i.e., delays in the milestones, socialization delays, speech delays, or others.
- There is evidence of severe language disorders, or severe learning disorders.
- There is a history of seizures or prior brain insult.
- There is a history of progressive decrement of intellectual and academic functioning.
- There is a recent history of regressive behavior with rapid loss of adaptive functioning.
- Emergence of psychosis in a child without previous psychiatric or neurological history.

The consultant neurologist may order further tests as he or she deems necessary. These may include EEGs, imaging studies, electrophysiological testing (evoked potentials),[2] or others. If the deficits or changes are considered to be associated with substance abuse, a consultation with chemical dependency experts for assessment and treatment recommendations is mandatory.

NEUROIMAGING

Imaging studies may be very helpful in the search for the diagnosis and etiology of psychotic disorders; findings vary with the condition(s) under investigation. Although imaging in schizophrenia and mood disorders is still beyond the realm of clinical practice, significant progress has been made in demonstrating structural abnormalities in disorders with childhood onset. Jacobsen and Bertolino (2000) summarize the functional imaging findings in child schizophrenia. Most of the available literature in this area comes from research conducted at the NIMH Childhood Schizophrenia Project. Imaging and functional imaging with children is very difficult and some of the findings are inconsistent. However, there is growing consensus regarding the following findings:

- There is significant decrease of total cerebral volume (9.7%) in patients with childhood schizophrenia; this finding is consistent with findings in adult schizophrenia. The reduction in cerebral matter is primarily a consequence of a reduction in gray matter volume.
- The temporal lobe structures and the lateral ventricles change over time. Rescanning of patients with schizophrenia show a progressive increase of the ventricular size in comparison to controls; there is a decrease of the right temporal lobe volume, in the superior temporal gyri bilaterally, and in the left hippocampus; the midsagittal thalamic area is also decreased in schizophrenic patients in comparison to controls.
- Functional studies (Cerebral Blood Flow (CBF) and glucose metabolism) have demonstrated evidence of hypofrontality in the same manner that this finding has been evidenced in adult schizophrenic patients.
- Childhood schizophrenic patients show lower metabolic rates (Cerebral metabolic rate of glucose-CMRGlu) than controls.
- Available data support a similarity of findings between adult and childhood onset schizophrenia suggesting a final common pathophysiology; however, studies so far fail to substantiate a straightforward relationship between early onset and the severity of the neurodevelopmental lesions.
- There is evidence of cerebellar hypermetabolism in childhood schizophrenia, consistent with a prefrontal-thalamic-cerebellar network dysfunction in adult schizophrenia (Jacobsen & Bertolino, 2000, pp. 192–198).

A meta-analysis reviewing 15 studies of voxel-based morphometric studies in adults, to identify structural brain abnormalities in patients with schizophrenia, revealed that of the 50 regions that have been reported to be significantly reduced in schizophrenic patients, the left superior temporal gyrus and the left medial temporal lobe were present in more than 50% of the studies (31% of the studies did not find volume deficits in the left medial temporal lobe). Fifty percent of the studies reported volumetric decreases in the parahippocampal gyrus, right superior temporal gyrus, left inferior frontal gyrus, and left medial frontal gyrus (Honea, Crow, Passingham, & Mackay, 2005, p. 2243).

Sporn et al. (2003) reported acceleration in the rate of gray matter loss during adolescence in patients with childhood-onset schizophrenia. This finding may not apply to all patients with early onset schizophrenia. A group of 16 patients with adolescent onset schizophrenia failed to display progressive brain abnormalities (p. 2187). There was a counterintuitive finding: Clinical improvement was associated with the rate of gray matter loss. The authors speculate that the paradoxical finding may reflect a compensatory pruning of malfunctioning neural circuits, consistent with neurodevelopmental model of schizophrenia (Sporn et al., 2003, p. 2188).

A bolder and more definitive assertion of the diagnostic value of neuroimaging is presented by Gogtay et al. (2004) who asserted that patients with childhood-onset schizophrenia (COS), in prospective brain MRIs, had significant gray matter loss (in frontal, temporal, and parietal areas) while a group of patients with atypical psychosis, associated with multidimensional impaired disorder (MDI), and healthy control children did not. The authors conclude that the gray matter loss is diagnostic specific for COS (p. 20).

This assertion was not supported by a study by Moreno, Burdalo, Reig, et al. (2005), who failed to demonstrate significant neuroimaging differences among a variety of first psychotic episodes (p. 1156). The diagnoses were confirmed at 12 months and revealed two distinct subgroupings: schizophrenia and "other psychotic disorders" (p. 1156).

Data regarding neuroimaging in mood disorders indicate that children and adolescents with familial bipolar disorder show significantly smaller amygdalae nuclei than controls, mostly in the right side, apparently due to gray matter reduction.

Frazier et al. (2005) reported that subjects with bipolar disorder had smaller hippocampal and cerebral volumes. This is particularly true for females. No significant hemispheric effects were observed (p. 1261, see note 2). There is significant overlapping in the neuroimaging studies findings between pediatric bipolar disorder (PBD) and major depressive disorder (MDD) patients. Parallel to the finding reported in PBD, Gabbay et al. (2005) reported a decrease in prefrontal cortex, a decrease in amygdala and hippocampal volumes, and a smaller corpus callosum (pp. 52–54), and Moreno et al. (2005) who reported overall increased CSF (cerebrospinal fluid) and increase of the CSF in the sulci of the left frontal and right parietal lobes as well as a decrease of the gray matter of the frontal lobes (p. 1154)

Cerebellar abnormalities are also present in bipolar disorders. Mills, Del-Bello, Adler, and Strakowski (2005) performed a MRI analysis of cerebellar vermis and substantiated that the vermal subregion-V2 volume was significantly smaller in multiple-episode bipolar disorder subjects than in first-episode patients and healthy controls. The vermal subregion-V3 was significantly smaller in multiple-episode bipolar disorder subjects than in healthy controls (p. 1530).[3]

It is interesting that adults with unipolar depression show decreased amygdalar size associated with increased amygdalar activity, suggesting that chronic amygdalar hyperreactivity could ultimately decrease amygdalar volume through toxic levels of glutamate neurotransmission (Altshuler, Bookheimer, et al., 2005, p. 569). Several laboratories report a reduction in hippocampal volumes in patients with adult major depressive disorder. This reduction is greater in patients with early onset, many prior episodes, longer duration of untreated illness, and childhood abuse history.[4]

Affective disorders also demonstrate evidence of neurodegeneration. Structural imaging studies of adults with major depressive episodes and bipolar disorders have evidenced a variety of neuroanatomic abnormalities, the most consistent being an increased rate of subcortical superintensities, increased ventricular size, decrease of temporal lobe volume, decrease of frontal lobe volume, and changes in basal ganglia structures (Kowatch, Davanzo, & Emslie, 2000, p. 210). Of interest is the finding of an association between white matter hyperintensities (WMH) and a history of suicidal behavior in MDD pediatric patients (12 to 18 years of age) with MDD (Gabbay et al., 2005, p. 54).

Controversy remains regarding the usefulness of neuroimaging to differentiate schizophrenia from bipolar disorder. Strakowski (2004) argued that such examinations are useful, stating that, "Although neuroimaging cannot currently be used to distinguish schizophrenia from bipolar disorder, recent findings suggest that the neural substrates of these conditions are indeed distinct, so that with continued advances, neuroimaging may some day differentiate these conditions" (p. 3). Strakowski added,

> Consequently, neuroimaging cannot yet be used diagnostically; however, as experience with these techniques grows and our ability to identify patterns of abnormalities among patient groups increases, we may well find the day when a relatively quick brain scan informs the diagnosis and treatment of these, and other specific psychiatric diagnoses (p. 14).

In contrast, Pearlson (2004) believes neuroimaging is not a useful diagnostic tool for differentiating these disorders. "Taken together, … data suggest potential overlap between etiologic and pathological mechanisms in psychotic bipolar disorder and in schizophrenia." Pearlson suggests that "future research should re-examine structural differences using psychotic/non-psychotic BPD subtypes rather than combining them into a collective diagnostic group" (p. 15). Neuroimaging is also playing an important role in schizophrenia prodromal research. For instance, studies on ARMS (At Risk Mental State) patients have found that larger left hippocampi volumes were predictive of transition to psychosis (Knowles & Sharma, 2004, p. 599). These and other emerging findings are not diagnostic for schizophrenia at this time. The primary role of laboratory tests and neuroimaging in the assessment of childhood-onset schizophrenia is to rule out other medical and neurological disorders (Tsai & Champine, 2004, pp. 387–388).

Positron Emission Tomography (PET) is a productive research tool that has illuminated a great deal of brain functioning activity. Single Photon Emission Computerized Tomography(SPECT) provides brain imaging that is clinically useful but is still used infrequently.

Positron Emission Tomography (PET)

PET provides a view of brain function by way of studies of brain blood flow and metabolism. PET images are often coregistered with MRI images to create an accurate map of brain structure for measurement of functional changes in the PET (Bremmer, 2005, p. 17). PET gives information about receptors and neurotransmitters. MRS (see below), a safer technique, uses similar principles and almost similar equipment as MRI. PET/SPECT studies play an important role in neurotransmitters research; these studies in schizophrenics were the earliest to show dopaminergic dysfunctions. PET/SPECT studies coupled with use of radioligands (radio tracers) permit assessment of the dynamics of receptor occupancy (density and distribution) of neurotransmitters (dopamine, serotonin, nicotinic, and others), as well as antipsychotic medications and other substances that affect the CNS (Wong & Brasic, 2005, pp. 58, 60).

Single Photon Emission Computerized Tomography (SPECT)

SPECT studies in MDD children (N = 11, 12–15 years of age) revealed reduced perfusion in the left antero-lateral and left temporal cortical areas compared to controls. These abnormalities were not found in follow up studies after the depressive symptom improved, suggesting that the abnormalities may be a state–dependent marker of this disorder (Gabbay et al., 2005, p. 55).

Even children at risk for the development of substance abuse disorders show neuroimaging findings. Subjects at the highest risk showed reduced right parietal PDE (phosphodiesters) concentration compared to other regions. This is likely to represent a heightened degree of synaptic pruning in the right parietal area because DPE signal is reflective of membrane catabolism (Yurgelun-Todd & Renshaw, 2000, p. 71).

Proton Magnetic Resonance Spectroscopy (H-MRS), Diffusion Tensor Imaging (DTI), and Magnetization Transfer Imaging (MTI), Magnetic Resonance Spectrography (MRS)

On the frontier of imaging studies, for the evaluation of schizophrenia and mood disorders, is the emergence of in vivo, noninvasive assessment of a variety of neurochemicals which reflect neuronal and glial integrity. H-MRS is suited to the early detection of neurochemical alterations, potentially assisting in the identification of individuals at risk. Among the metabolites that H-MRS quantifies are choline (Cho), which reflects membrane lipid breakdown, N-acetylaspartate (NAA), associated with neuronal integrity and viability, creatine (Cr) may indicate abnormal energy metabolism and decreased cellular density, gamma-aminobutyric acid (GABA), and glutamine (Gabbay et al., 2005, p. 55). So far, H-MRS results in MDD have been contradictory (pp. 55–56).

White matter imaging techniques such as diffusion tensor imaging (DTI) and magnetization transfer imaging (MTI) promise to provide new insights into a neglected area, the white matter (myelination) of brain tissue. DTI permits a visualization of the tractography (white matter tracts) of the brain. Schizophrenia is increasingly being considered as a syndrome of disconnection of brain circuitry; as a result, attention is being focused on the possibility that the integrity of the white matter is compromised in this illness. Emerging findings suggest disconnection between the frontal lobes and other regions of the brain. The degree of disconnectivity seems directly correlated with negative symptoms and impulsivity. In MTI, reduction of magnetization transfer reflects white matter abnormalities that may be correlated to abnormal myelinization (Diwadkar & Keshavan, 2003, pp. 30–31).

MRS is a promising technique for the diagnosis of bipolar disorder. MRS is a special form of imaging that allows the analysis of chemical properties of tissues. At the 2004 annual meeting of the Radiological Society of North America, Chicago, John D. Port made a preliminary report on the use of MRS for the diagnosis of drug naïve bipolar patients, using a 3 and longbore MRS scanner (twice the magnetic field strength used in previous studies). According to Port, "Unfortunately, traditional anatomical imaging has, for the most part, failed to be useful for the diagnosis and prognosis of psychiatric disease.... However, MRS, which measures brain chemistry, has shown promise...for the diagnosis of bipolar disease" (Port, 2005, p. 15). Port and colleagues identified significant differences between brain chemistries of people with and without bipolar disorder in the areas that control movement, vision, reading, and sensory information. The researchers hope to identify metabolic markers of bipolar disorders (*Primary Psychiatry, Psychiatric Dispatches,* February, 2005, p. 15).

Magnetoencephalography (MEG)

Magnetoencephalography (MEG) is the measure of magnetic fields generated by the brain. MEG is sensitive to the cells that lie tangential to the brain surface and that consequently have magnetic fields oriented tangentially. The EEG and MEG are complementary: the EEG is more sensitive to radial oriented cells (perpendicular to the brain surface) and fields. Whereas the EEG is "smeared" by different conductivities (skull, gray, and white matter, CSF), the MEG is relatively invulnerable to the media the fields traverse. MEG is a favorite technique for source localization. There have been very few studies about the use of MEG in schizophrenia (Gur, Andreasen, et al., 2005, p. 95).

EVOKED POTENTIAL STUDIES

Among evoked potential response findings, the reduction of the amplitude of the P-300 is one of the most robust and consistent markers in schizophrenia (Kuperberg & Caplan, 2003, p. 458). Another robust finding across studies is the increase of the N-400 latency, suggesting a delay of contextual integration of words in schizophrenic patients. The later finding is correlated with the presence of thought disorder in schizophrenia (pp. 458–459; for further evoked potential information as well as other electrophysiological data see chapter 8).[5]

PSYCHOLOGICAL TESTING

If the psychiatrist finds inconsistencies during the gathering of the patient's history or during her observations during the mental status examination, or if the clinician senses that the patient is withholding or misrepresenting information, or if the clinical picture is ambiguous or complex, further inquiry to clarify the issues is mandatory. In such situations, a psychological assessment referral may be beneficial. On occasion, the patient is guarded with information, and the child or parent, or both, provide partial or misleading information that precludes the psychiatrist from forming a coherent and integrated diagnosis and treatment plan. Psychological testing, and projective testing in particular, assists the psychiatrist in elucidating the patient's conflicts, the nature of the patient's defense structure, the affect regulatory capacity, the integrity of the reality testing function, the nature of thought processes (the presence of thought disorder), the quality of the child's interpersonal relatedness, and the child's coping capacities. When intellectual functions are not considered intact, that is, when cognitive deficits are suspected, an assessment of cognitive/intellectual functioning (verbal and nonverbal abilities) may be indicated.

Projective Testing

Projective testing (Rorschach, TAT, and others) in competent and expert hands is an invaluable aid in cases where the nature of the psychosis is uncertain or when the extent of impairment in a variety of personality dimensions is unclear. In every case, projective testing assists in the implementation of psychosocial interventions. The integrity of reality testing, the quantity and quality of human responses, the presence of peculiar or bizarre responses, the presence of thought disorder, and other findings may be very valuable in the diagnostic process. Patients undergoing an acute (confusional) psychotic state are not amenable to psychological testing. In these situations, testing is deferred until the patient's mental condition is more stable to obtain reliable results.

Projective testing is also an invaluable tool for the evaluation of the degree of recovery and relapse risk. Often times, after a psychotic break, and when the there is evidence of behavioral improvement, caretakers and even professionals may underestimate the underlying residual pathology and the degree of functional and emotional impairment. Equally, projective testing may give early indications of psychological and emotional decompensation and the growing risks of a psychotic relapse.

Neuropsychological Testing

Neuropsychologists have objectified consistent deficits in the neuropsychological performance of schizophrenic patients. Neuropsychological testing is useful when the patient's psychosis is controlled or stable, and further habilitation or rehabilitation plans are considered. Such testing is useful in identifying appropriate psychoeducational programming (commensurate with the child's intellectual strengths, learning preferences, or cognitive deficits), for appropriate school placement, academic remediation, or for vocational guidance. Testing results are not reliable when the psychosis is acute or reactivating.

Neuropsychological deficits have been consistently demonstrated in schizophrenic and bipolar disorder patients. Since some schizophrenic presentations produce a progressive decline in adaptive functioning, neuropsychological testing may be useful to assess the integrity and stability of the patient's neuropsychological and adaptive resources. Positive changes in the neuropsychological status substantiate the evidence of clinical improvement of the psychotic symptoms during longitudinal observations, and its decrement corroborates the patient's deterioration in adaptive functioning, frequently correlated with an exacerbation of the psychosis.

Both, neuropsychological and neuroimaging studies, have commonly indicated that not all the patients with schizophrenia exhibit the same pattern of cognitive abnormalities. The presence of heterogeneity raises the possibility that some patients with schizophrenia may have a cognitive profile that has characteristics of a frontal lobe syndrome, others may show a temporal lobe syndrome, while still others may display a pattern of deficits that is not suggestive of either frontal or temporal lobe dysfunction (Daniel, Goldstein, & Weiner, 2001, p. 8).

A substantial body of research since the mid-1980s has shown that patients with schizophrenia have poor performance on a wide range of neurocognitive function tests. The test batteries employed to objectify the neurocognitive deficits of patients with schizophrenia spectrum disorders are listed in table 5.2.

EVALUATION OF SUBSTANCE ABUSE

The SASSI-2 "is a brief easy-to administer, objectively scored, accurate, and cost-effective tool designed to screen for the presence or absence of substance use disorders in adolescents. As a screening instrument is designed to identify individuals who have a high probability of having a substance use disorder"

TABLE 5.2 Cognitive Tests

Cognitive domain	Tests
Executive function	Wisconsin Card Sorting Test
	Trail-making B
Attention/vigilance	Continuous Performance Test
	Verbal and Non-Verbal Span Tests
	(Attention Index of the Wechler Memory Scale)
Episodic memory	Rey Auditory Verbal Learning Test
	Rey Design Learning Test
	Rey-Taylor Complex Figure Immediate Recall Test
Verbal fluency and reasoning	Controlled Oral Word Association Test
	Similarities Subtest (Wechler Adult Intelligence Test Revised)
Psychomotor speed groove	Pegboard and Finger Tapping and Manual Dexterity tests
	Digit Symbol Subtest (Wechler Intelligence Test Revised)
Nonverbal fluency and construction	Design Fluency Test
	Hooper Visual Organization Test
	Rey-Taylor Complex Figure Copy Test

Source: Harvey (2003, p. 3).

(Miller & Lazowski, 1990, 2001, p. 1). The SASSI-2 has a number of subtle questions that assist in the identification of individuals with alcohol and other substance use disorders when they do not acknowledge substance misuse (Idem, p. 2). The adolescent SASSI-2 yielded an overall accuracy of 87% in identifying substance dependence (Idem, p. 4).

OTHER EVALUATIONS

Particular illnesses or neurological conditions found in children need to be followed on a regular basis by pertinent monitoring or by referral to the appropriate specialists. Children with gross and fine motor deficits or with coordination difficulties may require physical and occupational therapies and other adjunctive treatments. Language and speech deficits merit special considerations. First, these problems are common among children with psychiatric disorders, and among psychotic children in particular; second, these deficits are often not identified; third, language disorders create diagnostic difficulties because they simulate thought disorders, and fourth, the remediation of these deficits is frequently inadequate. There is a clear need for a timely identification of language and speech deficits, and for a more intense remediation of these disorders. Lack of a timely recognition and of adequate treatment of these disorders contributes to academic, learning, emotional, social, and behavioral consequences. It is not enough to agree on certain educational goals for children receiving special education. Frequently, the schools fall short in the implementation of objectives developed at the admission, review, and dismissal committees (ARDs). Parents need to advocate diligently for the implementation of the ARD recommendations.

CHAPTER 6

Differential Diagnosis of Psychotic Disorders
Medical Conditions Associated with Psychosis

This chapter deals with medical conditions associated with psychotic features; in some of these patients, the psychotic symptoms are rather isolated, whereas in others, the psychosis is more prominent and better organized, or has a more salient role in interfering with adaptive functioning.

According to the DSM-IV-TR (APA, 2000), in a psychotic disorder due to a general medical condition, the hallucinations and delusions are prominent and are judged to be a direct physiological result of a general medical condition (criterion A); there is evidence from history, physical examination, or laboratory findings that the psychotic features are the result of a general medical condition (criterion B); the psychosis is not better accounted for by any other mental disorder (criterion C); and the diagnosis is not made if the disturbance only occurs during the course of delirium (criterion D) (p. 334). The physician must demonstrate a temporal association between the onset, exacerbation, or remission of the general medical condition and the psychotic disturbance; the physician also needs to give consideration to the presence of atypical features for a primary psychotic disorder (atypical age of onset or presence of visual or olfactory hallucinations), and to the existence of literature support for the link between the demonstrated medical condition and development of the psychotic disturbance. Furthermore the psychotic conditions cannot be accounted for by other psychiatric or mental disorders (APA, 2000, p. 335). The psychotic disorder due to a general medical condition may be a single transitory state, or a recurrent or cycling condition with exacerbations and remissions of the underlying medical condition. Although it is not always the case, improvement of the medical condition results in the resolution or a significant improvement of the psychotic disturbance (p. 337).

The child and adolescent psychiatrist needs to be exhaustive in pursuing identifiable medical or neurological disorders that may be associated with psychotic disorders in childhood. To achieve the above objective the psychiatrist needs to:

1. Obtain a thorough background history that includes developmental, medical, family, and educational history,
2. Perform a comprehensive physical and neurological examination, or review the physical and neurological examinations done by other physicians.
3. Complement (1) and (2) findings by laboratory tests and other clinical and paraclinical examinations,
4. Obtain pertinent consultations.

These steps will assist the psychiatrist in identifying medical or neurological disorders that need appropriate workup, and additional consultation and pertinent treatment. Kendall and Jablensky (2003) raise serious questions as to the validity of categorical diagnoses in schizophrenia (the same may likely is true for other categorical diagnoses). In relation to diagnosis, they support a dimensional approach, meaning that, the genetic basis of illness encompasses a spectrum of other disorders, such as schizotypal and paranoid personality disorder, and even psychotic affective illness. They reason that, "signs and symptoms do not constitute the disease and that it is not until causal mechanisms are clearly identified that 'we can say we have 'really' discovered the disease'" (p. 6). Kendall and Jablensky (2003) quote Widiger and Clark (2000) who suggest that the variation in psychiatric symptoms may be better represented by an orderly matrix symptoms-cluster dimension" than by a set of discrete categories (p. 7). The diagnostic views of the present writer converge with those of Widiger and Clark. For clinical purposes the psychotic disorders in children and adolescents may be grouped in the following domains:

TABLE 6.1 Classification of Psychotic Disorders

1. Benign psychosis
2. Circumscribed psychosis
3. Psychosis associated with identifiable medical illnesses:
   Delirium
   Psychosis associated to medical illnesses
4. Psychosis associated with neurodevelopmental disorders
5. Traumatic psychosis
   Posttraumatic stress disorder (PTSD)
   Dissociative identity disorder (DID)
   Others
6. Affective psychosis
7. Schizophrenia and related psychosis
8. Psychotic disorders NOS
9. Factitious psychoses

TABLE 6.2 Benign Psychosis

Hallucinations and sleep deprivation
Hallucinations and sensory deprivation
Hallucinations and physiological states
Functional hallucinations
Sleep related psychosis
      Hypnagogic and hypnopompic hallucinations
Hallucinations associated with migraine
      Alice in Wonderland syndrome
Autoscopic hallucinations
Imaginary companions
Hallucinations associated with bereavement
Circumscribed psychosis
Isolated symptoms

BENIGN PSYCHOSIS

Benign psychosis refers to transient and circumscribed symptoms, not associated to lasting psychopathology. Symptoms are limited (in frequency and intensity) and the overall adaptive function is preserved. These symptoms emerge either from unusual physiological conditions or as result of extraordinary experiences or circumstances (see table 6.2).

Pilowsky (1998) labels the group of unusual perceptual experiences, *parahallucinations*. He includes in this category hypnagogic and hypnopompic hallucinations, eidetic imagery (instances of vivid imagination), imaginary companions, and other related experiences. Pilowsky considers night terrors (*Pavor nocturnus*) as parahallucinatory experiences. Determining if a child is hallucinating or not, is not always simple (p. 7).

Hallucinations and Sleep Deprivation

Sleep deprived children are prone to perceptual disturbances and to alteration of the sense of reality.

Hallucinations and Sensory Deprivation

The brain and the senses are entrained to receive and to process information; when that does not occur, the brain stimulates itself and "makes things happen" by creating false perceptions. These experiences are reported in persons who are under prolonged deprivation of food or fluids. "Phantom limb" experiences fall within this category.

Hallucinations and Physiological States

A state of exhaustion facilitates certain unusual perceptual experiences; thus, autoscopic hallucinations are more common when the organism has been subjected to prolonged stress. The so-called highway hypnosis, occurs under conditions of sleep deprivation, fatigue, and boredom (Boza, http://www.priory. com/halluc.htm).

Functional Hallucinations

Functional hallucinations are defined as those occurring when the patient simultaneously receives a real stimulus in the concerned perceptual field; for example, a hallucinated voice heard simultaneously with and specific to real water sound. In these cases, there is a clear relationship between the timber, prosody, and pitch of the environmental sound and the simultaneously perceived auditory hallucinations. Imaging studies have demonstrated activation of the auditory cortex; this activation may facilitate the misperception of environmental sounds (Hunter & Woodruff, 2004, p. 923).

SLEEP RELATED PSYCHOSES

Hypnagogic and Hypnopompic Hallucinations

Hypnagogic phenomena occur when the person is falling asleep. Hypnopompic phenomena occur when the person is awakening. These definitions do not have universal consensus. For instance, Reddy, Smith, and Robinson (2005) defined hypnagogic sleep phenomena as occurring upon awakening, and is experienced in a semiconscious state. According to these authors, the sleep phenomena involve vivid, auditory, visual, and tactile misperceptions or hallucinations. These authors believe that these experiences appear to represent the rapid transition from sleep stage into the state of wakefulness. Hypnagogic phenomena are rather common and far exceed the association with narcolepsy. Whereas, as much as 25% of college students and noninstitutionalized general population surveys of persons 15 or over endorse this phenomenon, only 0.04% of the same population qualifies for the diagnosis of narcolepsy (p. 11).

Hypnagogic experiences may be present in up to a third of children with narcolepsy and can be very frightening (Guilleminault, 1996, p. 323). These disturbances need to be differentiated from hallucinatory phenomena following a prolonged cataleptic attack (p. 322). Hypnagogic and hypnopompic hallucinations are also associated with narcolepsy (see pp. 148–149). The case of Jimma deals with related diagnostic issues.

This 16½-year-old Hispanic female was referred for a psychiatric evaluation due to a suicide attempt. She had overdosed on acetominophen, amoxycillin, and Claritin prior to the evaluation. She had previously tried to kill herself at age 9 and reported that she had regretted she had not succeeded. She reported a long history of depression. Her depressive features had become progressively worse over the previous few months. Jimma's mother reported a history of self-abusive behaviors since early childhood. The patient had felt emotionally abused by her mother for her underweight. Jimma had also abused alcohol and marijuana, and there was history of alcohol and substance abuse in the family. A sister was described as depressed and had experienced auditory hallucinations. Jimma's biological father had been in and out of jail for drug related charges. Her biological parents divorced when the patient was 9 years old and her mother had remarried two years prior to the examination.

Jimma endorsed severe neurovegetative symptoms and auditory hallucinations of people having conversations, sometimes in different languages. She also endorsed depersonalization phenomena; two months prior to the examination, she felt that she was a black man.

When she was interviewed again, to clarify the nature of hallucinations, she reported that the voices she heard only occurred during sleep: she heard songs in another language and she heard people talking among themselves in another language. She also endorsed other mild psychotic features such as seeing shadows, seeing red, and feeling that somebody touched her hair. Jimma also felt watched. From time to time, she felt that other people could read her mind, that she could read other people's minds, and that she had special powers. She also endorsed periodic feelings that her thoughts were racing and that she had lots of energy. Jimma did not endorse auditory hallucinations while she was awake. She only heard the voices at the time she was falling asleep. The auditory hallucinations were determined to be hypnagogic hallucinations.

There are times when the experiences reported by patients during sleep have the characteristics of perceptual disturbances (auditory and visual hallucinations) experienced during the day. These children rarely indicate spontaneously that these events occurred during sleep. Their narrative conveys the quality of an experience that happens during full state of wakefulness.

Hallucinations Associated with Migraines

Migraine variants represent a group of headache clinical presentations. Some special forms of migraine seen in childhood include conditions with disordered thought processes, such as confusional states, and the Alice in Wonderland syndrome with perceptual disturbances. Others include migraine stupor which sometimes gets prolonged for days, and transient global amnesia, which rarely occurs in children (Hockaday, 1996, p. 697).

Visual hallucinations are common in patients with migraine and narcolepsy. About half of the patients with migraine experience visual hallucinations, the most common being fortifications-type zigzag spectrum, often associated with scotoma. Fully formed hallucinations may also occur. A few patients with migraine experience persistent positive visual phenomena, including perceptions such as television static, snow lines, lines of ants, dots, or rain lasting months to years after a migraine attack. (Cummings & Mega, 2003, p. 190)

The rare Alice in Wonderland syndrome consists of bizarre visual illusions and spatial distortions occasionally associated with migraine headaches. Micropsias, macropsias, and other disturbances of perception are described. Children do not seem frightened when reporting their unusual experiences; children give detailed descriptions, often with a bemused facial look, or they may change body positions as if to get under a low ceiling. These patients are free from psychiatric symptoms between the attacks. These visual and perceptual abnormalities have also been reported with infectious mononucleosis, complex partial seizures, benign occipital epilepsy, and drug ingestions, as well as with psychiatric disorders (Rothner, 1999, p. 736).

Autoscopic Hallucinations

In autoscopic hallucinations the person sees a projection of the self outside of his or her real body. Some persons have this experience habitually without evidence of cerebral disease. Other times, autoscopic phenomena are associated with migraines or epilepsy. The emotional reaction to the experience is that of anxiety or of a quiet surprise (Lishman, 1998, p. 73). Less frequently, the patient relives a traumatic experience as illustrated in the following vignette.

> A 15-year-old adolescent female complained of seeing herself being raped. She was raped by three men two weeks before, and felt very dejected when experiencing these hallucinations (flashbacks?). She also experienced a number of feelings common in rape victims: felt dirty and had to take a number of showers a day. Furthermore, she experienced auditory hallucinations stating that she deserved what happened to her, that she was trash, a whore, and the like, that she deserved to die, and that she should kill herself.... This patient had been sexually abused before, and struggled with sexual abuse perpetrated against her when she was 8 years old.

The phenomena of the imaginary companion and of hallucinations associated with bereavement are discussed at the beginning of chapter 7; by and large, they are benign symptoms. Isolated psychotic features, which do not interfere with adaptive capacity and which do not disrupt the mental activity, should also be considered benign experiences. There are a number of isolated symptoms, either hallucinations or delusions that may be either associated with stress or associated with medical problems.

PSYCHOSIS ASSOCIATED WITH IDENTIFIABLE MEDICAL ILLNESSES

Most likely, all psychotic phenomena represent a physiological disturbance; as such, all psychoses have an organic foundation. *"Organic psychoses"*is still a useful term to refer to a group of psychoses related to demonstrable medical, neurological, or pharmacological causes. A better and more clinically relevant classification of psychosis is offered by Levenson (2005). He differentiates primary from secondary psychotic disorders. To the first group belong the schizophrenias (and related disorders) and the bipolar disorders (with psychoses). Secondary psychoses are related to medical conditions, delirium, dementia, substance abuse (intoxication or withdrawal), or medication side effects (p. 16; see table 6.3).

Even contemporary experts, like Biederman, Spencer, and Wilens (2004), consider that psychotic disorders in children, as in adults, can be functional or organic. According to them, functional psychotic syndromes encompass schizophrenia spectrum disorders and the psychosis associated with mood disorders. The organic psychoses are the result of lesions in the CNS as a consequence of a medical illness, brain injury, or drug use, either licit or illicit (p. 962). These disorders respond to timely identification and treatment of the etiologic disorders. It is the child psychiatrist's responsibility, when dealing with a psychotic disorder, to ensure that any identifiable medical condition or pharmacological reaction (i.e., medication side effects, drug interaction, etc.) is quickly identified (see "Delirium" section, below). The prompt identification of

TABLE 6.3 Differential Diagnosis Between Primary and Secondary Psychosis

Clinical signs	Primary psychosis	Secondary psychosis
Age of onset	Usually younger age	Usually older age
Family history of primary psychosis	May be present	Absent
Level of consciousness	Not impaired	Impaired
Cognitive impairment	Not impaired	Impaired
Focal neurological signs	Not present	May be present
Hallucinations	Auditory	Visual
Delusions	Complex (organized)	Simple
Thought disorder	Prominent	Not prominent
Incontinence	Usually absent	Common
Vital signs	Stable	Usually abnormal
Presence of medical conditions	Uncommon	Always present

Source: Levenson (2005, p. 16).

delirium is of utmost relevance; if not treated in a timely fashion the underlying condition may be fatal.

DELIRIUM

Wise and Brandt (1992) defined delirium as a transient and usually reversible dysfunction of the cerebral metabolism that has an acute or subacute onset and is manifested by an array of neuropsychiatric abnormalities. Even in its most protean manifestations, it is likely that delirium is underrecognized in childhood; the diagnosis of delirium is even more difficult in preschoolers. Schieveld and Leentjens (2005) state, "We fear that this child psychiatric emergency often goes unrecognized and is undertreated; the complex combination of a serious illness and polypharmacy in a young child often results in reluctance and delayed decision to add yet another medication to treat delirium (p. 394). The authors illustrated two cases in children younger than 42 months in a PICU.

Martini (2005) affirms that the hypoactive subtype of delirium is less likely to be recognized and is frequently misdiagnosed as depression (p. 395). Martini calls attention to delirium secondary to anesthesia with sevoflurane, and to anticholinergic delirium secondary to orphenadrine. Delirium should be considered when there are regressive and chaotic behaviors, anxiety and moaning in severely ill children (pp. 396–397). Children are not as prone to delirium states as are adults following a heart transplant. Delirium in children is sometimes confused with regressive and provocative behaviors (Williams, 1996, p. 345).

Delirium entails:

1. Disturbance of the level of consciousness (diminished awareness of the environment, and reduced attention and concentration) that cannot be accounted for by a preexisting medical condition or a dementing process.
2. Cognitive deficits (attention and recent memory impairments, disorientation, language and perceptual disturbances—threatening hallucinations or transient delusions—not related to previous deficits).
3. A rapid onset of the disturbance and a fluctuation of symptoms during the day, "sun-downing," that is, progressive decrement of sensorium as the day moves on.
4. Evidence by history, physical examination, laboratory, or other tests that indicate that the disturbance is a direct physiological consequence of an identifiable medical condition.

Delirum is frequently associated with a disturbance of the sleep–wake cycle, disturbances of the psychomotor behavior (restlessness or hyperactivity, or decrease of psychomotor activity, reaching sluggishness and lethargy); or evidence of emotional disturbance (anxiety, fear, depression, irritability, anger, euphoria, or apathy). These disturbances are particularly prevalent at night. The EEG usually shows generalized slowing (modified from DSM-IV-TR, APA, 2000).

5. In children, delirium may be associated with a sudden increase in psychomotor activity (agitation), disorganized, chaotic, or regressive behaviors, or with psychotic features. (pp. 136–138).

Differential Diagnosis of Delirium

The psychotic features associated with delirium are commonly of an acute nature, except when delirium evolves out of a chronic psychotic background. Wise and Brandt (1992) created an evocative mnemonic device for the different causes of delirium, "I WATCH DEATH" (see table 6.4).

Occasionally, there is a prominent confusional state in the presentation of primary psychoses: the patient appears disoriented to time, place, and even to person; he may also appear incoherent and contradictory in the responses to the examiner. The patient looks as if she or he were delirious. However, there is no fluctuation of the clinical state and, above all, there is no impairment of the autonomic nervous system (no impairment of pulse, blood pressure, no diaphoresis, and no sun-downing). The psychiatrist will also observe findings consistent with schizophrenia (i.e., stereotypes, negativism, or persistent negative and positive symptoms), or of a mood disorder (fluctuating mood, grandiosity, elation, irritability, pressure of speech, catatonia, etc). Moreover, in distinction to delirium, the neurological examination is noncontributory, EEGs and neuroimaging are negative.

PSYCHOSIS ASSOCIATED WITH PSYCHOTROPIC MEDICATIONS

Stimulants

Rarely is psychosis reported as a side effect of stimulant medications. Ross (2006) reports a frequency of 0.25% or 1 in 400 of psychotic-manic symptoms (toxicosis) in children treated with stimulants (p. 1150).

Guanfacine

Psychosis has been reported with guanfacine (Tenex).

TABLE 6.4 Mnemonics of the Causes of Delirium

"I WATCH DEATH"	
I	Infectious encephalitis, meningitis, syphilis, AIDS
W	Withdrawal: Alcohol, barbiturates, sedative-hypnotics, addictive drugs
A	Acute metabolic acidosis, alkalosis, electrolyte disturbances, hepatic and renal failure, porphyria[1]
T	Trauma: head trauma, heat stroke, postoperative state, severe burns
C	CNS pathology: abscess, hemorrhage, normal pressure hydrocephalus, seizure, stroke, tumors, vasculitis
H	Hypoxia: anemia, CO poisoning, hypotension, COPD, heart failure
D	Deficiencies of B_{12}, hypovitaminosis[2]: niacin and thiamine deficiences
E	Endocrinopathies: Hyper- and hypoadrenocorticism, hyper- and hypothyroidism, hyper- and hypoglycemia, hypoestrogenemia[3]
A	Acute vascular: hypertensive encephalopathy, shock, migraine
T	Toxic/drugs: medications,[4] pesticides, solvents
H	Heavy metals: lead, manganese, mercury

Source: Modified from Wise & Brandt (1992).

[1]Pies (2003), described a case of a 17-year-old white woman with a prior background of bipolar disorder, but with a clinical presentation of delirium, muscle weakness, abdominal pain, constipation, and paresthesias. The patient complained that "worms crawled through my guts." She also reported hearing, "shrieking in my head," and had expressed the view that teachers were trying to poison her. The CT scan showed cerebral atrophy; CBC, electrolytes, calcium, BUN, creatinine, and liver functions were all within normal limits. Serum ammonia, TSH, and ANA were also within normal limits. The lab technician informed the physician of the proverbial observation, that the urine sample that he had left on the windowsill turned amber after one hour. This alerted the physicians to the diagnosis of acute intermittent porphyria (AIP). Quantitative testing of 24-hour stool and urine samples showed elevated levels of porphobilinogen (PBG) and 5-aminolevulinic acid (ALA) consistent with AIP. AIP is an autosomal dominant disease with incomplete penetrance, which entails an inborn error of porphyrin synthesis. Most herozygotes remain asymptomatic until they are exposed to drugs such as barbiturates, carbamazepine, and valproic acid. Alcohol, food deprivation, and hormonal changes are also known precipitants.

[2]Psychosis and severe depression are very common in cobalamin deficiency. Cognitive loss and dementia have been documented consistent with subcortical dementia (Filley, 2003, p. 1002). Folate deficiency may actually be more closely associated with psychosis than cobalamin deficiency (p. 1011).

[3]A 23-year-old woman with no prior psychiatric history was admitted to a psychiatric hospital with florid psychosis with disorganized thinking, derealization, cenesthetic hallucinations, and delusions, fulfilling criteria for schizophrenia. The PANSS score was 65. Since puberty she had experienced fluctuating symptoms of derealization, mood swings, anxiety, and reduced interest in studying and social activities. Significant improvement of her psychiatric symptoms was noted after she began to take oral contraceptives at age 18. Gynecologic examination revealed a significant hypoestrogenemia (24 ng/L) while the levels of the other sex hormones were within normal range. Oral contraceptive treatment was instituted of 2 mg of estradiol/day for the first 11 days followed by 10 days of 2 mg estradiol/day plus 0.5 mg of norgestrel/day, and 7 days of no hormonal treatment. By the first week, the PANSS scores had decreased to 44, and by the third week, all the psychotic symptoms had remitted. At a 10-month follow-up the PANSS score was 20 (Ginsberg, 2004b, 13-14). It had been known that estrogen decreases D2 receptor sensitivity (p. 14).

[4]Drugs that most often cause psychotic symptoms include: antidepressants, anticholinergics, antiarrythmics, antimalarials, antivirals, anticonvulsants, corticosteroids, dopamine agonists, opiods, and sympathomimetics (Levenson, 2005, p. 16).

A 9-year-old child with a history of mental retardation had been receiving paroxetine 30 mg/day, lamotrigine 100 mg BID, and trazodone 50 mg q HS. Because of aggressive behaviors and possible Tourette's disorder, guanfacine 1 mg/day was added. The child developed auditory hallucinations (including command hallucinations), which resolved once guanfacine was discontinued. The patient had no prior history of hallucinations. There have also been reports of hallucinations with the use of clonidine.

In all the reported cases of guanfacine-associated psychosis, patients had been taking multiple medications, and a drug interaction is a possibility. The authors indicate that alpha-adrenergic medications can suppress the arousal by stimulating the autoreceptors in the locus ceruleus. A sudden change in arousal may lead to alteration in the mental state, causing anxiety and hallucinations (Boreman & Arnold, 2003, p. 1387).

Antidepressants

Bupropion

Available evidence suggests, that bupropion, in a dose related manner, pose a risk of creating or exacerbating psychosis in a fashion consistent with inferences from its mechanism of action. At particular risk are those who suffer with a primary psychotic disorder. Evidence also suggests that vulnerable patients may have the risk of exacerbating psychosis once they are stabilized with antipsychotics. But given the small sample of the studies reviewed, the side effects may have been understimated (Leard-Hansson & Guttmacher, 2004, p. 32).

SSRIs
See note.[1]

OTHER PSYCHOTROPIC MEDICATIONS ASSOCIATED WITH PSYCHOSIS

Disulfiram

In patients with alcohol abuse or dependency, disulfiran has been used with safety and some success to decrease alcohol use; it must be used with caution due to reports of increased psychosis (Brunette, Noordsy, & Green, 2005, p. 31).

Modafinil

Posmarketing, modafinil has been associated with mania and psychosis (Ginsberg, 2005c, p. 27).

Psychosis Associated with Anticonvulsant Medications

Barbiturates may also be associated with bizarre behavior and delusions, as well as with auditory and visual hallucinations (Fohrman & Stein, 2006, p. 38). For other anticonvulsants which may induce psychosis, see p. 263. See end note 3 for psychosis associated with topiramate.

Benzodiazepines

Benzodiazepines may cause bizarre behavior and delusions, as well as auditory and visual hallucinations (Fohrman & Stein, 2006, p. 38).

Psychotic Features Associated with Antipsychotics

Ginsberg (2005d) reviews data suggesting that aripiprazole may elicit or aggravate psychotic conditions (p. 30). It is unlikely this is an exclusive problem of aripiprazole, and that other antipsychotics may produce this paradoxically adverse reaction.

Antipsychotic Psychosis/Tardive Psychosis

Swartz (2004) discussed the concept of tardive psychosis (dopamine hypersensitivity psychosis or rebound psychosis). This psychosis was originally described as a superimposed clinical syndrome to schizophrenia, in patients undergoing long-term treatment with antidopaminergic agents. It is considered that this phenomenon is the result of hyperdopaminergic rebound secondary to an excess proliferation of postsynaptic dopamine receptors or receptor hypersensitivity to dopamine. This syndrome might also reflect cholinergic suppression. This psychosis is secondary to dopaminergic blockade, and is analogous to the tardive syndromes: tardive dyskinesia, tardive akathisia, and the like. These syndromes become manifested after dopamine blocking exposure decreases or ceases all together. Psychosis may be another tardive complication of dopaminergic blockade. There are reports of new onset psychotic symptoms attributable to antipsychotic drugs. Thus, in young adults followed prospectively, new onset of mood-incongruent psychosis developed after three or more years of dopamine-blocking antipsychotic agents for resistant nonpsychotic mania. The psychosis was breakthrough, not a withdrawal type. Tardive psychosis appeared while the patients were taking antipsychotic drugs and in spite of its effects, the psychotic effect was much stronger. New onset psychotic symptoms have also been observed on long–term antidomapaminergic treatment for patients with Tourette's disorder (p. 17).

Psychosis and Mania Associated with Herbal Agents

St. John's Wort and Ginseng, and other popular over-the-counter herbal products, may induce psychosis or manic behavior by themselves. These products
may also alter the CYP-450 metabolism of other medications causing untoward
side effects (Joshi & Faubion, 2005, pp. 56–57). Another plant, Ma-huang was
banned by the FDA in 2004 because of its association with anticholinergic
delirium (p. 59).

Psychosis Associated with Nonpsychotropic Medications

Fohrman and Stein (2006) list a multitude of medications that may be associated with psychotic features.[2]

OTHER PSYCHOTIC FEATURES OF NONPSYCHIATRIC ETIOLOGY

Perceptual Disorders Associated with Psychotomimetic and Prescribed Medications

Boza (http://www.priory.com/halluc.htm) identified a number of perceptual
experiences (in all the sensory modalities) and illusions that have as a cause an
identifiable drug, medication, a medical or neurological, or other nonpsychi-
atric etiology. Some of these interesting perceptual abnormalities, with exotic
and interesting names, are relevant in the differential diagnosis of psychosis
of children and adolescents.

It is essential to discriminate between visual hallucinations and visual
illusions.

Visual Hallucinations

- Alpha adrenergic agonists: clonidine [rare]. See above.
- Antiparkinsonian medications: bromocriptine, selegiline, and carbidopa.
- Anticonvulsants: carbamazepine [rare].
- Analgesics: pentazocine and fentanyl.
- Antivertigo medications: diphenidol.
- Psychotropic agents with robust anticholinergic effects, and SSRIs [rare].
- Histamine 2 blockers [rare].
- Antiarrhythmic agents: tonocaide (hallucinogenic in 12% of patients).
- Antiemetics: dronabinol (generates hallucinations in up to 5% of the
  patients).

Visual Illusions

- Chromatopsias, the environment is seen as uniformly tinted with a color:
    Xanthopsias (yellow vision) observed in patients on digitalis; purple vision observed in patients on Santonin (antihelmintic).
- Size hallucinations/illusions:
    In lilliputians and brodnignagian hallucinations people are perceived as either very small or as giants, respectively: Pregabalin may induce brodnignagian hallucinations.
- Metamorphopsias:
    Dysmegalopsia (alteration in the form of objects), micropsia, and macropsia (real percepts look smaller or larger). In teleopsia the object is seen far away, in pelopsia the object is seen nearer than it actually is. In allesthesia the object is seen in a different place, and in palinopsia, the perception continues even though the object is no longer present in the visual field. These events are associated with parietal pathology or a migrainous aura.

Other Hallucinations

- Haptic (Tactile), proprioceptive, somatic, and visceral hallucinations:
    Formicative hallucinations (patients complain of bugs crawling in their skin and may scratch themselves vigorously) may be drug related, such as in abuse of alcohol, methylphenidate, amphetamines, cocaine, or steroids. Amyl nitrate use may contribute to erotic sensations in the genital area (Boza, http://www.priory.com/halluc.htm).

Occasionally, there is a prominent confusional state in the presentation of schizophrenia-spectrum disorders, catatonia, and others. The patient appears disoriented to time or place, and even to person; he or she may also be incoherent and contradictory in responding to the examiner, and may appear as if delirious. However, there is no fluctuation of the clinical state and above all, there is no impairment of the autonomic nervous system (no impairment of pulse, blood pressure, no diaphoresis, nor sun-downing).

The onset of psychosis may be classified as acute or chronic. Occasionally, Acute psychoses may have a fulminating onset with sudden presentation of hallucinations, delusions, mood disorder or confusion; this requires immediate assessment and intervention. Youth who are acutely psychotic are often frightened, combative, and are potentially at significant risk of harming themselves or others. Signs and symptoms of psychosis are typically easiest to recognize during this phase, although determining the underlying cause may be difficult. Such youth may also present with other psychiatric features, such as aggression, destructiveness, suicidal behavior, functional deterioration, or regressive behaviors (Semper & McClellan, 2003, pp. 681–682).

CHRONIC PSYCHOSIS ASSOCIATED WITH MEDICAL ILLNESSES

The differential diagnosis of "organic psychoses" includes most of the etiological categories enumerated as causes for delirium. Following Wise and Brandt's (1992) delirium mnemonics, the child and adolescent psychiatrist should review the deliniated medical conditions to make a thorough differential diagnosis of chronic psychoses. We will review illnesses and medical conditions that are associated with some frequency with either acute or chronic psychotic symptoms in children and adolescents (for genetic/chromosomal abnormalities, see chapter 8)

Infections of the Central Nervous System (CNS)

There are a number of microbial (bacteria, spirochaeta, and others) and viral infectious agents that affect the CNS causing a variety of neurological signs and symptoms including psychotic features. The consultation from a psychiatrist is requested when the patient displays, behavioral or emotional abnormalities, and when the patient becomes aggressive and uncooperative with the medical team.

Encephalitis, Meningitis, and Other Infections of the CNS

Acute encephalitis occasionally falls within the purview of the child and adolescent psychiatrist, but rarely does the clinical picture of these CNS infections begin with prominent perceptual or delusional components. In 40% of the cases, acute encephalitis starts with mood related symptoms (apathy) or aggressiveness. Child and adolescent psychiatrists may be the first physicians to deal with these patients because of the nature of the latter symptom presentation.

Syphilis

The resurgence of syphilis throughout the world gives added importance to timely identification of acquired cases of neuropsyphilis in infancy and childhood (Maria & Bale, 2006, p. 503). Additionally, it is likely that incomplete treatments obscure the clinical presentations of tertiary syphilis. Juvenile paresis is the most common form of congenital tertiary syphilis that usually begins between 6 and 21 years, the average age of onset being around 13 years (p. 504).

A form of late active syphilis involves the central nervous system, with the most common being the meningovascular type. Paresis, a potentially dangerous form of CNS syphilis, occurs in juveniles, and may be detected in preparetic states by examining the CSF. If not treated, parenchimal involvement may be severe and eventually, irreversible. Juvenile tabes rarely occurs. Any form of congenital syphilis becomes spontaneously seronegative by the time the disease is recognized (Staat, 2003, p. 1005).

Among the neurosyphilitic syndromes, general paresis has the most psychiatric relevance. General paresis (dementia paralytica, paralysis of the insane) can develop any time from age 2 to 30 (usually 10 to 25 years after the primary lesion). It is more common in men than in women (3:1). About 60% of paretics present with progressive simple dementia; less than 20% display manic symptoms and megalomania. Faulty judgment, impaired memory, disturbed affect (depression or euphoria), or paranoia develops and progresses as the disease advances.

AIDS Encephalopathy

Children and infants with proven HIV infections are at a high risk of neurological problems. A great percentage of children with HIV (50 to 80%) get the virus from maternal–fetal transmission in utero, from tranfusions (20%), and the rest from sexual abuse. Two patterns of neurological disease have been established: (1) The most common, a progressive encephalopathy characterized by loss or a plateau of development, impaired brain growth, progressive atrophy, pyramidal track signs, and other neurological deficits. Apathy is common but seizures are rare. There is a progressive downhill course complicated by systemic infections leading to death within months or years. (2) Static encephalopathy occurs in 10 to 20% of children with AIDS. Nonprogressive motor and developmental impairments, microcephaly, and occasionally seizures may develop in children with AIDS. A small percentage of children, from 10 to 20%, are neurologically intact (Seay & De Vivo, 2003, p. 2311). Because children with HIV infection are living longer with highly active antiretroviral therapy, the risk of developing late-appearing disorders, such as HIV-associated dementia (HAD), may increase (Scharko, Baker, Kothari, & Lancaster, 2006, p. 107).

Other infections rarely associated with psychotic features include: Epstein-Barr virus (fever, sore throat, adenopathy, fatigue, poor concentration); Lyme disease (target lesion, fever; check for high risk geographic areas); malaria/typhoid fever (fever, mental status changes; check for endemic areas); mycoplasma pneumonia (fever, mental status changes; may occur in the absence of pneumonia); rabies (history of exposure) (Fohrman & Stein, 2006, p. 43).

Alcohol and Drugs of Abuse

Given the prevalence of substance abuse in the adolescent population, it is essential to consider that presenting psychotic or mood episodes may be secondary to substance intoxication, particularly CNS stimulants and hallucinogens. Careful history taking, often without the presence of parents or guardians, may reveal relevant information to shed light on this issue. Routine urine drug screening tests are unreliable and often are unable to screen for some of the new and popular synthetic "club drugs" such as ecstasy and gamma hydroxybutiric acid (GHB) (Semper & McClellan, 2003, p. 683).

Despite ample evidence demonstrating the neuropsychiatric effects of substance use and acute intoxication, there is little evidence that substance use or abuse directly causes persistent neuropsychiatric syndromes in children and adolescents (Bukstein & Tarter, 1998, p. 603). In spite of this, clinicians need to keep in mind that there is a significant rate of comorbid substance abuse in adolescents with bipolar disorder, other mood disorders and schizophrenia, reaching as much as 50%, in some studies (Tsai & Champine, 2004, p. 392).

Studies show that as many as one third or more of adolescents with schizophrenia or schizoaffective disorder have problems with substance abuse; those with substance abuse are more likely to fail at school, to come from dysfunctional families, and to require hospital sevices. Schizoaffective disorder is more common in dual-diagnosis cases. Substance abuse is common in youth with bipolar disorder. The risk of substance abuse was nine times higher in patients with bipolar adolescent onset, than those with childhood onset bipolar disorder, independent of the presence of comorbid behavioral or anxiety disorder (Reimherr & McClellan, 2004, p. 8). Psychosis caused by substances generally clears within hours to days, although there are reports of prolonged paranoid states caused by methamphetamine use (Semper & McClellan, 2003, p. 685).

Ethanol is a CNS depressant and the most commonly abused substance by youth (only second to tobacco abuse). Because of its depressing effects on inhibitory control mechanisms, alcohol can produce stimulation and excitement, and as a result, aggressive or abusive behaviors may occur. Accidental ingestion of alcohol (present in products, such as mouth wash) by toddlers and infants may induce hypoglycemia (Tenenbein, 2003, pp. 377–378).

Inhalant Abuse (Sniffing or "Huffing" of Volatile Substances)

Aliphatic and aromatic hydrocarbons, aliphatic nitrites, esters, and ketones, are the most common volatile organic compounds used for recreational and abuse purposes. These are available in countless consumer products. Up to 20% of pediatric abusers had experimented with inhalants, which are depressants and are related to anesthetic gases, also an important source of abuse. The physiological effects of inhalants are those of early stages of anesthesia, including stimulation, disinhibition, and impulsive behavior. Speech becomes slurred and the gait becomes staggered. Euphoria, frequently with hallucinations, is followed by drowsiness and sleep, particularly after repeated inhalation. The most feared adverse side effect from inhalants is sudden death as a result of ventricular arrythmias. White-matter degeneration, dementia, and cerebellar encephalopathy occur in chronic toluone (methylbenzene) abuse (Tenenbein, 2003, pp. 377–378). Paranoid psychosis has also been noted as a persistent problem in some individuals with toluene abuse (Filley, 2003, p. 1011).

Amphetamines and Related Drugs

Amphetamines and related drugs (such as cocaine), may be either illicit or pharmaceutical. Legitimate uses include treatment of ADHD, narcolepsy, and refractory obsesity. Medically prescribed medications include amphetamine, dextroamphetamine, methamphetamine, and methylphenidate. In the illegal drug world, caffeine, ephedrine, and phenylpropanolamine are commonly sold as if they were amphetamines. Methylenedioxymetamphetamine (MDMA or ecstasy) is a hallucinogenic amphetamine. Amphetamines stimulate the release of catecholamines, while cocaine blocks the presynaptic reuptake of these neurotransmitters. The effects of these drugs occur both within the central nervous system and peripherally. They produce changes in mood, excitation, tachycardia, hypertension, and even dysrhythmias. CNS manifestations include anxiety, agitation, confusion, psychosis, and seizures. Hyperthermia may be found in persons with moderate to severe toxicity (Tenenbein, 2003, p. 377). Stimulant abuse and dependence is common in bipolar disorder patients (Camacho, 2004, p. 43).

Hallucinogenics

Marijuana, LSD, Phencyclidine (Angel Dust or PCP), MDMA, and Ketamine

These substances induce sensory misperception, disordered thought processes, and mood changes. Marijuana is the most commonly abused hallucinogen. Children and adolescents consistently report that they seek the calming effects of marijuana, that this drug decreases their level of hostility, and that it, "makes [their] problems go away." Occasionally, hallucinogens elicit excessive, unpleasant, or persistent reactions, alterations of the mental state, agitation, panic, and anxiety reactions ("bad trips"), or acute toxic psychoses. PCP and MDMA can produce life-threatening toxicity. For a long time there has been an intense controversy regarding the role of marijuana in the development of psychosis, and of schizophrenia in particular. Rey, Martin, and Krabman (2004) state that taken together, a number of studies support the proposition that marijuana use increases the risk of psychosis; it is unclear if psychotic patients use cannabis for self-medication. The psychosis risk is dependent on the length and intensity of the drug use. Marijuana seems to increase the risk of schizophrenia (from 5 to 10 cases per 10,000 person years). It is unlikely that cannabis causes schizophrenia; it is more likely that cannabis brings forward the illness in persons with aggregated risks. Cannabis also exacerbates schizophrenic symptoms. Marijuana users with schizophrenia have an earlier age of onset, more psychotic symptoms, a poorer response to antipsychotic medications, and a poorer outcome compared to patients who do not use it (p. 1201).

Toddlers develop CNS depression after ingesting marijuana, toxic psychosis after ingesting LSD, and a very striking picture after intoxication with PCP, which is characterized by agitation, aggressiveness, coma, and seizures. Physical findings include hypertension, hypertonia, hyperreflexia, twitching, tremors, diaphoresis, and hyperthermia.

MDMA is associated with prolonged dancing parties, called raves. Beside hallucinogenic effects, this drug produces CNS stimulation and cardiovacular effects in overdose. Because of the increased level of physical activity and the decrease of fluid intake, adolescents ingesting amphetamines are at risk of hyperthermia, dehydration, electrolyte imbalance, and seizures (Tenenbein, 2003, pp. 377). Paranoid reactions and clinical pictures analogous to paranoid schizophrenia, secondary to cocaine, and amphetamines, PCP, and other drugs of abuse, are reported frequently.

LSD acts primarily on the serotonergic system, where it exerts both inhibitory and excitatory effects (Bukstein & Tarter, 1998, p. 599). Flashbacks from LSD and other hallucinogens sometimes spontaneouly occur weeks or months following an episode of drug abuse; they may be precipitated by stress, fatigue, or the ingestion of other substances such as marijuana. This experience is more common in frequent users. Flashbacks entail intensification of stimuli, apparent motion of fixed objects, and superimposition of geometric shapes in the field of vision (p. 603). LSD frequently produces cross-sensory and transensory experiences, such as hearing colors or feeling sounds. LSD occasionally elicits very dysphoric experiences, "bad trips."

Ketamine is classified as a dissociative anesthetic, and is primarily used by veterinarians and pediatric surgeons as a nonalgesic anesthetic. This drug causes a dose dependent dissociative episodes with feelings of fragmentation, detachment and what has been described as as a "psychic/physical/spiritual scatter." Ketamine induces a lack of responsive awareness not only to pain but to the general environment. Ketamine is a close chemical cousin of phencyclidine-PCP (McDowell, 1999, p. 299). This drug may induce tangential thinking and ideas of reference. At higher doses it distorts perception of the body, the environment, and time. At usual doses it stimulates illusions, and at higher doses, hallucinations and paranoid delusions can occur (p. 300). Ketamine substantially disrupts attention and learning. Retrieval, long-term recall, and consolidation of memory are all altered with ketamine use (p. 300). Sometimes, opioids are associated with psychotic symptoms (Fohrman & Stein, 2006, p. 38).[4]

Systemic Vasculitis with Central Nervous System Involvement

Systemic Lupus Erythematosus (SLE)

Neuropsychiatric complications develop in more than half of patients with SLE. Other neurological complications are present in 20 to 45% of children affected by the SLE (Legido, Tenenbaum, Katasos & Menkes, 2006, p. 628). Neuropsychiatric symptoms are the first manifestations of SLE in about 5% of the cases (There is a wide range of neuropsychiatric manifestations of SLE and the symptoms and signs are usually protean and progressive. The majority of patients present with mental changes including psychosis, mood disturbance (particularly depression), or confusion. A significant percentage of patients may also exhibit concomitant neurological manifestations (Legido, Tenembaum, Katsetos, et al., 2006, p, 630). Every form of psychiatric disturbance has been described with SLE, ranging from mood disorders to personality disorders and psychosis. SLE should be considered among possible causes of catatonia, even in young patients. Minimal investigations should initially include antinuclear antibody levels, followed by anti-DNA and anti-ribosomal P detection (Perisse et al., 2003, p. 499).

The following vignette raises the question of CNS lupus prior to the identification of the illness:

> Jeanna, a 10-year-old Hispanic female, consulted for depression and suicidal behavior. She had been feeling depressed and suicidal for the previous two years, coinciding with parental separation and divorce. She voiced that she could no longer cope with the stress of living at home. Jeanna, a very attractive and intelligent preadolescent, indicated that her mother was depressed, that her mother was not coping, and that her mother was not available for emotional support. Jeanna was participarly upset with the fact that her mother was attempting to reconcile with her biological father, who was coming home more often, and taking a progressive disciplinary role.
>
> One year before, she had suffered from incapacitating articular pain in shoulders, elbows, knees, and ankles; she could not get out of bed and was unable to attend school for a number of weeks. She was diagnosed with SLE. She stated that about one year before she was diagnosed with lupus, she started experiencing auditory, visual, and paranoid ideations. She had no prior history of physical or sexual abuse, and had not experimented with drugs. The auditory hallucinations consisted of voices which were derogatory, and the visual hallucinations related to a scary male figure; the paranoia was florid. She reported that she had experienced psychotic phenomenona all along.

Neurological Disorders

The developmental phase of the individual must be considered as part of the formula that determines the frequency and nature of neuropsychiatric syndromes occuring in conjunction with brain disease. When Huntington's disease, idiopathic basal ganglia calcification, metachromatic leukodystrophy, or temporal lobe epilepsy begins in adolescence, the patient is more likely to develop psychosis than when the disease begins later in life. In postencephalitic disorders following epidemic encephalitis, adults develop Parkinsonism and mood disturbances whereas children develop tics and conduct disorders. Thus, the developmental state of the brain is one of the determinants of the type of behavior disorder emerging with brain dysfunction. Gender also exerts important influences on neuropsychiatric symptoms: adolescent girls are more likely than adolescent boys to exhibit psychosis associated with epilepsy, and women are more likely to develop depression following stroke (Cummings & Mega, 2003, p. 64).

Cerebral Palsy

Autism and other psychotic syndromes are among the severest psychiatric symptoms associated with cerebral palsy. Although the identification of these disorders is not difficult, the management of these conditions is a big clinical challenge. Nonverbal tetraplegic patients may suffer from auditory command hallucinations. Physically and mentally handicapped persons have a high vulnerability to psychiatric disorders due to total dependency on others. Hallucinations may seriously interfere with communication between the patient and the caregivers, and loss of trust is apt to be a consequence (Lou, 1998, p. 1084).

White Matter Diseases

Adrenoleukodystrophy (ALD)

ALD belongs to a group of progressive, X-linked recessive, perioxisomal degenerative disorders of myelin (leukodystrophies); the responsible gene maps to Xq28. These disorders are characterized by deficiency of lignoceroyl coenzyme A synthatase (Pryse-Phillips, 2003, p. 20). Six phenotypes have been described; in the adult cerebral ALD, a rare, dominantly inherited variant, sometimes presents with psychosis; another curious phenotype is the X-linked Addison's disease without neurological involvement (p. 21). ALD is the most common and clearly defined form of sudanophilic cerebral sclerosis, with an incidence of 1 in 10,000 male subjects. It is also the most common peroxisomal disorder, the enzymatic deficiency results in an accumulation of very long chain fatty acids in tissues and plasma. The condition is characterized by visual and intellectual impairment, seizures, spasticity, and a more or less rapid progression to death. ALD is often accompanied by adrenocortical insufficiency (Menkes, 2000, p. 212). The first symptoms are usually an alteration of behavior ranging from a withdrawn state to aggressive outbursts (Fenichel, 2005, p. 146). Psychiatric symptomatology analogous to schizophrenia has been reported in this disease as far back as 1975 (Powell et al., 1975, p. 254; Schaumburg et al., 1975, pp. 579–580). The case of Roger, a 7-year-old boy, suffering fron ALD, with prominent regressive symptomatology was described (Cepeda, 2000, pp. 262–263). Bone marrow transplantation is an option for boys and adolescents who are in early clinical stages and have MRI evidence of brain involvement (Fenichel, 2005, p. 146).

Metachromatic leukodystrophy (MLD)

MLD belongs to a group of recessively inherited lysosomal storage diseases caused by a deficiency of arylsulphatase A which leads to intralysosomal storage of cerebroside sulfate in the white matter of the CNS and periphreal nerves. Clinically, the disease is heterogeneous and different forms are classified according to the age of onset of symptoms (late infantile, juvenile and adult) (Pryse-Phillips, 2003, p. 581). In children, there is a progressive deterioration toward a vegetative state and death within a few years; later age onset of the illness has a less severe course. In older children and adults, dementia is the predominant manifestation. A frequent tendency for psychosis to herald the onset of the illness has been reported, possibly because of the disruption of cortico-cortical connections between the frontal and the temporal lobes (Filley, 2003, p. 997).

The clinical picture of two slow virus diseases, human inmunodeficiency virus and subacute sclerosing panencephalitis, include symptoms of psychosis prior to the emergence of progressive dementia (Cummings & Mega, 2003, p. 174).

Multiple Sclerosis in Childhood

Multiple sclerosis is usually a disease of young adults, but up to 3 to 5% of cases occur in children less than 6 years of age (Fenichel, 2005, p. 225). Psychosis in MS, probably secondary to fronto-limbic disconnection and temporal demyelination, is rare (Filley, 2003, p. 999).

> In the late 1970s, while training at a major mid-western university, this author became aware of a 12-year-old white girl with a complex behavioral and emotional syndrome; this adolescent had complained about visual problems and dysesthesias in the arms, regressed behavior, and psychotic features. These symptoms had been interpreted as manifestations of a conversion disorder. As the vision appeared to deteriorate, and evidence of probable brain compromise continued to emerge, a neurological consultation was requested. The consultant found evidence of neurological illness and requested a brain CT scan. Findings of demyelinization were compatible with MS.

In adults, multiple sclerosis may display a pure neuropsychiatric presentation (Asghar-Ali, Taber, Hurley, & Hayman, 2004). Two cases with manialike presentation and psychosis were discussed. It is reported that the percentage of patients with T2-weighted white matter hyperintensities (WMH; 0.83%), consistent with the diagnosis of multiple sclerosis, is 15 times the reported prevalence of multiple sclerosis in the United States (0.058%). Affective disorders (depressive and bipolar) were the most common psychiatric findings in these patients; that is, affective illness due to multiple sclerosis (pp. 226–228).

Basal Ganglia Diseases

Yu (2004) alerts physicians to the psychiatric presentations, including psychosis, of illnesses that ordinarily do not have a primary psychiatric manifestation. Such is the case of Huntington's, Wilson's, and Fahr's diseases.

Huntington's Disease
Huntington's is an autosomal disorder that causes basal ganglia degeneration. The genetic defect consists of an abnormal trinucleotide repeat on chromosome 4, leading to the abnormal production of the protein huntingtin. It is estimated that up to 24 to 79% of Huntington's disorder patients may have a psychiatric disorder as an initial manifestation, and that psychotic symptoms may be present in as much as 5 to 17% of these patients. Affective symptoms are the most common, though. Psychosis was more common in Huntington's patients whose first degree relatives had suffered from psychosis. The so-called childhood onset Huntington's disease, characterized by rigidity instead of chorea, cerebellar signs, and rapidly progressive dementia should not be confused with a first schizophrenic break (pp. 69–70).

Wilson's Disease
This disorder of copper metabolism (hepatolenticular degeneration), is an autosomal recessive genetic disorder with more than 100 identified mutations on the 13 chromosome. The age of onset ranges from childhood to adulthood with a mean onset of 17 years of age. Timely identification is essential to arrest the progression of the hepatic (and portal hypertension) and neurological disease. In up to one third of patients, psychiatric symptoms, without hepatic or neurological signs, are the earliest manifestations. In up to 2% of the patients, psychosis is diagnosed. Psychiatric symptoms include behavioral and personality changes, affective symptoms and psychosis (Yu, 2004, pp. 70–71).

Fahr's Disease
This familial, idopathic, basal ganglial calcification is associated with psychiatric symptoms in up to 40% of the cases. Psychosis may be present in patients 20 to 40 years of age. Classic schizophreniclike symptoms have been described. Unusual symptoms not associated with schizophrenia have been reported,

including musical auditory hallucinations and complex visual hallucinations (Yu, 2004, p. 71).

Seizure Disorders

Complex Partial Seizures

Complex partial seizures (CPS) originates locally in a limited area of one of the cerebral hemispheres; it presents most often in adolescence or adult life. These seizures involve motor, sensory, or psychological manifestations, and there is always some impairment of consciousness. Seizures usually last for 1 minute but occasionally for up to 15 minutes and are seldom preceded by aura. No single EEG manifestation has been described (Pryse-Phillips, 2003, pp. 212–213). The following vignette illustrates some clinical behavioral complexities of CPS.

> A 10-year-old Hispanic male complained of a persistent foul odor, "like a fart." He kept on asking his mother if she smelled it. The perception of the bad smell was so strong that he showered many times during the day to get rid of the bad smell; he also changed clothes up to eight times a day. This child also complained about stomach pain, headaches, and pain in the arms (it would have been reasonable if this child had been misdiagnosed as suffering from an obsessive–compulsive disorder)
>
> This child had a long history of behavioral and emotional disturbance; he had displayed and endorsed strong suicidal and homicidal ideation, and was very paranoid. He was also markedly anxious and feared that other children were going to beat him. Furthermore, he had history of enuresis and encopresis.
>
> A referral to the pediatric neurologist was done to ascertain the presence of complex partial seizures. The neurologist requested an MRI and performed a spinal tap. The MRI was normal. The CSF was within normal limits. A previous EEG had been unremarkable. A second EEG showed definite temporal paroxysmal activity. The child was placed on carbamazepine. Ten days after the carbamazepine initiation, mother and child reported significant improvement: the smells were infrequent and the frequency of showering and clothes changing was markedly reduced.

This vignette exemplifies an important caution regarding the detection of complex partial epilepsy: one or more normal EEGs do not exclude the presence of this disorder. Often a number of EEGs are necessary. At times, telemetry or extended EEG recording is necessary.

Psychosis is rare in children with epilepsy, and when present, is associated with significant cerebral abnormalities. Psychosis has been reported in children with complex partial seizures, perhaps more commonly with left temporal lobe foci (Weisbrot & Ettinger, 2001, p. 134). Psychosis is a rare phenomenon among patients with neocortical extratemporal epilepsy. Some studies report a higher frequency of psychosis with focal seizures that involve the mesial temporal structures, particularly those involving the left temporal lobe, but the relationship between lateralization of seizure focus and psychosis is in need of further clarification (Doval, Gaviria, & Kanner, 2001, p. 266).

Complex partial seizures (CPS), formerly termed *temporal lobe* or *psychomotor seizures* are among the most common seizure types encountered in both children and adults. Automatisms (involuntary motor activity such as facial grimacing, gestures, chewing, lip smacking, finger snapping, and repetitive speech) are frequent during the period of impaired consciousness; there is no recall of this activity following the seizure. Seizures last from 30 seconds to several minutes and most patients experience some degree of postictal lethargy or confusion (Holmes, 1996, p. 225).

Here is another interesting example of an adolescent female with florid symptoms associated with complex partial symptomatology:

> Ruby, a 17-year-old blond and attractive female, was referred by the Immigration and Naturalization Service (INS) for a psychiatry evaluation due to concerns with suicidal risk and progressive depression. Ruby, a native from Central America, had crossed the border illegally, and had been detained and interned in a juvenile center in the Southwest area while her disposition was determined.
>
> Ruby reported she was very depressed; she felt very sad and did not want to live any more. She had been depressed for a number of years, and a year before she had been hospitalized for depression and suicidal behavior (she had attempted to poison herself). Ruby felt hopeless and useless. She saw no purpose in life. Ruby felt extremely angry with her mother for her predicament. She blamed her mother for her situation and for her eventual extradition to her native country. Ruby felt so angry with her mother that she felt like strangling her. The anger and hatred went beyond this: the hatred got so vehement that she voiced that she felt like killing her mother, and more. Ruby indicated that she would kill her mother, cut her to pieces, degut her, and the like. She also reported suffering from a very unstable mood, a low energy level, and she also complained of a periodic sense that her thoughts went very fast.
>
> Ruby denied any health problems and endorsed no history of seizures, head trauma, or a history of physical or sexual abuse. She was a chain smoker, claiming that she smoked up to three packs of cigarettes a day. She also had experimented with cocaine for six months in a row, and had smoked marijuana about three times in the past. Ruby stated she did not like to be around peers or people, in general. When queried about sexual feelings she voiced that she had a sense of repugnance about sex, that she experienced a great deal of disgust or aversion about sexual issues; she avoided being around boys. However, she denied any homosexual feelings.
>
> Ruby endorsed poly-sensory hallucinations and florid paranoid ideations (she felt that people talked about her, that people watched her, that there were cameras taking pictures of her, that people followed her, and that somebody was persecuting her). She stated that she had heard voices for a very long time. Ruby heard many voices that deprecated her, and told her that she was worthless, that she was "shit," that she did not deserve to be alive, that she should kill herself. The

voices also told her to kill other people. The voices were tormenting and relentless. She saw dead people, and reported awful olfactory hallucinations: she smelled "feces," and like "stinky feet." She added that the smells made her feel nauseous and somewhat confused. Ruby periodically felt that she was somebody else (depersonalization), "that somebody had changed my spirit." She expressed a desire to leave her past behind. She also reported autoscopic phenomena. Moreover, Ruby reported déjà vu and jamais vu experiences (dyscognitive states), and even expressed fears that somebody could put thoughts in her mind. She stated that she could not concentrate.

The mental status examination revealed that Ruby was distant and difficult to engage. However, she was alert and cooperative. Ruby's mood was moderately to severely depressed, and her affect was very constricted. Even though she reported pleomorphic hallucinations and florid delusions, she did not display any thought disorder; strikingly, she was disoriented as to day, date, and month; this is more striking if we realize that she seemed very intelligent and spoke five languages. The disorientation was an additional factor suggesting complex partial status.

Neurological consultation confirmed the presence of bilateral spiking in the temporal fields (complex partial symptomatology). She was treated with carbamazepine and responded satisfactorily to it. Ruby was followed up for about three months before she was deported to her Central American native country.

Ruby displayed elements of the psychomotor triad (motor changes, automatisms, and alterations of psychic function). According to Victor and Ropper (2001), the clinical pattern (phenomenology) probably varies with the precise location of the lesion and the direction and extent of the spread of the electrical discharge. Complex partial seizures show an increased incidence in the adolescent and adult years. The history of febrile seizures seems to be associated with it. Two thirds of the patients with complex partial seizures also have generalized tonic-clonic seizures or have had them some time earlier in their lives (p. 340).

Psychomotor epilepsy refers to the automatic behavior originating in the temporal lobe. The automatisms are stereotyped from seizure to seizure. Autonomic symptoms may occur during a temporal lobe episode; such is the case of abdominal epilepsy, unpredictable in its presentation, and lasting 10 to 15 minutes. The episode may be accompanied by other autonomic phenomena such as sweating, salivation, and flatus. Emotional changes before, during, and after the episode may be observed: irritability, silliness, fear, agitation, sadness, embarrassment, or laughter. Gelastic (laughing) seizures have been reported. Less frequently, alterations of perception, in the form of illusions and hallucinations, may be reported including macropsias, micropsias, macroacusia and microacusia. Hallucinations may be somatosensory, visual, auditory, olfactory, or gustatory (p. 227).

It has long been observed that some patients with temporal lobe seizures also exhibit a number of behavioral abnormalities and personality changes during the interictal period. Often these patients are described as slow and rigid in their thinking, verbose, circumstantial, and tedious in conversation; they are inclined to mysticism and are preoccupied with religious and philosophical ideas. Often they are prone to outbursts, bad temper, and aggressiveness. Personality traits commonly described include: obsessive traits, humorless sobriety, emotionality (mood swings, sadness, and anger), and a tendency to paranoia. Diminished sexual interest and potency in men have also been described. Geschwind proposed a triad of behavioral abnormalities in patients with complex partial symptomatology: hyposexuality, hypergraphia, and hyperreligiosity. Attempts at localization of this proposed syndrome have been controversial (Victor & Ropper, 2001, pp. 341–342). This syndrome has rarely been observed in adolescence.

Young patients with complex partial seizures are prone to display more illogical thought patterns, hallucinations, and delusions compared to children with generalized epilepsy. Caplan believes that the, "[P]athology of the mesial limbic system might, therefore, underline illogical thinking and its association with cognitive dysfunction and a schizophrenia-like psychosis in pediatric CPS (complex partial seizures)" (Caplan, Arbelle, et al., 1997, p. 1291). Only 20% of children with CPS displayed schizophrenialike symptoms; none of these children had loose associations. On the contrary, loose associations were found in 71% of schizophrenic children (p. 1291). Children with CPS do not display loose associations or negative signs characteristic of schizophrenic children.

Many cases of complex partial seizures may be identified with systematic exploration of perceptual disturbances. Seizures originating in the frontal lobe last 30 seconds or less, and commonly begin and end suddenly. These episodes may not involve total impairment of consciousness and some degree of recall may be possible. Arrest of motor activity associated with a blank stare and loss of contact may be commonly observed as initial manifestations of frontal lobe seizures. Whereas speech arrest may hint to the Broca's area or to the supplementary motor area, other phonatory disturbances such as cries, moans, or grunts may involve the inferior frontal gyrus and the anterior part of the midfrontal gyrus. Tonic head turning, often with conjugate eye deviation, partial motor tonic and clonic seizures, and automatisms are motor behaviors sometimes observed in frontal lobe seizures. The automatisms may be complex and bizarre; sexual automatisms have been reported (Holmes, 1996, pp. 228–229).

A variety of visual distortions (macropsias, micropsias, and metamorphopsias) also occur as an ictal phenomenon, either without hallucinations or concomitantly with them. Ictal hallucinations are more frequently associated with right- than with left-side lesions (Cummings & Mega, 2003, p. 190). Psychosis, depression, anxiety, and emotional lability may occur after temporal lobectomy, the treatment for intractable epilepsy. Most studies have found that after lobectomy; one third to one half of patients develop de novo psychiatric symptoms including suicide, which accounts for 22% of postoperative deaths.

These complications account for many readmissions and psychiatric hospital-izations (Lambert, Schmitz, Ring, & Trimble 2003, p. 1114).

Of significant clinical relevance is the substantiation of interictal psychosis, alternative psychosis (forced normalization, postictal psychosis), or interictal personality changes.

The Phenomenom of Forced Normalization

Forced normalization describes the tendency for patients with partial epilepsies to develop schizophrenialike psychosis when they achieve better seizure control; the EEG tends to a more normal pattern at those times and conversely, the EEG reverts to its former abnormal state as the psychosis clears (Pryse-Phillips, 2003, p. 364). The concept of forced normalization was first described in the 1950s by Landolt and stems from the puzzling observation that as the epileptic patient's EEG looks less and less abnormal, the patient's thinking and behavior becomes more and more bizarre (Pies, 2002, pp. 17–18).

Pies reported on an interesting case of forced normalization.

The patient was a 17-year-old female who had been admitted to the psychiatric service for the evaluation of a "rapid onset psychotic illness." Her symptoms had become florid over the preceding week. The patient had a documented history of temporal lobe epilepsy (TLE) since age 12, but her symptoms had been under good control. The presenting "psychotic" disorder differed markedly from the usual TLE symptoms and, in addition, the patient showed some features of a depressive quality, including the thoughts, "I might be dead...I don't deserve to be here." Her parents also described episodes in which the patient seemed to think she was somebody else. There were no focal neurological signs. All the lab blood studies were within normal limits except the brain CT, which was read as "minimal mesial temporal sclerosis on the left side, unchanged from the study three years ago.

Previous TLE episodes had been described as consisting of "tummy tickles" (abnormal epigastric sensations), repetitive and stereotyped movements of her right arm (e.g., picking up a pen and putting it down repeatedly), and a period of "staring at people and hearing them but not really understanding them." The patient had poor recollection of these episodes. She also reported déjà vu phe-nomena. In contrast, in the most recent symptoms, the patient complained that, "she may be dead," and that, "she wants to be with Uncle Fred." Occasionally, the patient would say, "My name is Fred T," which was the name of an uncle who had died two months before. She believed that her heart had been replaced by a mechanical one

Since dissociativelike phenomena occur in patients with TLE, Pies considered the diagnosis of dissociative identity disorder in the differential diagnosis. The patient seemed to be identifying with her deceased uncle and spoke of herself in the third person; however, in dissociative identity disorder the patient rarely assumes the personality of an actual individual, and the alters are usually fictitious or fabricated personas. Pies also considered the diagnosis of a psychotic depression associated to a grief reaction, and the possibility of a nonconvulsive status epilepticus mimicking ictal psychosis, among others. After informed clinical reasoning he reached the logical conclusion that this patient suffered from a forced normalization syndrome.

Hypothesis regarding the relationship of schizophrenia and epilepsy are emerging, and are summarized by Pies:

1. Chronic paranoid (hallucinatory psychosis very similar to schizophrenia) does occur more often than chance in some epileptic patients, particularly in TLE.
2. There may be a distinct subgroup of schizophrenia-like psychosis, in which psychotic episodes are transient and self-limiting, often increasing when seizures are diminishing and tending to subside when fits return.
3. Some intermediate forms may exist. (pp. 16–18)

It is important to keep in mind that antiepileptic medications produce many adverse neuropsychiatric events including psychosis. Such is the case with phenytoin, carbamazepine, vigabatrin (in up to 12% of patients), topiramate, tiagabine (up to 2% of cases), and oxicarbazepine. Some of the psychoses associated with antiepileptic medications may be the result of forced normalization. No association with psychosis has been observed with valproic acid, and psychosis is rarely seen in patients treated with lamotrigine. Psychosis may also occur when anticonvulsants are withdrawn (Lambert et al., 2003, pp. 1111–1113). Kober and Gabbard, 2005, reported the case of a man who experienced a topiramate-induced psychosis; the patient had no prior history of psychotic episodes.[4]

Cerebellar Lesions

Deviant and aberrant behaviors in individuals with cerebellar anomalies have been observed since the 1800s, Further clinical experience strengthened the observations of a relationship between cerebellum and personality, aggression, and emotion; psychosis, and schizophrenia in particular, is associated with structural cerebellar abnormalities (Rizzo & Eslinger, 2004, pp. 578–579). The cerebellum is typically associated with motor coordination and also plays a pivotal role in synchronizing motor and cognitive activities (Ho, Mola, & Andreasen, 2004, pp. 1146–1153). Patients with cerebellar signs have poorer premorbid social adjustment, more severe negative symptoms, and greater deficits in a variety of cognitive domains. These patients have smaller cerebellar volumes in the MRI (pp. 1146–1153).

The cerebellar cognitive affective syndrome (CCAS) in children is characterized by impairments of intelligence, memory, language, attention, academic skills, and psychosocial function. These symptoms are present in children who have cerebellar tumors or who undergo cerebellar resection or radiation (Rizzo & Eslinger, 2004, p. 576). Adults and children with CCAS display altered regulation of mood and personality, obsessive-compulsive tendencies, and psychosis. Patients may display paranoid ideation, bizarre illogical thinking, and even stereotypical rituals (p. 578).

The Posterior Fossa Syndrome

An intriguing neurobehavioral syndrome that has many catatoniclike features has been described in children who undergo resections of midline tumors of the cerebellum. Mutism develops within 48 hours of the tumor resection. Patients develop dysarthria and buccal and lingual apraxia some months after the surgery. Children also display regressive personality changes, apathy and poverty of spontaneous movements, and there is marked emotional lability (Rizzo & Eslinger, 2004, pp. 576–577).

Traumatic Brain Injuries (TBI)

Persons are a greater risk for TBI between their midteens and mid-20s, before the onset of most psychotic disorders, and males have several-fold higher risk for TBI than females. There is extensive evidence of an association between TBI and psychosis: psychotic symptoms are consistently found to occur more frequently in individuals who had a TBI (posttraumatic psychosis), and patients with psychotic disorders are consistently more likely to have a prior history of TBI. Although psychosis is not the most frequent complication of TBI, it is a disturbing and disabling outcome with great comorbidity and cost. Key brain regions implicated in the etiology of psychosis –and schizophrenia-, such as the prefrontal cortex, temporal lobes and hippocampus are particularly vulnerable to TBI (Corcoran, McAllister, & Malaspina, 2005, p. 213). Phenomenologically, posttraumatic psychosis may be indistinguishable from a primary mental disorder, such as schizophrenia (p. 215). Many patients have features characterisitic of deficit symptoms of schizophrenia: loss of social contact (68%), lack of interest (55%), lack of spontaneity (53%), slowness (53%), and speech abnormalities (p. 216). Major predictors of posttraumatic psychosis were a positive family history of schizophrenia and the length of loss of consciousness (p. 217). Having a first degree relative with a psychotic disorder was found to be among the strongest predictors for posttraumatic psychosis (p. 219). For factors predictive of posttraumatic psychosis (see table 6.5).

"A more recent large study of the association of multiplex schizophrenia,

TABLE 6.5 Factors that Predict Posttraumatic Psychosis (PP) in Brain Injured Individuals

1. Location of the injury
2. Severity of the injury
3. Other features of the injury
4. Inherent vulnerability to psychosis
5. Gender
6. IQ/Cognition
7. Substance abuse
8. Prior neurological disorder
9. Posttraumatic epilepsy

Notes:

1. Left hemisphere and particularly left temporal injuries.
2. Duration of coma, imaging evidence, and cognitive deficits predict PP.
3. No association with type of injury (close or open).
4. Genetic vulnerability is one of the strongest predictors of PP.
5. PP is more common in men; they have higher TBI prevalence.
6. Lower IQ, impaired verbal and nonverbal memory, and significant language deficits, reflecting diffused neuropsychological impairment, have higher likelihood of PP.
7. History of substance abuse is more common in patients with PP.
8. Persons with a previous neurological disorder are at a higher risk for PP.
9. Recent studies do not support an association of PP and posttraumatic epilepsy.

Source: Corcoran, McAllister, & Malaspina (2005, pp. 218–220).

and multiplex bipolar pedigrees found that rates of TBI were significantly higher for those with a diagnosis of schizophrenia, bipolar disorder, and depression than for those with no mental illness" (Max, 2005, p. 485). Within the schizophrenic pedigree, TBI was associated with a greater risk for schizophrenia consistent with synergistic effects between genetic vulnerability for schizophrenia and TBI (p. 486).

Posttraumatic epilepsy (posttraumatic seizures) is a common complication of moderate to severe brain injury. Many psychiatric disorders, secondary to TBI with seizures have been described: mood disorders (dysphoria, euphoria, rapid cycling, and mixed); irritable-impulsive disorders; schizophreniform disorders (paranoid, delusional, and hallucinatory); anxiety disorders (panic, phobic, and generalized); amnestic-confusional disorders; somatiform disorders (pseudoseizures and pain); and personality disorders (viscous, hyperemotional, and changes in sexual behavior) (Tucker, 2005, p. 314).

Aphasias

Developmental and language disorders and aphasias sometimes create diagnostic difficulties. Psychoses manifest disturbed verbal output in content and in form. Spontaneous verbalizations of psychotic patients with a thought disorder may reveal loosening of associations, thought blocking, condensation, illogicality, neologisms, incoherence, and perseveration.

Aphasia may be mistaken for psychotic speech, and some fluent aphasics tend to develop paranoid syndromes resembling schizophrenia, making the differentiation more difficult. The two disorders share some features including fluent output, poverty of information content, relative preservation of syntax and phonology, paraphasia, perseveration, incoherence, and impairment of the pragmatic aspects of discourse. There are some differences: schizophrenics tend to have more extended replies than do fluent aphasics; they are less aware of their communication deficits, and are less engaged in communicational exchange. Schizophrenic content tends to be bizarre and repetitive. Neologisms and paraphasia are common in fluent aphasics and rare in schizophrenia. Neologisms in schizophrenia are ideosyncratic. Aphasics rarely repeat the same substitutions. Language abnormalities are more prominent in schizophrenics with salient negative symptoms. Negative symptoms are not characteristic of aphasics. Language testing is contributory: naming ability, comprehension, and repetition may be impaired in aphasics but seldom in schizophrenics. The same is true for word generation, reading, and writing. Bizarre content may emerge in the answers of schizophrenic patients (Cummings & Mega, 2003, pp. 90–92).

Narcolepsia

In up to 7% of patients with the diagnosis of schizophrenia, the psychotic symptoms may represent a psychotic variant of narcolepsy (Bhat & Galang, 2002, p. 1245). Hypnagogic and hypnopompic hallucinations are present in 20 to 50% of patients with narcolepsy. These hallucinations are mostly visual but they can also be auditory and somesthetic; macropsias and micropsias have also been reported. The hallucinations are present during the EEG REM sleep and represent intrusion of the dream state into the drowsy state. Hypnagogic hallucinations may occur in a variety of psychiatric disorders (schizophrenia, depression, paranoid state, and puerperal psychosis (Cummings & Mega, 2003, p. 190).

Multiple Cavernoma and Schizophrenia

Israeli and Zohar (2004) suggest that multiple cavernous hemangiona (MCH) may be associated with schizophrenia. MCH is a developmental defect of the small blood vessels that causes diffuse honeycombing of vascular spaces in the brain. This causes sedimentation, thrombosis, and calcifications which can be detected in MRI studies. Familial cavernoma is an autosomal dominant disorder with incomplete penetrance, apparently associated with the q7 gene locus.

Common clinical signs of multiple cavernoma include neurological deficits, seizures, and hemorrhage (p. 924).

PSYCHOSIS ASSOCIATED WITH NEURODEVELOPMENTAL DISORDERS

Pervasive developmental disorders (PDDs) are a group of neurodevelopmental disorders that usually affect children before 5 years of age. Pervasive developmental disorders include five distinct disorders: autistic disorder, Rett's disorder, childhood disintegrative disorder, Asperger's disorder, and PDD-NOS (Tanguay, 2000, p. 1079–1095). A variety of undefined brain abnormalities are considered the cause of PDDs.

Autism

Autistic disorder is characterized by (1) A qualitative impairment of reciprocal social interactions; (2) a qualitative impairment of verbal and nonverbal communication and imaginative play; (3) markedly restricted repertoire of activities and interests; and (4) onset during infancy or childhood (before 30 months). Indications of lack of reciprocal interactions include: (1) marked impairment in the use of nonverbal behaviors to regulate social interactions; (2) a failure to develop peer relationships appropriate to developmental level; (3) a lack of spontaneous seeking to share emotions or activities with other people; (4) a lack of awareness of the existence or feelings of others, and no or abnormal seeking of comfort from others. Indications of impairment of verbal and nonverbal communication include: (1) no communicational mode (communicative babbling, facial expression, gestures, mime, or spoken language); (2) in an individual with adequate speech, marked impairment in the ability to initiate or to sustain a conversation with others; (3) stereotyped, repetitive, or idiosyncratic language; (4) lack of varied, spontaneous, make-believe play or social imitative play appropriate to developmental level. Behaviors that indicate restrictions in activities and interests include: (1) preoccupation with stereotyped or repetitive pattern of interests that is abnormal either in focus or intensity; (2) adherence to inflexible nonfunctional routines or rituals; (3) stereotypic or repetitive motor mannerisms (flapping, twisting, whole-body movements); (4) persistent preoccupation with parts of objects. The disturbance is not better accounted for by Rett's syndrome or childhood disintegrative disorder (DSM-IV-TR, 2000, p. 75). For the differential diagnosis of autism see table 6.6. Psychosis may be a comorbid condition in autistic children (Green et al., 2003, p. 531).

TABLE 6.6 Differential Diagnosis of Autism

- Rubella
- Phenylketonuria
- Lactic acidosis
- Purine and calcium disorders
- Congenital toxoplasmosis
- Cytomegalovirus infection
- Herpes encephalitis
- Hydrocephalus
- Hypothyroidism
- Fragile X syndrome
- Tuberous sclerosis
- Neurofibromatosis
- Hypomelanosis of Ito
- Rett syndrome
- Mobious syndrome
- Williams syndrome
- de Lange syndrome
- Lawrence–Moon–Biedl syndrome
- Muchopolysaccaridosis
- Coffin Lowry syndrome, and others

Source: Green et al. (2003, pp. 505–506, 531).

Disintegrative disorder (improperly called disintegrative psychosis) is a neurodevelopmental regressive syndrome, rarer than autism, starting after an apparently normal period of development (the first 2 to 3 years of life). The regression in cognitive and behavioral fuctioning is progressive, including communicative and self-care skills and associated affective and behavioral symptoms. There is absence of obvious signs of neurological dysfunction, and children have a normal appearance (Volkmar, 1994, p. 120). Apoptosis has been proposed as an explanation for this baffling disorder.

A 3-year-old white male was brought for a psychiatric evaluation after he lost developmental acquisitions. Mother reported the child had developed normally until the second year. The child spoke two languages: English and Serbian, his mother's native tongue. The child's mother relocated to the United States while his father completed a military assignement in Europe. By the second year, the child began to withdraw and to lose adaptive functioning, including self-care skills. He stopped talking and became progressively unresponsive to verbal communication. His mother felt that the child was missing his father and thought that this explained the child's changes. Progressively, the child grew more indifferent and self-absorbed. A neurological examination ruled out the presence of a progressive neurological disorder. MRI and EEG were noncontributory. One year after the initial evaluation the child had not changed in spite of psychosocial treatments.

Tsai (2004) asserts that in only a few cases there is progressive loss of intellectual capacity as seen in the various types of degenerative neurological disorders (p. 334). It has been reported that up to 40% of children with childhood disintegrative disorder regain a capacity to speak in words, and that up to 20% of patients regain a capacity to speak in sentences. Up to 77% of the patients develop seizures, and in 50% of them the seizures are psychomotor (p. 326).

Asperger's Syndrome

Asperger's syndrome (AS) is a pervasive developmental disorder belonging to a family of congenital conditions characterized by marked social impairment, communication difficulties, play and imagination deficits, and a range of repetitive behaviors and interests (Klin & Volkmar, 2003, p. 1). In the DSM-IV-TR (2000), there is a significant overlap in A and B, diagnostic criteria between Autism and AS. In Asperger's, criterion C, specifies that the disturbance causes significant impairment in social, occupational, or other important areas of functioning; criterion D, indicates there is no clinically significant general delay in language, and criterion E, establishes that there is no significant delay in cognitive development or in the development of age appropriate self-help skills, adaptive behavior (except for social interactions), and curiosity about the environment (p. 84).

Asperger's disorder lacks definitional boundaries and the distinction of this syndrome with high functioning forms of autism is not clear-cut. Although Asperger's and high functioning autism could be initially differentiated from a developmental perspective, as patients grow up the distinctions fade and the clinical characteristics of the syndromes merge. Towbin (2003) places together the high functioning patients from either group under the designation *high functioning autism/Asperger syndrome* (p. 24). Although some Asperger's children show obvious oddities and dysmorphic features, some do not display any physiognomic abnormalities.

Clinical examination often reveals the presence of thought disorder (tangentiality, perseveration, cognitive rigidity), ritualized behavior, and many peculiarities (eccentricities) in verbal and nonverbal interpersonal communication. Issues associated with language disorders, described in the section on aphasias, may play a role. Children's peculiarities and eccentricities may be misinterpreted as negative symptoms or as an indication of a thought disorder; bizarre behaviors and relatedness problems associate this condition with schizophrenia. As a matter of fact, up to 10% of grown-up Asperger's patients receive the diagnosis of schizophrenia at some point in their lives (Tantam, 2003, p. 156).

Rett's Disorder

Regressive behavior, self-abusive behavior, and peculiar stereotyped hand movements are charateristic of Rett's syndrome; they need to be differentiated from other regressive-psychotic disorders.[5]

PSYCHOTIC SYMPTOMS AND REGRESSIVE BEHAVIOR

In patients with psychosis and significant regression a decisive search for the presence of an organic disorder needs to be undertaken. Goodman (1994) recommends initiating an investigation to detect organicity and to seek appropriate referrals when the following conditions exist:

1. Child loses well-established linguistic, academic, or self-care skills and performs below previous levels.
2. There is emergence of symptoms suggestive of a brain disorder.
3. There is presence of risk factors for genetic or infectious disease (Huntington's disease, a mother with AIDS, and others).

The most common dementing disorders in childhood,, which cause regressive and psychoticlike behavior in children and adolescents, are listed in table 6.7.

TABLE 6.7 Neurological Illnesses and Developmental Disorders Associated with Regressive and Psychotic Behaviors

---

Ceroid-Lipofuscinosis: Batten's & Spielmeyer-Vogt Disease

Disorders of Lysosomal Enzymes: Gaucher & Krabbe diseases, juvenile-onset Metachromatic Leukodystrophy, muchopolysaccharidoses (Hunter syndrome, Sly disease, Niemann-Pick sphingomyelin lipidosis

Infectious diseases: Subacute sclerosing panencephalitis, HIV encephalopathy, syphilis

Pervasive developmental disorders

Rett's syndrome

Lesch-Nyhan disease

Wilson's disease

Huntington's disease

Adrenoleukodystrophy

Xeroderma pigmentosum

Seizure disorders

Head injury

Mitochondrial encephalopathies

Cerebrotendinous xanthomatosis

Source: Goodman (2002, pp. 179–181); Fenichel (2005, chap. 5).

CHAPTER 7

Differential Diagnosis of Psychotic Disorders
Psychiatric Disorders Associated with Psychosis

Psychotic symptoms are present in many psychiatric disorders. The presence of psychosis adds severity to the psychiatric diagnosis and prognosis, and complicates the psychiatric treatment. Identification of psychosis is fundamental to establishing a thorough diagnostic formulation and a comprehensive treatment plan. Most of the time, the dimension of psychosis requires specific treatment.

PSEUDOHALLUCINATIONS

Pseudohallucinations are defined as hallucinations that the patient knows are not real. Although, the experiences may be vivid and crisp, the patient knows (has the insight) that those experiences have no foundation in reality (Boza, http://www.priory.com/halluc.htm). In incipient psychosis, or when psychosis is about to relapse, the patient may have some degree of awareness that the experiences are not real or may not be real; sometimes patients are able "to fight the hallucination or delusions" or "to keep them in check."

IMAGINARY COMPANIONS

Imaginary companions are rather common childhood experiences between 3 and 6 years of age. Companions that start after this range of age should be viewed with apprehension and should be evaluated critically. Imaginary companions are by nature supportive emotional experiences, and are always under the child's full control. If the so-called companions become unsupportive, and, worse, if they frighten or tell the child bad things, to misbehave or even to do bad things, this ought to be viewed as a malignant psychotic experience.

HALLUCINATIONS ASSOCIATED WITH BEREAVEMENT

After the death of a loved one, it is not uncommon for children to experience a feeling of the presence of the deceased person. At times, seeing the deceased one or hearing his or her voice may fall within the range of normal experiences of mourning. These experiences are usually comforting, or at least emotionally neutral. If the child hears the deceased telling him or her to do bad things or if the dead one asks the child to join him or her in the other life, the experience is most likely psychopathological. The following vignette illustrates many features related to perceptual experiences associated with bereavement.

> Tony, a 10-year-old Hispanic boy, had lost his father to a metastatic cancer, a month prior to the psychiatric evaluation. Mother brought the child for a psychiatric assessment due to increasing depression and suicidal ideation.
> Tony heard his deceased father telling him, "I love you...I miss you...come with me." Tony reported that he did not feel frightened by the voice; on the contrary, he experienced a positive feeling. He also felt that his father was around him. When the examiner asked Tony what his father meant when he said, "come with me," he stated that his father meant that someday, he and all his family will join him in heaven. Tony felt supported by these experiences and liked them.

In true psychotic features, the child is usually scared of what he hears (or what he sees) and does not want to repeat the experience again.

CIRCUMSCRIBED PSYCHOSIS

The term *circumscribed psychosis* refers to psychotic states that are pathological but circumscribed; the psychotic features have an identifiable adaptive function and create limited degradations of the adaptive capacity. Symptoms are related to a specific event or to an identifiable developmental stressor.

> A 5-year-old white male child was brought in for a psychiatric evaluation due to disruptive and aggressive behaviors and deterioration in academic performance. His mother reported the onset of problems a year earlier, a short time after the child's half-sister was born. His mother also stated that afterward, he had become more irritable and prone to anger, and had started talking back and raising his voice and his fists. He had temper tantrums when he did not get his way. His mother reported that the child had become more attention seeking.
> Coinciding with the birth of his half-sister, the child learned that the person

he thought was his biological father, was not. The biological father, who had not been involved with the child, unexpectedly demanded contact with his son.

Although, not overtly aggressive toward his baby sister, the patient took her toys away frequently when the mother was not attending to her. The child had a good relationship with his cousins.

Developmental and medical histories were unremarkable. The child had not received any prior psychiatric treatment. Mother reported episodic soiling that she attributed to the child's carelessness when he wiped himself. The child was very competent and independent in his self-care skills. The mental status examination revealed the presence of a small but engaging, talkative child who wore glasses. He was euthymic. He stated that he loved his sister and that he was never mean to her. When the examiner explored perceptual disturbances, the child endorsed hearing growling noises made by monsters that hid behind the bushes near his home. He reported that he heard the noises day and night. He said that the monsters couldn't enter the house, and that he was ready to defend his sister, claiming that the monsters intended to do bad things to his sister. Oftentimes, he dressed as a power ranger to fight the monsters with his sword. He got involved in intense imaginary fights with monsters to keep them at bay. Exhaustive exploration did not reveal any other perceptual disturbance or any delusional beliefs.

The child was expressing anger toward his baby sister in a covert manner, and by the mechanisms of projection and reaction formation he was coping with his aggressive sibling rivalry. At the time of the evaluation, the defenses against his aggressive impulses were somewhat effective. Since the psychosis was circumscribed, it was monitored on a regular basis. The psychodynamics of this circumscribed psychosis are rather transparent.

A number of children and adolescents report hearing their name being called; this by itself, without other symptoms, lacks psychopathological significance. Other children report isolated hallucinations or paranoid symptoms with limited maladaptive impairment. These symptoms need to be monitored; some of them vanish and leave no trace. Other psychotic features persist and become associated with maladaptive behavior.

The following psychiatric conditions may be associated with psychotic symptoms:

ATTENTION DEFICIT HYPERACTIVITY DISORDER (ADHD)

Hyperactivity, impulsivity, and concentration difficulties may be caused by a variety of psychiatric disorders including bipolar and psychotic disorders. Mania (frequently associated with psychotic features) may resemble ADHD or may co-occur in children with ADHD more often than previously thought. Stimulant medications may unmask or activate manic symptoms, and because of the danger of inducing mania with the use of antidepressants, a thorough mood disorder assessment is required (prepubescent major depression carries a 50% lifetime risk of developing mania). Pediatric bipolar disorder goes undetected for a long time because children tend to present with different phenomenology than the one described in the DSM-IV-TR. For pertinent diagnostic criteria, the reader is referred to the DSM-IV-TR (APA, 2000, pp. 388–389). Children present with more mixed states, less distinct periods between episodes, more grandiosity, irritability, and a continuous course (Fuller & Fuller, 2005, p. 78).

Differentiating preschool ADHD from preschool mania is very difficult. Preschool mania is particularly controversial. Detractors of this diagnosis believe that the preschool mania (under 5 years of age) is no more that a severe manifestation of a "bad" ADHD. The diagnosis of mania shares a number of criteria with ADHD combined type: psychomotor activation, impulsivity, irritability (common in hyperactive preschoolers) (Dilsaver, 2005a, p. 3). Opponents of the diagnosis question the validity of grandiosity at a preschool age and assert that the two classic features of mania, euphoria and grandiosity, cannot rationally be applied to preschool age children (pp. 3, 14). Opponents of the diagnosis of preschool mania, also express strong reservations against stigmatizing preschoolers with such a severe diagnosis (p. 14). On the other hand, Dilsaver (2005b), also takes the other side of the argument, and defends the diagnosis of preschool mania. Dilsaver states that superb clinicians do not seek the diagnosis of preschool mania, that they consider this possibility in the differential diagnosis of complex presentations (p. 15), that mania is a more severe and pervasive entity than ADHD, and that the concept of kindling supports the concept of early identification and treatment; actually, mania should be aggressively treated in preschool age children whenever it is strongly suspected. Dilsaver notes, however, that the literature on preschool mania suggests that it is an intractable, treatment-resistant disease with poor outcome (p. 15). With these propositions, the present writer agrees. Although, treatments for mania do not worsen ADHD, treatments for ADHD sometimes worsen mania. This justifies the predilection of the diagnosis of mania when it and ADHD have equal footing in the differential diagnosis.

Pressured speech, flight of ideas, and decreased need for sleep in well documented in cases of preschool mania, are not ADHD diagnostic features (p. 15). The irritability of mania is a prolonged, abiding, unyielding state of affect that frequently emerges without apparent provocation (Dilsaver, 2005b, p. 16). Dilsaver asserts that both euphoria and grandiosity in preschool can be inferred by clinical observation (p. 16).

Akiskal (2005), commenting on Dilsaver's articles (2005a, 2005b), states that there is a consensus that preschool mania exists, that children with this disorder have families loaded with bipolar disorder, are frequently male, and that despite irritable and mixed features, the euphoria and grandiosity are unmistakable (p. 17).

CONDUCT DISORDER

There are a number of reasons to include conduct disorders in the differential diagnosis of psychosis:

1. Conduct disorders are frequently associated with multiple comorbid psychopathologies including psychosis. Unfortunately, the comorbidity is frequently overlooked during the diagnostic assessment. "Clinicians are obliged to attempt to overcome the negative feelings toward the child that may be aroused by the child's frightening or obnoxious behaviors. Psychiatrists and clinicians must embark in the evaluation of a behaviorally disturbed child with curiosity and an open mind (Otnow Lewis, 1996, p. 571). Unfortunately, the child's obnoxious behavior tends to deter clinicians from conducting a comprehensive evaluation necessary for identifying underlying complex psychopathology (p. 566).

2. In conduct disorder populations, psychotic disorders (including paranoid disorders) are common.

3. In conduct disorder patients, history of abuse and subsequent PTSD-related symptomatology (including psychosis) is present.

4. In conduct disorder patients, a history of brain trauma secondary to physical abuse is common; seizure disorders, caused by brain injury, may induce psychotic-related psychopathology. On the other hand, because of impulsivity and risk taking behavior, conduct disorder children and adolescents are prone to suffer from head trauma with some of the consequences noted above.

5. Conduct disorder youth abuse mind-altering drugs that elicit psychotic behavior.

6. In addition, Biederman, Mick, Faraone, and Wozniak (2004) highlight the frequent association of conduct disorder with bipolar disorder, which is frequently associated with psychotic symptoms. Conduct disorder is quite common in bipolar disorder youth (up to 69% of patients); in manic patients, the most common mood disturbance, affective storms (prolonged, aggressive, or violent temper outbursts) are common. These symptoms may be due to bipolar behavioral disinhibition, irritability, or low frustration tolerance common in pediatric bipolar illness (p. 38). The association of bipolar disorder and antisocial behavior is supported by epidemiological data: Kennedy et al. (2005) found on a 35-year epidemiological study, a strong association between childhood antisocial behavior and early onset of mania and bipolar disorder (p. 260). Antisocial behavior (behavioral difficulties) in childhood could represent a manifestation of neurodevelopmental abnormalities or even early onset bipolar disorder (p. 260).

Jensen (2004) articulates many of the psychopathological issues prevalent in conduct disorder children:

> In clinical settings, adolescents and children with poor conduct [conduct disorder] may experience the impulse control problems of ADHD; the impulsivity and rapid mood swings, including aggressive acting out, of bipolar affective disorders; the aberrant thinking and sudden changes in mood with resulting unpredictable behavior of childhood psychosis, including schizophrenia; the irritability and temper outbursts of adolescent [and preadolescent] depression; and the rages, self-destructive behavior, and somatic responses of adolescents with reactive attachment disorders and borderline personality disorder (BPD). (p. 104)

Jensen emphasizes the importance of assessing conduct disorder patients in residential centers in unmedicated conditions; in these settings, careful and methodological observation can be made, control of detrimental environmental influences may be accomplished, and compliance and medication monitoring can be achieved under supervised conditions (pp. 104, 107).

PERSONALITY DISORDERS

The DSM-IV-TR (2000) defines personality disorder as an enduring pattern of inner experience and behavior that deviates markedly from the expectations of the individual's culture; the pattern is pervasive and inflexible, has an onset during adolescence or early adulthood, is stable over time, and leads to distress and impairment (p. 685). The DSM-IV-TR also defines personality traits as enduring patterns of perceiving, relating to, or thinking about the environment and oneself that are exhibited in a wide range of social and personal contexts (p. 686). The DSM-IV-TR also asserts that personality disorder categories may be applied to children or adolescents in those unusual instances in which the individual's particular maladaptive personality traits appear to be persistent, pervasive, and unlikely to be limited to a particular developmental stage or to an episode of Axis I disorder, and that the personality disorder should be present for more than one year, except for antisocial personality disorder which cannot be diagnosed before 18 years of age (p. 687).

Schizotypal Personality Disorder (SPD)

There is significant clinical overlap between children diagnosed with schizotypal personality and those diagnosed with schizophrenia. The groups differ in the severity of the symptoms. Schizotypal children have perceptual disturbances or bizarre preoccupations; schizophrenic children display frank hallucinations or delusions. There is no difference in the frequency of illogical thinking and loose associations between these two groups (Caplan, 1994b, p. 20; DSM-IV-TR diagnostic criteria for schizotypal personality disorder, p. 701; DSM-IV-TR differentiation between SPD and schizoid personality disorder, pp. 697, 701).

Not all children presenting with the diagnosis of schizotypal personality disorder will develop full-blown schizophrenic syndromes. Follow-up of 12 SPD children revealed that 92, 75, and 80% of the sample showed continuing schizophrenic spectrum disorder during the first, second, and third year after the initial assessment, respectively. SPD was the most common follow-up diagnosis: 67% in year 1, and 50% in years 2 and 3. One child developed full-blown schizophrenia during the third year (Asarnow, Tompson, & McGrath, 2004, p. 181). Consistent with other data, a subgroup of patients who initially met criteria for schizophrenia later developed bipolar disorder or schizoaffective disorder. Actually, in the SPD follow-up group, schizoaffective disorder was diagnosed in 20% of the sample (p. 181).

> Individuals with Asperger disorders have more severe impairment in social interactions, emotional reciprocity, and communicational skills, have more stereotyped behaviors and unusual interests than children that later develop schizoid disorder or schizotypal personality disorder (Tsai, 2004, p. 321).

Genetically, SPD is associated with schizophrenia spectrum disorders. There are elevated rates of SPD among biological relatives of patients with schizophrenia, and research suggests that schizotypal symptoms such as social isolation and signs of thought disturbance may be early precursors of schizophrenia (Asarnov & Asarnov, 2003, p. 474). A somewhat discrepant view regarding the association of SPD with schizophrenia is expressed by Adler and Strakowski (2003): the increased rate of SPD versus schizophrenia in first degree SPD relatives suggests that the disorder overlaps only partially with schizophrenia. There is data suggesting genetic concordance between SPD and affective disorders and schizophrenia. Studies support the possibility that SPD includes, but is not limited to patients with a mild form of schizophrenia; these studies note distinct heritability patterns for syndrome subsets (p. 13). Longitudinal studies indicate that 20 to 40% of youth with schizotypal features eventually show an Axis I schizophrenia spectrum disorder (Walker, Kestler, Bollini, et al., 2004, p. 413). Furthermore, adolescents with SPD manifest some of the same functional abnormalities observed in patients with schizophrenia, including motor abnormalities, cognitive deficits, and an increase of cortisol (p. 413).

Borderline Disorders of Childhood (BPD)

The so-called borderline children usually present with a rapid, unpredictable, regression in thinking, reality testing, and affective control. These children are very vulnerable to stress and as a result, develop sudden suicidal and homicidal behaviors or psychotic features (including hallucinations and delusions). In general, these children reintegrate rapidly when the stress subsides. Conversely, children may be chronically regressed (Lewis, 1994, p. 33). Symptoms such as rage, temper outbursts, violent fantasies, regression, and impulsivity occur frequently, sometimes mimicking or representing comorbid conditions, including ADHD, anxiety disorders, and depression (and bipolar disorder) (p. 33). Transient or persistent psychotic features are common in these children.

This disorder has received the more recent denomination of *multiple complex developmental disorder and multidimentional impaired disorder* (MDI). Some experts consider that this syndrome is a variant of schizophrenia (Kumra et al., 1998). MDI children present with a history of prominent disruptive behaviors and transient psychosis. These children are considered to have a psychotic disorder NOS. Although, these patients report hallucinations and delusions, the symptoms are usually brief (occuring a few times a month) and usually in reponse to stress. The psychotic features are distressing but the impairment is mostly attributable to affective instability and associated aggressive behaviors. These patients resemble children with childhood onset schizophrenia (COS) in the similarity of developmental profiles, the history of recurrent, lengthy psychiatric hospitalizations, and the long history of exposure to psychotropics, particularly antipsychotic medications (Gogtay et al., 2004, p. 18).When compared to children with schizophrenia, children with MDI had earlier cognitive and behavioral abnormalities, and an onset of psychotic symptoms. Regarding outcome, about half of the sample developed a defined diagnosis like schizoaffective, bipolar, major depressive disorder, and others; in the other half, disruptive disorders were common, and the majority showed remission of the psychotic symptoms (p. 182). When some of these atypical children reach adolescence, the psychopathological profile resembles more and more the symptom cluster of adult borderline personality disorder. Borderella's case is illustrative.

> Borderella, a 17-year-old African-American woman was referred to the partial hospitalization program due to lack of response to outpatient treatment. She had no prior psychiatric hospitalizations. Presenting complaints centered on chronic depression, psychosis, and bulimia. She felt overwhelmed and unable to cope; she felt her body "couldn't take any more." She stated she was "delusional" and complained that she "hallucinated." She said she was hearing and seeing people. She claimed that she was seeing serial killers and what they did. She had these experiences for over a year, and had seen the referring psychiatrist for the previous six months. She had been on Tegretol 200 mg BID, Risperdal 1 mg q HS, and Serzone 150 mg/day, but there had not been any changes on her symptoms. Borderella was a senior high school student; she complained of difficulties concentrating and her grades had slipped. She had frequent school absences.

Her medical history was positive for allergies and asthma. She denied being sexually active or being on drugs. She denied any history of rape or of any prior history of sexual abuse but reported that she had suffered bad beatings by her parents. She reported worsening of depression with her periods. Her mother had a history of depression and had received psychiatric treatment.

Borderella reported depression since age 12 and had received the diagnosis of bipolar disorder for the previous six months. She also had received the diagnosis of borderline personality disorder. The family had been told that Borderella could suffer from seizures. She was very concerned with her weight.

Borderella showed poor compliance with medications and the family had difficulty procuring them. She had been prescribed Wellbutrin SR 150 mg BID; lamotrigine 50 mg BID, and quetiapine 25 mg q AM and 75 mg q HS. She had decided to take only 18.75 mg of quetiapine, that is, three quarters of a 25 mg tab a day. She lost 12 pounds over a few months, and since the psychotic symptoms had diminished the treatment with quetiapine was discontinued. Because of issues of affordability, Topomax (that had been prescribed as a weight-reducing agent) was also discontinued.

Borderella was a very attractive and a very dramatic adolescent; although she sounded very psychotic, she was very likable and displayed a broad range of affect. She displayed no thought disorder during the interviews. The family was advised to ignore her regressive behavior and to demand and expect that Borderella act her age. The psychiatrist enforced the same principles.

Two years after the initial evaluation Borderella was markedly better. She finished high school and was planning on attending college. She endorsed no hallucinations or delusions; overall, she appeared more mature, and the relationship with her parents had improved. Her compliance with medications had improved. Borderella's differential diagnoses had included: psychosis NOS, dissociative disorder, borderline personality disorder, and complex partial seizures.

REACTIVE ATTACHMENT DISORDER (RAD)

According to the DSM-IV-TR (2000), the essential feature of RAD is markedly disturbed and developmentally inappropriate social relatedness in most contexts; it usually begins before age 5 and is associated with grossly pathological care. In the inhibited type, the child persistently fails to respond to most social interactions in a developmentally appropriate manner. In the disinhibited type, there is a pattern of diffuse attachments; the child displays indiscriminate sociability or lack of selectivity in the choice of attachment figures (pp. 127–128). According to this definition RAD is secondary to abusive or neglectful parental behavior (grossly pathological care). It should be stated, however, that most of the children who suffered from pathological parenting do not develop RAD.

Swain, Leckman, and Volkmar (2005) describe a case of RAD in a 15-year-old boy who exhibited animal-like behavior including walking on all fours, growling, barking, and even digging holes in the ground. He would also nibble at his mother's legs. He behaved like a dog most of the time but at times he also behaved like a gorilla. The child had a secluded life and had no friends. Apparently animal behavior emerged about one month after a traumatic incident in which he fell into the rapids while on an outing with his father. He became overtly aggressive toward mother, often requiring up to three to four adults to restrain him. The child came to believe he was a werewolf. The authors indicate that this condition should be differentiated from lycanthropy (pp. 56–61). This case is a carbon copy in multiple dimensions to a case seen by this writer. She was a 15-year-old intelligent female who conspicuously behaved like a dog and who from time to time believed she was a werewolf. She had also been diagnosed with Tourette's, and had been considered a very difficult student due to her extreme defiance and refusal to do schoolwork. Although, this patient would not hold to the belief that she was a werewolf or dog, her reality testing was compromised, she "could not help" acting either like dog or a werewolf.

TRAUMATIC PSYCHOSIS

Psychoses are common in traumatized individuals. Commonly, the psychotic features are isolated, and yet painfully disturbing; there are other situations when the trauma produces complex and perplexing organizations as in cases of dissociative identity disorders (see below).

Posttraumatic Stress Disorder (PTSD) Related Psychosis

Frequently, PTSD-associated psychosis does not respond well to neuroleptic medication; sometimes, patients respond better to sensitive psychosocial interventions (Lohr & Birmaher, 1997, p. 1604). The hallucinations and delusions of traumatized children and adolescents connect rather directly to the traumatic situations and to the perpetrators in particular. Traumatized children and adolescents hear the perpetrators frightening them, and making derogatory remarks to them, or announcing or threatening new victimization. Victims see the perpetrators, smell them, and fear that the victimizer would follow them, or feel that the perpetrators will come to hurt them again. Abused children frequently hear command hallucinations (by the perpetrators) telling them to harm themselves or others. These hallucinations are frequently nocturnal, and most of the affected children complain of recurrent and frightening nightmares.

PTSD associated hallucinations are present in about 9% of abused children in pediatric clinics or in children recruited from juvenile courts. Up to 20 to 76% of PTSD children in inpatient psychiatric units endorse hallucinations. Psychosis is present in up to 75 to 95% of those diagnosed with dissociative disorders.

Often, hallucinations resolve rapidly in response to sensitive and safety assuring interventions. Psychotic symptoms are frequently associated with impulsive, aggressive, and self-abusive behaviors; traumatized patients display trancelike states but intact social relatedness (Lohr & Barmier, 1997, p. 1604). It is important to identify triggers for the hallucinations and to evaluate safety issues to safeguard children against repeated traumatization, to avoid any further contact of the child with the perpetrator, and to build an emotional supportive network around the child.

Dissociative Identity Disorder (DID)

For the differential diagnosis of DID, see table 7.1. For pertinent criteria regarding the diagnosis of DID, the reader is referred to the DSM-IV-TR (2000, p. 529).

Dissociation is defined as the segregation of any group of mental processes from the rest of the psychic organization. In dissociation, there is a loss of the usual interrelationship among various groups of mental processes. Terms or concepts related to dissociation are splitting (of personality functions), isolation of content (discontinuity of mental contents), and isolation of affect (disconnection of affect from narrative discourse). The results of these operations can induce transient changes in memory or, in the most severe form, long-standing alterations of personality functioning (Steiner, Carrion, Plattner, & Koopman, 2003, p. 231).

Dissociation and splitting seem to be relatively common experiences in youth. Dissociation as a defense is as common as reaction formation, acting out, and withdrawal, and more common than conversion and projection (p. 235). Dissociative symptoms, common in acute stress disorders, pose a risk for PTSD and can be comorbid with PTSD, or be present in dissociative disorders: dissociative amnesia, depersonalization disorder, dissociative identity disorder (multiple personality), and others, such as dissociative fugue and others.

TABLE 7.1 Differential Diagnosis of Dissociative Disorders

1. Delirium
2. Seizure disorders
3. Central nervous system lesions (e.g., brain tumors, congenital malformations, and head trauma)
4. Neurodegenerative disorders (e.g., Huntington's chorea, lipid storage disorders)
5. Metabolic disorders (e.g., endocrinopathies, Wilson's disease)
6. Toxic encephalopathies (e.g., substances of abuse such as amphetamines, cocaine, hallucinogens, phencyclidine, alcohol, marijuana, and solvents; medications such as stimulants, corticosteroids, or anticholinergic agents; and other toxics such as heavy metals) and
7. Infectious diseases (e.g., encephalitis; meningitis; Lyme disease, with punctuated lesions in the frontal lobes) and viral immunodeficiency related syndromes

Source: McClellan & Werry (1994).

The clinical presentation of dissociation is pleomorphic. It can manifest in a variety of disturbances including problems of memory, affect, and disturbances of mood and self-regulation, anxiety and PTSD symptoms. Conduct disturbance, difficulties with attention, learning, and concentration difficulties may also be present, and finally, disturbing hallucinations and thought process difficulties (confusion, disorganization, tangentiality, and shifts in thought content) have also been observed (Steiner et al., 2003, p. 241). Behavioral disorders, impulsivity, homicidal, self-abusive, and suicidal behaviors are rather common in patients with DID.

All psychotic children and adolescents displaying problems in the continuity and integrity of the self, as well as alterations in the level of self-awareness, should receive a thorough pediatric and neurological evaluation to rule out a variety of identifiable organic mental disorders. The following are a number of potential organic etiological factors, among others, that need to be considered in the differential diagnosis of dissociative disorders (see Table 7.1).

Many patients with dissociative features have concomitant psychotic symptoms. Some patients with DID or dissociative symptoms are incorrectly diagnosed as schizophrenics. Children who report dissociative symptoms immediately after disclosure of abuse are at a greater risk for later PSTSD symptoms. Dissociation appears to be the strongest predictor of PTSD symptoms. It has been proposed that dissociation prevents the open expression of emotions and cognitions associated with trauma, thus interfering with the processing of trauma. Dissociation may also represent an adaptive response to buffer the impact of a traumatic experience.

AFFECTIVE PSYCHOSIS

Affective psychoses are the most common psychotic conditions in childhood and adolescence. Affective disorders are frequently associated with psychotic features. In affective disorders the mood disturbance is paramount and, in general (but not always), the psychosis is associated in content and tone with the prevailing mood disorder. Thus, patients with severe depressions commonly report derogatory auditory hallucinations while grandiose features are common in patients with psychotic mania. Clinical pictures are not always clear-cut, and, at times, the mood is not too obvious, and in other cases the psychotic features dominate the clinical presentation.

Psychotic features in children and adolescents with mood disorders have been reported in higher frequency than the correspondent frequency in adults. Auditory hallucinations have been observed in one third to one half of preadolescent depressed children, and up to 31% of inpatient depressed adolescents. Delusions in depressed children and adolescents are less common (Hammen & Rudolph, 2003, pp. 236–237). Geller, Warner, Williams, et al. (1998) reported a frequency of psychoticl symptoms in up to 60% of bipolar manic children, 87% had elated mood, 85% of grandiosity, 55% had grandiose delusions, 26.7% had suicidality with plan and intent, and 83% were ultra-rapid or ultradian cyclers (p 97).

Weinberg, Harper, and Brumback (1998) state that "Children or adolescents who have evidence of hallucinations or delusions usually have these symptoms as a result of a disorder of mood and affect (depression or mania), and [that] the hallucinations or delusions resolve with the improvement of the mood disorder" (p. 201).

Somatic complaints, psychomotor agitation, and mood-congruent hallucinations are considered to be more prevalent in prepubertal children with major depressive disorder. These children also frequently have comorbid anxiety disorders (Weller, Weller, & Danielyan, 2004, p. 413). In psychotically depressed children, auditory hallucinations are more common than delusional symptoms. Delusions are more common in psychotically depressed adolescents (p. 414). As children with a history of prepubertal major depression grow up, they have higher rates of mood disorders and other comorbid disorders than children without a history of depression: bipolar disorder I (33.3% vs. 0.0%), any bipolar disorder (48.6 vs. 7.1%), major depressive disorder (36.1 vs. 14.3%), substance use disorder (30.6 vs. 10.7%), and suicidality (22.2 vs. 3.6%) (p. 416).

The clinical picture may be altered by psychotropic medications and this may be a source of diagnostic confusion. Although psychosis associated with mood disorders commonly responds to antipsychotics, in a number of cases, psychosis is resistant to them. As far back as 1979, Akiskal and Puzantian postulated that affective psychoses could take many forms, even psychotic presentations that were previously considered schizophrenic. In general, bizarre delusions with content of thought control, thought insertion, and disturbances of thought processes are more characteristic of schizophrenia than affective psychosis in childhood (Caplan, 1994b, p. 20). However, studies have failed to detect language coherence differences between manic and schizophrenic patients (Kuperberg & Caplan, 2003, p. 454).

Cumming and Mega (2003) argue that there are some clinical differences between manic and schizophrenic patients' discourse. Mania and schizophrenia have different effects on verbal output. Both disorders affect discourse trajectory and coherence. Manics have better preservation of hierarchical structures, more structural linkages, and they are more successful at communicating complex ideas. Schizophrenic utterances are shorter than those of manic patients. Loss of coherence in the two disorders reflects different underlying abnormalities: schizophrenics tend to have less structure in their discourse whereas manics shift more rapidly from topic to topic. Schizophrenics are less able to anticipate the needs of the listener and to structure the conversation accordingly. In a small percentage of schizophrenics, the verbal output resembles jargon aphasia and it is difficult to differentiate from it (p. 91).

Swaan (2006) states that bipolar disorder as we know it today, is a recent construct. About 100 years ago, Kraepelin described a recurrent affective disorder, but bipolar disorder was not differentiated from major depressive illness until the work of Leonhardt 50 years later. Bipolar disorder is now recognized as a potentially treatable psychiatric disorder that has substantial mortality and high social, economical, (and developmental) impact. Every aspect of its definition, boundaries, mechanisms, and treatment, however, is the subject of debate (p. 177). We are far from a rigorous definition of bipolar disorder. Our current definition is syndromal and based on affective symptoms (DSM-IV-TR), and is highly unreliable. The requirement of manialike states is clearly problematic because for most patients, the disorder starts with depressive episodes, and a depressive first episode predicts a more severe course of illness. Neither overdiagnosis nor underdiagnosis of bipolar disorder provides a service to patients and their families. There is limited information on what predisposes patients to manic or depressive episodes, or the factors that determine the course of illness. It needs to be understood that there is no objective measure that can determine that one has bipolar disorder or not (Swaan, 2006).

Bipolar disorder differs in clinical presentation according to the age of onset. Early onset subjects (with and age of onset before the age of 21) had higher indexes of comorbid substance abuse, suicidality, rapid cycling, increased episode frequency, and a greater risk for eating disorders, in comparison to subjects whose disorder started between 21 and 28 years of age, or in subjects whose disorder started after age 28 (Lin et al., 2006, pp. 243–244). Siblings of probands with age of onset before 21 were about 10 times more likely to have drug abuse problems than siblings of probands whose disorder started after 28 years of age (p. 244).

Pediatric bipolar disorder is associated with higher rates of psychosis than is found in subjects with an onset of bipolar disorder later in life. This clinical feature may put these individuals at higher risk for poor long-term outcome (including suicidal behavior). Adolescents suffering from adolescent mania with psychotic features requiring hospitalization, have a poor short-term prognosis than adult-onset mania (Pavuluri, Herbener, & Sweeney, 2004, 19). Childhood physical or sexual abuse is associated with higher frequency of bipolar episodes. Early abuse is associated with an early age of onset of bipolar disorder, serious suicidal attempts, and comorbid drug-abuse and anxiety disorders. It is likely that early traumatic experience may contribute to a later adverse clinical course (Kupka et al., 2005, p. 1278).

Schizophrenic children are odd and have poor levels of sociability, peer relationships, scholastic achievement, school adaptation, and interests before the onset of their illness (Caplan, 1994b, p. 20). Youth with bipolar disorder in contrast to youth with early onset schizophrenia and psychotic disorder NOS, demonstrated the highest functioning premorbidly, with better academic and social interactions. These youth also showed high rates of behavioral disorders and substance abuse (McClellan, Breiger, McCurry, & Hlastala, 2003, p. 670).

The diagnosis of bipolar disorder now includes what was previously defined as manic–depressive psychosis; because psychosis no longer needs to be mood congruent, the term *bipolar disorder* covers a spectrum of symptoms ranging from eccentricity to mood-congruent symptoms to paranoia, to bizarre delusions and hallucinations (Carlson & Kashani, 2002, p. xviii). Early onset preadolescent psychotic depressions are considered forerunners of bipolar disorder: "Although it is difficult to predict who will develop bipolar disorder, the presence of psychosis, psychomotor retardation, pharmachologically induced hypomania or mania, and a family history of bipolar disorder have been associated with increased risk of a manic episode" (Birmaher, Arbelaez, & Brent, 2002, p. 631).

Bipolar disorder in young children (preadolescent mania or juvenile mania) commonly has a mixed affective presentation (mixed mood). Instead of mania, young children display irritability, affective storms, and prolonged and aggressive temper outbursts. They also display moodiness, worsening of disruptive behaviors (impulsivity, hyperactivity, concentration difficulties), and explosive anger followed by remorse, depression, and poor school performance. Then, mixed features, rapid cycling features, psychotic features, high rate of externalizing disorders, and significant psychosocial impairments are common in bipolar preadolescents (Weller, Weller, & Danielyan, 2004, p. 415).

Carlson (2005) uses the acronym HIPERS in the diagnosis of pediatric mania:

H-Hyperactivity (goal oriented and pleasure seeking) and High Energy
I- Irritability
P-Psychosis—Grandiosity
E-Elated Mood
R-Rapid Speech, Racing Thoughts, Flight of Ideas
S-Sleep Need reduced (pp. 4–5; for the DSM-IV-TR [2000] diagnostic criteria for bipolar disorders, pp. 388–392).

Bipolar disorder in children (juvenile mania) has a high degree of comorbidity with ADHD and conduct disorder, and has an atypical presentation (chronic course, pervasive irritability, and affective storms or prolonged aggressive outbursts). Furthermore, this condition is highly comorbid for anxiety disorder and psychosis (Wozniak & Biederman, 1996, pp. 826–827). Early onset affective aggression is often predictive of a chronic course; such children have high rates of school drop-out, delinquency, and substance abuse (Carlson, 2005, p. 3). The assertion that juvenile mania has a continuous course is being disputed by observations in Amish populations. The pattern of episodic

TABLE 7.2 Selected Causes of Secondary Mania

Medical conditions

> Brain tumors
> Strokes
> Traumatic brain injury
> Psychomotor seizures
> Multiple sclerosis
> Huntington's disease
> CNS infection, including HIV
> Hyperthyroidism
> Hyperadrenalism

Medications

> Anabolic steroids
> Antidepressants
> Cocaine
> Corticosteriods & corticosteroid withdrawal
> Dextromethorphan
> Dopamine agonists like amantadine, bromocriptine and others
> Hypericum (St John's Wort)
> Isoniazide
> Stimulants
> Sympathomimetic amines like ephedrine
> Zidovudine

Source: Levenson (2005, p. 17).

symptoms does not seem to be unique to the Amish people (Egeland et al., 2003, p. 794). For consideration of preschool mania see the ADHD section above. In the differential diagnosis of mania, the following medical conditions and medications produce secondary mania (see table 7.2).

Differentiating depression from negative symptoms may be difficult, but there are subtle distinctions. For example, patients with negative symptoms appear more emotionally flat and unconcerned about the lack of motivation and diminished social and role functioning; depressed persons, on the contrary, often verbalize their demoralization, hopelessness, and desire to feel and behave differently (Correll & Mendelowitz, 2003, p. 66). Outcome is generally poor in the presence of negative symptoms in both schizophrenia and bipolar I disorder. However, negative symptoms in first episode bipolar I disorder did not endure over 18 months and had limited prognostic value compared to the prognostic significance of negative symptoms in schizophrenia (Pavuluri, Herbener, & Sweeney, 2004, p. 25).

Premorbid social withdrawal and isolation may represent early manifestations of schizophrenic illness, and stem from whatever pathophysiological processes ultimately become manifested as negative symptoms. Premorbid history of social withdrawal and schizoid personality style increases the likelihood that the diagnosis will be schizophrenia. Academic and behavioral abnormalities are not helpful predictors (McClellan, Breiger, McCurry, & Hlastala, 2003, p. 670).

The two to six years follow-up of 33 cases initially diagnosed as mood disorders with psychotic features, evaluated by blind interviewers confirmed the diagnosis. None of these cases developed schizophrenia. Originally, 13 of 15 cases with major depression had experienced mood congruent or derogatory hallucinations. None of the patients with depression or bipolar disorder had a history of grossly disorganized behavior or negative symptoms (Sporn & Rapoport, 2001, p. 2).

Finally, Duffy (2003) warns that the current practice of basing treatment of bipolar disorder on psychiatric diagnosis alone is not sufficient for most patients. Family history is essential to understanding the present illness, and can help in determining the best course of action with respect to treatment. There are cases of children of lithium-responsive bipolar parents manifesting mixed psychopathology; these children respond well to lithium. It has been proposed that lithium response is a familial trait. It has also been demonstrated that patients who respond to lithium do not respond as well to anticonvulsants. Patients with comorbid anxiety disorders and substance abuse respond better to lamotrigine, and patients with incongruent psychotic features, unremitting course, and a positive family history of psychotic disorders respond well to antipsychotic monotherapy (pp. 2–3). Some experts believe that schizophrenia and mood disorders belong to the same category of illness. This controversy is overviewed in chapter 8.

ANXIETY DISORDERS

Severe social phobias and related anxiety disorders sometimes present with confusing clinical pictures, more so, if long-standing patterns of interpersonal avoidance have been established. Patients appear as displaying prominent negative symptoms, and bizarre and disorganized behaviors. Werry, McClellan, and Chard (1991) reported 30% of anxious personality type, as one of the premorbid variables of schizophrenia (p. 461). The case of Weer exemplifies features that may create diagnostic confusion.

Weer, a 15-year-old Asian-American male, was referred to an acute psychiatric hospital for progressive isolation and persistent refusal to attend school. The initial mental status examination revealed the presence of a bizarre looking adolescent male, disheveled and with poor hygiene. As he entered the room he crawled up in his chair, gave the back to the examiner, and remained downcast throughout the initial examination. He also went down on the floor and began to "draw circles" on the wall. When asked questions, his answers were muttered. The examiner often had to repeat the questions and got short responses that frequently were difficult to understand. He refused to make eye contact. His mood appeared depressed and anxious, with marked affect constriction, if not flatness of the emotional display.

When Weer was queried as to the presence of perceptual disturbance he denied auditory, visual, and olfactory hallucinations. However, he endorsed broad paranoid ideation, such as feeling that people talked about him, watched him, and followed him. He reported that he felt depressed and scared. Weer was started on an SSRI and an antipsychotic medication. In the acute program, he frequently isolated himself from peers, and it was common to see him in a corner, away from peers and staff. When he went to the cafeteria it was observed that he rarely ate. Some staff members were able to talk to the patient and surmised that he was awfully shy and anxious.

As the SSRI was increased his demeanor began to normalize. Progressively he was able to make better eye contact and became more engaging. He revealed that he was very anxious around people and, that when around people, he felt that others would talk about him and watch him; he stated he could not eat in front of others, and added that he felt uncomfortable being around people; he had that problem for a long, long time. He could not go to malls, to the movies, or crowded places. He reported occasional panic episodes. He added that he did not trust anybody. He had been skipping school and cutting classes because he could not tolerate sitting in the classroom, surrounded by other people. New queries corroborated his lack of perceptual disturbances, and confirmed the broad paranoid ideation he had initially endorsed.

Weer's biological father was in prison for molesting Weer's younger sister; Weer blamed his mother and sister for his father's imprisonment, and had threatened to kill both of them. Apparently, Weer's biological father also had problems with drugs and alcohol. As Weer became better able to communicate, the examiner explored other areas of the patient's past. In particular, a thorough exploration of prior abuse, legal and drug history was pursued. Weer had been physically abused by his biological mother in the past and did also reveal that he had been using drugs extensively. Weer had used marijuana and cocaine for the previous two years. He stated that he used marijuana frequently, many times during the day, and had used cocaine at least weekly. Furthermore, he acknowledged he had sold drugs. He had never had any legal problems and had never been in juvenile detention. Weer had been in psychiatric hospitals twice before, the first time, eight months prior to his most recent admission for suicidal behavior.

What ostensibly appeared like a schizophrenic presentation turned out to be a very severe case of social phobia with prominent avoidant features, associated with paranoia, and complicated by drug dependence.

Anxiety disorders (separation anxiety, panic disorder, OCD), in preadolescence and early adolescence, are frequently observed in children who later develop bipolar disorders. There are severe OCD presentations in which the reality testing seems to be compromised; these clinical pictures have been named schizo-obsessive disorders or schizo-obsessive conditions. Psychotic features are very common in severe OCD manifestations in preadolescents. In general, these children are extremely dysphoric, prone to anger outbursts, intense and prolonged temper tantrums, and are markedly oppositional both at home and school. Academic and behavioral problems at school are quite common. OCD preadolescent children display prominent compulsions and are very ritualistic; frequently they pick at their skin, particularly nose and limbs. OCD children have also problems communicating and relating; they rarely get along with other children. Psychotic features, auditory hallucinations, and referential ideation are not uncommon. The examiner will rule out Tourette's disorder, present in about a third of cases, in this neuropsychiatric condition.

SCHIZOPHRENIA AND RELATED DISORDERS

Schizophrenia is still considered one of the most severe and malignant mental illnesses, and its prognosis is still guarded due to its chronic, and often unremitting or deteriorating course. Intermediate forms such as schizoaffective disorders are quite incapacitating, sometimes to a lesser degree.

Tsai and Champine (2004) defend the use of adult criteria for the diagnosis of children: (1) there is convincing evidence that autism and schizophrenia are two distinct entities; (2) schizophrenia as described in adults can begin in childhood, and, (3) children and adolescents display the same symptoms as adults diagnosed with schizophrenia (p. 379; for the DSM-IV-TR diagnostic criteria of schizophrenia, see pp. 312–313).

Very early onset schizophrenia (VEOS) and childhood onset schizophrenia (COS) produces such a profound disorder of mental functioning, "that external behavior seems bizarre to observers, and internal mental experiences are incomprehensible and frightening to the patient…. Thinking, feeling, perceiving, behaving, and experiencing operate without the normal linkages that make mental life comprehensible and effective" (Nasrallah & Smeltzer, 2002, pp. 7, 8). "COS and VEOS usually presents with poor premorbid functioning and insidious rather than acute onset of illness, thus resembling cases of adult onset schizophrenia with poor outcome" (Sporn & Rapoport, 2001, p. 1).

There is clear evidence that schizophrenia with childhood onset can be reliably diagnosed via the same criteria employed with adults, and that, in many cases, childhood onset schizophrenia continues into adulthood. Similarities between children and adults with schizophrenia in such diverse domains as genetics, brain imaging, neurocognition, thought disorder, treatment response, outcome, and family patterns suggest continuity between the childhood and the adult onset forms of the disorder. There are differences, though: the atypical onset of the childhood presentation, and current findings suggesting that these children may be characterized by poor premorbid adjustment, increased family loading for schizophrenia-spectrum disorders, higher rates of insidious rather than acute onsets, and a greater loss of cortical gray matter over time, with possibly poorer outcomes (Asarnow & Asarnow, 2003, p. 479).

The current standard within the field is to use systematic diagnostic interviewing and procedures to elicit data on symptoms and functioning and to formulate diagnoses using the same criteria used in adults (Asarnow, Tompson, & McGrath, 2004, p. 180; see chapter 5).

Etiology

For a review of some of the issues regarding etiology, including genetic factors, the reader is referred to chapter 8.

Issues Related to Diagnosis

There is no laboratory test to determine with certainty that a person has schizophrenia. This leads to a number of diagnostic dilemmas and ambiguities when attempting to diagnose children and adolescents who present with symptoms suggestive of schizophrenia and schizophrenia-spectrum disorders (Asarnow, Tompson, & McGrath, 2004, p. 181). The problem is complicated by the developmental variations in the presentation of the illness. Clinicians are frequently confronted with questions of when the disorder began as opposed to when the diagnostic data is sufficient to establish the diagnosis (p. 181). Difficulties related to the diagnosis of VEOS and EOS are discussed in an endnote.[1]

COS may be overdiagnosed; Werry, McClelland, and Chard (1991) rediagnosed 61 cases of COS, after a period of follow-up from 1 to 16 years (mean, 5 years); 35 patients had received the diagnosis of schizophrenia; 13 had been considered schizophreniform; 1 schizoaffective; and 9 bipolar disorder. At follow-up, 30 subjects received the diagnosis of schizophrenia; 23 of bipolar disorder; and 6 were diagnosed as schizoaffective (all bipolar type). Up to 55% of the children that previously had been diagnosed as schizophrenia spectrum disorders, were rediagnosed as mood disorders (p. 461).

A view expressed for adult schizophrenia is also applicable to schizophrenia with an adolescent onset.

> More than 80% of persons with schizophrenia have no affected relatives within the first degree of kinship (parents, children, or siblings), and more than 60% have family histories that are completely negative. Nevertheless, it has been established beyond a doubt that schizophrenia is a familial (genetic) disease, and only a few skeptics remain unconvinced that this is determined more for genetic transmission than by environmental factors. (Nasrallah & Smeltzer, 2002, pp. 31–32)

As reported by Schaffer and Ross (2002), delusions and hallucinations are not frequent initial symptoms in very early onset schizophrenia: 3 out of 17 (18%) and 2 out of 17 (12%) children respectively, presented delusions or hallucinations as initial symptoms. The most common presentations were developmental delays, school problems, and learning disabilities, present in 11 of 17 cases (65%), and oppositionality, violence, aggression, rages, temper tantrums, and fighting which were present in 6 of 17 children (35% of the cases). These observations parallel Sporn and Rapoport's descriptions, cited above.

Observational data suggest the likely continuity for psychotic disorder between childhood and adulthood, but highlight the difficulties differentiating between schizophrenia and affective psychoses in childhood, as well as the potential importance of examining such clinical features as onset patterns and depressed mood (Asarnow & Asarnow, 2003, p. 478). The confusion in differentiating a major depressive episode with psychotic features from schizophrenias stems from a number of factors: (1) Up to a third of schizophrenic patients qualify for the diagnosis of depression. (2) Psychotic withdrawal and negative symptoms may be misinterpreted as depression. (3) Severely depressed unconventional children with atypical attire and unusual demeanor may be misinterpreted as showing evidence of schizophrenia. (4) There are phenomenological phenocopies of schizophrenic symptomatology: psychomimetic drugs, anxiety disorders, DID, and many others. The present and previous chapters expand on this subject.

Prevalence

Childhood schizophrenia is a rare disease The National Institute of Mental Health (NIMH) received 1,300 referrals for the evaluation of this disorder; after telephone screening, 700 medical records, that is 54% of the referred cases, were requested for review. Out of 700 cases, 550 (79%) cases were excluded due to lack of documented presence of psychotic symptoms, onset after age 12, or other exclusion criteria, such as medical illness or mental retardation. Of 213 subjects screened in person, 83 were admitted to the inpatient unit with the diagnosis of schizophrenia. Only 62 out 1,300 patients received the diagnosis of childhood schizophrenia. This represents less that 5% of a severely psychotic referral cohort (Sporn & Rapoport, 2001).

VEOS is a rare illness indeed. VEOS is about 50 times rarer than EOS and probably about 50 times rarer that OCD in early childhood. This is not an absolute diagnosis, however; it is likely that, over the years, even for the NIMH narrowly selected cohort, some of the children diagnosed with COS may evolve into schizoaffective or mood disorder diagnoses. Louis's case illustrates a childhood schizophrenia onset (VEOS), with a severe regression and a chronic course in a preadolescent child with previous neurodevelopmental difficulties, including mutism.

> Louis was a 10-year-old white boy, in second grade (note the academic retardation), first evaluated for complaints that he was "retarded and withdrawn." There were also complaints that no one "could get to him." Louis was the third of four children. He had two older brothers, age 13 and 12, and one younger sister.
>
> A few months before the psychiatric assessment, Louis had received an inpatient psychiatric evaluation at a child and adolescent psychiatric program at a major university program. From this evaluation came the strong presumption of childhood psychosis or childhood schizophrenia. Upon termination of the diagnostic admission the university program recommended long-term residential psychiatric treatment. The organic workup for this child, including imaging studies and EEGs, had been unremarkable.
>
> One year before, this child had been referred to child protective services because of his steady regression. Louis had two years of kindergarten and two years of first grade, and had made no academic gains in second grade; he was not going to be promoted at the end of the school year. The school psychologist had recommended special education placement, but Louis's parents had rejected the recommendation. Apparently, as the schoolwork became "harder" he withdrew and refused to complete any assignments. Louis was reported as being progressively withdrawn and self-absorbed. Now, none of Louis's teachers ever heard him speaking out loud any more. He stopped communicating with other students and he did not seem to be aware of his activities or their activities. Retrospectively, Louis was most likely either profoundly regressed or catatonic at that time.
>
> His behavior in the classroom became quite stereotyped. Sometimes he spent the day circling his desk or rocking back and forth. Other days he would sit and stare at the ceiling or stare straight ahead. He frequently smiled or cried inappropriately but he would respond to simple directions such as "sit down," "go to bed," or "eat." If he were not told what to do, he would tend to do nothing.
>
> Louis had been removed from his parents due to medical neglect. His parents appeared bitter, hostile, and paranoid about social agencies. Four months prior to the psychiatric evaluation, Louis was placed in a foster home where his behavior continued without any significant change. Louis's family did not admit that there was anything wrong with him and were unwilling to cooperate with any psychiatric or psychological evaluation. When the family revealed that Louis had started talking at age 5, and as the examiner attempted to explore this, the family became defensive. The father stated that, "Lots of children don't start talking until they are 10." The family felt the child had been "kidnapped" from them, and believed that the CPS intervention was, "just another example of the communist takeover in this country." The parents refused to provide any information regarding the child's background or any family history.
>
> Louis would recognize the examiner's presence and would respond to greetings, but when he was told to go with the examiner he would nonverbally indicate, on a regular basis, that he did not want to go with him. He would stare at the psychiatrist and smile in a silly, childish, and inappropriate way. He would stare at the examiner or keep either rocking and isolating himself. When he was

observed in a group,with other children, he did not relate to them. A number of times he was found on the playground standing by himself, rocking and smiling, as if involved in some other world, or as if responding to internal stimuli; he seemed to be lost in his own world. To most of the questions or verbal suggestions he would respond with very short phrases or would not respond at all. He was oppositional (negativistic?): for instance, on one occasion, when he was on the playground rocking and after climbing on the slide, the examiner asked him to come down. Louis would not slide down, but kept fidgeting and moving his arms in a peculiar way, like flapping, or moving the little fingers of both hands in a peculiar manner (stereotypes). When he was asked to come to the office, he indicated by nodding, that he did not want to. In general, his verbalizations were minimal, he would assume unusual postures, all bent over, sometimes smiling and sometimes staring; at other times, he seemed preoccupied in his own world, oblivious of other people or of whatever was going on around him.

Louis was a blond, handsome boy with blue eyes and an intense gaze. Very readily he would display a childish demeanor. His verbalizations were minimal; sometimes he did not speak in full sentences and sometimes he would not respond at all. There seemed to be a persistent smiling with some silliness and inappropriateness. Louis seemed to be slightly underdeveloped for his age, but his physical appearance was otherwise unremarkable. There were times when he appeared to be happy and enjoying himself; at other times he appeared puzzled, bewildered, and lost, and still other times, he appeared estranged or rather confused. His attention was very erratic, and he needed repeated prompting to perform a task, and to bring him away from his inner world. There were no spontaneous behaviors. Louis did not display any form of behavioral organization.

Since verbal communication with him was very limited the examiner resorted to obtaining some information from drawings (see chapter 4). Louis's drawings were very primitive, dereistic, and puzzling, and the figures he produced were very atypical. There was extraneous material, indicating ego disruptions and regression into primary process thinking. There were times when he seemed unable to represent some visual images and he resorted to writing or drawing peculiar and stereotyped letters or words. In the family kinetic drawing, he drew a set of five seats with a strong pencil pressure, and over those he drew what appeared to be some faces without any bodies or any other corporal elements; after that, he sketched some idiosyncratic figures and continued doing so in a persistent (perseverative) manner. He appeared to be preoccupied with the letters *f* and *g* and at times he incorporated them into his picture. This preoccupation with the letters *f* and *g* seemed to represent a ritualistic and magical quality, and appeared in many of his drawings. When he was asked to draw a tree, he drew a very unsophisticated, simple tree, and with some violation of reality principles, he put the name *Hoover* on the tree and began to be so preoccupied with the letters *Rg* along with the letters *Fg* that he transformed them into an entangled drawing with meaningless scribbles. This was another example of ego disruption and of intrusion of primary process ideation (peculiar, idiosyncratic content erupting into consciousness). When he was asked to draw a car, the picture was more visually accurate and reality based than the previous drawings, except by the location of the muffler, windows, and doors. Even in this picture, that he called a Mercury, he wrote under the car the letters "moven" (moving?) and then changed the vowel *e* for *i* and later on for an *a*, and under this he wrote some enigmatic graphisms. After doing this, he tried to sketch a house, he wrote on the wall of the house *Vvg*, then transformed the *g* into an arched concave figure; he also transformed the *v* into an arrow after which he drew a signpost of a big arrow indicating "east and west." These nonverbal observations seem to be parallel to verbal productions indicating of looseness of associations, and thought incoherence, thus of a thought disorder.

With significant prompting, Louis was able to draw himself producing a square face wearing a cap with the body fragmented into a disjointed upper and lower part. He called the part corresponding to the chest both a bone and a body, and the part that would correspond to the abdomen, he called a penis.

In summary, apparently, Louis underwent a massive regression; he lost ability to communicate, to relate to others, and to maintain contact with reality. The background information is sketchy due to the paranoid attitude of family. Neurological and neuroimaging studies, including EEG, were negative. The drawings indicated that this child had at least a low average IQ. It appeared that it was very hard for Louis to keep in touch with reality and that he continuously withdrew into fantasy and primary process ideation. It was hard to establish if Louis experienced perceptual disturbances. His reality testing seemed very erratic and he had tremendous difficulty focusing and maintaining attention. There was some evidence of fragmentation of thought and of frequent intrusion into consciousness of idiosyncratic ideation. Louis's verbal language was very impaired and he seemed to have lost any interest in communicating. Catatonic symptoms were prominent. Nonverbally, his demeanor appeared to be very regressed, infantile, childish, and stereotyped; sometimes he displayed autistic and hebephrenic features. Progress of this child in the residential program was limited. Louis's response to antipsychotic medications was marginal.

Affective disorder with psychotic features remains the major differential diagnosis of VEOS and COS. Statistically a child with psychotic symptoms has a 70 to 80% chance of suffering from an affective disorder. Affective features in schizophrenic children cloud the diagnosis. Asarnow, Tompson, and Goldstein (1994) pointed out that in their schizophrenic cohort, 56% of children displayed significant depressive features; 39% of these children qualified for the diagnosis of dysthymic disorder before the onset of schizophrenia, and 44% of patients met diagnostic criteria for major depressive disorder in addition to schizophrenia (p. 606). Differentiating schizophrenia from mood disorders poses a major clinical challenge. The case of Uranus, exemplifies these complexities.

Uranus, a 10½-year-old white boy, had been admitted to an acute preadolescent hospital program for the first time, 18 months before a psychiatric evaluation was required for aggressive and delusional behaviors. He had participated in a partial hospital program prior to the admission to the acute care program. This had been precipitated by the patient's assault on his 5½-year-old brother, believing he was laughing at him. His grandmother had to pull Uranus from his brother, and his mother had overheard him saying that his brother was the devil.

Uranus believed he was an alien from another planet (Uranus); he had an elaborate story as to how he landed on earth, and how he was born. He was convinced he was 19 years old, and would become enraged when confronted with his real age. He also believed that "Chip" (his teddy bear) was his son. He also was markedly irritable and his parents felt unable to control him. Uranus also complained of racing thoughts.

Uranus consistently denied auditory, visual, or olfactory hallucinations. He consistently denied suicidal or homicidal thoughts. He was a very intelligent child, but suffered from dysgraphia. He was quite provocative and immature, but otherwise, he was somewhat engaging.

In one occasion he stated that he "was taking over the world." He had asked his mother if she was his real mother. He had strong negative feelings against his stepfather, and innumerable times, had asked his mother to divorce him. Uranus had accused stepfather of being abusive to him, a charge that mother adamantly denied. Uranus was frequently goofy, silly, agitated, irritable, and prone to angry outbursts when he did not get his way. Uranus's mood would change drastically from one moment to the next at minor frustrations of his wants. At times, he would rapidly regress into a whiny, childish, and pathetic state. He was markedly inflexible in his reasoning. Prior to treatment with antipsychotics he was unflinching in his peculiar beliefs.

During the psychiatric examination he acknowledged that "Chip" talked to him; he frequently blamed Chip for his misbehavior. On one occasion mother found Uranus enacting sexual acts between Chip and "Chip's girl friend," (Chiperella).

Uranus had been followed in outpatient treatment over five years. He had shown inconsistent progress and erratic stability; however, mother said that he was progressively more manageable, less aggressive and argumentative, and that he displayed a more stable mood with antipsychotics and mood stabilizers. He has also been progressively more mature. His regressive episodes had become less frequent than before, but major difficulties at school remained. Uranus complained about his peers and teachers, and about the limit-setting and discipline that were imposed on his oppositional and regressive behaviors. Silliness and giddiness decreased over time. However, he remained prone to tantrums and regressive behavior when he felt frustrated.

Uranus was for a long time on quetiapine 400 mg q AM & 600 mg q HS; divalproex 1000 mg q HS, guanfacine 1 mg BID, and trazodone 100 mg q HS. In spite of that regime, he remained irritable and hypomanic. On one occasion, he started vomiting a great deal for many days so the divalproex was discontinued. In spite of the GI symptoms, he continued taking quetiapine and guanfacine at the same doses. Since he remained significantly symptomatic and previous attempts to improve therapeutic effects with lithium and lamotrigene had been ineffective, oxcarbazepine at a dose up to 300 mg q AM and 600 mg q HS was implemented with limited results.

Augmentation with aripripazole 7.5 q AM had a very clear favorable stabilizing effect. Mother reported that tantrums, which had been a major problem before, had improved considerably; along with this beneficial effect the patient continued losing weight. He had been overweight before. On the combination of

Oxcarbazepine (300 mg BID), guanfacine (1 mg BID), quetiapine (400 mg q AM and 600 mg q HS), and 7.5 mg aripiprazole, his weight normalized.

Although Uranus displayed mood and thought disorder features, the mood/affective components seemed more predominant than the thought disorders features. The diagnosis of schizoaffective disorder or bipolar disorder, provisional, seemed appropriate.

Three years after the first contact, and when Uranus was more stable, he was asked to reflect on his previous beliefs. He was asked to explain his belief that he was from Uranus. He explained, comfortably and coherently, that he had learned that he had scored very high on intelligence tests; because this made him different from other children, he thought he was an alien from another planet. He added that he had stopped believing that for a long time. When he was asked to talk about issues with his age, he said that he was convinced, then, that he was 19; he said he no longer believed this.

When he was asked to discuss his belief about Chip, he said that because that teddy bear had been with him since infancy, that is, because they "had grown together," he had special feelings toward that teddy bear. He explained that when a child has a teddy bear he feels that the teddy bear understands him. He always felt that Chip was special, that he could understand him. Since the patient had said that Chip talked to him, he was asked to expand on this. He indicated that Chip never talked to him with words, but he always had the feeling that Chip understood him. He was told that he had stated that his brother was the devil. He pointed out that mother used to say that his brother was a "demon," that is why he felt he was the devil. Furthermore, he said his brother used to "torture" him, and claimed that his brother used to make his life very unhappy. He stated that he loves his brother now, but he still resented that his brother refused to play with him. Surprisingly, Uranus kept his composure during this query, and never got upset by these challenges. Previously he used to cry easily, and would begin to act in a regressed and immature manner; nothing of this sort was observed this time. In the past, he threw tantrums, became upset, and had difficulties calming himself. He also added that he had made major progress in controlling his anger; he said that his "mood swings" were better, and that he was able to sleep better. Uranus was most happy to see that he was no longer obese.

Differentiation of pediatric bipolar disorder and schizophrenia is critical and is based on type of symptoms and course of the illness. The chances of correct differentiation are increased by: (1) systematic acquisition of history and mental status examination; (2) consistent use of DSM-IV-TR (2000) diagnostic criteria; (3) characterizing the mood congruent and incongruent delusions and hallucinations; and (4) determining the overall course and level of function (Pavuluri, Herbener, & Sweeney, 2004, p. 24). The present writer is in agreement with these propositions.

Prepubertal or early onset bipolar disorder has higher rates of mixed presentations (including ultra rapid cycling) and also has a higher prevalence of grandiose and paranoid delusions than the adolescent onset bipolar disorder. Adolescent onset bipolar disorder, like adult onset bipolar disorder, can have complicated presentations with marked thought disorder and severe behavioral disturbance, including comorbid substance abuse (Pavuluri, Hebener, & Sweeney, 2004, p. 22).

Adler and Strakowski (2003) indicate that the gradual decline in function that has been attributed to schizophrenia since Morel's initial characterization does not differentiate schizophrenia from bipolar disorder. Many patients with bipolar disorder do not return to baseline between affective episodes, and some studies suggest that bipolar disorders may show a gradual deterioration in function that is accompanied by an increased likelihood of further symptoms and decrements in neuropsychological testing (p. 3). For the epigenesis and illness progression, as well issues related to etiology and pathogenesis of schizophrenia, the reader is referred to chapter 8.

The prepsychotic period of psychotic disorders like COS and adult onset schizophrenia can be divided into two phases: (1) The "premorbid phase" is a stable phase during childhood, and usually, part of adolescence, in which emotional, cognitive, and behavioral functioning is not progressively or persistently impaired. (2) The "prodromal period" or "at-risk mental state" is characterized by a sustained and clinically important deviation from the premorbid level of experience and behavior (Amminger, McGorry, & Leicester, 2002, p. 2). Prodromal criteria of inclusion in an Australian research group are discussed in an endnote.[3]

Longitudinal MRI analysis of patients with childhood-onset schizophrenia, from the NIMH cohort, demonstrated striking anatomical profiles of accelerated gray matter loss. Although, there was some increase of the amount of cortex during adolescence, these cortical structures demonstrated the greatest abnormalities over time. In this regard, the Asarnows (Asarnow & Asarnow, 2003) quote Thompson et al. (2001); they state that the earliest deficits were found in parietal regions supporting visuospatial and associative thinking whereas adult deficits are known to be mediated by environmental (nongenetic factors). Over five years, these deficits progressed anteriorly into temporal lobes engulfing sensorimotor and dorsolateral cortices, and frontal eye fields. These emerging patterns correlated with psychotic severity and mirrored the neuromotor, auditory, visual search, and frontal executive impairments of schizophrenia. In temporal areas, gray matter loss was completely absent early in the disease but became pervasive later. The latest changes included dorsolateral prefrontal cortex and superior temporal gyri, deficit regions found consistently in adults studies (Asarnow & Asarnow, 2003, p. 470; for issues related to neuroimaging in schizophrenia, see chapter 5).

Risk Factors for COS

In the background of schizophrenic subjects, research has consistently demonstrated the following findings: poor premorbid functioning; increased family history of schizophrenia spectrum disorders; language impairment; smooth eye movement abnormalities; obstetrical complications are well-known risks for adult onset schizophrenia (this latter finding was not supported in the NIMH studies in VEOS/COS..

Higher rates of schizophrenia "spectrum" disorders (schizoaffective, schizotypal, or paranoid personality disorder) have been reported in first-degree relatives of children with COS, even higher than in cases of adult onset schizophrenia. For more information regarding the etiology and neurobiology of schizophrenia the reader is referred to chapter 8 (pp. 235–236).

The importance of obstetrical complication as a major causative factor of VEOS/COS is controversial. The rate of obstetrical complication for identified psychotic adolescents was not elevated above the rate for their siblings in the NMIH studies.

Premorbid Abnormalities

Premorbid abnormalities are neither sensitive nor specific of schizophrenia. The vast majority of children with developmental impairments do not develop schizophrenia in adolescence or adulthood. Neurodevelopmental studies may permit the initiation of earlier interventions, with the expectation of altering the outcome of these disorders. Earlier interventions may improve outcomes in a number of ways: (1) protecting patients through high risk periods; (2) enhancing developmental progression; (3) improving environmental interaction; (4) preventing kindling and sensitization; and (5) promoting healthy neurodevelopment (Asarnow & Asarnow, 2003, p. 6). For more information regarding biomarkers and premorbid abnormalities see chapter 8. For criteria regarding inclusion in an Australian prodrama study, see endnote 2.

As has been said before, there are no pathognomonic signs of schizophrenia. Even affective psychosis may present with first rank Schneiderian symptoms, and some children who display clear thought disorder in childhood may convert or evolve into schizoaffective or mood disorder diagnoses later in life. Paranoid delusions, catatonia, and Schneiderian first rank symptoms are often observed in manic episodes (Pavuluri, Herbener, & Sweeney, 2004, p. 24). Clinicians need to exercise caution against hopeless prognostications.

Schizophrenia Outcome

Werry, McClellan, and Chard (1991) reported the poorest outcome results (see table 7.3); remission was described in only 3% of the sample, with a follow-up from 1 to 16 years (mean interval, 5 years); 90% of the sample showed either chronic schizophrenia or two or more schizophrenic episodes. Approximately, 1 in 8 (13%) had committed suicide, underscoring the lethality of schizophrenia. The precise nature of those deaths was not ascertained. Only 17% (1 in 6) of the sample was in school full time or had full-time employment. Eggers reported better outcome figures (Eggers 1989; Eggers, Bunk, & Burns, 2002) on 57 patients diagnosed as schizophrenic prior to age 14. Evaluation at an average of 16 years after initial assessment showed that 27% (1 in 4 patients) of the sample was in remission; 24% (1 in 4) showed slight defect; and 49% (1 in 2) showed severe defect. Forty-two years after the initial evaluation, one third (33% of the sample) suffered from continuing psychotic symptoms; 27% were unable to work; 59% were unmarried and living alone; and only 7% (less that 1 in 12) of the sample were in stable relationships. Asarnow's data, from follow-ups on a COS sample initially identified between 7 to 14 years of age, overlap with outcome data from Eggers. The rates of schizophrenia evolved from 100% to 78%, 67%, and 73% at one, two, and three years follow-up, respectively. Over a three-year follow-up 61% of the sample showed continuing schizophrenia, and 67% showed continuing schizophrenia or schizoaffective disorder; 56% (approximately, 6 of 10 patients) of the sample showed some improvement in functioning over the course of the follow-up and 44% (4 of 10 patients) showed minimal improvement or deteriorating course. Twenty-eight percent of the sample (more than 1 in 4 patients) showed fairly good psychosocial adjustment based on GAF scores of 60 or above (table 7.3 gives an overview of relevant outcome studies).

In summary, there is significant consistency of outcome results across studies. First, it is likely that even when using strict diagnostic parameters, in up to 20 to 40% of patients, the diagnosis will change at follow-up. It is likely that no more than 20 to 25% of schizophrenic patients will experience remission; another 20 to 25% of patients will experience some degree of functional improvement; and another 15 to 20% of patients will experience a deteriorating course. About 40% or more of schizophrenic patients will experience no significant adaptive or functional change. Finally and sadly, the rate of suicide in VEOS/EOS populations may be as high as 15% or more.

Cultural Biases in the Diagnosis of Schizophrenia

In adults, cultural biases complicate the diagnosis of schizophrenia. African-American and Hispanic males (and to a less extent females) are more frequently diagnosed as schizophrenic than comparable white peers (Strawkowski, 2003a, p. 74). African-American patients are more likely than their white counterparts to receive antipsychotics, and less likely to receive psychotherapy (p. 75). Four factors may contribute to African-Americans' and other minorities misdiagnosis (see table 7.4).

It is clear that cultural diagnostic biases may also vitiate the field of child and adolescent psychiatry. The child and adolescent psychiatrist needs to be attentive to these potential threats to diagnostic objectivity.

TABLE 7.3 Outcome Studies in Childhood Schizophrenia

	Sample	Follow-up period	Remission	% DX SCZ at Follow-up		Doing well	Other
Werry et al., (1991) (Westermeyer & Harrow)	59	1–16 y M: 5 y	3% 25%	90%		17%	15% dead
Eggers (1978) Eggers (1989; Eggers et al. (2002)	57	16 y (6–40)	20% 27% (31% in schizoaffective disorders)		24%: slight defect; 49%: sev. defect.		7% stable relation
Asarnow et al. (1) (1994,1999)	21 (18)	1,2,3 y 3–7 y	33% 22% of SZ remitted without medications	78%, 67%, 73%, (11% schizo- affective	56%: better, 44%: no better worse	28%***	61%**
Hollis (2000)	110 (93) [2]	11–17 (14.9 y)	12%****	80%			

*   1, 2, and 3 years after initial assessment.
**   Schizophrenia continued at 3–7 years of follow-up.
***   Fairly good psychosocial adjustment: GAF of 60 or above.
****   Patients with history of VEOS or EOS had a poor prognosis.
Source: Werry, McClellan, & Chard (1991).
50% of bipolar patients had been diagnosed as schizophrenic Eggers (1989).
In about 28% of schizophrenic children, chronic course is preceded by short depressive, manic or manic–depressive episode(s).
Source: Eggers, Bunk, & Burns (2002); Asarnow, Tompson, & Goldstein (1994).
(1) Sample consists of very early onset schizophrenia cases (onset below 12 years of age). In 20% of patients diagnosis, changed during follow up. 38% of patients had history of suicidal attempts; other 38%, had history of suicidal ideation.
Source: Asarnow & Tompson, & Goldstein (1999); Hollis (2000).
[2] Of the 93 followed-up patients, 51 (55%) were still schizophrenic, 12 (13%) were schizoaffective, 23 (25%) had an affective psychosis, and 7 (8%) had an atypical psychosis.

Hebephrenia

This uncommon form of schizophrenia may also become a source of diagnostic confusion both in its acute and insidious manifestations.

Jabs, Verdaguer, Pfuhimann, Bartsch, and Beckmann (2002) traced the development of the concept of hebephrenia since Esquirol (1838) and Morel's (1860) case reports that resembled descriptions of hebephrenia. Kahlbaum introduced the concept of hebephrenia in 1863. Kahlbaums's pupil, Hecker, published the first meticulous reports of hebephrenia in 1871. Hecker observed a marked affective dulling and an "unrestrainable inclination toward laughter

TABLE 7.4 Sources of Racial and Cultural Bias in the Diagnosis of Schizophrenia

---

- Differences in symptom presentation as compared to whites are more common in African-Americans' mood disorders.
- Failure to identify affective symptoms in African Americans (and other minorities)
    Same symptoms were recorded but received different diagnostic criteria—criterion variance—and different information was recorded which led to diagnostic discrepancies—information variance.
- Minority patients' wariness with health services
    Depressed African Americans are more distrustful of clinicians than whites; this puts them at risk of being perceived as paranoid, and as being diagnosed as paranoid schizophrenia.
- Racial stereotyping.
    African Americans more often are committed involuntarily, and are referred to social and legal agencies rather than to medical services. They are perceived to be violent—which may lead to excessive medication and restraints.

Source: Strakowski (2003, pp. 76–77).

and fatuous jokes." These patients seldom had authentic delusions and often display "rudimentary elements of delusions," constituting fundamentally fatuous, uncritical, and infantile interpretations of objective facts. Episodes of marked "fury" could be triggered by sexual excitement or irritation of peripheral nervous structures (i.e., toothache). Hebephrenia was the basis for Kraepelin's initial concept of dementia praecox, and hebephrenia became a subtype of dementia praecox (1899; pp. 2000–2001). The concept of hebephrenia was submerged with Bleuler's (1911) categorization of schizophrenia, and hebephrenia became then, a form of the "group of schizophrenias," and with Schneider's (1980) reconceptualization, the concept of hebephrenia disappeared. In the DSM-IV (1994), the concept of hebephrenia was replaced by the label of disorganized subtype of schizophrenia (p. 2002).

The authors, following the approach of Kleist and Leonhard, propose that hebephrenia is a reliable diagnosis for a clinical homogeneous entity with well-defined cross-sectional symptomatology and course and, in their view, "[T]his highly operationalized and empirically well confirmed concept of hebephrenia elaborated by Leonhard seems to provide useful heuristics for future research" (p. 205).[4] Background information regarding the classical view and relevant clinical aspects of hebephrenia are discussed in an endnote.[5]

Eddy exemplifies many of the "classical" hebephrenic features described above:

Eddy, a 15-year-old Hispanic youth, was seen for the first time at the age of 12 for aggressive and destructive behaviors. At the time of the initial evaluation, he had attacked two peers and a teacher. He also had recently pinched his baby nephew. It was reported that Eddy was often found laughing and crying without any apparent reason.

Eddy's mother reported a marked decline in adaptive and appropriate social behavior for more than a year. He had become progressively withdrawn, silly, impulsive, aggressive, irritable, and sexually inappropriate both at school and at home. Eddy's mother began to receive progressive complaints about Eddy's behavior at school. It was reported that school felt unable to handle Eddy, and that there were also concerns that he posed a risk to the safety of teachers and other students.

Eddy did have a long history of aggressive behavior and self-abusive behaviors including, head banging, self-hitting, picking at his skin, and removing the scabs; he had also threatened to hurt himself with scissors, and had been destructive to home property including doors and windows. At some point, he pulled a knife on his sister and had threatened to kill her. There was also history of cruelty to animals.

Eddy was disinhibited: he exposed himself, masturbated openly in the classroom and at home. He displayed severe problems with boundaries, and would touch peers and adults indiscriminately; he would grab breasts and touch female teachers inappropriately. He had attempted to molest his 7-year- old sister, and did not seem to show any regard for urinating in his pants but was not enuretic at nighttime. Eddy had problems sleeping at night. Family reported that he was frequently found grinning, laughing, and talking to himself.

Relevant medical history: Eddy had been hyperactive all his life; he fell from a roof at age 5; there was no loss of consciousness and no evidence of skull fracture. There was a history of seizures, and the last episode had occurred one year before. He also had appendicitis a year before, and had a prior psychiatric hospital admission three months before the initial evaluation.

His biological parents had a common law marriage. There were six children; at the time of the initial psychiatric examination, the oldest child, a girl, was 16 years old, and the youngest, another girl, 7. From a previous marriage mother had five children, all girls. The oldest was 30 and the youngest 21. It was reported that Eddy's father had neuropsychiatric difficulties. Allegedly, Eddy's father had history of speech developmental problems and ADHD.

The initial mental status examination revealed the presence of an overweight male who displayed regressive behavior and some stereotypes: he rocked, and displayed inappropriate laughter. He was distant but inappropriately friendly; he kept satisfactory eye contact. Eddy seemed to have problems communicating, mostly problems in understanding verbal communication and verbal expectations. The mood was shallow and moderately elated, and the affect was inappropriate. There was evidence of thought disorder: he was not coherent, logical, or goal directed. He endorsed hearing a number of people (three persons talking to him). It was unclear if he was paranoid. He did endorse homicidal ideation toward his sister. Judgment, insight and superego functioning were considered severely impaired. During the evaluation, he passed gas on one occasion; instead of excusing himself, he grinned.

The physical examination was positive for the presence of obesity, gynecomastia, and soft neurological signs: there was some degree of tremor, choreathetotic movements, right–left disorientation, and constructional apraxia. He could not read nor write. He was disoriented to day, date, month, and year, and was unable to do very simple calculations. Vital signs were within normal limits. Urinalysis showed blood and significant amount of bacteria.

Relevant values in the comprehensive metabolic: SGPT 137 (normal values: < 40), SGOT 79 (normal values: <35). These abnormal levels of hepatic enzymes could be secondary to obesity. Alkaline phosphatase was 616 (normal values: < 200) (alkaline phosphatase is elevated in growing children); ceruloplasmin: 43 (normal value: 25–63). Urine drug screen was negative. An EKG was read as normal sinus rhythm, short PR interval; atypical EKG. An EEG showed evidence of paroxysmal activity originating in the left temporal region indicating cortical seizure activity at that area. An MRI showed no gross abnormalities. The psychologist desisted in her attempts to test Eddy due to the child's severe comprehension difficulties.

With the workup results the diagnosis was changed to Axis I, impulse control disorder, ADHD, developmental language disorder, with profound receptive deficits. Axis II mental retardation, mild; Axis III, static encephalopathy; complex partial symptomatology, Landau-Kleffner syndrome.

Two months after the initial evaluation, Eddy was seen in an inpatient setting after he became unmanageable at school. He continued having difficulties sleeping at night and had persistent aggressive, self-abusive, and inappropriate behaviors. He had attempted to throw a chair to a teacher. There were concerns with his lack of progress. The mental status revealed again the presence of a low functioning, overweight male who required repeated redirection due to his persistent attempts to touch the examiner. He was sloppily dressed and displayed poor hygiene. He would give selective one-word answers, and at other times, he became selectively mute. Previous findings of the mental status were unchanged. During the hospital stay, Eddy was on a one to one staffing, most of the time, for impulsive and inappropriate behaviors. At the time of this reevaluation, Eddy's 16-year-old sister had overdosed.

One year after the psychiatric reevaluation Eddy had a hospital readmission for aggressive behavior toward mother and peers, and for the persistent inappropriate sexual behavior. His self-abusive behavior had continued and he did not seem to respond to redirection nor limit setting. The school called mother on a daily basis to pick Eddy up because they could not cope with his misbehavior. He endorsed auditory command hallucinations. Mother reported that on one occasion while she was taking a nap, and in the twilight of consciousness, she sensed that somebody was getting on top of her. She thought her husband was "getting amorous." To her horror, when she opened her eyes, she saw Eddy making sexual movements on her.

In the ensuing two years, Eddy had multiple subsequent acute psychiatric admissions, including a referral to the local state hospital adolescent program. Eddy remained a very dysfunctional and inappropriate adolescent; even with the multiple medications, he maintained silly and inappropriate laughter; he remained profoundly regressed; he rocked continuously and also displayed other stereotypes. Eddy continued farting in groups without any concern. The progress of this child was very limited and the prognosis remained poor. Also see the related case of Louis, above.

Psychotic features are often associated with bipolar disorder and may be more common in adolescent onset mania than in adult onset (Kafantaris, Coletti, Dicker, Padula, & Kane, 2001, p. 1448). Bhangoo, Dell, et al. (2003)

found that the cardinal symptoms of mania (elation, grandiosity, pressured speech) and episodicity are strongly correlated. Psychosis, depressive episodes (meeting full DSM-IV criteria), and suicide attempts are all more common in the episodic group than in the chronic group (p. 512). Children in the episodic group are more likely to have a parent with bipolar disorder (p. 513). In affective psychosis, the psychotic features (hallucinations and delusions) are commonly congruous with the mood, there is no evidence of thought disorder, and in general the relatedness is intact. Some clinicians argue that when in doubt, one should diagnose a mood disorder rather than schizophrenia, because the latter has a less favorable prognosis and is less responsive to treatment (Weller, Weller, & Danielyan, 2004, p. 447).

Mental Retardation and Schizophrenia

Since the time of Kraepelin mental retardation has been considered a risk factor for schizophrenia. Under the term *Pfropfschizophrenia* he included 3.5 to 7% of cases of dementia precox he felt were "engrafted" in mental retardation (Mack, Feldman, & Tsuang, 2002, p. 1104). The current literature supports the idea that psychiatric disturbances are more common in patients with mental retardation than in persons with normal intelligence (p. 1107). Some authors suggest that the presence of low IQ might represent a general risk for psychopathology and psychosis rather than a specific risk for schizophrenia (Tsai & Champine, 2004, p. 387).

SCHIZOAFFECTIVE DISORDER

Jacob Kasanin introduced the term *schizoaffective* in 1933. Its specific meaning remains unclear. Patients who meet criteria for this diagnosis usually have a confusing blend of mood and psychotic symptoms. This disorder may encompass multiple etiologies (Strakowski, 2003, p. 23), and the diagnosis remains poorly validated (p. 27).

Four explanatory concepts regarding this condition have been advanced: (1) Schizoaffective disorder is a variant of schizophrenia. (2) Schizoaffective disorder is a variant of mood disorder. (3) Schizoaffective disorder represents a heterogeneous combination of schizophrenia and mood disorder (real schizoaffective disorder). (4) Psychotic disorders share a genetic vulnerability and exist on a continuum (p. 28).

Schizoaffective disorder appears to be an unreliable diagnosis. The term is often used to describe schizophrenic patients with mood symptoms or youth with active psychosis in the context of mood episodes. Many youths with emotional and behavioral dysregulation problems exhibit psychoticlike phenomena and are characterized as schizoaffective; their psychotic symptoms may be atypical and associated with chaotic social and abusive histories (Reimherr & McClellan, 2004, p.6). The DSM-IV-TR (2000) diagnostic criteria for schizoaffective disorder include:

> An uninterrupted period of illness during which, at some time, there is either a Major Depressive Episode, a Manic Episode, or a Mixed episode concurrent with symptoms that meet Criterion A for schizophrenia.[5]
> During the same period of illness, there have been delusions or hallucinations for at least 2 weeks in the absence of prominent mood symptom.
> Symptoms that meet criteria for a mood episode are present for a substantial portion of the total duration of the active and residual periods of the illness.
> The disturbance cannot be explained by the influence of a substance (drug of abuse or medication) or by a general medical condition (p. 323).

In most recent studies, neither first-rank symptoms nor other subtypes of psychotic symptoms (mood incongruent delusions or hallucinations) have been shown to specifically identify patients with schizophrenia. In fact no psychotic symptoms are considered pathognomonic for any specific disorder at this time (Strawkoski, 2003, p. 27). Clinicians will also be attentive to symptom switching during the patient's follow-up. Such a switch, changes the diagnosis and treatment orientation as illustrated in the following vignette:

> The "physicist," a 17-year–old, overweight male patient, had been followed for more than two years for chronic depression and a sense of futility and alienation. Frequently, he had felt that there was not a reason for him to live and had been hospitalized twice for suicidal behavior. A major source of internal pain was his sense of being ostracized by peers (feeling that peers disliked and hated him), and he had a deep inner sense that he was weird and abnormal. He also felt misunderstood and unappreciated; he felt frustrated that people did not pay enough attention to his quest for the solution of serious unsolved problems in the realm of physics. In particular, he was preoccupied with breaking the barrier of the speed of light, issues related to matter and antimatter, and other profound astrophysical enigmas. He carried with him notebooks filled with diagrams and designs of machines he dreamed would solve the problems physicists had been unable to resolve. When he made a presentation of his ideas, the psychiatrist felt that this adolescent was talking over the physician's head; the ideas did not look overtly bizarre, and he expounded on his ideas with significant coherence and enthusiasm. He claimed that he had presented his ideas to a real physicist who had responded to his ideas with some degree of interest; apparently, the physicist expressed that the patient's ideas were "plausible."
> The "physicist" had complained of a number of psychotic features for many years. He heard mumbling voices that impaired his concentration, and experienced florid paranoid ideation (he felt that people talked about him, watched him,

followed him, and that somehow, people were against him). He had difficulties attending school on a regular basis, because of his feeling of a lack of fitting in with his peer milieu. The "physicist" had insomnia for many years. He would stay up till 1 or 2 a.m., and the limited sleep that he achieved was interrupted by frequent awakenings. He felt continuously tired and unmotivated. Because of his obesity, a sleep study was requested; the study confirmed the presence of a severe sleep apnea. He began to use the PAP machine with some positive results. The "physicist's" clinical symptoms met DSM-IV-TR (2000) diagnostic criteria for a schizoaffective disorder, depressed type.

One day, the "physicist" came to his outpatient appointment in a frank state of mania: he was euphoric, hyperactive, and hypertalkative with obvious pressured speech. He declared to his psychiatrist that he had never felt "that good" in his life. He reported that he felt an unusual degree of energy, and that his thinking was very active; as a matter of fact, he endorsed that his thoughts were going very fast. He believed he had found the solutions to the conundrums that had preoccupied him. He brought a couple of bags in which he carried a number of contraptions he had created, one that purportedly extended the reception radius of a walkie-talkie, and the other, an engine he had constructed from discarded parts.

The diagnosis was changed; mood stabilizers were added to the antipsychotics he was receiving, and his antidepressants were tapered off. His mania subsided, his mood became more stable, and his paranoia decreased. He continued in outpatient treatment for several years and remained in a satisfactory level of adaptation.

PSYCHOTIC DISORDER NOS

Psychosis NOS comprises a sizable second group of patients commonly confused with VEOS and COS. In these children, the psychosis and disorganized behavior is transient and infrequent, and often occurs under stress. At times, the psychotic features are enduring. Adaptive functioning is not so globally impaired as in cases of schizophrenia. Affective dysregulation and aggressive behavior are quite common in these patients. The DSM-IV-TR (2000, p. 343) describes a number of issues related to the diagnosis of psychosis NOS. The case of Ivan is illustrative of a case of psychosis in a preadolescent boy:

Ivan, an 11-year-old white male, was seen for the first time 6 years before for disruptive and aggressive behaviors. Hyperactivity, impulsivity, and difficulties with temper tantrums became a problem by age 3. There were concerns about the rate of his learning. He had history of severe sleep problems for the first three years of his life. He walked at 15 months of age and had a background of speech and language delays: he started talking by the end of the second year. 6 years prior to the psychiatric evaluation, he received the diagnosis of developmental expressive and receptive language disorder and ADHD. This background is consistent with risks for VEOS/COS.

During the first psychiatric evaluation, when he was 11 years old, it was noticed that he was illogical, and made bizarre statements: he claimed that, "my tummy talks to me." Psychological testing, two years before, revealed a WISC-III Full Scale IQ of 81, VIQ of 72, and PIQ of 94. Mixed receptive expressive language disorder, learning disorder NOS, ADHD, and conduct disorder were diagnosed.

Ivan claimed he had been hearing voices for the previous six years. One year earlier, he reported auditory hallucinations mocking him and commanding him to do bad things. About that time, his mother found him trying to stab himself with a stick. He disclosed experiencing voices threatening him if he didn't do what they told him to do. The voices had told him to kill his sister, his parents, and to harm himself. He also heard the voices cursing. He became frightened at night, fearing that somebody could get into his room and kill him. When he was challenged as to the reality of the hallucinations, he claimed that the hallucinations were very real to him.

Months later, Ivan was admitted to an acute care hospital because of suicidal behavior; this followed his fabricated story that he had been having sex with his sister, three years his senior, "to get her in trouble." At that time Ivan revealed that he had been sexually penetrated by an older adolescent male one year before. He displayed strong paranoid ideation at that time: he felt that there were cameras everywhere taking pictures of him, and he was terrified of having AIDS or other serious illnesses. Command hallucinations were corroborated, as well as persecutory delusion of people coming to kill him.

Ivan claimed that there were times when the voices made him laugh, and even with treatment with antipsychotics he continued complaining of paranoid ideation, that he still felt that somebody followed him, and that he still felt that people were after him.

Ivan was a likable and engaging child. He was somewhat insightful and he displayed an appropriate, though somewhat constricted affect. There was no evidence of thought disorder. The diagnosis of psychotic disorder NOS was appropriate. Comorbid traumatic and anxiety disorders were likely.

There is an association between PTSD and psychosis NOS: there is a high frequency of PTSD and abuse histories in children with a diagnosis of psychosis NOS. This suggests that some of the atypical psychotic symptoms are posttraumatic phenomena. In one study, a high percentage of the sample characterized as having psychosis NOS also had significant mood and behavioral dysregulation, and many of these patients met criteria for borderline personality disorder. Transient psychotic symptoms are one of the characteristics of that disorder (McClellan, Breiger, McCurry, & Hlastala, 2003, p. 670).

Both the experience of abuse before age 18, and its frequency (dosing) were highly correlated with the development of psychosis (auditory and visual hallucinations, and paranoid ideation). Subjects who reported abuse in the highest frequency had an estimated 30 times greater chance to develop the diagnosis of psychosis than those without any exposure to childhood abuse (Krabbendam, Hanssen, Vollebergh, et al., 2004, p. 41). Furthermore, in both clinical and nonclinical populations, the diagnostic group with the highest rate of childhood abuse consistently reported the most Schneiderian symptoms (p. 39). The authors suggested that reported childhood abuse predicted psychotic symptoms in adulthood in a dose-response fashion. The association between childhood abuse and psychotic symptoms was robust and remained significant after adjustment for possible confounders (p. 42).

Confusingly, children diagnosed with psychosis NOS have high familial rates of schizophrenia and schizophrenia spectrum disorders, enlarged ventricles, and smooth pursuit eye tracking abnormalities, similar to those with COS.

A two- to six-year follow-up of 27 cases with the diagnosis of psychotic disorder NOS revealed that none developed schizophrenia; 50% developed a defined mood disorder (3, schizoaffective disorder; 4, bipolar disorder; 6, major depression (Nicolson, Lenane, Brookner, et al., 2001).

Postpsychotic Adjustment State (PPAS)

A condition described in adults is also likely to be present in children and adolescents. The postpsychotic adjustment state (PPAS) is a phenomenon more than a diagnosis; it denotes a change in mental state after the experience of a psychotic episode. Proponents of this condition consider that a psychotic episode is a traumatic experience, and that PPAS is often misdiagnosed as a relapse or as an exacerbation of schizophrenic symptoms. PPAS is characterized as intense feelings of fear (that symptoms may return and of inability of regain or maintain control), a sense of failure, humiliation, shame, anxiety, and anger associated with the psychotic episode. Fear is probably the most debilitating component of the condition. Patients undergoing PPAS begin to lose interest in treatment and in trying to recover. They may appear depressed and undergo a number of medication changes. By the end of the first year many patients feel overwhelmed and give up. After the second year the changes are permanent; the patient loses interest in life goals, and what appears to be apathy represents a loss of courage or persistence. Profound sadness, reluctance to move forward, and hopelessness are common. Whereas illness exacerbations require medication adjustments, PPAS requires psychotherapy and psychosocial support (*Clinical Psychiatric News*, October 2003, p. 28).

OTHER PSYCHOTIC DISORDERS

Catatonia

Taylor and Fink (2003) propose that catatonia be classified independently from other syndromes, similar to the identification and classification of delirium (p.

TABLE 7.5 Selective Causes of Secondary Catatonia

Medical conditions

>   Brain tumor
>   Cerebral anoxia
>   Cerebrovascular disease
>   Closed head injury
>   CNS vasculitis
>   Encephalitis (acute or post-infectious)
>   HIV encephalopathy
>   Neurosyphilis
>   Normal pressure hydrocephalus
>   Seizure disorders
>   Uremia
>   Parkinson's

Medications or toxic substances

>   Carbon monoxide
>   Corticosteroids
>   Cyclobenzaprine
>   Disulfiram
>   Ecstasy
>   Neuroleptics
>   Sedative-hypnotic withdrawal
>   Phencyclidine
>   Tetraethyl lead poisoning

Source: Levenson (2005, p.18).

1238). For selected causes of secondary catatonia, related to medical conditions or medications, see table 7.5.

Stupor or catalepsy, mutism, negativism, posturing (waxy flexibility), grimacing, stereotypies, echolalia and echopraxia, or pronounced hyperactivity, are the most prominent clinical features of catatonia; this syndrome is seen in adolescents and less commonly in preadolescents. The retarded or stuporous variety is the most common form of catatonia. The excited form is less common but is more malignant and frequently overlooked. The excited form is often accompanied by fever and autonomic imbalances, and needs to be differentiated from the neuroleptic malignant, serotonin syndrome, delirium, akathisia, mania, schizophrenic agitation, and severe ADHD.

Prior to 1970, catatonia was closely associated with schizophrenia; currently, catatonia is more commonly aligned with mood disorders. Many psychiatric disorders present with catatonia: mania and depression; neurological and medical illnesses; autism and developmental disorders; mental retardation and schizophrenia. The catatonic syndrome is most often associated with affective disorders. It is considered that catatonia is present in about 10% of patients admitted to acute psychiatric services (Fink, 2002, p. 28).

Only 10 to 15% of patients with catatonia meet criteria for schizophrenia;

25% or more of manic patients met diagnostic criteria for catatonia, and more than half of catatonic patients have manic–depressive illness (Taylor & Fink, 2003, p. 1237). Pediatric catatonia is more often found in boys than in girls, with similar characteristics, similar precipitants, and the same response to treatment as adult catatonia (Fink, 2002, pp. 28–29). Exposure to either typical or atypical antipsychotics usually worsens catatonia or induces a malignant form (Taylor & Fink, 2003, p. 1237).

Fink considers that catatonia is, "sufficiently frequent among children and adolescents that any young patient with stupor, unexplained excitement, or persistent motor signs should be formally assessed for it. The differential diagnosis (in order of decreasing frequency) is mood disorders, seizure disorder, developmental disorder and autism, and schizophrenia (p. 29). The case of Glenda illustrates some complex issues related to catatonia in preadolescence.

This 9½-year-old white child was readmitted to an acute preadolescent psychiatric program after she began to bang her head at school, stating that she wanted to kill herself. That same day, she lost control and started hitting, screaming, and biting; she also scratched one of her teachers. The night prior to the readmission she shaved her eyebrows and cut her arms. She also swallowed buttons with the intention of killing herself. She ran out of the gym into traffic, putting herself at great risk. Five days before, she alleged that her "grampa" James had fondled her "vagina."

The prior admission had been less than a month before, and had been precipitated by a severe anger outburst at school: she refused to go into the classroom, had started yelling, became self-abusive (head banging, stabbing her arms with a pencil), and had threatened to kill a classmate. Glenda also had expressed a suicidal plan, saying she was planning to kill herself with a kitchen knife by cutting her throat.

Glenda had demonstrated difficulties with anger control for the previous three months, and had become progressively defiant and oppositional at school. She reported experiencing nightmares about women getting raped by a man. Glenda had a long history of ADHD. She also cried easily and had stated that she was ugly; actually, she was a pretty blue-eyed young girl. She had a history of hematuria, and apparently she had a urinary reflux. Glenda had right hearing loss and had been in special education.

Glenda's rearing environment had been unstable: some time in the past Glenda accused father of throwing rocks at her, and because of physical abuse and neglect by her biological mother, she had lived with her biological father for nine months. Glenda's mother believed that her biological father had physically and sexually abused Glenda and her older sister, one year her senior. Maternal grandmother had taken care of the children while their biological mother was in prison for nine months. Glenda's mother had remarried 18 months before, and her stepfather was described as strict; apparently, he was the main disciplinarian in the family. During the earlier hospitalization her mother did not visit Glenda and did not attend any scheduled family appointments.

According to her biological mother, Glenda had a severe problem with her temper. The girl had called 911 (when mother and her boyfriend were fighting). Mother reported that she had to sleep by the front door to prevent Glenda from running out at night. Glenda had verbalized that her mother's boyfriend was scary, that he called her mother names, and that, "he screamed and spanked the girls." Glenda complained of nightmares "of two girls being raped by a man at school." She also reported hearing voices telling her to kill her mother. Child protective services had been involved with this family due to allegations of abuse. Glenda had been removed from the mother at least one time before.

Apparently, Glenda witnessed her biological father abusing her mother. Her mother was in prison for nine months for "writing hot checks" and had been treated with Paxil in the past. There was a history of depression in the maternal grandmother. The biological father was in prison for robbery. He is said to have suffered from anxiety attacks. A biological sister was on Celexa for depression and had a prior psychiatric hospitalization, and a maternal uncle was also in treatment for depression and had been hospitalized for severe depression when he was 16 years old.

Glenda's mental status examination revealed the presence of a very attractive but nonrelating female preadolescent. She appeared to be her stated age. She was markedly withdrawn and displayed a marked decrease in psychomotor activity. She was very difficult to engage; her eye contact was poor. She did not utter any spontaneous verbalizations and refused to answer any questions. She appeared self-absorbed and internally preoccupied. At times, she seemed to stare. The mood appeared depressed with blunted affect. With some encouragement and efforts at engagement, Glenda began to respond in short sentences. She endorsed that she was hearing voices telling her to run away and to kill her mother. She did not respond to questions regarding orientation and her intellectual functions were difficult to assess.

During the hospitalization, a number of observers noted that Glenda was very withdrawn and that she stared a lot. The author once observed that Glenda was mute, akinetic, negativistic, and blunted. At that time, she displayed cereas flexibilities: when the examiner raised one of her hands, she kept the hand raised for a very long time, apparently indifferent to her body sensations, and also seemingly neglectful of her surroundings.

Because of the staring, an EEG was requested; results showed nonfocal paroxysmal bilateral activity. Benzodiazepines failed to provide a visible improvement in her catatonic picture. She was started on valproic acid, sertraline, and risperidone. With this combination there was a progressive improvement in her depression and withdrawal; she reported that the psychotic features, both hallucinations and paranoid feelings, disappeared. Glenda's relatedness and capacity for engagement improved markedly; she was able to relate in a warmer manner, to maintain better eye contact, and to communicate verbally with a natural discursive speech.

This vignette is interesting because of the association of catatonic behavior with epilepsy and a mood disorder. The next two vignettes describe first, a very severe catatonia in a preadolescent, and then a periodic catatonia in an adolescent.

> An 11-year-old Hispanic girl was admitted to an acute preadolescent program for severe withdrawal. She had stopped communicating with the family, began to neglect herself to the point where she didn't care about her hygiene, and most importantly, she had stopped eating. She would remain motionless for long periods of time; she needed to be encouraged, even assisted, in her most basic care. She would stare indifferently for long periods of time. She would stay in a place without change of position for extended periods of time. She displayed cereas flexibilities. The neurological evaluation, including an EEG was noncontributory.
>
> She was started on progressive doses of clonazepam, which brought about a decisive change in her demeanor and emotional state. As the clonazepam dose was increased her clinical state became progressively better. This patient received up to 12 mg of clonazepam a day; at this dose her catatonic symptoms vanished and she showed no evidence of sedation.

> Bert, an 18-year-old Hispanic male, with history of previous catatonic episodes, was readmitted to an acute care program for progressive withdrawal. His family, familiar with symptoms due to two previous similar episodes, began to notice progressive withdrawal and inability to communicate with him for the previous 72 hours. He had started a job two weeks previously, and apparently had been doing well.
>
> Bert had his first catatonic episode the first day of his senior year of high school, one year before. His family believed that this was the first time in Bert's life that he was not around his older brother, two years his senior. The family felt he had panicked. At the time of the readmission, he was unresponsive, and akinetic. His speech was incoherent, and his affect was blunted. He stared all the time. He revealed he had heard voices but was unclear as to the nature of the auditory hallucinations. At times he looked self-absorbed and confused.
>
> Neurological evaluations were not contributory. Bert showed distinct deterioration in his clinical state every time he was exposed to antipsychotics. He responded readily to benzodiazepines and a SSRI. Upon the remission of the catatonic state, Bert was a high functioning individual and in between his catatonic episodes, there was no appreciable residual pathology. He was advised to remain on prophylactic benzodiazepines. The last time the author saw Bert, he came to the office with his fiancée to announce he was getting married and was moving out of state.

Up to 50 to 70% of catatonic patients respond to lorazepam or amobarbital (Taylor & Fink, 2003, p. 1235). The neuroleptic malignant syndrome and malignant catatonia (see pp. 408–410), cannot be differentiated either clinically or by laboratory testing. Currently, the neuroleptic malignant syndrome is considered a specific form of malignant catatonia (Taylor & Fink, 2003, p. 1236). Benzodiazepine and ECT are the standard treatments for malignant catatonia; these treatments have proven to be equally successful with the neuroleptic malignant syndrome (p. 1236). Exposure to either typical or atypical antipsychotics usually worsens catatonia or induces a malignant form (p. 1237).

Perisse et al. (2003) reported the case of a 16-year-old adolescent hospitalized for depression and catatonic features who had been diagnosed with systemic lupus erythematosus (SLE) six months before. She displayed florid catatonic features. MRI and CSF were unremarkable. Labs corroborated the diagnosis of SLE. Catatonia did not respond to benzodiazepines. Because her condition became life-threatening, plasma exchange was implemented (pp. 497–498). The authors stated that etiopathogenic investigations are mandatory when dealing with catatonic presentations, even in young people (p. 499).

It is interesting to note that catatonialike behavior can be feigned. The author observed a case of catatonia factitia that could fool experts.

> One Saturday morning during weekend rounds, when the examiner was documenting on another child, he overheard a staff commotion regarding an 8-year-old Hispanic female who was unresponsive to repeated stimulation. The examiner went to the child's room to examine her. The girl did not respond to verbal commands, or to strong physical stimulation. The vital signs were: P, 72, regular; BP, 80/60; T, 37.5; R, 12. Auscultation: Normal sinus rhythm, no murmurs; good ventilation sounds. Patient had a good color and a good state of hydration. The patient did not respond to painful stimulation such as the squeezing of the Achilles tendon. No evidence of spasticity or meningeal signs. Tendon reflexes were symmetrical, ++, throughout. No abnormal reflexes. Plantar reflex: no Babinski signs. There was one finding that seemed peculiar: when the examiner attempted to examine the patient's eyes, it appeared that the she made an effort to move the eyes upward making it difficult for the examiner to check her eyes.
>
> The examiner ordered hourly neurological checks, monitoring of input and output, and ordered a stop of all the psychotropic medications. The examiner went back to his desk to document the contact. While doing this, the head nurse asked the examiner if he had seen what the patient had just done. The examiner responded in the negative. The head nurse saw the patient sitting up on the bed putting her socks on! Half an hour after the examination, the patient woke up and began roaming the unit. The examiner was very intrigued by the patient's behavior and attempted to get some verbalization. When the patient was asked how many times she had done this, she smiled. When she was asked to tell how long she had done it, she did not respond. She remained quiet and guarded regarding the incident. She was a very attractive girl and displayed a nice and innocent smile.
>
> She had been hospitalized for anger outbursts, physical aggression, and self-abusive behavior that included self-biting and self-scratching. The caretaker also complained that she did not want to wake up in the mornings. There were complaints that she tended to isolate and to withdraw. Some staff members in a previous group home had observed that she laughed inappropriately. She had a prior hospitalization in another facility. The patient had been removed from her mother three weeks before due to neglect and physical abuse. Sexual abuse by mother's boyfriend had also been suspected.

Last but not least, neuroleptic medications (typicals and atypicals) may induce catatoniclike side effects. If the patient under investigation is receiving antipsychotic medications, this possibility should be considered in the differential diagnosis.

Shared Psychosis (folie à deux)

Shared psychosis is an infrequent phenomenon. Two presentations of shared psychosis are commonly observed in children and adolescents: shared psychosis between intimate siblings (twins in particular), and shared psychosis between a disturbed parent and a child. In both instances there is a particularly close relationship between the subjects and a marked degree of isolation from alternative views or influences. The couple or group that participates in a shared psychosis, share a distorted worldview that lacks consensual validation by the society at large. In shared psychosis, a pathological system is maintained and supported by the parties involved. This can be the case with twins, for example, much more so if they are identical, because of a very close, intimate, secretive, and exclusive relationship. See the DSM-IV-TR (2000) diagnostic criteria for shared psychotic disorder (p. 334).

A disturbed (psychotic) parent, due to the position of power, influence, and control over the child, may exercise overpowering effects over the child's perception of reality or over the way the world or other people are viewed. Two examples of shared psychosis will be presented. The first is a case of shared psychosis in monozygotic, 10-year-old twins, and the second, a case of shared psychosis between a mother and her adolescent daughter.

> Ten-year-old twin sisters required emergency evaluation due to aggressive, regressive, and psychotic behavior. The oldest twin (A) had lit a fire in the home bathroom and had burnt her sister's nose (B) while she slept. Twin A had been aggressive toward peers and had threatened to kill her sister. This twin bickered and fought a great deal. Apparently, the older twin was physically abusive toward her younger one when she did not do what the older twin wanted. The older twin also appeared to be sexually preoccupied: she was found in the boys' bathroom and had been observed kissing boys. It appeared she had started kissing boys a couple of years before. Prior to the evaluation mother had found the twins naked in their room; on that occasion, the older twin had been found on top of the younger one. Mother also found twin A with a vibrator on the floor. Mother stated that twin A was constantly dancing like a stripper. Mother also complained that twin A did not seem to have any sense of fear, that she was full of energy, and that she had a big problem sleeping. She would not fall sleep until 2 a.m., and would be back on her feet by 4 a.m. She would climb up to the second floor and would jump onto electrical boxes. She was constantly restless and on the go. Mother stated that this twin seemed to believe that "she ran everything and that she talked too much."

A younger sister had died in a house fire when the twins were 3 years old and it was alleged that the older twin had witnessed the burning of the younger sister. Both twins had witnessed physical abuse in the household. Apparently, father had been brutally abusive to the twins' mother in the past. It was not clear if the twin had suffered physical or sexual abuse, but twin A overreacted every time her father was mentioned, and would scream: "I would kill him for what he has done." Contact between the twins and the biological father was limited. It was alleged that biological father had a history of incarceration and that he was a mob member. There was strong family history of mood disorders, and of bipolar disorders, on both parental sides.

The older twin also had history of antisocial behavior such as stealing, extortion from peers at school, lying, fighting, and bullying. She was failing fourth grade. This twin frequently complained of stomach pain. A complete GI series had been completed, and the results were unremarkable. There had not been a prior psychiatric treatment before.

Mother had divorced the twins' father 8 years before, and had remarried. This was an unsuccessful marriage, too; there was discord and fighting, "all the time." Mother had separated from her second husband six months before, and seemingly, the twins had displayed behavioral deterioration since.

Both twins claimed that the dead sister was talking to them, that she was asking them to join her. Both twins also claimed that they saw the dead sister, that they saw her intermittently around the house, playing. The twins' mother spent an undue amount of time outside the house leaving the children under the care of a sickly maternal grandfather and a close friend.

During the mental status examination the older twin expressed a prominent fascination with fire and indicated that she had almost burnt the house down with a fire she had started at home, the day before. She claimed she had visions of her dead sister and asserted that she heard her voice, and that her sister told her to come to her. She indicated that she had an angel on one shoulder and a devil on the other, adding that the devil told her to do bad things.

The younger twin (twin B) had suffered from depression for about six months, had become progressively withdrawn, and had a very poor appetite. This twin slept all the time. She had stated she wanted to die to be with her sister; apparently, she had also witnessed her sister being burned. Twin B had aggressive control problems at school, displayed temper tantrums and crying spells. She had a history of suicidal ideation and had attempted to jump from the second floor balcony the day before. She also had visual hallucinations regarding her dead sister. She had been quite clingy and had sought physical contact with her mother more frequently. She was described as very dependent, slept in a fetal position, and sucked her finger; she slept with her mother, and couldn't sleep on her own. Mother stated that this twin saw and heard her dead baby sister who apparently was very close to her. Mother reported that the younger twin was not interested in sex, but she liked to play with boys and play a "boy's" role. Her twin sister ran her life. She endorsed being depressed for years and cried a lot; when feeling sad she felt like going to sleep. She reported that she heard her baby sister telling her to kill herself and to come and be with her. She revealed that she had tried to kill herself before; from time to time, this twin's behavior was very regressed.

The twins shared a pathological system of beliefs regarding their dead sister; their psychotic symptomatology had a striking similarity. The twins had parallel behavioral and emotional problems.

The adult–child example follows:

A 16-year-old adolescent female needed an emergency evaluation due to a suicide attempt; she had taken many pills because she wanted to kill herself; she had felt overwhelmed. She had been self-abusive and had overdosed six months before. She also felt homicidal every time she felt angry. There had been a number of unexplained events, which the adolescent found uncanny, if not mysterious, very hard for her to explain. According to her, those events defied rational explanations. She felt that people were spying on her, and had other paranoid and unusual experiences; she felt guilty for "hanging around" friends her mother disapproved of. She had a history of school truancy and school suspensions. She had initiated sexual behavior five months before but the circumstance of that initiation was unclear. Mother believed that her daughter had been coerced to have sex; as a matter of fact, she had started counseling at the rape crisis center. This adolescent had been involved with marijuana, cocaine, acid, and alcohol.

When the adolescent attempted to explain the baffling experiences, her mother supported her irrational beliefs. This adolescent had been depressed for more than three years. and she had a background of self-abusive behavior, skipping school, and drug abuse. Mother had a prolonged history of mental illness with multiple hospitalizations including admissions to the local state hospital. Mother had received a variety of diagnoses including paranoid schizophrenia, bipolar, and schizoaffective disorder. She had discontinued psychiatric treatment for the previous two years and had received disability payments the previous two years. The adolescent patient had never known her biological father and there was no contact with her extended family. Mother and daughter had cut contact with the extended family.

This patient was an attractive, depressed looking adolescent, anxious and hesitant; she constantly sought her mother's support as well as confirmation of her assertions. In particular, mother attempted to give credence to her daughter's distorted beliefs. The adolescent endorsed florid paranoid ideation: felt that people talked about her, watched her, felt followed, and felt that somebody was after her. Furthermore, she felt that people could read her mind, believed that people could put thoughts in her mind, and that people could take thoughts away from her mind. The patient felt she had special qualities and felt that other people were jealous of her.

During the conjoint interview of child and the mother, and when the examiner was documenting that there was history of mental illness in the family (the examiner was subvocalizing while he was transcribing), the mother began to expresses fear and concern. She wondered if the examiner was going to take her daughter away, because he had made it a point to emphasize that, "she was mentally ill" (mother). By the end of the interview, after the examiner asked the mother if she was dating anyone, she wondered if the examiner had seen that in her eyes!

It became clear that in this enmeshed relationship, mother and daughter partook of abnormal beliefs and that mother had a pathological influence on her daughter's reality testing; furthermore, mother supported her daughter's abnormal beliefs and rationalizations.

POSTPARTUM PSYCHOSIS

It is estimated that the prevalence of postpartum psychosis is approximately 1 case per 1,000 births and it is important to consider this condition when adolescents have recently given birth. Symptoms start rather abruptly, and include confusion, hallucinations, and delusions, labile mood, and mixed affective states (dysphoric mania). About half of the cases start in the first week, and about 75% of the cases occur within the first two weeks after delivery (Chaudron, 2003, pp. 54–55).

Three theories predominate in the literature on postpartum psychosis: (1) It is a variant of bipolar disorder. (2) It is a unique diagnostic entity. (3) It is not associated with any specific psychotic illness. It is considered that childbirth triggers postpartum psychosis and other various psychotic illnesses. The greater part of the evidence supports a link between bipolar disorder and postpartum psychosis (Chaundron, 2003, p. 56). Women with bipolar disorder are at a higher risk for an episode during the postpartum period than during any other time in their lives, much more so if they had a prior puerperal episode. Longitudinal studies indicate that women who have an initial diagnosis of puerperal psychosis are at increased risk of developing further affective episodes both puerperal and nonpuerperal. In an Australian study it was found that 86% of women with puerperal psychosis met criteria for bipolar disorder.

ANOREXIA NERVOSA (AN)

Anorexia nervosa patients seem to be delusional about their body image including shape and size. These misperceptions have been considered a body image disturbance or body dissatisfaction. Some patients report hearing an anorexic voice, coming from an external source; other female anorexics describe hearing a male voice telling them not to eat. Anorexics also share with schizophrenics, cognitive deficits and neuroimaging findings such as enlarged cerebral ventricles and a decrease in white and gray matter (Powers, Simpson, & McCormick, 2005, p. 40).

FACTITOUS DISORDERS

Children, and adolescents in particular, may feign psychotic symptoms for ulterior motives. The author has observed manipulation of the claim of the presence of psychotic features in the following circumstances:

> Adolescents in detention centers make up psychotic or other psychiatric symptoms, to seek a transfer to less restrictive settings. Manipulative adolescents know that the courts tend to divert juveniles to mental health settings rather than to detention centers when there is indication of psychiatric illness. The reasons behind the feigned catatonia described above were unclear. Some children attempt to avoid responsibility for their own behavior by "blaming the voices" for aggressive, antisocial, or other acting out behaviors.
>
> Children and adolescents feign psychotic illness or other symptoms to seek a safe haven when they want to escape abusive and neglectful environments.
>
> Deprived mentally ill children seek the caring and structure of the hospital setting when they do not find satisfaction of those needs at home.
>
> Addicted adolescents make up symptoms, including psychotic symptoms, in an attempt to obtain mind-altering medications.
>
> Occasionally, adolescents feign psychotic symptoms to buttress their claim for psychiatric disability.

Resnick and Knoll (2005) distinguish malingering from factitious disorders; in malingering there is an intentional production of false or greatly exaggerated physical or psychological symptoms, motivated for external circumstances. In factitious disorders, the patient's motivation is internal or psychological and centers on assuming a sick role (p. 14). However, Samuel and Mittenberg (2005) state that there is a false dichotomy between factitious disorders and malingering, and that in clinical practice these conditions often overlap (p. 61).

Clinicians will find inconsistencies in the pseudopsychotic claims: when these adolescents are asked to explain the "symptom," the elaborations show lack of consistency and are discrepant from known psychotic experiences; furthermore, the alleged symptom is not accompanied by the correspondent affect. The examiner, sooner rather than later, will detect evidence of manipulation and other sociopathic traits. On the other hand, the content of the "psychotic symptoms" do not explain the degree of distress or impairment that the patient alleges. The clinician learns in the course of the interview(s), that the patients attempt to "force the symptom," upon the examiner, often stressing the presence of the "symptom," though being unable to reveal clinically meaningful and consitent details. The more the clinician challenges the symptom the greater might be the person's attempts to convince the examiner of the factuality of the fabulation. This is consistent with Resnick and Knoll (2005), who indicate that the malingerer attempts to "thrust forward" the illness whereas persons with genuine schizophrenia are reluctant to discuss their symptoms. Furthermore, the malingerer attempts to take control of the interview and behaves in an intimidating and hostile manner (p. 20).

In forensic cases, the presence of psychotic features has significant importance in the attribution of legal responsibility and in the sentencing phase. Forensic psychiatrists use a multimodal approach for data gathering (including extensive interviews, collateral information, extended observations, psychological testing, and others) to assist the court in ascertaining legal responsibility over the action or behaviors in question.

CHAPTER 8

Etiology and Pathogenesis

The nature of causality of mood and psychotic symptoms is complex and evolving. Investigations from different perspectives are under way to elucidate the nature of the origins and maintenance of these disturbances. There is increasing evidence that primary psychotic disorders (bipolar disorder and schizophrenia) are expressions of altered neurobiology. Progress is being made at the genetic and molecular level in the identification of fundamental factors underlying the cause of the major psychotic disorders. Impressive progress has been made at the neurochemical, electrophysiological, and imaging fields.

There is a lack of understanding of how endophenotypes and other factors determine the initiation, course, and perpetuation of the disease processes; however, significant progress has being made in the genetic field. It is progressively evident that multiple factors including genetic, constitutional, gestational/obstetric, developmental, environmental, psychological, and family experiences, among others, may be involved in the disease process of chronic psychotic disorders. The controversy of nature vs nurture has lost the intensity of former years, and a more integrative thinking continues evolving to explain why persons at risk may become clinical cases by adverse experiences or circumstances. Scientific efforts focus in the identification of biological markers that could assist in early identification and intervention of severe psychotic disorders.

The elucidation of the genome promises to advance the understanding of genotypes and how phenotypes evolve, and will also assist in the clarification of the pathophysiology of these disorders. A better understanding of the genome will provide new opportunities for the understanding of the basic vulnerabilities and the development of new psychopharmacological treatments for mood and psychotic disorders. There is also an expectation that the expression of these disorders may be forestalled if early detection is assured.

In relation to bipolar disorders, Swann (2006) advises that:

> [W]e must question our assumptions about bipolar disorder." Is affective disturbance basic to bipolar disorder? Is affect an epiphenomenon of a more fundamental disturbance in regulating functions like motivation, arousal, or reinforcement? Are there potential physiological or behavioral markers that can be used clinically

to identify a bipolar disorder before an individual becomes manic? It is not appreciated enough that the basis of bipolar disorder is not depression or mania; rather, bipolar disorder is an illness that confers abnormal susceptibility to these mood states (p. 177).

ARE MOOD DISORDERS AND SCHIZOPHRENIA SPECTRUM DISORDERS DISTINCT ENTITIES?

For decades, a clear distinction between schizophrenia and affective disorders was emphasized. In 1989, Eggers "concluded that the simple classification of functional psychosis into schizophrenic and affective is highly questionable and certainly oversimplified" (p. 340). The view of opposition between these disorders is changing. Early behavioral genetic studies led to the conclusion that there were separable genetic liabilities for schizophrenia and major affective disorders (bipolar disorder and psychotic depression). More recent evidence indicates that this is not the case. Researches have shown that there is a significant overlap in the genes that contribute to schizophrenia, affective disorders and manic syndromes (Walker, Kestler, Bollini, & Hochman, 2004, p. 409). Buckley, Gowans, et al. (2004) stated that recent literature on the course and outcome of schizophrenia and bipolar disorders, as well as several historical reviews, have strengthened the perception that the boundaries between schizophrenia and bipolar disorders are far from clear-cut even when cases of schizoaffective disorder are discarded (p. 50).

Adler and Strakowski (2003) summarize the apparent similarities between schizophrenia and bipolar disorders. They indicate that several lines of evidence support suggestions that schizophrenia and bipolar disorders represent aspects of a single larger illness or group of overlapping disorders. Schizophrenia and bipolar disorders may be indistinguishable in clinical presentation, may include a spectrum of cognitive deficits that seems to increase with severity over time, and may be treated with similar psychopharmacological agents. There is an impressive demographic overlap and there are also pronounced similarities in the proposed causes. Both disorders involve suggestions of environmental insults, although the evidence for developmental abnormalities is greater for schizophrenia. Both disorders are postulated to involve genetic susceptibility and there is even overlap in the proposed susceptibility loci. Schizophrenia and bipolar disorders may be associated with abnormalities of diffuse, largely overlapping brain regions (p. 9).

Mortensen, Pedersen, Melbye, Moors, and Ewald (2003) support an overlapping of conceptualization between schizophrenia and bipolar disorder. These authors found a strong association between the risk of bipolar disorder and a history of bipolar disorder (as well as other psychiatric disorders, including schizophrenia and schizoaffective disorder) in parents and siblings. The authors also found an association between the death of the parent in early childhood (before age 5) and bipolar disorder, implicating nongenetic and genetic risk factors (p. 1214). These conclusions are qualified by the authors' assertion that schizophrenia and bipolar disorders are at least partially separate etiological entities (p. 1214).

Adler and Strakowski (2003) also emphasized the dissimilarities between schizophrenia and bipolar disorders: epidemiology does not support the view that schizophrenia and bipolar disorders represent a single disorder or a group of interrelated disorders. There is limited convergence of the two disorders within single-family lineages, and in instances in which there is family concurrence, schizophrenic patients with first-degree relatives diagnosed with bipolar disorders seemed to be qualitatively different from patients with schizophrenia who did not have such a relative (p. 9). In relation to this controversy, Buckley, Gowanset, al. (2004) concluded that the extent of the overlap evidence is not overwhelming and that is not consistent across studies, and that the current classifications of distinction between schizophrenia and mood disorders should be kept as a benchmark until more satisfactory neurobiological based systems or grouping emerge (p. 54).

ETIOLOGY, GENETIC FACTORS

A variety of family, twin, and adoption studies have demonstrated significant genetic influences on susceptibility to major depressive disorders and to bipolar disorders (Todd & Botteron, 2002, p. 500). The same is true for the schizophrenic spectrum disorders.

How genetic factors get ultimately expressed in an identifiable phenotype is unclear. It is plausible that genes exert a determining role in a number of ways: first, density and sensitivity of the receptors; second, levels and ratios of the neurotransmitter systems; third, the nature of the mitochondrial enzyme systems (i.e., CYP-450, and other metabolic pathways); fourth, pharmacokinetics and related issues; fifth, temperament; sixth, resilience to stress; seventh, the integrity of the CNS; eighth, neural connectivity; ninth, variation of biorhythms; tenth, immunological variables, and others.

Increasing attention is being paid to the elucidation of endophenotypes, which have a fundamental role in the elicitation of the disease process. Endophenotypes relate to basic structural or functional defects that ultimately have a decisive role in illness expression. Endophenotypes may be identified long before a prodromal or frank disease state is expressed.

Modern studies suggest that, on the average, parents, siblings, and offspring of individuals with schizophrenia have a risk of illness, about 12 times greater than that of the general population (Gur et al, 2005, p. 101). Parents of childhood-onset schizophrenia patients have an over tenfold increased risk for the development of schizophrenia (p. 101). Neuromotor difficulties, attentional and memory deficits, and other executive deficits are consistently observed in longitudinal studies of at risk children (p. 145). Neuromotor dysfunction in early childhood predicts the presence of attentional impairments under high processing demands during early adolescence; also, neuromotor dysfunction and attentional difficulties during adolescence predict the development of schizophrenia-related psychoses. Cortico-striatal pathways are implicated in the pathophysiology of schizophrenia. Striatal dysfuction results in impaired sequential motor performance and difficulties in the chunking of action sequences. Impairments in a variety of attentional functions, including self-shifting and self-monitoring, are also associated with striatal dysfunction (pp. 149–150).

According to Hirshfeld-Becker et al. (2006), behavior disinhibition might be elevated among the offspring of parents with bipolar disorder. Accumulating evidence suggests that: (1) the trait of behavioral disinhibition is related to a number of behavior outcomes (such as, oppositional defiant and conduct disorders, comorbid mood disorders), common prodromes or associated features, of bipolar spectrum disorders in affected individuals and at risk offspring; longitudinal studies suggest that early externalizing or affective symptoms precede the onset of bipolar disorder; (2) studies support links between bipolar disorders and specific personality styles suggestive of personality disinhibition (including, "hyperthynic personality"), novelty-seeking, extroversion, and the approach of novelty. In summary, offspring at risk for bipolar disorder may show a trajectory from behavioral disinhibition in the preschool years to disruptive behavior and bipolar disorder in childhood and adolescents (p. 265).

Follow-up studies suggest that only 50% of early psychosis patients go on to develop a chronic schizophrenia form with poor level of functioning and intellectual deficits (Hirschfeld-Becker et al., 2006, p. 100). Excessive pruning may occur before or around the illness onset.

Neurodevelopment, neurodegeneration, adolescent changes, and environmental stressors, individually or in combination converge to produce the psychotic syndrome. It is being accepted that most people or even every person who develops the psychotic syndrome may have had a developmental vulnerability, although this may not have seemed obvious before the syndrome became overt (Gur et al., 2005, p. 141). "[I]t can be genuinely debated whether it will ever be possible, regardless of technological advances, to trace in a clear and unambiguous fashion a complete set of causal links from DNA base-pair variation to a complex biobehavioral phenomenon such as schizophrenia or depression" (Kendler, 2005, p. 8).

Genetic epidemiology has clearly demonstrated heritability of psychosis in studies of concordance in monozygotic twins: "The morbidity risk estimates with a 95% confidence interval (CIs) were 0.82% (95% CI = 0.69–104) for the schizophrenic syndrome, 0.35% (95 % CI = 0.25–0.51) for the schizoaffective syndrome, and 0.38% (95% CI = 0.27–0.55) for the manic syndrome" (Cardno, Rijsdijk, Sham, et al., 2002, p. 540). These authors proposed that there are

> significant genetic correlations between the schizophrenic and the manic syndromes. These results would be in keeping with the suggestion, based on a review of genetic linkage studies, that schizophrenia and affective disorder share some susceptibility genes. In addition, these results support an overlap in environmental risk factors for the schizophrenic and manic syndrome.. (cited in Nicolson & Rapoport, 1999, p. 542–543)

Family studies indicate that in relatives of bipolar probands, there is an increase in the prevalence of bipolar disorders, schizoaffective disorders, and unipolar depression, the latter having the highest prevalence among bipolar proband relatives (Badner, 2003, p. 248). Early onset bipolar disorder probands had the highest prevalence of bipolar disorders. The early onset bipolar disorder group had more psychotic symptoms, more mixed episodes, were more likely to have panic disorder, and were less likely to respond to lithium as compared to the late onset bipolars (p. 248).

Chromosomal Abnormalities

Microdeletion Syndromes

The 22q11 deletion syndrome (22qDS), also known as DiGeorge syndrome, Sprintzen syndrome, velocardiofacial syndrome (VCFS), is characterized by cleft palate, absent thymus, and congenital heart disease (CATCH-22 syndrome) (Carey, 2003, p. 736). The 22qDS represents the second most common human chromosomal anomaly after the 21 trisomy (Kendler, 2003, p. 1549). Of particular relevance is the frequent association of schizophrenia with velocardiofacial syndrome. Murphy reported that 30% of 22qDS children have psychosis, of which the most common type is schizophrenia (24%). Schizotypy was also quite common (Murphy, 2002, p. 427).

Higher rates of 22qDS may be present in subtypes of schizophrenia with childhood onset or in dual diagnosis of schizophrenia and mental retardation. The genetic risk for schizophrenia is related to the deletion occurring spontaneously (de novo mutation) even in the absence of family history of psychotic illness. The highest risk for the development of this illness is present in individuals with schizophrenia in both parents, and in monozygotic twins affected with schizophrenia, followed by 22qDS patients (Bassett et al., 2003, p. 1550).

On the other hand, patients with schizophrenia have a high prevalence of 22q11 deletions. Results of molecular genetic studies suggest that schizophrenia susceptibility locus maps to chromose 22q11. VCFS and deletion of chromosome 22q11 represent the highest risk factor for the development of schizophrenia identified to date (Murphy, 2002, pp. 428–429). Children with 22q11 syndrome display lower prepulse inhibition (see below) in comparison to their normal siblings. Information regarding ongoing specific genes under investigation is presented in an endnote.[1]

Another deletion, an 8q21 deletion, has been reported as associated with psychosis and mental retardation (Urraca et al., 2005, pp. 864–866).

Considerations Regarding Genetic Studies

Malhotra (2005) expressed reservations regarding a number of gene disbinding studies; these reservations could be extended to other genetic studies: (1) Many of the studies have not demonstrated that the same form of the gene increases the risk for schizophrenia. Thus, the actual causative variant has not yet been discovered. (2) Even in studies that report a correlation, the prevalence of the high risk form of the gene is still relatively low and not that dissimilar from that found in the general population. (3) The association may not be specific (pp. 18–19).

The state of flux of gene research is exemplified by a publication of disconfirmation of the purported gene COMT haplotype influence for the development of schizophrenia. Williams et al. (2005) in two large study groups, found no support for the hypothesis that valine/methionine polymorphism in the COMT gene influences susceptibility to schizophrenia or the hypothesis that a COMT haplotype influences susceptibility to schizphrenia in Ashkenazi and Irish subjects (p. 1736).

In relation to the state of gene research and its clinical applications, Malhotra (2005) makes a number of cautionary statements:

> Despite the success of these initial gene-finding efforts, their implications for the treatment of schizophrenia are less clear. The mechanisms by which these genes predispose to illness development are not known; the specific genotypes associated with risk remain to be fully established; and the relationship of disease and genes and the relevance to treatment is under of investigation. (p. 18)

Kendler (2005) is even more definitive:

> The strength of the association between individual genes and psychiatric disorders is weak and often nonspecific. Genes do not appear to contain all the information needed for the development of psychiatric illness, since environmental factors for several disorders have been shown to have causal specificity.... The causal chain from genes to psychiatric disorders is probably long and complex. The appropriate level of explanation for gene action is much more likely to be basic biological or mental processes that contribute to psychiatric disorders rather than the disorders

themselves....Although, we may wish it to be true, we do not have and are not likely to ever discover "genes for" psychiatric illness. (p. 1250)

The precise steps by which constitutional endowments gained expression in the clinical phenotypes are not known at this time. The accepted view is that severe mental disorders have an underlying polygenic cause (*influence* is probably a better term) coupled with developmental and other adverse experiential influences. Ultimately, persons with major psychiatric disturbances demonstrate, among other things, abnormalities in a variety of CNS functional systems, and other abnormalities.

Advances in pharmacogenetics are more promising to the psychotropic therapeutic field. "Pharmacogenetics can be used to individualize drug therapy, using molecular genetics to predict the likelihood of a response and the risk for toxicity before the medication is dispensed" (Nnadi, Goldberg, & Malhotra, 2005, p. 194). Ready availability of accurate methods to predict therapeutic response to psychiatric medications is more important nowadays due to the wide range of medications that have been introduced since the early 1950s (p. 194). Is the response to psychotropics genetic? "Taken together, the pharmacoepidemiologic studies on antipsychotic, antidepressant, and antibipolar medications provide strong preliminary evidence that the response to psychotropic drugs is heritable" (Nnadi et al., 2005, p. 198).

ETIOLOGY, TRAUMATIC BRAIN INJURY (TBI)

Psychosis following a TBI is not rare. The neurobiology of psychosis associated with TBI overlaps with corresponding findings in primary psychosis. A history of TBI has been found in 11% of patients with schizophrenia, compared with 4.9% of patients with mania, 1.5% in patients with depression, and 0.7% in surgical control subjects (Corcoran, McAllister, & Malaspina, 2005, p. 220). Right hemispheric injury is associated with specific misidentification delusions, such as Capgras's syndrome (the belief that loved ones are replaced by identical appearing impostors), the Fregoli's syndrome (the belief that the persecutor is able to change appearances and appears as different people), and in reduplicative paramnesia (the belief that there are similar familiar places existing in two different places at the same time) (p. 220).

Schizophrenia and TBI patients have similarities in neurocognitive functioning: deficits in insight, executive functioning and memory, which indicate similar neuroanatomical pathological sites (orbitofrontal region, dorsolateral prefrontal cortex and hippocampi). In addition, common deficits in sensory gating (see below), in both conditions, may indicate abnormal connectivity between various parts of the brain (Corcoran et al., 2005, p. 222). Finally, a history of child abuse was reported in 57% of first episode psychosis and in

44% of patients with chronic psychosis (p. 224). The authors concluded that up to 17% of schizophrenia cases are secondary to TBI (p. 226).

Mood disorders (mania and schizoaffective symptoms) have been reported in patients after a TBI. Many of these patients exhibit psychotic symptoms; in a series of 20 patients, grandiosity was present in 90%, pressured speech in 80%, and flight of ideas in 75%. None of the patients in the series had a genetic loading for bipolar disorder (Corcoran et al., 2005, p. 224). Incidentally, patients with TBI have a higher incidence of suicidal behavior than those without TBI history (Robinson & Jorge, 2005, p. 208).

PRENATAL AND POSTNATAL FACTORS ASSOCIATED WITH THE DEVELOPMENT OF PSYCHOTIC DISORDERS

In the section, "The Origins of Vulnerability" (Walker et al., 2004), the authors state that schizophrenia (and probably other primary psychoses) is a complex disorder. From the level of overt behavior, to intracellular processes, primary psychoses have defied scientific explanations (p. 402) and that despite the advances in diagnosis we still do not know the diagnostic boundaries of schizophrenia; also, the boundaries between schizophrenia and mood disorders are still obscure (p. 405). See below. Based on cumulative findings, it appears that genetic and prenatal factors give rise to a constitutional vulnerability, and that this risk is present at birth (p. 407), but it is not clear how that vulnerability interacts with external factor to cause the disease. Sussman (2005) asserts that, "In the end, no single factor adequately explains why people become mentally ill. Genetic predisposition[s], environmental factors, and events during development, all play a role, with genetics probably being a dominant force" (p. 11).

Events that adversely affect fetal development are considered to be potentially environmental triggers of genetic vulnerability. It is even likely that these factors by themselves may produce vulnerability for primary psychoses. Obstetrical complications (OC) and infections (like rubella and other viral infections) are examples of adverse events. Hypoxia is a consequence of OC. The odds of schizophrenia increase linearly with an increased number of hypoxia-related OCs (Walker et al., 2004, p. 410).

Animal studies demonstrate that prenatal maternal stress interferes with brain development. In humans, there is evidence that stressful events during pregnancy are associated with greater risk of schizophrenia and other psychiatric disorders in the offspring (p. 411). Risk is also increased in women whose spouses died during pregnancy. "It is likely that prenatal stress triggers the release of maternal stress hormones, disturbing fetal neurodevelopment as well as disrupting subsequent functioning of the hypothalamic-pituitary-adrenal axis, which in turn influences behavior and cognition" (Walker et al., 2004, p. 411).

Stressful events can worsen the course of schizophrenia, and precipitate a schizophrenic relapse. Patients have a greater risk of relapse if they live in families whose members express more negative attitudes and emotions (p. 414). See, Expressed Emotion, chapter 9. Evidence indicates that stress exposure can contribute to the onset of symptoms in vulnerable individuals and that the negative impact of adverse events may be cumulative. For instance, the offspring of schizophrenic parents displayed higher levels of maladaptive behaviors if they were also victims of neglect or abuse (p. 414).[2]

It is well established that stress exposure impacts brain functioning; these effects are mediated by activation of the HPA axis, culminating in the release of cortisol. This hormone has a negative impact on brain function and alters a number of neurotransmitters systems; cortisol also promotes an increase in dopamine activity (p. 414). The role of head injury as a risk factor for the development of major psychosis was discussed above.

GENDER DIFFERENCES IN THE EXPRESSION OF PSYCHOTIC SYMPTOMS

In reference to schizophrenia, some studies have demonstrated significant gender differences in its clinical expression: the illness is more frequent and more severe in males than in woman. Schizophrenia starts at an earlier age and has more prominent symptoms in males than in females. There are also significant neuroanatomical differences: male subjects display greater structural brain abnormalities, including larger ventricular–brain ratios, larger reduced gray matter volume, and a lack of normal asymmetry shown in healthy subjects. There are also differences in regional cerebral blood flow and high temporal resolution measures such as EEG; evoked potentials, functional brain connectivity, and others have also been observed (Slewa-Youman et al., 2004, p. 1595–1596).

PSYCHOSOCIAL FACTORS AND PSYCHOTIC DISORDERS

It is doubtful that psychosocial factors have a prominent etiological valence in the production of schizophrenia or bipolar disorders. The NIMH studies have not found support for the psychosocial factors having an etiological role in the development of schizophrenia. Psychosocial factors, on the other hand, play a role in maintenance and relapse of the schizophrenic and bipolar disorder.

Contrary to assertion that psychosocial factors do not have any significant role in the elicitation of schizophrenia, Wicks, Hjern, Gunnell, Lewis, and Dorman (2005) indicate that the diagnosis of schizophrenia and other psychoses is more frequent among children from households with more adverse groupings (p. 1653). In addition, a stronger association was found between socioeconomic adversity and the risk of psychoses, with an increasing number of exposures indicative of a dose-response relationship (p 1655). The authors proposed that in genetically vulnerable individuals, adverse socioeconomical circumstances could be of significance in developing schizophrenia and other psychosis (p. 1656).

Papolos and Papolos (2002) believe that the genetic information inherent in the cells unfolds in the context of the internal and external environment, and that certain vulnerability genes predispose certain individuals to disturbances in the regulation of emotion and behavior (p. 206). Family intactness and maternal warmth serve as a mediator in the outcome of bipolar children (Shaw, Egeland, Endicott, Allen, & Hostetter, 2005, p. 1109) and, on the other hand, adverse life stresses, including personal loss, such as a death or the end of a relationship, often initiate depression in a predisposed individual (Sussman, 2005, p. 11).

There are a number of psychosocial factors associated with the development and maintenance of mood disorders. Reinherz, Paradis, Giaconia, Stashwick, and Fitzmaurice (2003) highlight the importance of biological-genetic and environmental factors in the family domain as forces determining the manifestation or maintenance of depression. Thus, parental and sibling depression, and sibling substance abuse, present by the time the subjects reach 15 years of age, are relevant factors. Family violence and lack of family cohesion characterize the households of depressed subjects. In the same manner, family composition and birth order within the family are significant: later born children in large families perceive their families as punitive and unsupportive. Later born children are also at the risk for the development of depression, anxiety, and lower self-concept (p. 2145). Furthermore, a chaotic and unsafe family environment (history of family violence reported by age 15) is the most salient predictor for development or perpetuation of depression during the transition to adulthood. Internalizing problems emerged as the most important behavioral-emotional factor (p. 2145).

Cultural habits and food availability have an important protective factor against the development of bipolar spectrum disorders. Noaghiul and Hibbeln (2003) reported lower rates of lifetime prevalence of bipolar I disorder, bipolar II disorder, and bipolar spectrum disorders in association with greater rates of seafood consumption (p. 2225). The authors clarify that their findings do not demonstrate a causal relationship; however, their findings are consistent with the hypothesis that insufficient dietary intake of omega-3 essential fatty acids increases the risk of affective disorders. Results are also consistent with the results of a controlled, double-blind study that reported a reduction in the number of severe affective episodes and a reduction in depression scores in bipolar patients receiving 9.6 g/day of EPA (eicosapentaenoic acid) and DHA (docosahexaenoic acid). It appears that omega-3 fatty acids are more affective in reducing depressive than manic symptoms.

DEVELOPMENTAL CONSIDERATIONS
IN THE ORIGIN OF PSYCHOSIS

Since the mid-1960s, neurobiology has played a dominant role in the conceptualization of the etiology of the major psychiatric illnesses: bipolar disorders and schizophrenias. Issues of development and the impact of early life experience have been relegated to the periphery of causal explanations. Although that bias, if not neglect, may be inconsequential to the practice of adult psychiatry, development and early experience, unfolding of capacities and dispositions, personality formation, the role of dependency and the impact of family life, among others, are issues at the very core of the child psychiatry experience. Furthermore, child psychiatrists are interested in the elucidation of the origin of psychiatric disorders with the goal of prevention and early intervention. Greenspan and Glovinsky (2005), attempted to integrate neurodevelopment with psychosocial development in the context of family experience. They use the term *patterns* rather than *disorder* when discussing bipolarity in children. This seems to agree with Kowatch et al. (2005), who stated that pediatric bipolar disorder children "are best conceptualized as having a severe mood dysregulation with multiple, intense, prolonged mood swings each day. This 'mixed' type of episode frequently includes short periods of euphoria and longer periods of irritability" (p. 214).

Greenspan and Glovinsky assert that these "patterns" are best understood within a developmental biopsychosocial model. The authors propose that children with bipolar patterns suffer from severe emotional dysregulation and difficulties of executive functioning that involve interrelated features including genetic and biological, interactive, and family interactions (p. 1). Bipolar patterns are pervasive in that they affect all areas of the child's functioning, bearing little resemblance to the adult bipolar disorder. The authors suggest that the conceptualization of bipolar patterns needs to be integrated in the context of the relationship with significant others in the child's life. According to these authors, "Intervening Developmental Organizations," mediate between genetic-biological, experiential factors, and presenting symptoms, and behavior. Even genetic-biological differences (sensory reactivity, sensory processing, sensory affective processing, and motor functioning) need to be seen in the context of the child–parent interactions, and through a sequence of emotional developmental levels (pp. 2–3). For Greenspan and Glovinsky, the "developmental signature" of bipolar patterns involves: (1) Sensory overreactivity and sensory craving. (2) Most children are highly purposeful and relational. (3) Children are creative and imaginative but emotionally constricted. Children have problems containing emotional states and representing them in higher symbolic and communicable levels. (4) Children have difficulties with reflective thinking, and are unable to modulate emotionally charged situations such as aggression, and loss; these children have a high level of emotional vulnerability (pp. 4–5).

Based on the above premises, the authors offered a series of intervention recommendations to guide significant others in the process of "up or down regulation" of the dysregulated offspring (p. 5; see chapter 9).

Among a population of high-risk Amish children, there were high levels of rejection sensitivity and crying in the younger cohort, preschool through age 12. As the youth aged, there was a clear shift from internalizing symptoms to symptoms associated with maniclike behaviors: high energy, decreased sleep, excessive, loud talking, and problems of concentration (Shaw et al., 2005, p. 1108). It was also interesting that, in children under age 12, the investigators did not found cases that fulfilled the diagnostic criteria of pediatric bipolar disorder (p. 1109).

Greenspan and Glovinsky (2005) state that the diagnosis of bipolar disorder in childhood is highly controversial and that the developmental components make it difficult to determine what is age-typical versus pathological in young children. The prevalence data on this disorder is quite limited and there is marked variability in the presentation of the disorder (p. 1).

Cognitive deficits (besides hallucinations and delusions) have received strong recognition as factors associated with psychosis, particularly, in relation to schizophrenia; the same deficits are being progressively demonstrated in bipolar disorder. Pavuluri, Schenkel, et al. (2006) demonstrated the presence of neurocognitive deficits in pediatric bipolar disorder in areas such as sustained attention, working memory, verbal memory, and executive functions (p. 290). Illness status (acutely ill or euthymic) and medication status (lithium plus risperidone versus divalproex sodium plus risperidone) appears to have a minimum role in influencing the severity of or the nature of cognitive deficits associated with bipolar disorder; that is, in the pediatric group, treated euthymic patients performed no better than acutely ill unmedicated patients. In other words, medicated and unmedicated patients display the same pattern of neurocognitive deficits (p. 291). Pediatric bipolar disorder patients with comorbid ADHD demonstrated greater neurocognitive deficits than the counterparts without ADHD (p. 291). These findings suggest that the prefrontal and mesial temporal lobe circuitry that underlies working memory and verbal memory may be specifically affected in pediatric bipolar disorder because these impairments were associated with pediatric bipolar disorder regardless of the ADHD status.

The role of emotional deficiencies in the development of psychosis is beginning to be examined. Investigators assessed emotional processing traits of affect intensity, attention to emotions, and clarity of emotions. Participants who reported high intensity, high attention, and low clarity were labeled as overwhelmed since they appear to overregulate their moods and be more influenced by them. Schizotypy was associated with overwhelmed traits in 62% of the studied subjects contrary to 28.6% of controls. Investigators proposed that people at risk of psychosis have a difficult time understanding their emotions during stress, a necessary first step in the process of mood regulation. Improving this recognition may constitute an important treatment goal for patients with psychotic illnesses. These results support previous findings that emotional influences on cognition might contribute to the development of odd beliefs and experiences, and other psychotic symptoms. Understanding emotion-processing deficits may lead to improved early detection and prevention of psychosis for at risk patients (Croog, Naccari, & Wong, 2005, pp. 13–14).

In summary, a longitudinal and developmental perspective is absolutely necessary for the understanding of early-onset bipolar and schizophrenic disorders.

NEUROBIOLOGY OF CHRONIC PSYCHOTIC DISORDERS

Regarding the neurobiology of schizophrenia, current data support the view that: (1)Schizophrenia is a brain disease with complex etiological sources involving biological, environmental, and cultural factors. A similar conclusion, although with less supporting evidence, is accumulating in the field to bipolar disorders. (2) Childhood onset schizophrenia may represent a severe variant of schizophrenia, in which etiological pathways and the biological substrates for the disorders may be more clearly discernable; similarly, early onset bipolar disorder is considered a more virulent form of the illness than the adult counterpart. (3) There is some degree of heterogeneity in childhood onset schizophrenia (COS) like the one present in adult schizophrenia. There is also heterogeneity in bipolar disorder expression. (4) Childhood-onset bipolar disorders share family factors in common with adult-onset affective disorders and do not represent an etiologically distinct group (DelBello, Axelson, & Geller, 2003, p. 4). However, the pediatric and adult forms may have different pathogenesis, may represent variants of the same vulnerability, or may represent different disorders. Similar comments could be said about childhood schizophrenia-spectrum disorders of childhood and adulthood.

Keshavan (2005) speaks for many investigators when he asserts that while schizophrenia starts in early childhood, adolescence, or adulthood, "its seeds are planted early in a long-term neurodevelopmental process eventually leading to deviant brain functioning. It is also evident that multiple and sequential etiological factors may interactively and additively contribute to the emergence of the illness" (p. 25).

Hollis (2001) proposes a model that attempts to dispel the assumption that schizophrenia has a single onset,

> Rather, there may be a sequence of onsets, starting with a "biological onset" in fetal life, followed by a "preclinical onset" with the development of premorbid behavioral changes during childhood, and finally a "clinical onset" coinciding

with the emergence of positive and negative psychotic symptoms, typically in late adolescent and early adult life... the model embodies the principle of developmental vulnerability in symptoms (developmental heterotypy)—with premorbid impairments conceptualized as age specific manifestations or underlying neuropathology (pp. 86–87).

NEUROANATOMICAL, VOLUMETRIC AND IMAGING ABNORMALITIES IN PRIMARY PSYCHOSES

In bipolar disorder subjects, the following evidence has been demonstrated:

1. Neuroimaging studies show a decrease in brain volume (with increase in the lateral ventricles size) suggesting neuronal (gray matter) atrophy or loss in the prefrontal and temporal cortices. These findings are similar to corresponding findings in schizophrenia spectrum disorders.
2. Hyperintensities in subcortical white matter are consistent findings.
3. Alteration in basal ganglia and cerebellum has also been demonstrated, with less consistency, suggesting cortical-limbic dysfunction. There is also evidence of glucose hypometabolism and blood flow abnormalities in cortical and subcortical areas (Frey, Rodrigues da Fonseca, Machado-Vieira, Soarese, & Kapczinski, 2004, pp. 181). Hwang et al. (2006) demonstrated major striatal shape differences in the right side of adult bipolar disorder drug-naïve patients (the right hemisphere is known to process and operate on nonverbal material and intrinsic functions, whereas the left hemisphere mainly mediates language related functions). In bipolar disorder patients the performance IQ is lower than the verbal IQ, and nonverbal and visuospatial and abstraction abilities have been found to be more severely affected than verbal skills, indicating a right or nondominant dysfunction. Findings correlate with metanalysis of volumetric studies reporting that the right side ventricle enlargement was one of the most consistent findings in bipolar disorders. The pattern observed in drug-naïve patients was not observed in drug-treated patients. It appears that caudate and putamen shape abnormalities observed in this disorder may be modulated with treatment (p. 283).
4. Glial density is decreased. Glial cells take part in the development, maintenance and remodeling of the synaptic connections by releasing trophic factors. Decrease of glial density, therefore, may indicate a decrease of functional synapses in bipolar patients. Low density of glial cells in Broadman area 24 has been shown in schizophrenics but not in bipolar disorder patients. However, in area Broadman 10, of the dorso-lateral prefrontal cortex (DLPFC), glial cell density was decreased for both bipolar and schizophrenics. Glial cells are also decreased in the hippocampal region

(CA2), in both bipolar and schizophrenics, suggesting a decrease of the GABAergic inhibition. (Frey et al., 2004, pp. 181).

5. Cingulate cortex abnormalities have been recently demonstrated in bipolar disorder children (Kaur et al., 2005). Children with bipolar disorder evidenced smaller mean cingulate volumes compared to controls for the left anterior cingulate, left posterior cingulate, and right posterior cingulate but not for the right anterior cingulate (p. 1639). The meaning of these finding is unclear.

For related issues related to volumetric finding and other neurobiogical abnormalities in primary psychoses (see chapter 5, "Neuroimaging," pp. 197–203).

A recent study, Nierenberg et al. (2005) demonstrated that in first-episode schizophrenic patients, the normal left-greater-than-right angular gyrus asymmetry is reversed. The left angular gyrus was 14.8% smaller in first-episode schizophrenic patients than in normal subjects. None of the other regions measured showed any significant volumetric or asymmetrical differences. The authors suggested that the angular gyrus may be a neuroanatomical substrate for the expression of schizophrenia. This finding is consistent with previous reports of parietal-lobe abnormalities in chronic schizophrenia. (p. 1540). There were correlations between asymmetry measures for the angular gyrus and the planum temporale (part of the superior temporal gyrus), structures intimately related to language in the left hemisphere. The authors had previously demonstrated that the planum temporale had reverse asymmetry at first hospitalization (p. 1541).

ALTERED CORTICAL INTERNEURONAL CONNECTIVITY

Elaboration of brain circuitry is a lifelong process, especially the connection between cells in circuits within and between different regions of the cortex; this process is particularly active during adolescence and early adult life (Gur et al., 2005, p. 98). Adolescence is a time of explosive growth and development of the brain. While the number of nerve cells does not increase after birth, the richness and connections between cells do, and the capacity of these networks to process increasingly complex information changes accordingly.

Abnormalities in Frontal-Temporal Circuits

The frontal and temporal cortices are considered abnormal in schizophrenia. Injury to these areas (by trauma, stroke, or neurological illness) is more likely to be associated with psychosis than is damage to other regions. Neuroimaging techniques suggest that a malfunction in the frontal and temporal lobes processing relationship best characterizes the problems of schizophrenic patients. Language is highly dependent on the fronto-temporal circuitry; this is impaired in schizophrenia and causes the known disturbance of thought disorder, characteristic of the illness. Whereas normal subjects, when asked to generate a list of words beginning with a particular consonant, activate the frontal lobe and suppress the temporal one, schizophrenic patients do the opposite. Also, schizophrenic patients show a different pattern of fMRI activation for semantically encoded words: less inferior frontal lobe activation and a significant increase of the activation of the superior temporal cortex (Gur et al., 2005, p. 98). Other fMRI activation abnormalities in schizophrenia are discussed in an endnote.[3]

In bipolar disorders, Krüger et al. (2006) demonstrated a decrease in rCBF in the orbitofrontal cortex coupled with an increase of rCBF in the dorsolateral cingulate. Orbitofrontal hypoactivity is linked to shifts between euphoric and dysphoric mood states, and the inability to differentiate between relevant and irrelevant emotional stimuli findings; these areas seem to underlie the biological correlates of emotional vulnerability in both patients and siblings. The contiguous but more dorsal and rostral medial frontal regions are involved in mediating self-referential processing of emotionally saliency and reward assessment. The close reciprocal connection of the orbitofrontal cortex to the dorsal anterior cingulate (implicated in attention to emotional salience and monitoring the extent of the emotional response to various stimuli), suggests that the interplay of these regions is involved in bipolar disorder patients' greater vulnerability to emotional provocation. Although, siblings did not meet criteria for any psychiatric diagnosis, when emotionally provoked, they showed changes in brain activity consistent with those of bipolar family members (p. 261).

Diffusion tensor imaging has demonstrated white matter connectivity abnormalities between the frontal and temporal lobes in schizophrenic patients (Krüger et al., 2006, pp. 98–99). Schizophrenics also demonstrate connectivity problems in other brain regions and it is unlikely that any particular cortical area in schizophrenic patients is normal under all conditions. This suggests that schizophrenia could be characterized as a "disconnectivity" disorder (Gur, et al., 2005, p. 99).

In adolescents experiencing their first manic episode, Adler, Adams et al. (2006) showed decreased prefrontal fractional anisotropy consistent with white matter abnormalities; this may reflect axonal disorganization and may represent an early marker of bipolar disorder (pp. 322–333). These findings support the hypothesis of a loss of network connectivity indicating evidence of neuropathology of bipolar disorder (p. 3240).

Abnormalities in Prefrontal Striatal Circuits

Research in animals has conclusively demonstrated that abnormalities in pre-frontal function disrupts a tonic brake on dopamine neurons in the brainstem, leading to a loss of the normal regulation of these neurons and to their excessive activation (Gur et al., 2005, p. 99). It is considered that the prefrontal cortex helps guide the dopamine reward system toward reinforcing of contextually appropriate stimuli. Neuroimaging studies show overactivity in the striatum in schizophrenic patients, and this overactivation, is strongly correlated to abnormal prefrontal cortex dysfunction. The prefrontal cortex plays an important role in how other brain systems function. Behavioral disturbances in schizophrenia involve dysfunction of diverse and interconnected brain systems (Adler et al., 2006).

PSYCHOSIS AND CEREBELLAR ABNORMALITIES

Anatomical and functional studies indicate that the human cerebellum plays a wider role in many cognitive functions, such as language, executive functions, and spatial cognition. A number of neurological and psychiatric conditions have been associated with cerebellar dysfunction, including autism, ADHD, mood disorders, and schizophrenia (Tamminga, 2005, p. 1253).

There is accumulating evidence that the cerebellum plays an important role in cognitive functioning that is impaired in schizophrenia. Positron emission tomography studies have revealed cerebellar blood flow abnormalities while patients carry out cognitive tasks. A model of schizophrenia as secondary to disrupted development in a cortico-cerebellar-thalamic-cortical circuit has been labeled "cognitive dysmetria," referring to incoordination in the processing, prioritization, retrieval, and expression of information.

The excess loss of brain tissue during adolescence seen in a variety of studies may be a trait marker for schizophrenia, especially since there is also evidence of reduction of cerebellar volume in relatives of adult patients with schizophrenia compared with normal control subjects (Keller et al., 2003, p. 132). Patients with cerebellar lesions display cognitive deficits similar to those seen in patients with schizophrenia: impairment in working memory, abstract reasoning, verbal memory, and executive function. Smaller vermis volumes and reduced linear density and Purkinge cells size in the vermis has been found in postmortem studies of patients with schizophrenia. Findings of a deficit in cerebellar inhibition compared to healthy controls provide confirmation in vivo evidence of either abnormalities in Purkinje cell output or of disrupted cerebellar-cortical connectivity. It is proposed that in schizophrenia, aberrant cerebellar activity may result in altered activity of the inhibitory interneurons of the cortex (Daskalakis, Christensen, Fitzgerald, Fountain, & Chen, 2005, pp. 1203–1204; for other psychotic syndromes associated with cerebellar pathology, see chapter 6, pp. 263–264).

EVIDENCE OF NEURODEVELOPMENTAL IMPAIRMENT IN PRIMARY PSYCHOSES

Contemporaneous thinking considers schizophrenia a neurodevelopmental disorder. It is proposed that noxious events cause initial neurodevelopmental cortical impairment and that this impairment causes susceptibility thereafter for the later emergence of neurodegenerative process (Buckley, Mahadik, Evans, & Stirewalt, 2003, p. 46). Children at high risk for schizophrenia, show evidence of neurodevelopmental disturbance since birth: in infancy (from 0–2 years) they display motor impairment and high or variable sensitivity to sensory stimulation, abnormal growth patterns, short attention span, and low IQ. During this age, these children display a difficult temperament, look quiet, passive, or inhibited, lack fear of strangers, display low communication competence in child–mother interactions and less social contacts with their mothers. In early childhood, these children show low reactivity, poor gross and fine motor coordination difficulties, and variable performance in cognitive tests. During this age, these children show anxiety and depression, display anger, a hostile disposition, low reactivity and schizoid behavior, and are more likely to receive the diagnosis of a developmental disorder. In middle childhood and early adolescence, those children show soft neurological signs (poor fine motor coordination, delayed motor development, and isolated sensorory perceptual signs), poor social adjustment, attentional deficits under overload conditions, anxiety, and scatter or variance in intellectual tests. During this period, these children show poor emotional control, withdrawal, poor interpersonal relation-ships, cognitive slippage, mixed internalizing and externalizing symptoms, fear, and ADHD-like symptoms. The birth cohort studies corroborate the observations described above (Gur et al., 2005, p. 145).

In relation to childhood onset schizophrenia, findings of an association with spectrum disorders in relatives, supports a model in which specific disease-related factors interact with a general liability or, could indicate that genes involved in the etiology of schizophrenia also interfere with the neurodevelopment of language-related brain regions (Nicholson & Rapoport, 1999, p. 1423).

Children and adolescents who later developed schizophrenia as adults have higher than expected rates of abnormal speech and motor development, poorer social development, lower intelligence and worse educational perfor-mance (Nicolson, Lenane, Singaracharlu, et al., 2000, p 794; also see chapter 6).

Aberrant neurodevelopment may be even more salient in cases of schizophrenia with very early onset.

Young bipolar patients appear to have a decreased level of N-acetylaspartate (NAA), a putative marker of neuronal integrity, in the dorsolateral prefrontal cortex, similar to findings described in adults. These findings seem to reflect an underdevelopment of dendritic arborization and synaptic interconnectivity and do not seem to be the result of long-term degenerative processes (Sassi et al., 2005, p. 2109). Interestingly, lithium administration at therapeutic doses, increases brain N-acetylaspartate; imaging studies have demonstrated that lithium increases the brain gray matter (Bachmann, Schloesser, et al., 2005, p. 51).

EVIDENCE OF NEURODEGENERATION IN PRIMARY PSYCHOSES

Longitudinal MRI analysis of patients with childhood-onset schizophrenia, from the NIMH cohort, demonstrated striking anatomical profiles of accelerated gray matter loss (GML). Giedd et al. (1999) demonstrated progressive brain changes in child-onset schizophrenia (COS) subjects in comparison to controls. For the COS group but not for controls, there were significant changes in the total cerebrum (decrease), lateral ventricles (increase), and hyppocampus (decrease) (p. 895). For schizophenic children, for whom follow-up scans were available, there was a significant correlation between ventricular volume (increase) and changes in the SANS and between changes in the hippocampus (decrease) and changes in the SAPS (p. 896). In this regard, the Asarnows quote Thompson et al. (2001), who indicated that the earliest deficits were found in parietal regions supporting visuospatial and associative thinking. See above. Over five years, these deficits progressed anteriorly into temporal lobes engulfing sensorimotor and dorsolateral cortices, and frontal eye fields. These emerging patterns correlated with psychotic severity and mirrored the neuromotor, auditory, visual search, and frontal executive impairments of schizophrenia. In temporal areas, GML was completely absent early in the disease but became pervasive later. The latest changes included dorsolateral prefrontal cortex and superior temporal giri; these deficit regions are consistently found in adults studies (Asarnow & Asarnow, 2003, p. 470). Neurodegenerative brain changes can be demonstrated by neuroimaging techniques (see chapter 5).

Cummings and Mega (2003) consider that schizophrenia is a dysfunctional limbic syndrome that,

> may involve dysfunction in the implicit integration of affects, drives, and object associations, supported by the orbitofrontal limbic arm, with explicit sensory

processing, encoding, and attentional/executive systems, all supported by the hyppocampal limbic arm and the dorsolateral prefrontal cortex. Functional imaging studies of patients with [chronic] psychosis have implicated dysfunction in temporal and limbic regions as well as in dorsolateral frontal cortex bilaterally. (p. 18)

The authors add that, even though schizophrenia has undeniable biological underpinnings, for a comprehensive understanding of this neuropsychiatric illness, a careful developmental history and an integration of the life span is required (p. 2).

In the following vignette, a progressive unfolding of the negative and positive psychotic symptoms in a boy is illustrated.

Jimmy was followed up for more than five years for a deteriorating psychotic disorder with severe behavioral and conduct difficulties. As Jimmy grew older, his symptomatology became more in line with adult psychotic symptomatology; this was particularly true of his paranoid pathology.

Jimmy was 11 years old when he was first hospitalized for regressive and psychotic features. Six months before, he had been attacked by a group of children and he became very upset by the incident. Jimmy had been school homebound for the previous three months because of behavioral difficulties. He alleged that a teacher had tried to kill him because of his school problems. Six months before, he had attempted to stab himself with a butcher knife, and because of that, his mother decided to hide all the household sharps. Jimmy had lost five pounds over the previous year.

Psychological testing performed the previous year was consistent with the diagnosis of childhood schizophrenia. Projective data did not indicate the presence of depression.

During the previous six months, Jimmy had complained of a number of somatic problems; he had been nauseous and had vomited a number of times. From time to time he appeared anxious. He had been regressing progressively, and had even started to baby talk.

During the initial psychiatric evaluation, Jimmy came across as an odd looking preadolescent; he displayed mild dysmorphic features: he had antimongoloid eyes, synophris (the eyebrows joined in the midline), and exhibited very elongated eyelashes. He was slim and small for his age. He also carried a teddy bear and displayed a regressive posture and demeanor.

Jimmy walked in an unusual manner, and cried and whimpered childishly. He reported hearing voices: he indicated that Oddie, a teddy bear, talked to him and told him multiple things. Apparently, Oddie told him, "to massage his butt with peanut butter" and "to keep on trying." Jimmy had seen a shadow he believed represented his guardian angel playing a trick on him. He verbalized fears of being in danger and reported that at times he couldn't control his mind. Throughout the initial evaluation, he showed low motivation and displayed no insight.

Jimmy was readmitted six months later for increasingly aggressive and destructive behaviors. The day prior to his readmission he had a major episode of dyscontrol in which he broke a curtain, flipped over a rocker and a chair, and overturned a bookcase. He also cursed at the teacher and had to be restrained.

Jimmy had a recurrent difficulty waking up in the mornings. It was a daily struggle to get him out of bed. He got mad when he was awakened. His parents reported that he had been violent and destructive at home and that he had run from the house. His parents also reported persistent irritability over the previous week. Jimmy continued being unable to attend a regular classroom and had needed a highly modified special education program. He denied feeling depressed but had attempted to jump from his parents' car some time prior to the readmission. He denied hallucinations or paranoid ideation, and also denied suicidal and homicidal ideation (these denials were questionable). Jimmy seemed very preoccupied with his penis and asked many questions about it. Although he had initially objected to going to the hospital for the second time, he requested to stay longer because he did not want to lose the new friends he made there. He claimed that at home, nobody wanted to be his friend.

At age 12, Jimmy needed a new hospital admission for impulsive and unpredictable behavior. At that time, he reported that, "my dark side is coming to get me." Jimmy had told his father that a bad man was coming after him. He also said that his "good side" was talking to his "bad side," and claimed that the evil side was telling him to do bad things like hitting the teacher, touching the teacher's buttocks, etc. He revealed that the bad side had told him to kill himself by running into traffic or by cutting his veins. Jimmy had asked his family if they had seen people being run over by a car. He claimed that the evil side had told him to do many other things that he did not care to discuss. He acknowledged experiencing suicidal ideation and stated that he banged his head against the wall to help him sleep. Jimmy felt unwanted and believed that nobody liked him. He had started hitting himself in the face, stating that he wanted to die.

Jimmy acknowledged auditory hallucinations once more but was secretive about them; he endorsed broad paranoid ideation, feelings that people talked about him, watched him, followed him, and that people were after him. Jimmy disclosed that he had made some inventions but did not want to discuss them because he feared that the psychiatrist would steal them. He expected to make lots of money from his creations. Short-lived pressured speech was observed occasionally.

Jimmy became irritated with his doctor because he did not support Jimmy's demand, "to be sent to a special school where my gifts could be nurtured." He became upset when he was asked if he had special powers.

At age 16, Jimmy was hospitalized again. The police took Jimmy to an acute adolescent facility because he became aggressive and destructive at home. He claimed that he got mad and that he had destroyed multiple things in the house. On the day of admission, he overturned a computer and had tried to beat his father and mother with a broomstick. The day before, he twisted his mother's arm and pushed her against the wall. He had been angry with his parents because they were taking him to the doctor and were making him take medication. He also threatened to burn the house down if he were taken back to the hospital. Preceding the new admission, Jimmy smashed a window of his parents' car and forced his mother to eat a piece of paper he had torn.

Jimmy claimed he was hearing things. The night prior to the latest admission he heard television voices when the set was off; this made him very angry. He claimed that he got messages from the TV and believed that people could read his mind. The fear that people could read his mind became so strong that he opted to stay in his room for prolonged periods of time. He also indicated that he could predict the future. He would stay in his room and avoided going outside, believing that people would laugh at him, fearing that people would talk about him. He avoided going to school and continued refusing to get up in the mornings. Jimmy claimed he had difficulties sleeping at night due to "problems with my brain"; and stated that his head hurt and that his mind felt tense.

Jimmy blamed the medications for his increased sleepiness during the day and for his increased appetite. Jimmy endorsed that he felt very angry, but he identified his anger as coming from the devil. He stated that he hated his psychiatrist because he gave him medications. Jimmy had lost 16 pounds during the previous four months. He stated that hated Depakote because it made him eat but his parents reported, however, that he had been eating infrequently. Jimmy's parents reported that he had left the house and wandered off in the middle of the night. On one occasion, the sheriff apprehended him for walking across a busy highway. He had verbalized to his mother that he could not tolerate his life anymore and had made threats to kill himself, again.

The mental status examination revealed the presence of a reserved male adolescent with decreased psychomotor activity. Occasionally, Jimmy displayed a rhythmic rocking. His speech was decreased in rate and intensity. There were prominent negative symptoms: Jimmy appeared downcast, displayed blunted affect, and was very negativistic, and difficult to engage; he was asocial (he said he was trying to stay away from people to avoid people from reading his thoughts). He stated he did not want to participate in any activity. His mood was moderately depressed and his affect was constricted and inappropriate. A number of times, Jimmy expressed that he would be better off dead. His thought processes were coherent and goal directed but illogical. No looseness of associations was detected. He revealed that he had thoughts, "I can't put into words and can't make them to go away." Jimmy endorsed auditory hallucinations but was vague and reserved as to their content. He hinted that his brain was talking to him; reluctantly, he acknowledged that he thought of mocking people and reiterated his fears that people could read these thoughts. He revealed that he saw things, too. Jimmy acknowledged that he believed he had special powers. He felt very strongly that people could read his mind and that he got messages from the TV. He was very suspicious and endorsed broad paranoid ideation believing that people talked about him, watched him, and followed him. He believed that medications did bad things to his body. He was obsessed with germs and washed his hands for 15 to 30 minutes at a time; his pillow had to be washed if somebody touched it. He changed his clothes many times during the day because he felt dirty and wanted his clothes washed. He had frequent suicidal thoughts but denied any suicidal plans. He also endorsed homicidal ideation toward the family. His judgment and insight were considered poor.

Jimmy felt very intimidated by the future and stated he was not sure he could manage. He persistently rejected medications and other psychiatric treatments.

The family admitted to the presence of a close relative (patient's first cousin) with history of severe mental illness, possibly schizophrenia. Jimmy's adaptive functioning had been poor for the previous four to five years, there had been progressive unfolding of negative and positive symptoms and he had become progressively withdrawn and unable to control himself.

This is a very complex clinical vignette. Beside the florid psychotic symptoms there are strong mood and affective symptoms; furthermore, there was evidence of significant comorbidity: ODD, mood symptoms, and OCD features, among others. The onset and progression of Jimmy's illness is compatible with the diagnosis of very early onset schizophrenia (VEOS).

In Jimmy's case, there was strong developmental psychotic history and clinical findings were compatible with the diagnosis of paranoid schizophrenia. This child's paranoia extended over many aspects of the psychiatric treatment including medications, and the interactions with the psychiatrist. Jim's case exemplifies the process of continuity of childhood schizophrenia to an adult form.

ELECTROPHYSIOLOGICAL STUDIES IN PRIMARY PSYCHOSES

Prepulse Inhibitory Deficits

Lower prepulse inhibition has been shown among children with disorders characterized by a failure of inhibitory brain mechanisms, that is, impairment of sensory filtering, selective attention, and inhibitory control. These deficits are present in Tourette's syndrome, postraumatic stress disorder, fragil X syndrome, and among boys, nocturnal enuresis and ADHD (Sobin, Kiley-Brabeck, & Karayiorgou, 2005, p. 1091).

Children with 22q11 syndrome display lower prepulse inhibition in comparison to their normal siblings, 26 and 46%, respectively. There was greater group effect for boys than for girls. Also, the mean percentages of prepulse inhibition for children with and without subsyndromal symptoms associated with schizophrenia, were 9 and 34%, respectively. Neuropsychological testing in these children demonstrate specific impairments in working memory, selective and executive visual attention, and sensorymotor functioning (Sobin et al., 2005, pp. 1094–1096).

Event Related Potentials (ERPs)

Event-related potentials provide a functional window on many aspects of brain processing; these include, (1) the most elementary ones, gamma band activity, involved in early, simple signal detection and gating (P50), and (2) automatic detection of changes in the environment—mismatched negativity activity (MMN), a more complex activity involving a conscious updating of expectations in view of unusual events (P300). Data support the hypothesis that schizophrenia involves abnormalities in brain processing from the most simple to the most complex, and that the anatomical substrates of auditory processing in the neocortical temporal lobe (superior temporal gyrus), correlated with a reduction of the gray matter volume (Gur et al., 2005, p. 89).

The following are some relevant electrophysiological findings in primary psychosis:

Gamma Band Activity

This deficit is present in about 50% of first-degree relatives of schizophrenia. Patients with affective disorders also show gating deficits, but these are state-dependent, that is, the deficits disappear when the abnormal mood is resolved. This is not the case in schizophrenics in which the deficits persist even when the patients go into remission. It is proposed that early sensory gating and P-50 deficits result in "sensory flooding" (Gur et al., 2005, pp. 89, 90).

Mismatched Negativity (MMN)

The MMN amplitude is consistently reduced in chronic schizophrenia. It is likely this is a traitlike (endophenotype) phenomenon; this characteristic persists even when the patient enters into remission. Of significance, the MMN is frequently normal at the time of the first psychotic break but becomes abnormal over time (1.5 years on the average), reflecting a probable neurodegeneration (Gur et al, 2005, pp. 90–91).

P300 and Failure to Process Unusual Events

Reduction of the P300 amplitude, at midline sites, is the most frequently replicated abnormality in schizophrenia. However, this abnormality is also evidenced in other psychiatric disorders. The P300 reduction also seems to be a trait-like (endophenotype) illness feature and endures regardless of the disease state. Atypical antipsychotics increase the P300 amplitude but not to the extent of normal levels (pp. 90–91). It is also interesting that there is an asymmetry in the P300. First-episode schizophrenics display smaller voltage over the left temporal lobe than over the right. There is a direct association between the degree of the amplitude abnormality and the severity of the psychopathology, reflected in thought disorder and paranoid delusions. The left temporal deficit is not found in affective psychosis. The greater the reduction of gray matter volume in the posterior superior temporal gyrus (STG), the greater the P300 amplitude reduction. The posterior STG on the left, in right-handed individuals, involving part of the Wernicke area, is an area intimately involved with language processing and thinking (Gur et al., 2005, p. 92). Finally, ERPs may be used to track the progression of brain abnormalities. As discussed above, MMN is normal at the onset of first schizophrenic break but becomes abnormal in the course of the illness; such a development is associated with gray matter loss in the auditory cortex (p. 95).

Contingent Negative Variation (CNV)

Diminished Np amplitude is the earliest consistent ERP index of schizophrenia related information processing deficit in the UCLA studies. The UCLA studies consistently demonstrated smaller P300 amplitude in both schizophrenic children and adults in span, CPT, and idiom recognition tasks. The earliest reliable electrophysiological correlate of impaired discriminative processing in schizophrenia is the Np component. Children and adolescents with schizophrenia are deficient in the allocation of attentional resources necessary for efficient and accurate discriminative processing. Diminished Np visual processing may be specific to schizophrenic pathology (this is another likely endophenotype). Further details of EPRs in schizophrenia and bipolar disorder are discussed in an endnote 3. In the same manner, absence of right-lateralized P1/N1 amplitude in visual ERPs has been another consistent finding in the UCLA studies (Gur et al., 2005, p. 94). For more information regarding electrophysiological issues related to schizophrenia, see note.[4]

NEUROENDOCRINOLOGICAL FINDINGS IN PRIMARY PSYCHOSES

A large body of research suggests a link between psychosocial stress and relapse or exacerbation of schizophrenia (see "Expressed Emotion," chapter 9, pp. 465–466); this effect appears to be mediated by the HPA axis. Dysregulation of the HPA axis is frequently found in unmedicated schizophrenics and higher levels of cortisol are associated with more severe symptoms (Gur et al., 2005, p. 97). Increase of cortisol levels increases dopamine activity, implicated in the etiology of schizophrenia. Adolescents with schizoid personality disorder, genetically linked to schizophrenia, show elevated levels of cortisol; the degree of the elevation appears to be directly related to the severity of the symptomatology, in the same manner that has been reported in unmedicated schizophrenics; see above.

DISTURBANCE OF BIORHYTHMS AND IMMUNOLOGICAL PROBLEMS IN PATIENTS WITH AFFECTIVE AND PSYCHOTIC DISORDERS

Patients with mood disorders show desynchrony in the biorhythms, sleep–wake, specifically. Sleep is considered to have a depressogenic influence but sleep deprivation produces a transient antidepressant effect in both unipolar and bipolar depressed patients. There seems to be a close association between sleep loss and the onset of bipolar disorder, mainly, those with rapid cycling illness. Extended sleep, therefore, may be helpful in preventing manic episodes and rapid cycling.

Temperature, REM sleep (a cholinergic mechanism), and other neuropeptide and neuroendocrine factors may be dysregulated in patients with mood disorders. Melatonin, a neuroptide, is secreted at night and inhibited by light. Bipolar patients appear to be sensitive to light and manic episodes have been precipitated by phototherapy. Among the neuroendocrine disturbances, the hypothalamic-pituitary-adrenal (HPA) axis dysregulation and hypercortisolemia, with insensitivity to dexamethasone administration has been demonstrated. Patients with mood disorders show nocturnal secretion disturbances of TSH and a blunted TSH response to thyrotropin-releasing hormone (Rao, 2003, pp. 223–230).

Several conditions that result from immune dysfunction are known to present with symptoms of mania or depression such as multiple sclerosis, lupus, Lyme disease, HIV infections, and steroid therapy (Soto & Murphy, 2003, p. 203). In the major psychiatric disorders, cytokine elevations, lymphocyte subsets alteration, and antibodies to viruses and self-proteins have been demonstrated. Increase of the level of interferons and interleukins (cytokines) have been evidenced in individuals of schizophrenia and bipolar disorder. Patients with rapid cycling bipolar disorder and seasonal affective disorder show lymphocyte activation. These finding are not consistent, however. Increased levels of antibodies to many viruses, especially retroviruses and Borna viruses have been demonstrated in patients with bipolar disorders and schizophrenia. Other findings that are coherent with the proposition that there is an immune alteration in patients with bipolar disorder include the neuropsychiatric symptoms triggered by group A streptococcus, the pediatric autoimmune neuropsychiatric disorders associated with streptococcus (PANDAS) (Soto & Murphy, 2003, pp. 202–203, 204).[5]

OBSTETRICAL ISSUES AND PSYCHOTIC DISORDER

The importance of obstetrical complication as a major causative factor of VEOS/COS is controversial. The rate of obstetrical complication for identified psychotic children was not elevated above the rate for their siblings in the NMIH studies. In the NIMH studies, neither obstetrical complications, socio-conomic stress, nor psychological trauma were related to COS when compared with community samples. These findings are in clear opposition to a large body of adult studies showing a consistent correlation between obstetrical complications and the development of schizophrenia.

A meta-analysis revealed three groups of obstetrical complications potentially associated with schizophrenia: (1) pregnancy complications (bleeding, diabetes, rhesus incompatibility, preeclampsia); (2) abnormal fetal growth and development (low birth weight, congenital malformations, reduced head circumference; and (3) complications of delivery (uterine atony, anoxia, emergency cesarean section). The pooled estimates of effect size were generally less than 2 (Cannon, Jones, & Murray, 2002, p. 1080). The links between these complications and the genetic factors remain elusive. In line with the above, Rosso et al. (2000) propose that fetal hypoxia associated with obstetrical complication is a risk factor for early onset schizophrenia and not for adult onset schizophrenia (p. 805).

Genetic factors, brain insult at birth, neurodevelopmental, neurodegenerative issues, and probably other environmental and experiential factors converge in the expression of impaired brain functioning; this has been consistently demonstrated in schizophrenic patients and is increasingly recognized in mood disordered subjects

NEUROCOGNITIVE DYSFUNCTION IN PRIMARY PSYCHOSES

In a pioneer study, Keshavan et al. (2003) demonstrated that demanding cognitive and perceptual tasks are more frequently impaired in first episode schizophrenics than in other psychotic disorders, and in normal controls. These abnormalities seem to have neurological specificity. The authors found correlations between the cognitive and perceptual abnormalities and neuroimaging findings in the heteromodal association cortex (dorsolateral frontal cortex, superior temporal cortex, and inferior parietal cortex) and the cerebellum; the neurological abnormalities have a localizing value. In light of these findings, the diagnostic examination of psychotic disorders needs to include tests that examine the neuroanatomical intactness of the cerebellum and the left heteromodal association cortex (p. 1302; see chapter 5).

Neurocognitive deficits are also being progressively demonstrated in mood disorders. McClure et al. (2005) reported that the pediatric bipolar disorder group scored significantly lower than controls on the comprehensive assessment of spoken language pragmatics judgment test and made significantly more errors on the Diagnostic Analysis Nonverbal Accuracy scale child facial expression and adult facial expression (p. 1648). These results indicate deficits in social cognition and motor flexibility in patients with narrow phenotype pediatric bipolar disorder. The bipolar disorder group performed more poorly on tasks of involving facial emotional identification and formulation of social appropriate responses to interpersonal situations (p. 1649). Performance on social-cognitive tasks correctly classified 86% of the study participants. The bipolar group also showed deficient response flexibility when required both to inhibit a propotent behavior and to execute an alternative response (the stop–change test) (McClure et al., 2005, p. 1649); see also Pavuluri, Schenkel, et al., 2006 for a demonstration of neurocognitive deficits in pediatric bipolar patients independent of the clinical state or of the nature of the psychopharmacological treatment.

Bipolar patients in a euthymic state fail to activate brain regions associated with performance of an interference task; this may contribute to impaired task performance (Adler, Holland, Mills, et al., 2005, p. 1697). Bipolar patients exhibited significantly poorer performance than healthy subjects on the counting Stroop interference task. The pattern of impairments in bipolar patients suggests an impulsive response bias that was associated with more incorrect responses (false hits) and a failure to slow down during the interference condition in order to improve performance, as healthy subjects did. The bipolar disorder patients' tendency to impulsive response may be reflected in brain activation differences (p. 1701).

ROLE OF NEUROTRANSMITTERS IN PRIMARY PSYCHOSES

A variety of neurotransmitters have been implicated in the pathophysiology and neurochemical mechanisms underlying primary psychosis. For a long time dopamine remained supreme as the exclusive biochemical explanation for psychotic disorders. Overtime, other neurotransmitters (acetylcholine, serotonin, norepinephrine, GABA, and others), have been recognized as important contributors of the biochemical basis of aberrant thinking, feeling and behavior. Moreover, more recent conceptualizations have moved away from ascribing specific and exclusive roles to a single neurotransmitter to a proposition of unbalance among a number of neurotransmitters systems.

Dopamine Role in Schizophrenia

The dopamine hypothesis remains the predominant explanation of how antipsychotics work. The evolution of antipsychotic therapy has led to further refinements of the dopamine hypothesis, including selective (D4) antagonism, rapid dissociation of dopamine receptors, dopamine-serotonin receptor system interactions, dopamine-GABA system interactions, and now, with aripiprazole, the one of partial agonist effects at the dopamine (and selective serotonin) receptors (Buckley, Sebastian, Sinha, & Stirewalt, 2003, p. 71). The NMDA receptor hypofunction represents an alternative or a complementary hypothesis to the dopamine one, see below. In a very elegant and integrative theoretical work, Kapur (2003) articulates the presumptive role of dopamine on symptom formation in schizophrenia, and the presumptive dopaminergic role of antipsychotics in the treatment of this illness. The fundamental proposition is that dopamine mediates motivational salience.

According to Kapur, the role of dopamine in psychosis and schizophrenia should be placed in perspective. First, it is quite likely that the dopaminergic abnormality in schizophrenia is not exclusive (as other systems are probably involved, and it may not even be the primary one). Second, the dopaminergic disturbance is likely a "state" abnormality associated with the dimension of psychosis in schizophrenia, as opposed to being the fundamental abnormality in schizophrenia.

The mesolimbic dopamine system has as a critical role the "attribution of salience," a process whereby events and thoughts come to grab attention, drive action, and influence goal directed behavior because of the association with reward or punishment. This neurochemical aberration usurps the normal process of contextually driven salience attribution and leads to aberrant assignment of salience to external objects and internal representations. Thus, dopamine, which under normal conditions is a mediator of contextually relevant saliences, in the psychotic state becomes a creator of saliences, albeit aberrant ones (pp. 13–15; italics in the original text).

Other issues related to dopamine theory of action are discussed in an endnote.[6]

Interactive Balance of Dopamine and Other Neurotransmitters

The role of the dopamine (DA) system in schizophrenia is currently in a state of reappraisal; other neurotransmitter systems are considered as having a role in the pathogenesis of schizophrenia. A number of interacting models are being proposed: DA-glutamate, DA-acetylcholine, DA-norepinephrine, for example. Although these models still accord DA a significant role in schizophrenia pathophysiology, they suggest that an altered balance between DA and one or more neurotransmitter systems underlie the production of schizophrenic features (Tandon, Taylor, et al., 1999, p. s189).

Role of Cholinergic System

Indirect evidence from several lines of research suggests that the cholinergic system may differentially influence positive and negative symptoms in schizophrenia (Tandon, Taylor, et al., 1999, p. s190). These authors propose that:

1. A disruption of the DA-Ach balance is of central importance in the expression of schizophrenia;
2. Increased dopaminergic activity in the psychotic phase of the illness is accompanied by increased cholinergic activity as a homeostatic response to restore balance;
3. The compensatory increase of cholinergic activity is in turn, accompanied by an intensification of negative symptoms during the acute phase of the illness (pp. s190–s191).

It is reported that the use of 10 mg of trihexyphenidyl a day, reduced the severity of negative symptoms, as assessed by the Scale of Assessment of Negative Symptoms (SANS), in five chronic schizophrenics treated with neuroleptics. The use of biperiden produced similar results, that is, significant increase of positive symptoms and a significant reduction of negative symptoms. Collectively, the data suggest that cholinergic augmentation can play an adjunctive role to neuroleptics in the pharmacological treatment of positive and negative symptoms of schizophrenia. Augmentation with cholinesterase inhibitors, M1 agonists, or partial agonists could prove to be an effective treatment for otherwise neuroleptic-refractory positive symptoms (p. s197).[7]

Muscarinic Receptors

A number of observations suggest that the availability of multiple muscarinic receptor subtypes is reduced in schizophrenia. This is also compatible with the results of neuropathological studies, which have shown a decrease in different muscarinic receptors subtypes (e.g., M1 and M2/M4) in patients with schizophrenia.

Recently, the role of muscarinic system in schizophrenia has been evaluated as a potential novel pharmacological approach for the treatment of psychosis. PTAC is a muscarinic receptor-ligand with partial agonistic effects on M2 and M4 receptors and antagonistic effects on M1, M3, and M5 receptors. PTAC selectively inhibits dopamine cell firing as well as the number of spontaneously active dopamine cells. Since this substance proved to have functional dopamine receptor antagonistic properties in animals, it may be further investigated as a novel approach for the treatment of schizophrenia (p. 125).

In analysis of receptor availability for different neurotransmitters in the frontal cortex, in two samples of patients with schizophrenia and normal comparison subjects, it was found significant lower 3H-QNB binding in patients with schizophrenia. A significant reduction of M1 receptor density in the caudate-putamen of patients with schizophrenia compared with normal subjects has been reported (Raedler et al., 2003, p. 123).

N-Methyl-D-Aspartate (NMDA) Receptor Hypofunction in Primary Psychotic Disorders

NMDA receptors have been the most studied and most broadly distributed in the brain. The NMDA transmitter system is thought to have an important role in memory and cognition, and in sensory information processing, among others. Underexcitation of NMDA receptors (NRHypo), induced by even low doses of NMDA antagonistic medications, produce memory dysfunction; severe NMDA hypofunction produces core features of psychosis as well as euphoria and excitation (Farber & Newcomer, 2003, p. 132). Ketamine and PCP are two NMDA antagonists.

In the proposed hypothesis, glutamate (Glu), acting at the NMDA receptor, functions as a regulator of inhibitory tone. This is accomplished by the tonic stimulation of NMDA receptors on GABAergic interneurons, which in turn inhibit excitatory projections that converge in vulnerable cerebrocortical neurons; this results in a loss of inhibitory control over two major excitatory projections to the cerebral cortex: the cholinergic that originates in the basal forebrain, and the glutamatergic that originates in the thalamus. In addition, NRHypo interferes with inhibitory control over serotonergic and noradrenergic neurons, and also produce underinhibitory Glu control. Simply, disinhibition of this circuitry can trigger psychotic reactions, because the glumatergic neurons lose control of their own firing due to interference with the inhibitory feedback loop (p. 134).[8] GABAergics, alpha-2 agonists, clozapine, and lamotrigine that prevent NRHypo toxicity, fit well within this explanatory model (p. 138). It is further proposed, that dopamine (DA) is increased by the NMDA antagonists, and that this produces psychosis; this is obviously congruent with the familiar hyperdopaminergic theory of psychosis and with PCP and ketamine psychomimetic properties (p. 138).

In the frontiers of clinical research, there is ongoing work on Glutamate receptor modulators and in glycine transport inhibitors (*Clinical Psychiatric News,* August 2005).

THE ROLE OF SECOND MESSENGERS

Frey et al. (2004) reviewed the second messengers' role in the neuropathology and neurochemistry of bipolar disorder (BD). In summary, there is increasing evidence of an alteration of the second messenger systems in BD, reflecting neurobiological changes in this disorder. An increase in the activity of G proteins and cAMP and PIP pathways, have been demonstrated. These alterations disturb the regulation of DNA synthesis, which modifies the proteins involved in protein plasticity, neurogenesis, and the conformation of the cytoskeleton I (p. 185).

Intracellular Signaling Systems

Second messengers like cyclic adenosine monophosphate (cAMP) and phosphatidylinositol (PIP2), exercise their effect via the G proteins. The G protein modulates multiple CNS receptor systems.

Role of the G Proteins

An increase of G8 proteins in the frontal, temporal, and occipital cortices has been reported in bipolar patients (Frey et al., 2004, p. 181). These and related studies seem to indicate a possible association of the role of G proteins in the pathophysiology of bipolar disorders (p. 182).[9]

Role of the cAMP Pathway

Adenilate cyclase (AC) is an effector protein regulated by G proteins; this enzyme catalyzes the formation of CAMP from ATP to produce cAMP. Several studies demonstrate a significant increase in the activity of basal and activated AC among BD subjects. Related studies consistently suggest an increase of cAMP-PKA (protein kinase A) pathway in several brain regions of BD subjects.

Phosphatidylinositol (PIP2) Pathway Role

Several neurotransmitters systems use the PIP2 through the activation of G proteins. In this pathway, G protein stimulates the phospholipase C effector protein (PLC) which hydrolyzes (PIP2); two important second messengers are formed: diacilglycerol (DAG) and inositol triphospohate (IP3). IP3 has a receptor at the endoplasmic reticulum which releases Ca2 stocks when activated. DAG activates protein kinase C (PKC)[10] (Frey et al., 2004, pp. 182–183). Lithium is a potent inhibitor of IMPase (inositol monophosphatase), thus regulating the PIP2. It is likely that this is the basis of lithium mood regulating function (p. 183). In one study, using magnetic resonance spectroscopy (MRS), lithium reduction of inositol concentration in depressed bipolar subjects in the right frontal cortex was demonstrated.

Wnt (Wingless/Glycogen Synthase Kinase 3 [GSK3]) Pathway Role

Therapeutic concentration of lithium and valproate decrease the activity of the GSK3 protein. GSK3 phosphorilizes an extensive array of metabolic, signaling, and structural proteins, and genetic transcription factors, including the regulation of apoptosis, that is stimulated by GSK3. It has been suggested that the neuroprotective effects of neurotrophines, neurotrophic growth factor (NGF) and brain derived neurotrophic factor (BDNF), and lithium are secondary to the inhibition of the GSK3 (p. 184).

Role of Intracellular Calcium (Ca++)

Intracellular calcium levels (Ca++i) modulates synaptic plasticity, cell survival and death. Ca++i signaling interacts with other signaling cascades (cAMP and PIP) and other regulatory proteins (such as calmoduline), which modulate other enzyme systems. Studies suggest that variation in mood state is correlated to Ca++i levels and that these alterations may be reverted with the remissions of the crisis (Frey et al., 2004, p. 184).

Regulation of Gene Expression and Neuroplasticity

Recent studies have shown that lithium, valproate, and carbamazepine may exert therapeutic effects by means of regulating gene expression through transcription factors. Lithium reduces the expression of miristoylated alanine-rich C kinase substrate (MARCKS) protein, involved in the regulation of neuroplastic events, by altering the conformation of the cytoskeleton through actine filaments. Lithium also acts by regulating the proteins genic transcription (dependent in inositol concentration) and on the activation of the receptor linked to the PIP2 cascade. Valproate is capable of inducing similar effects (Frey et al., 2004, p. 185).

BIOMARKERS AND PREDICTOR FACTORS

There is increasing interest in early identification of severe neurodevelopmental disorders with the aim of blocking the expression of incapacitating disorders. The study of neurodevelopment seeks an understanding of the early stages of mental illness and of the process of disease progression. Early interventions pursue outcome improvements in a variety of ways: to protect patients through high-risk periods; to enhance developmental progression, to improve environmental interactions, to prevent kindling and sensitization, and to promote or create healthy neurodevelopment. This is only possible if neurodevelopmental disorders are studied and followed up with a dimensional rather than a categorical approach (Hendren, 2003, p. 6).

The search is on for molecular genetics or imaging signs that will make diagnosis and prediction of clinical course more accurate (Cornblatt, 2003, p.

15). Loci of vulnerability seem to be represented by some phenotype characteristics: physical anomalies, so called minor physical anomalies (MPAs) (such as high-arched palate, low set ears; see p. 5), neurological soft signs (such as difficulties with rapid alternating movements), and developmental instability (such as body asymmetries) (p. 7). Subtle behavioral signs also begin to emerge gradually over the course of development, beginning with early negative symptoms such as increasing social isolation, depression, and anxiety (p. 15).

In the New York High Risk Project, early attentional deficits, which could be reliably identified by age 12, were valid predictors of later schizophrenia-related illness. The strongest predictors for the development of schizophrenia 1 to 10 years later, in apparently normal Israeli children, are the presence of deficits in social functioning, organization ability, and intellectual ability at age 16 and 17 (Lee & McGlashan, 2003, p. 36), which are followed by the emergence of attenuated positive symptoms (Cornblatt, 2003, p. 15). Symptom severity must be considered in the choice of medications. Antidepressants may be as effective as antipsychotics in early phases of the disorder (p. 18). For the definitions of risk, vulnerability, and related concepts, see Table 10.3b.

TABLE 8.1 Therapeutic Implications of Cellular Neurobiological Studies for the Long-Term Action of Mood Stabilizers

Phosphodiestarese inhibitors increase the levels of cyclic adenosine monophosphate (cAMP) response element binding protein (CREB) and the mitogen-activated protein kinase (MAPK) cascade modulators to increase the expression of B-cell lymphoma-2 (Bcl-2) protein, a major neuroprotective protein, and brain-derived neurotrophic factor (BDNF), and inhibit pro-apoptotic signals.

Metabotropic glutamate receptor (mGluR) II/III agonists modulate the release of excessive levels of glutamate; Riluzole and felbamate act on $Na+$ channels to attenuate glutamate release.

Alpha-amino-3-hydroxy-5-methyl-4-isozalopropionic acid (AMPA) potentiators enhance neuroplasticity and upregulate the expression of BDNF.

N-methyl-D-aspartate receptor (NMDAR) antagonists: memantine enhances plasticity and cell survival by decreasing the excess of glutamate

Drugs that increase glial release of neurotrophic factors and stimulate removal of excessive extracellular glutamate might have antidepressant effects

Corticotropine-releasing hormone (CRH) antagonists may reverse the depressogenic and anxiogenic effects of excessive CRH.

Glucocorticoid antagonists might attenuate the deleterious effects of hypercortisolemia, often observed in depression

Agents that upregulate Bcl-2 or other neurotrophic factors can have antistress and antidepressant actions.

Glycogen synthase kinase-3 (GSK-3). Increased activity of GSK-3 is pro-apoptotic. GSK is a primary mediator of the effect of neurotrophic factors such as BDNF and a target of the drug lithium. Lithium reduces GSK-3 activity.

Source: Bachmann, Schloesser, Gould, & Manji (2005, p. 50).

CHAPTER 9

Psychosocial Interventions for Chronic Psychoses

This chapter provides a succinct overview of treatment approaches to the main psychosocial issues confronted by psychiatric clinicians in dealing with psychotic symptoms and chronic psychosis in daily practice. The main premises of this chapter are summarized in the following propositions:

- There is limited evidence-based information to guide clinicians in the choice, intensity, or length of psychosocial interventions for children and adolescents suffering from psychotic spectrum disorders.
- To a large extent, interventions in children and adolescents are based on psychotherapeutic and psychiatric experience with adult patients, with sensitive attention to developmental and family interaction issues.
- Psychosocial interventions are important components of the comprehensive treatment plan of psychotic disorders.
- Research has consistently demonstrated that combined psychopharmacological and psychosocial treatments improve the therapeutic effect size, and that in general, pharmacological interventions have effect size superiority over psychosocial interventions when their therapeutic impact is compared.
- The psychotic child needs a variety of integrated psychosocial, educational, and vocational interventions.
- The psychotic child benefits from applied individual psychotherapeutic techniques aimed at improving subjective states and functioning skills.
- Family interventions aid family members to understand the child's issues, improve parental consistency in the provision of effective discipline, and assist parents in the prevention of regressive behaviors in psychotic children.
- Parents are a key factor in achieving medication compliance and adherence to other components of the treatment plan.

- At all times, psychiatrists will monitor substance abuse, suicide and homicide risks, as well as the risk for endangerment of the living or cultural environment.
- The risk of terrorism and of school massacres is becoming an unfortunate reality that neither the schools nor mental health professionals can ignore. Psychiatrists need to be on the alert for the identification and timely intervention of these possibilities.

This chapter highlights issues relevant to psychotherapeutic goals and objectives for the child and the family of the psychotic child. Issues related to the specifics of the psychotherapeutic modalities are beyond the scope of this presentation; relevant issues will be addressed in a general fashion as they pertain to the comprehensive treatment of psychosis. This chapter is schematic by design.

The child and adolescent psychiatrist needs to monitor a number of specific issues in the lives of acute and chronically psychotic children. In the current mental health delivery of care, psychiatrists rarely become directly responsible for carrying out psychosocial interventions. At best, psychiatrists are assumed to provide an oversight or integrating role regarding all interventions the patient and family receive.

Patients and families do not parcel out professional roles in the same way managed care systems do. Parents tend to see the child and adolescent psychiatrists as the foremost experts in the field, and expect that psychiatrists will provide medical, pharmacological, and psychosocial guidance. The greater the psychiatrists' knowledge and expertise in psychosocial treatments, the better they will be able to serve their patients, even when those services are provided by other mental health practitioners. Even in cases where other individual or family therapists are involved, patients and families still consult the child and adolescent psychiatrist about a number issues going on in their lives and in the psychotherapeutic relationship in particular. Moreover, there are circumstances in which the child or the family asks the psychiatrist opinions about issues that transpire in therapy or about the way therapy is being conducted. Occasionally, the child or adolescent needs to address these concerns with the therapists; rarely, the psychiatrist needs to recommend a change of individual or family therapist(s).

GENERAL PRINCIPLES OF PSYCHOSOCIAL TREATMENTS FOR PSYCHOTIC CHILDREN

Siris and Bermanzohn (2003) propose two models of psychiatric rehabilitation: medical (treatment) and educational (training). The first model deals with biological defects that need to be diagnosed and rectified. The second attends to the strengths or abilities that constructively can be modified through skills acquisition to maximize the patient's potential (in the process of habilitation or rehabilitation). The authors suggest that a thoughtful combination of the two models is the most useful approach to serve the patients (p. 171). The present author subscribes to this combined model.

Whereas in adult psychiatry, rehabilitation (restoration of a lost function) is the predominant approach, in children and adolescent psychiatry, both habilitation (building of functions or skills) and rehabilitation are necessary. In children and adolescents, control of regressive behavior is also a major therapeutic goal. All psychotherapeutic goals need to address interferences with social and academic learning and the loss of adaptive functioning. Based on a comprehensive assessment and auxiliary diagnostic tests (laboratory examinations and pertinent consultations), the psychiatrist constructs a comprehensive treatment program for the child and family.

TREATMENT GOALS FOR THE PSYCHOTIC CHILD

Although medications are important in the treatment of most chronic psychotic disorders, careful consideration must be given to the psychological and social aspects of this population (Bryden, Carrey, & Kutcher, 2001). Medications are not a substitution for psychosocial treatments but a different and complementary approach to assist the child and the family in the process of adaptive growth. Medications render children more amenable to psychosocial interventions by controlling positive symptoms and by decreasing the negative ones; medication may also improve patients' cognition, and indirectly may also assist in improving self-esteem.

WORK WITH FAMILIES OF PSYCHOTIC CHILDREN

Once the psychiatrist has gathered the evaluative data and has made a diagnostic formulation, he shares his or her findings and formulation with the family and the child. The psychiatrist will indicate the biological and relevant psychosocial factors that relate to the presenting problem and the disorder(s) in question. When the child has shown persistent developmental deviation, in spite of a caring and consistent parenting, the psychiatrist will call the parents' attention to intrinsic biological factor that may have a significant bearing in the presenting problems. With few exceptions, parents are prone to attribute to themselves, to blame themselves, for the child's dysfunction. Sometimes parents may have contributed to the child's symptoms; many times, they have not. Guilt-prone parents may take responsibility for whatever goes wrong with their children. On the contrary, self-centered parents tend to disregard or minimize the impact that parenting has on the child.

Chronic psychiatric disorders promote developmental deviations resulting in difficulties in many areas of adaptive functioning. The chronically psychotic child usually manifests difficulties at home and school; these problems are secondary to the child's inability to relate appropriately, to exercise effective impulse control, or to the lack of resilience in coping with the daily narcissistic injuries that every child goes through. Intruding psychotic ideation in the classroom interferes with concentration and task orientation. Moreover, many chronically psychotic children and adolescents suffer from demoralization and amotivation resulting in a lack of school work interest and academic underperformance. Cognitive deficits should be underappreciated.

It is helpful for the psychiatrist to indicate to the parents the dimensions of the child's dysfunction that need special attention or that will become the target of intervention, rather than giving them global explanations that disconnect them from the child. Thus, telling parent that the child evidences difficulties with anger control, getting along with others (making or maintaining friends), focusing attention in class, or the like, is more understandable and helpful than telling them, "your child is bipolar, Asperger's, pervasive developmental disorder," or the like.

In adults, "For persons with schizophrenia, the combination of psychoeducational family therapy and antipsychotic medication produced dramatic improvements in the relapse rate compared to either modality alone" (Gabbard & Kay, 2001, p. 1957). There is no reason to think differently about the impact of combined interventions in the field of child and adolescent primary psychosis (schizophrenia and bipolar disorder).

Remschmidt, Martin, Hennighausen, and Schultz (2001) recommend a number of practical goals with the families of schizophrenic children; these recommendations may be extended to children with other psychotic disorders psychoses. (1) Development of a therapeutic alliance. (2) Psychoeducation. It is important to inform the family about the prevailing views of the illness (the role of "organicity," the role of genes and inheritance, issues related to the role of brain structure and dysfunction, developmental delays and deviations, as well as vulnerability to environmental stresses). Families should be informed of the clinical course, prognosis, and available treatments with due emphasis on antipsychotic medications. The information related to the disorder needs to be presented in a gradual and timely manner (and in understandable terms).

1. Psychoeducation should emphasize the severity of the illness, its long-term course, and the need for uninterrupted treatment. Parents need to be encouraged to keep a long view of the treatment process; they need to be given hope, and support and encouragement for adhering to psychopharmacological treatment, complementary psychosocial treatments, and the provision of consistent discipline and limit setting.
2. Priority objectives for family therapy interventions are the neutralization

of parents' negative emotions (mostly, guilt for "causing the child's illness") and to disconnect the family from feeling responsible for the child's problems. Efforts should be made at reducing guilt and decreasing "expressed emotions," particularly criticism and hostility (see below). Conflicts and emotional vicious circles of blame and guilt developed around the disorder need to be interrupted. Children's symptoms need to be disconnected from putative family interactions. Broader family goals should only be pursued until the child achieves a significant reduction of symptoms and a good therapeutic alliance has been established.

3. To build positive and supportive relationships among the family members, and to assist the family to avoid overinvolvement (pp. 240–243). To these objectives we add,

4. The families will be made aware of suicide risk, as well as the risk for violence, and the risk of unfolding comorbidities, like anxiety disorder, drug abuse, or others.

Psychoeducational family interventions (PFIs) are the only family therapy modalities with international evidence support. PFIs present a diathesis stress model of chronic psychosis, and address family needs for education, support, behavior management techniques, and problem solving strategies. Available psychoeducational models differ significantly in structure and content (Lefley, 2004, p. 70). Culturally sensitive interventions maximize the effectiveness of family psychoeducation.

Multimodal treatments offer some promise for treatment of children and families with psychotic conditions in childhood. These interventions incorporate various treatment approaches, and select a number of foci or dysfunctional sectors for intervening directly with the youth and the family (Farmer, Dorsey, & Mustillo, 2004, p. 864).

Among multimodal interventions, multisystemic therapy (MST), with demonstrated effectiveness and replicable results, offers applications for the treatment of psychotic disorders of children and adolescents. MST has strong evidence-based research and has strong ecological underpinnings; it focuses on the fit between youth and the environment, and concentrates on interventions and modifications that improve this fit with the goal of improving targeted behaviors. MST can be individualized.

Suicide and Homicide Risk

Schizophrenia (and related disorders) and bipolar disorders (and other mood disorders) carry the highest lethality risk: both conditions are associated with the highest suicide risk among all other psychiatric illnesses. The suicide risk for bipolar disorder (and related conditions) is slightly higher than the risk for schizophrenic disorders: 15 and 12%, respectively. This means, that approximately one in six patients with bipolar-related disorders will end up inducing his or her own demise, and that up to one in eight schizophrenic patients will end up killing themselves. The homicide risk for both conditions is considerably less, but, this eventuality is above the potential risk of other psychiatric conditions and of the general population at large. Basil, Mathews, Sudak, and Adetunji (2005) state that according to the Epidemiological Catchment Area survey, about 13% of schizophrenia patients engage in violent behavior. The authors added that violence is more common during acute psychotic episodes, and that people with mental illness who come from violent backgrounds are often violent themselves (p. 60). It is likely that the rate of violence in mood disordered youth is higher that the cited schizophrenic one.

Families need to learn to identify any increase in the suicide or homicide risk, and to take appropriate steps to decrease that risk. Changes in mood, increased irritability, changes in the quality of relating, increased level of hostility, evidence of substance abuse, deterioration of adaptive functioning, and a lack of compliance with psychotropic medications should raise the level of concern and increase surveillance over possible suicide and homicide risk.

Any suicide or homicide threats should not be taking lightly. The risk is more serious if the child has already made an attempt against his life or that of others. Signs of inner tension or of increasing turmoil may be presumed when the level of adaptation or prosocial behaviors deteriorates, when there are indications of emotional or behavioral dyscontrol, when there are problems with reality testing, paranoia, or indications of substance abuse.

The psychiatrist will be exhaustive in the exploration of imminent risk and will not be satisfied with the patient's denials. It is wise to assume that the risk will remain until the level of adaptation and the interpersonal rapport improves. In like manner, any homicidal verbalization or threat, or any terroristic verbalization should be given the seriousness of exploration that it deserves.

All along, the clinician will alert the family about the patient's risks and of the need to keep a watchful eye on the patient's behavior and emotional lability. The family will also be reminded of the risks of comorbid conditions, mainly, depression, conduct problems, and of alcohol/substance abuse. For the specifics of the assessment of suicidal and homicidal risks, as well as a therapeutic approach for these constellations of behaviors, the reader is referred to appropriate, current, and pertinent texts in the child and adolescent psychiatry field.

Self-abusive behavior creates concern and alarm for most families. Any kind of self-abusive behavior requires expert evaluation. Response to chronic self-abusive behaviors rests on expert advice. In general, the family will be advised to develop a zero tolerance toward suicidal and homicidal behavior, and to decrease the level of fear and preoccupation toward chronic self-abusive behaviors.

Expressed Emotion

The importance of controlling expressed emotion within the family cannot be overemphasized. Expressed emotion is a pernicious factor for the vulnerable child and for the family as a whole. Although expressed emotion has gained notoriety in relation to schizophrenia relapse, the concept has broader implications for the maintenance and reactivation of a number of psychiatric illnesses such as schizophrenia, affective disorders, eating disorders, and probably others. Actually, expressed emotion is a more reliable predictor for relapse of affective disorders and eating disorders than for schizophrenia. It is possible that children affected by expressed emotion become more sensitive to its effects as the illness continues, probably akin to the process of kindling implicated in the progression of seizure and affective disorders (Butzlaff & Hooley, 1998).

Other family therapy objectives include:

1. Up and Down Regulation

For parents of a "bipolar pattern child," Greenspan and Glovinsky (2005) recommended work on affective signaling, including more effective and sensitive patterning of up and down regulation (p. 5). They also recommended engaging the child in problem solving discussions (strategies) to think about the upcoming day and to anticipate and describe feelings associated with positive and negative expectations. They stated that the home program focuses on providing a stable, nurturing caregiver relationship and firm, persistent guidance but not punitive limit setting (see next item.). This intervention is in line with found emotional processing deficits, in addition to cognitive deficits in patients at risk for psychosis (Croog, Naccari, & Wong, 2005, pp. 13–14). "Doctors might want to spend some time with patients and families discussing the identification of feelings during stressful situations so that patients can better regulate their moods and cope with those stressful situations" (p. 14).

2. Promotion of Consistent Limit Setting

Family therapy interventions strive to assist the family in the provision of sensitive and consistent limit setting. The psychological handicaps created by overindulgence (infantilization) and inconsistency are frequently more incapacitating than the illness itself. Whereas schizophrenic children need optimum prompting and encouragement, bipolar psychotic children need firm and consistent limits due to impulsivity and their limited controls over aggressive and sexual behaviors.

Viewing treatment as long-term in nature, as a transition from one developmental stage to another, and helping child and family to work at each particular stage, helps children and parents to focus attention away from simply problematic behaviors, to issues that are in need of refinement and improvement through transitional stages. Having the family "map out" where they are now, where they are headed, how they will get there, and how to check their progress as they "travel" in treatment is crucial to ongoing success.

TABLE 9.1 Factors That Influence Parental Inconsistency

Lack of parental alliance
Parental discord
Complex attachments to grandparents and others relatives
    The role of the absent and undermining parent
    Unresolved divorced issues
    Issues related to adoption

3. Promotion of Sensitive Developmental Guidance

As psychotic children mature and reach adolescence, parents feel uncertain about how to deal with the child's growing strivings for independence or with their increasing sexual interests. Parents need to be reminded of the risks of drugs, unwanted pregnancies, and the need for birth control, as well as the need to be vigilant about medication compliance, exploitative peers, and antisocial acting out.

4. Attention to Other Children's Needs

As a result of the parents' efforts to help the identified patient, the family's emotional and financial resources are seldom evenly distributed. Because of this, siblings resent parental devotion to the identified patient. Parents need to be reminded to attend to the needs of their more adaptive children, and to make special efforts to spend quality time with them. Unintended neglect and its unforeseen consequences often cause resentment and create maladaptation and psychopathology in other siblings and family members. It is lore in family therapy that when the identified child improves, other children's problems begin to surface. It is likely that the family will be able to attend to other children's needs when the identified child's needs are resolved.

5. Promotion of Independence

Parents stimulate the exercise of increasing autonomy by making the child progressively responsible over a number of life tasks. The delegation of autonomy should be commensurate with the child's demonstrated capacities and judgment. It is very hard for a handicapped youth who reaches adult age to accept fewer privileges than his nonhandicapped siblings or peers; it is equally complicated for parents to curtail privileges or to increase supervision over young adults who lack reliable judgment or who are not quite capable of protecting themselves.

The impaired child needs to take progressive responsibility over his own basic needs; he (as well as she) needs to learn to prepare meals (basic cooking), to launder and iron, and to develop the habit of keeping the living environment tidy and clean. The child also needs to learn to use money, to budget, to keep a checkbook, and to save.

More challenging issues arise around curfews and car use. If there are reservations about permitting so-called normal children to drive before the age of

18, there are greater concerns in the exercise of this privilege for children with problems of reality testing or sustained concentration difficulties, and for those suffering from unstable mood, impulsivity, and faulty judgment.

6. Support of Independent Living

Parents need to support and encourage the child's efforts for independent living; parents need to support the child's highest possible levels of autonomy and independent functioning. Parents promote independent functioning by allowing children to take charge of their daily care activities: hygiene, toileting, dressing, and eating. Sound nutritional and eating habits are of major relevance in psychotic children since they carry an intrinsic risk for DM and metabolic syndrome, more so if they receive antipsychotic medications that promote weight gain; ditto for the need of having an active physical life, and for striving to maintain a healthy level of fitness.

Sedentary habits, excessive Internet use, and TV viewing need to be discouraged. Since many psychotic children are psychologically vulnerable, and their reality testing is unstable, it is important to be vigilant over Internet use, TV programming, and being aware of the movies they watch. Since most children navigate the Internet, it is important for parents to monitor the sites their children visit. Inappropriate Internet sites expose children to misinformation and encourage children to maladaptive behaviors.

Issues regarding sleep hygiene are important to most psychotic children; this is particularly relevant to children with bipolar disorder for whom sleep difficulties may bring about reactivation of the mood disturbance. Sleep difficulties are major indicators of incomplete stabilization or of deterioration of the clinical course.

Limit Setting and Boundary Enforcement

Limit setting and enforcement of boundaries are problematic areas for many parents, more so for parents with chronically psychotic children. Thinking they are responsible for the child's illness, parents feel that the child deserves special considerations and special concessions; in consequence, parents compromise, allowing children to bend or to break the rules, thus permitting children to be inconsistent in meeting expectations. Enforcing the rules requires firmness and constructive assertiveness. Setting limits and imposing consequences requires firmness, determination, and consistency, a sine qua non of good parenting.

Guilty parents feel that if they are firm and determined they will be perceived as mean and unyielding. As a result, they become inconsistent and erratic with limit setting and with the enforcement of consequences. Even worse, some parents undermine the discipline or the consequences appropriately set by the other parent, the school, or other authority figures.

A critical issue for psychiatrists to convey to parents is the need for them to train themselves to look at the results of the misbehavior rather than just at the misbehavior itself (Dinkmeyer, 1989). A practical guideline for parents as to how to sort out the nature of the child's misbehavior and how to approach an appropriate response (limits or consequences that need to be imposed) is provided by Dreikurs and Gray (1970). They classify the motives of misbehavior into four broad categories: Attention, Power, Revenge, and Display of Inadequacy. It is important for the parents to learn to understand what motive is being activated by their child's acting out. When they do so, their interventions will be sensitive and developmentally sound. Psychiatrists would do well to point out to parents that their feelings about the child's misbehavior can often point to the category of the motive that is fostering the child's misbehavior.

In some cases, parents infantilize their children by interfering with the children's emerging strivings for separation-individuation and with their progressive efforts to gain autonomy. Some parents are apprehensive about the children's strivings for separation and increasing sexual interest. The end result is that many children become completely handicapped by the time they reach adulthood. When these adolescents reach maturity, they have not learned to take care of themselves and many reach adult life without the most basic self-care skills: they do not know how to take care of their most basic needs.

Regressive Behavior

Psychological and behavioral regression occurs when the child or adolescent resorts to ways of thinking or behaving that were appropriate to prior developmental phases. Specifically, regressed children attempt to solve conflicts and developmental demands using coping mechanisms characteristic of prior, infantile developmental states.

Developmental regression differs from the concept of developmental arrest. The latter involves the lack of developmental progression secondary to trauma (physical, sexual abuse, a medical insult, etc.), or for lack of environmental stimulation (neglect) needed for the achievement of higher levels of psychological, emotional, and interpersonal adaptation. When stress is overwhelming and children cannot cope with developmental demands, the regressive pull is inevitable. Developmental arrests create fixation points that operate as forces that pull development back to immature and infantile levels of adaptation. Simply, when a children regress they go back to the fixation points, where less demands and autonomy are required, that is, to the fixation points that create the illusion they will be protected from further demands.

Regressions can be transitory or permanent. The transitory ones are common and even expected in the developmental course (i.e., increased attention seeking behavior on the part of a 2½-year-old upon the arrival of a sibling, or lapses in bowel or bladder control in a 6-year-old when the family moves to new neighborhood). With sensitive support children regain mastery of the functions they had temporarily surrendered. Permanent regressions, on the other hand, are stable, enduring, passive-dependent adaptations in which the individual no longer struggles to achieve mastery or a higher level of autonomy. The "child's ego" no longer strives to master conflict or environmental demands but goes back to states of lesser psychological demand. It could be said that in stable regression the ego has surrendered to dependency and passivity, and that "the ego feels" overwhelmed with attempts to achieve higher levels of adaptation.

Psychotic children lack inner resources to cope with developmental expectations and environmental demands. Instead of attempting to master conflicts or to resolve demands, they regress to prior developmental states where the stress and the demands are less. In these regressive states, the ego is passive and autonomy is relinquished. At those levels, children want to be cared for and expect to be passively satisfied. Some regressed children activate primitive grandiosity and feel entitled to make irrational demands. Stable regressions have a great deal of adhesiveness; frequently, regressed children are reluctant to give up the secondary gain extracted from passive gratifications, dependency, magical thinking, and power and control they exercise over their parents. Parents assist in solidifying the regression when they accept and nurture the passivity and dependency of their regressed children. Many immature and needy parents accept and hold onto the regressed children for their own narcissistic gratifications; worse, some parents block their children's attempts to move forward in the developmental timeline.

When examining regressed patients, it is suggested that the psychiatrist contrast the behavioral age with the chronological age as a preliminary intervention (Cepeda, 2000, pp. 210–211). The main goal of this intervention is to call the child's attention to the regressive behavior, to create dystonicity with the maladaptive behavior, and to encourage and reinforce an adaptive, age-appropriate demeanor. Regressive behaviors are common in patients undergoing malignant decompensations, such as acute psychotic states, schizophrenias, bipolar disorders, trauma, and other severe disorders.

Handling regression is a very difficult task for the parents: they need to meet the child's immediate needs, but at the same time they need to expect and demand from the child that he or she be more autonomous, act more maturely, and be less dependent. This is a difficult and trying endeavor.

Parents are advised to expect children to behave their age all the time; this expectation prompts children to gain mastery and to pursue active means to fulfill gratification of their needs. Children need to be rewarded for acting adaptively and need to be discouraged (they need to be given consequences) for acting regressively (immaturely). The ongoing prompting and stimulation serves as a counterbalance to the regressive tendencies. Regressive behavior requires a coordinated approach: all the interventions (individual, group, family therapy, and others) need to target regression as a major therapeutic objective.

Support for Families of Psychotic Children

The need to provide ongoing support for families with chronically psychotic children should not be underestimated. Children with chronic psychiatric illnesses put a great deal of stress on their families. There is increased risk of parental exhaustion (parental burnout) with the associated risks of parental abuse and neglect. Stressed families tend to fragment. For parents with a history of psychiatric illness or alcohol or substance abuse, the stress of dealing with a difficult child puts the parent at risk for relapse of the psychiatric illness, chemical dependency problem, or both. Marital conflict, separation, and divorce are common in families with chronically ill children. As previously stated, neglect, and physical and sexual abuse are common in stressed families.

Clinicians will assess the degree of support the family receives from the previous generation; stressed families may require the restoration of broken emotional ties with their prior generations. Clinicians will uncover the nature of the family estrangement and how previous emotional bonds were prematurely "cut off." Therapists will create opportunities for the stressed family members to reconnect, to "make amends," with the family of origin; that is, to restore intergenerational communication and emotional bonds. When the reason for the estrangement is justified (e.g., the grandfather is a pedophile or a chronic criminal), the clinician will attempt to encourage alternative sources of emotional support.

When the psychiatrist observes significant marriage conflict or evidence of psychopathology in other family members, he will refer the parent(s) for a psychiatric evaluation, or to a marriage counselor or family therapist, to address the identified difficulties.

Parents Support Groups

Multifamily groups are helpful in resolving issues of blame regarding the cause of the disorder; parents feel less alienated when they learn that many other parents struggle with children with psychotic and other chronic dysfunctions. Furthermore, parents may receive help with their own parental and family issues, and at the same time, they may provide assistance to other parents in problem solving as to how to deal with particular challenges related to raising chronically psychotic children.

Issues Related to the School and the Parents

The family needs to know how the school deals with students' acting out or aggressive behaviors. Families need to know how the school will deal with behavioral crises. Commonly, parents are called every time the child acts up, and are asked to pick up children when they misbehave. Commonly, the school resorts to suspending a student when the school considers that the child's safety is at risk, when the child gets out of control, when the child endangers others students, or when the child is disruptive to the learning environment for other students. Such interventions cause a great deal of disruption in the parents' work responsibilities and add further stress for them. Frequently, parents need to make unexpected arrangements to procure babysitting or adult supervision when the child is dismissed. Some parents are terminated from their jobs due to the ongoing work disruptions; unemployment adds a further stress to emotionally and financially overtaxed families..

Respite Services

A comprehensive program for stressed families caring for children with severe psychotic disorders and its associated disabilities needs to include respite services. Respite services are defined as the provision of temporary care to persons with disabilities, with the primary purpose of providing relief to caregivers. Respite has been common in the field of developmental and physical disabilities (Farmer, Dorsey, & Mustillo, 2004, p. 872). This service is particularly helpful for families caring for children with severe neurodevelopmental difficulties that demand intense care and supervision, to avoid parental burnout, and to deescalate negative child–parental practices.

Career and Vocational Goals

Realistic career options and vocational goals need to be established. There are parents who set unrealistic goals for their children by disregarding the children's limitations; other parents have very low expectations for their children, in spite of their intellectual or academic potential; they fear that children with chronic psychotic illnesses will never be able to achieve any major goals in life. Psychoeducational programming that achieves a good integration of cognitive and personality strengths with the child's abilities, aptitudes, and attitudes, are likely to promote optimum academic and vocational goals.

Governmental agencies like the Texas Rehabilitation Commission, and its equivalents in other states, are a great resource for parents and youth to access services of vocational assessment and training, and other assistance in the process of rehabilitation (or habilitation) of chronically psychotic youth.

Communication with Professionals

Parents will be encouraged to develop a network of supportive resources for ongoing care and eventual crises. Parents need to feel they can communicate with their child's psychiatrist and therapist(s) at moments of crisis; they need to know that psychiatrists and therapists would like to be informed of any unusual development in the patient's life, of any negative development in the clinical course, of the emergence of a medical illness, or of development of medication side effects.

It is likely, that children with chronic psychosis will receive case-management services that will assist in appropriate, timely, and cost-effective utilization of medical and psychiatric services. See table 9.2 for a summary of goals of parental and developmental guidance. Parents need to keep in close communication with the school to monitor the child's progress in academics and his or her deportment with teachers and peers. The quality of the child's socialization needs special attention. Regular contact with the school psychologist or school counselor is expected. When the child has social deficits, he or she is expected to receive social skill training as part of the special education curriculum. It is very desirable that prior to each psychiatric appointment the parent communicates with therapists, the school counselor, teachers, and other professionals who are working with the child; the better the overview the child psychiatrist receives, the better he or she will be able to make pertinent decisions and recommendations to the child and family.

Role of Medications and Other Treatment Modalities

Medications are not panaceas to deal with the multiplicity of issues related to child and adolescent psychosis. Most of the available antipsychotics are effective in ameliorating major psychoses. It is difficult to say that one medication is better than a competing one. In practice, what ultimately matters is the practitioner's experience with a number of antipsychotics and mood stabilizing medications, and the physician's familiarity with each medication's clinical applications, pattern of response, tolerance, and their side effect profile.

Different children react differently to the same medication, and the same medication elicits different responses and side effects in different patients. More often than not, antipsychotic or mood stabilizers are changed because of unfold-

TABLE 9.2 Goals of Parental and Developmental Guidance

1. General goals
   - Monitoring of the implementation of the treatment plan
   - Monitoring of parents' working through of the diagnosis and their commitment to treatment goals
   - Monitoring of the implementation of treatments (individual and family therapies, medical work-ups, neurological follow-ups, etc.)
2. Monitoring of adherence to psychotropic medications
   - Is the family certain that the child is taking the medications?
   - What habits or routines have the child and family developed to insure medication intake?
3. Pertinent issues that need to be monitored in the families include:
   - Parental alliance
   - Consistent limit setting
   - Consistent discipline
   - Setting consistent consequences

   Other issues that need special discussion with parents include,
   - Curfews
   - Internet use, TV viewing, phone and cellular use, etc.
   - Dating
   - Car use
   - Allowances
   - Chores and work
   - Friends
   - Sexual behavior
   - Birth control
   - Alcohol and drug use monitoring

ing undesirable side effects rather than for a lack of therapeutic effectiveness. If a particular side effect develops, a different mood stabilizer or antipsychotic with less likelihood of bringing about the same side effects is usually tried. This is a more sound practice than sticking to a particular medication and adding additional drugs to counteract emerging side effects.

School plays a major role in the identification of neuroleptic and other psychotropic medications' side effects. In the classroom, sedation, concentration difficulties, disturbances of memory, interferences with language, and other obstacles to learning can be identified, monitored, and communicated to parents and the psychiatrist. School can also assist with the monitoring of negative symptoms and emergence of extrapyramidal side effects.

Issues Related to Medication Compliance

The clinician will assume that problems of medication compliance will become an issue for all patients and with all families. Medication is an indispensable component in the treatment of children with chronic psychosis. Parents need to be extensively educated on the role of antipsychotic and other psychotropic medications. The idea that a child may need to take medications for years is a difficult reality for many parents to accept. Even before a child begins antipsychotic treatment many parents ask, "How long will my child need to be on this medication? What are the long-term effects of this antipsychotic?" These and related questions are frequent worries for many parents.

Parents need to be told that before concerns with long-term side effects could be addressed, the short-term issues related to medication effectiveness and tolerance take immediate priority. If the child responds well and tolerates a given mood stabilizer or antipsychotic, issues related to the long-term consequences of the medication(s) will be addressed at that point. Target symptoms and potential side effects will be reviewed and documented. A comprehensive review of common medication side effects and of serious long-term untoward side effects must be discussed with the parents and should be documented. Health risks, neurological side effects, hormonal difficulties, cognitive interferences, and other adverse events, should be discussed and documented on a regular basis.

Clinicians underestimate the extent of their patients' nonadherence (lack of compliance). Adherence to treatment in general and medications in particular, is generally low, even in patients who attend appointments on a regular basis. Low compliance has been reported even for medications that are considered "vital" or indispensable, such as antiepileptic, antidiabetic, antibiotics, and many others. Clinicians need to learn the patient's medication routines and should make suggestions to develop habits to insure compliance. The clinician will consider lack of compliance, or of partial adherence, a serious breach of the working alliance, prompting the family and the child to review the treatment plan.

Clinicians will strive to understand the frequency of partial compliance or the lack of participation in other treatment modalities, and will strive to elucidate why the patient does not follow through with the recommended treatments. When patients do not take their medications, the psychiatrist needs to suspect the presence of undesirable side effects; in sexually active adolescents, the possibility of sexual side effects or feared side effects, deserves serious consideration. Rarely, if ever, do patients stop medication to prolong the secondary gain of their illness. More often, patients "give up" on the medications because they do not feel any relief from their distressing symptoms.

Compliance with individual and family therapy, psychoeducational interventions, and other medical–neurological or psychotherapeutic recommendations need consistent monitoring. The attentive clinician will help the child and family to avoid crises and will assist parents to identify and cope with inevitable life problems and adversities.

In all cases, the physician will pay attention to the family's style of discipline and will promptly intervene at first evidence of abusive practices. The mental health professional should not hesitate to involve the child protective services (CPS) if he or she suspects that abuse has occurred or is ongoing. In general, families have a negative perception about the role of CPS, but CPS has many positive things to offer to stressed families. CPS may provide needed supervision and may also facilitate access to a number of community and psychotherapeutic resources for families in distress.

Illness Management

Chronically psychotic children need to learn to take progressive responsibility in managing their psychiatric illness. These children need to learn to communicate to their families issues related to their disorder and its treatment: reappearance of psychotic features, reemergence of mood difficulties, increased anger, sleep difficulties, dysphoria, restlessness, EPS, or the emergence of other untoward medication side effects.

Psychotic children need to take progressive initiative in taking their medication on a regular basis, in alerting the family that the medications need to be refilled, or that blood for laboratory tests needs to be drawn. They also need to take initiative in accelerating appointments with the psychiatrist when symptoms reemerge or when untoward side effects become manifest.

TREATMENT GOALS WITH THE CHRONICALLY PSYCHOTIC CHILD

Skills Building

For children with major neurodevelopmental problems, including psychosis or mood dysregulation, adaptive skills will be promoted in those areas identified as neuropsychologically deficient. Skills that take preeminence as treatment goals include:

Anger Control

Anger management problems are major issues of maladjustment in psychotic and mood dysregulated children. They are the cause of serious disciplinary measures by schools, including recurrent suspensions, alternative schools, and expulsion. Schools are intolerant of aggressive behavior and intervene promptly following even minor signs of lack of anger control. More often than not, any student who displays anger difficulties is required to undergo a psychiatric evaluation. After an episode of dyscontrol, if the student is allowed to continue schooling, it is likely that he or she will be referred to an alternative school program prior to reintegration into a special education program at his or her home school.

Children with difficulties in anger control frequently display violence toward family members, typically siblings and parents. Parents become targets and victims of the psychotically or labile-mood and uncontrolled child. The family is usually more tolerant than school of the child's aggression, but persistent victimization of family members forces parents or caretakers to seek psychiatric assistance, to ask the police to intervene, or to consider placing the child outside of the family. When the family takes this difficult step, reintegration of the child into the family system will be contingent upon the child's demonstration that it is safe for him or her to be around family members again. Skills in anger management and improvement of problem-solving techniques are important objectives in the treatment of the aggressive psychotic children.

Cognitive processes influence the child's response to interpersonal conflicts or frustrations with environmental obstacles. These processes involve perceptions and attributions of the problematic events and a cognitive plan as to how to respond to those events. It is proposed that children's cognitive and emotional processing of the problem and their chosen response determine the nature of the behavioral response (aggression, assertion, passive acceptance or withdrawal) (Lochman, Barry, & Pardini, 2003, p. 264).

Components of the anger coping and coping power programs designed for aggressive children with conduct difficulties may be adapted for the treatment of aggressive psychotic children. These programs include group sessions addressing issues such as anger management, perspective taking, social problem solving, emotional awareness, relaxation training, social skill enhancement, positive social and personal goals, and dealing with peer pressure. There is also a parent component designed to address such issues as social reinforcement and positive attention, importance of clarity of house rules, behavioral expectations and monitoring, the use of appropriate and effective discipline strategies, family communications, positive connection to schools, and stress management (p. 265).

Self-removal from provocative situations, self-breaks, self-talk, distraction, and relaxation techniques are methods to deal with aggressive feelings and behaviors as they arise. Steiner (2004) summarized the evidence-based nonpharmacological treatment options for aggressive behavior in children and adolescents as follows:

Contingency Management
Anger Management

Cognitive Problem-Solving Skills Training
Parent Management Training
Functional Family Therapy
Multisystemic Therapy

Frustration Tolerance

Easy reactivity and recurrent emotional flareups (affective storms) that overwhelm ego controls are common problems in chronic psychosis and mood dysregulated patients. The ability to delay frustration and to assess the implications of personal actions is a fundamental developmental acquisition. This is a mature executive function. The capacity to modulate aggression and to apply appropriate problem solving measures to cope with challenging and frustrating situations are high level adaptive behaviors.

Elements of the anger coping program have applicability in dealing with psychotic children who are aggressive, lack social competence, or display low frustration tolerance; this program works by way of modeling, role-playing, group problem solving tasks, and feedback reinforcement of children's social behavior with peers and adult group leaders (Lochman, Barry, & Pardini, 2003, p. 268).

Motivation

"Motivation" and "will" are considered energizers of thought and behavior, providing them with spontaneity and strength against opposing inner psychic or outer environmental forces (Souza, Moll, & Eslinger, 2004, p. 59). Disorders of motivation and will stand out as the most disabling symptoms in clinical practice. Disorders of will comprise a heterogeneous family of symptoms and abnormal behaviors with discrete neural correlates. They have been described under the rubric of "abulia" or "avolition" and may result from many different diseases affecting the body or the brain (p. 59). The differential diagnosis of amotivation includes depression (lack of interest, withdrawal), drug abuse, neurological impairment (frontal lobe syndromes), schizophrenic disorders, and others. Demoralization and pervasive hopelessness resulting from a defective self-concept such as the sense of being internally damage, "crazy," or "incurably mentally ill" need to be considered.

Amotivation causes disregard for the self in relation to others and the abandonment of goals and ambitions with a future orientation. Serious psychotic illnesses cause a core disorganization of the personality functions that strive to utilize and coordinate adaptive resources to reach individual satisfying goals. Amotivation undermines personal care and social behavior as well as educational and vocational objectives. Any of these areas may require special attention in the rehabilitation of the psychotic child. Improvement of motivation is one of the most complex and difficult habilitation and rehabilitation tasks. These efforts are facilitated by the amelioration of positive and negative symptoms.

Speech and Communication Deficits

If the child reports a history of speech delay or if there is evidence of speech comprehension or of expressive language difficulties, a thorough speech and language evaluation is mandatory. If suggested by expert evaluations, the child should receive regular, intense, professional speech and language remediation. Since language is the basis for most cognitive and sociocognitive functions, parents will be advised to advocate for the implementation of speech/language therapy intervention at an optimal level of competence and intensity. Timely identification of speech/language disorders improves the quality of the relationship between the child and the family, and interferes with the parent's negative perception of the child. It is common for receptive language disorder children, who can't understand commands or expectations, to be labeled as oppositional or defiant, when in reality, the child is unable to process the parents' verbal demands. It is important to insure that children with speech defects or language delays have an intact auditory function; speech pathologists frequently request audiological evaluations prior to a speech and language assessment.

School criteria for implementing speech therapy differ from the criteria that speech pathologists consider needing remediation. Schools disregard types of speech pathology that actually have a major impact on the social and psychological functioning of the child. School considers its main responsibility to remediate deficits that interfere with learning. Stuttering and other speech disorders are seldom considered an area of school responsibility. Even in children whose speech pathology the school considers within its domain, the quality and intensity of the interventions often leaves much to be desired. Sometimes, parents are advised to seek complementary speech services outside of the school. The same is true for other additional services the child might need. Particular emphasis should be placed on improving the child's communication pragmatics, a fundamental factor for successful socialization. See below.

Social Skills

For those children with significant socializing deficits, interventions should be geared to improve social skills, and to improve the pragmatics of human communication. These include:

Improving eye contact and social demeanor
Attention to social graces
Attention to hygiene, grooming, and attire
Improvement of rules of verbal exchange

Effort will also be made to:

Decrease developmental deviations
To correct abnormal posture
To decrease mannerisms (stereotypes)
To eliminate socially alienating behaviors such as nose picking, thumb sucking, bone cracking, and others.

Parents can do a great deal regarding neurological deficits, developmental deviations, and regressive behaviors of their children. For instance, for children who have difficulties with eye contact, pragmatics of communication, and other social skill deficits, parents can teach children to maintain eye contact every time they are talking to them, and provide feedback when children display gazing difficulties while interacting with siblings and friends. Parents can also foster accepted norms of social behavior (greetings, handshakes, and other social pleasantries).

Parents can do a great deal to improve the communication pragmatics of their children as well. They can teach basic rules of communication: respecting turns, noninterrupting, keeping to the topic of the conversation under discussion, avoidance of non sequiturs. Furthermore, if the child has dysprosody (expressive aprosody) the parent can teach the child to repeat what he said in a different tone and with a different melody, and to adjust any gesturing to the verbal communication and to the emotion that has been activated or to the emotion that wants to be conveyed. For children who have difficulties decoding emotions from social communication (receptive aprosody), parents can teach their child to learn to read prototypical emotions and other implicit messages.

Parents will be made aware of their child's receptive language difficulties or of other information processing problems. Parents will be encouraged to use redundant verbal and nonverbal language with their children. These parents need to understand that when their children fail to follow expectations it is not because they are oppositional but because they do not understand what is expected from them.

THERAPEUTIC APPROACHES TO DEPRESSION AND OTHER MOOD DISTURBANCES

For therapeutic approaches to depression, see below; for mood disturbances related to bipolar disorders and related disorders, refer to pertinent areas in this book (chapters 4, 5, 7, 8, 9, and 11).

Cognitive Behavioral Therapy (CBT)

CBT has two major applications in psychotic children and adolescents: treatment of depression and treatment of psychotic features.

Cognitive Behavior Therapy for the Treatment of Depression

CBT shows substantial advantage in reducing the rate of MDD when compared to nondirective supportive therapy (NST), 42 versus 17%, respectively, and its principles may be utilized in the treatment of depression associated with psychosis. Adolescents with MDD who were treated with CBT had a recovery rate of 65%, compared to those treated with systemic-behavioral family therapy (SBFT), 38%, and (NST), 39%. Anxiety disorders, a high level of cognitive distortions, and a strong sense of hopelessness at the beginning of treatment, predicted a more limited treatment outcome. At two years of follow-up, there was no statistically significant difference among the treatment groups (Gallagher, 2005, p. 35). The author concluded that CBT was probably effective during the MDD in accelerating patients' recovery even though adolescents receiving other treatment modalities showed similar recovery in the long run (p. 35).

Primary and secondary control enhancement therapy (PASCET), shares many qualities of CBT but makes a greater emphasis in skill development and personal effectiveness. PASCET is designed for youths between 8 and 15 years of age. Two kinds of skills are fostered in depressed children: ACT and THINK; these acronyms stand for:

Activities or Actions that solve problems
Calm yourself, demonstrate confidence
Talent building to gain confidence

Think positively
Help is around. Seek help from a friend to gain perspective on problems
Identify goodness in even difficult situations
No replaying of negative events
Keep thinking to insure that all alternatives have been considered. (pp. 35–36)

On self-report measures, youths who participated in the PASCET program had decreased rate of depression without necessarily meeting diagnostic criteria, when compared to controls immediately and at nine months follow-up (p. 36).

How did psychosocial treatment for depression compare to antidepressant medications? Four treatment conditions were randomly compared in a 12-week treatment protocol on 439 adolescents who met diagnostic criteria of MDD:

placebo, CBT alone, fluoxetine alone, and CBT plus fluoxetine. The results indicated that both medication conditions were superior to CBT alone and to placebo in facilitating the clinical improvement of depression. CBT was not significantly different from placebo, while the combined treatment and fluoxetine alone was significantly superior that placebo in facilitating the improvement on a broad range of depressive symptoms (Gallagher, 2005, pp. 36–37).

Cognitive Behavior Therapy for the Treatment of Psychosis

Kingdon and Turkington (2005) in their excellent text, *Cognitive Therapy of Schizophrenia*, challenge a number of erroneous assumptions about psychotherapy of schizophrenia and other chronic psychotic illness; they challenge widely held assumptions that symptoms are incurable and inaccessible to understanding. These authors assert that psychotic symptoms (hallucinations, delusions, and negative symptoms) can be understood by the therapist and patient, and that symptoms respond to cognitive behavioral therapy. In adults, there is a growing evidence-based research to support this intervention as a complementary modality for patients who receive psychopharmacological treatment. Cognitive therapy makes understandable many strange and bizarre psychotic symptoms and assists patients to feel understood; at the same time, this treatment modality promotes improvement of level of adaptation and decreases patients' level of subjective suffering by helping them to understand and to cope with their symptoms better. The book contains many concepts regarding assessment, formulation, treatment planning, as well as approaches and strategies to deal with positive and negative symptoms in a broad variety of psychotic patients and clinical situations (including associated comorbidities); these strategies may be sensitively applied to the field of child and adolescent psychosis.

In bipolar disorder children, dialectic behavioral therapy (Lehan), to deal with affective storms, overreactivity (overarousal), and impulsivity may offer optimal therapeutic opportunities. These children need to modulate the affective arousal to develop appropriate adaptive responses. CBT is not beneficial for patients with acute symptoms and either new onset or in the postacute illness phase (Bender, 2005, p 36).

Sudak (2004) states that in the United Kingdom cognitive behavior therapy is mandated as an adjunct intervention in the treatment of individuals suffering from schizophrenia. "Randomized controlled trials have demonstrated that patients who receive cognitive-behavioral therapy along with their medications have significant improvements in both positive and negative symptoms of schizophrenia, and these improvements are sustained in follow-up" (p. 331). There are no such studies in the child psychiatric field. Sudak recommends the application of cognitive-behavioral therapy principles in three specific areas in the treatment of schizophrenia (chronic psychoses) in adults. These recommendations have relevance for the treatment of psychosis in children and adolescents.

1. Medication adherence. The emphasis in this area takes several forms, including psychoeducation, engaging the child and family in issues related to medication concerns (target symptoms and side effects), development of routines to insure their intake, and identifying concerns that may promote nonadherence. Sudak indicates that adherence problems are frequently associated to dysfunctional beliefs related to the nature of the illness, the medications or the physicians.
2. To develop an explanatory model for the development of the disorder, emphasizing a stress-diathesis model (also, see expressed emotion, above). The model includes exploration of stressors at the time of the disorder onset, genetic and biological vulnerabilities, and attempts at coping with the disorders, including maladaptive resources such as substance abuse. The patients and families are given the opportunity to discuss the nature of the positive and negative symptoms, and to understand the nature of the disorder better. Therapist will attempt to normalize unusual perceptions or beliefs, to develop a plan of coping, and strategies to deal with the disturbing symptoms.
3. Sudak, as with Kingdon and Turkington (cited above) support the process of guided discovery and behavioral experiments to help the patient challenge delusional beliefs and perceptual distortions. The exploration of symptoms with the patients and their families, in their historical contexts and the meaning of their symptoms, strengthens the therapeutic alliance and the collaborative attitude between child and family and the psychiatrist or therapist, helping them to deal more effectively with the illness.

Examples of how to use cognitive therapy techniques in dealing with delusional symptoms (symptom management) is exemplified by Pinninti and Sosland (2004), who suggest use of cognitive techniques on five symptom related areas (questions):

1. How strong is your belief? The authors advice psychiatrists to engage patients in evaluating evidence for the belief before reaching definitive conclusions.
2. How long have you had this belief? Psychiatrists may reinforce initial doubts patients had about their unusual beliefs.
3. How the belief has affected your life. Writing down the pros and cons about the belief may discourage the belief.
4. How have you coped with the negative aspects of the belief? The psychiatrist reinforces the adaptive aspects of symptom coping and highlights the symptom adaptive cost.

5. What if the delusion is/is not true? Patients may develop depression after abandoning a delusion. Steer patients toward various activities and ask them to rate their enjoyment and mastery of them (p. 98).[1]

Dialectical Behavioral Therapy with Bipolar Children and Adolescents

For bipolar children with borderline personality organization traits, application of dialectical behavioral therapy (DBT) complemented with psychosocial skills training, as devised by Linehan (1993), seems to offer opportunities for children and adolescents with prominent mood and affect dysregulation, and a number of significant interpersonal deficits. Linehan integrates CBT with interpersonal therapy.

Linehan asserts that the form of DBT that has demonstrated effectiveness with borderline patients is a combination of individual psychotherapy and psychosocial skills training (p. 1). Dialectic therapy focuses in the immediate and larger context of behavior as well as in the interrelationship of individual behavior patterns. With respect to skills training, therapists need to take into account the interrelatedness of individual deficits (pp. 1–2). Learning psychosocial skills is difficult if the person's immediate environment, or the culture at large, do not support this learning (p. 2). A basic principle of DBT is that the fundamental nature of reality is change and process rather than content and structure. Therapy does not focus on maintaining a stable, consistent environment but rather aims at helping the patient to be comfortable with change (p. 2).

According to biosocial theory, the core dysfunction in borderline personality disorder is emotional dysregulation. This deficit is considered a joint outcome of biological disposition, environmental contexts, and the transactions of the two throughout development. It is postulated that borderline individuals have difficulties regulating several if not all emotions resulting in emotional vulnerability characterized by, (1) hypersensitivity to emotional stimuli; (2) intense response to emotional stimuli; and (3) slow return to emotional baseline once emotional arousal has occurred. BPD subjects have difficulties in emotional modulations as reflected by an inability to (1) inhibit inappropriate behavior related to strong positive or negative emotions; (2) organize oneself for coordinated action in the service of an external goals—not mood dependent goals; (3) self-sooth; and (4) refocus attention on long-term goals in the presence of strong emotions (Linehan, 1993, p. 2).

Linehan postulates that the crucial developmental circumstance in producing the deficiency of emotional dysregulation is the experience of an "invalidating environment," that is, the tendency to respond erratically and inappropriately to private experiences—beliefs, thoughts, feelings, or sensations. In an optimal family environment the child's preferences (e.g., the color of the room, clothes, activities, and other choices) are taken into account, the child's beliefs and thought are elicited and responded to seriously, and the child's emotions are viewed as important communications. This is in contrast to invalidating environments where the child's painful experiences are trivialized and attributed to negative traits such as lack of judgment or impulsivity; in these settings, the child's demands and preferences are restricted, and excessive punishment or control are exercised over them (p. 3).

The development of self-regulatory capacities, especially the ability to inhibit and control affect, is one of the most important acquisitions in the child's development. Absence of this capacity leads to the disruption of behavior, mostly goal directed and other prosocial behaviors. The inability to regulate emotional arousal interferes with the development and maintenance of the sense of self because of emotional inconsistency (p. 4).

Linehan recommends continuing efforts to reframe suicidal and other dysfunctional behaviors as part of patient's learned problem solving repertoire, and to focus therapy in active problem solving strategies, balanced by a corresponding emphasis on validating the patient's current emotional, cognitive, and behavioral responses just as they are (p. 5). Linehan puts emphasis on four areas in the treatment of borderline individuals:

1. Emphasis on acceptance and validation of behavior as it is in the moment.
2. Emphasis on treating therapy-interfering behavior of both client and therapist.
3. Emphasis on the therapeutic relationship as essential to the treatment process, and,
4. Emphasis on dialectic processes (Linehan, 1993, p. 5).

DBT goes one step further than standard cognitive-behavioral therapy in emphasizing the necessity of teaching clients the need to fully accept themselves and their world as they are at the moment. Four skill-training modules are aimed to deal with the major BPD dysfunctions:

1. Emotional regulation skill.
2. Interpersonal effectiveness skills.
3. Distress tolerance skill, and,
4. Ability to consciously experience and observe oneself and the surrounding events (1993, pp. 6–7).

ROLE OF THE THERAPEUTIC ALLIANCE

Multimodal treatments have demonstrated therapeutic superiority over isolated treatment approaches across a broad spectrum of psychiatric disorders. This has been true even in circumstances where particular interventions produce a robust impact in the course of a given disorder. This is especially applicable in the treatment of chronically mood dysregulated and chronic child and adolescent psychoses.

The therapeutic alliance is a fundamental pillar for successful interventions with children and adolescents. The term refers to the family and the child's effort in working together with the psychiatrist in the process of reducing disturbing symptoms and overcoming psychosocial obstacles that interfere with the achievement of optimal adaptive functioning. The therapeutic alliance with children and adolescents also implies the promotion of an optimally supportive and stimulating psychosocial environment. The younger the child is, the greater the importance of the parents and other significant others' roles (teachers, relatives, and others), in promoting and maintaining the therapeutic alliance.

By paying attention to the individual's subjective distress (including, that reflected in nonverbal behavior), the psychiatrist attempts to understand the child or adolescent's subjective world and the nature of the distressing emotional conflicts. These conflicts could be approached by a variety of psychotherapeutic interventions and by a sensible combination of psychosocial and psychopharmacological approaches.

GOALS OF INDIVIDUAL THERAPY

The treatment objectives should not create any undue stress for the individual child or the family. After a major psychotic break ("mental breakdown") enthusiasm about the initial recovery or denial as to severity of the illness, may pressure parents or even therapists and psychiatrists to set high and untimely expectations for the recovering patient. Kingdon and Turkington (2005) utilize the concept of *convalescence* and use the analogy of the broken leg in dealing with the process of recovery after a psychotic break: "Such injury needs rest, protection, and time to heal—usually less time than after an acute psychotic episode. But taking it out of the plaster cast too early or not immobilizing it in plaster in the first place just builds up problems for the future. Similar to immobilization, a peaceful relaxation, is needed to heal a mind that has been traumatized" (pp. 139–140).

There is no contradiction in the clinical application of the concepts of convalescence and the one dealing with the approaches to improve regression. The first relates to a process of restoration or recuperation after a sudden or acute loss of adaptive capacity; the second refers to efforts to decrease chronic patterns of maladaptive behavior that interfere with optimal adaptation or illness management. These concepts demand a sound clinical differentiation. Chronic patterns of maladaptive and ineffectual behaviors induce severe demoralization and a pervasive sense of hopelessness. For patients with ego strength, or for

TABLE 9.3 Targets of Individual Therapy

Promotion of optimal adaptive behavior
Decrease of regressive behavior
Improvement of reality testing
Decrease of the impact of productive symptoms:
      hallucinations and delusions
        improvement of negative symptoms
Improvement of impulse control
Improvement of frustration tolerance
Improvement of problem solving
Improvement of affect modulation
Improvement of interpersonal relationships
Attention medications and psychosocial compliance

those with ego dystonic symptomatology and introspective capacity, individual psychotherapy may be attempted when the positive symptoms are well controlled. A number of areas may be selected for intervention, see table 9.3.

With psychotic bipolar patients, insuring safety and dealing with issues of impulsivity and lack of judgment take precedence over other issues. Compliance with medication is a universal problem with bipolar adolescents; these problems require persistent focus and a very active but sensitive deconstruction of denials and grandiosity.

With schizophrenic and psychotically disorganized patients, issues of reality orientation and assistance in coping with daily demands, as well as dealing with the negative impact of perceptual or delusional symptoms are major therapeutic priorities. Issues of compliance with antipsychotics are of foremost importance. Paranoid fears of being poisoned or being controlled by external sources are frequent fears that interfere with medication intake, and that need to be identified.

GROUP THERAPY

Group therapy may play a useful role when the patients have achieved a significant degree of stabilization. When patients are acutely ill and in crisis, they frequently are unable to process what is going on in groups and often become disruptive to the therapeutic work of other patients. Some groups may deal with general issues of mental illness and on how to cope with reality demands; other groups have a more circumscribed focus and address specific issues, such as how to deal with suicidal behavior or self-abusive behaviors, anger management, symptom management, or drug abuse. With psychotic patients it is helpful to limit the focus of the group process to issues of how to deal with hallucinations or delusions, medication compliance, family issues, anger problems, or others.

PSYCHOEDUCATIONAL PROGRAMMING

The Admission, Review, and Dismissal (ARD) committee is the legal authorized forum for decision making regarding any change in any student's educational programming. The ARD officially decides and approves special education for any student considered in need of it. Technically, the ARD committee defines the student's placement, the nature of the student's programming, the degree of structure needed, and the intensity of the remediation that the student requires. The ARD also decides on the need for additional services that a particular student may demand. Parents may bring to the ARD meetings recommendations from the psychiatrist and other experts, or even bring ombudsman or legal representation to promote the implementation of special education or to procure special education services that parents considered necessary.

The quality and intensity of the structure as well as the intensity of academic support need to be commensurate with the child's needs and developmental level. In general, special education programs fail in achieving a comprehensive diagnosis of the learning or emotional issues of the impaired students, and in implementing comprehensive programs to deal with the identified deficits. Many special education recommendations do not transcend the good intensions of the ARD; that is, many of the psychoeducational goals and objectives agreed upon (in these legally binding meetings) are only partially implemented, at best. It could be said, that in general, the ARDs make promises that are not delivered. Parents need to diligently monitor the school implementation of the ARDs' decisions, and advocate for the fulfillment of objectives established in them, as well as demand further programs if new needs emerge throughout the child's development and academic progress.

The current trend to "mainstream" all the special education students could be construed as a deceptive measure to short-circuit school responsibilities with special education students.[2] For psychotic children with severe disruptive behaviors, highly structured and even self-contained programming is indicated.

What Special Education Programs Ought to Provide

1. *Universal interventions* with the goal of enhancing protective factors and preventing or minimizing future difficulties.
2. *Selective interventions* designed to meet the needs of students who respond insufficiently to high quality programming.

TABLE 9.4 Psychoeducational Goals for Chronically Psychotic Children

- Comprehensive diagnosis of student's emotional and learning difficulties
- Determination of optimal learning environment structure
- Determination of optimal classroom placement for appropriate intellectual, academic, and social stimulation
- Optimal remediation of learning and language deficits
- Promotion of optimal academic functioning
- Promotion of appropriate social skills

3. *Indicated interventions* designed to meet the needs of an estimated 1 to 5% of students who fail to respond to universal or *selected interventions*.

Universal evidence-based interventions are geared to all the student body; selective interventions are targeted to those students who display more significant risk factors, involving 10 to 15% of the student population, and who are in need of more intense interventions (Kratochwill, Albers, & Shernoff, 2004, pp. 891–892).

See a summary of psychoeducational goals in table 9.4.

The family needs to diligently advocate for the provision of comprehensive diagnostic and remediation services. These may include: psychological and neuropsychological testing, and other evaluations that may be necessary to better ascertain the child's neuromotor, intellectual, academic and psychosocial needs.

Neuropsychological Testing

This testing is useful for identification of deficits in information processing and to objectify optimal learning avenues; testing findings may be indispensable for determining the most appropriate psychoeducational programming and will also assist in the provision of sound vocational guidance.

Occupational Therapy Assessment

This assessment is important in identifying fine or gross motor deficits as well as difficulties with balance or coordination that require pertinent remediation.

THE ROLE OF THERAPEUTIC PROGRAMS

Case Management

For children and families with multiproblem presentations, case management is a commonly used strategy to increase access to and coordination of services. Case management mobilizes, coordinates, and maintains an array of services and resources to meet individual and family needs. Case management is often seen as the lynchpin of a system of care because it provides the central function of bringing together the disparate interventions and practitioners into a coherent whole to meet children's and family needs. Case management includes various functions to meet those needs, including assessment, service planning and implementation, service coordination, monitoring, evaluation, and advocacy (Farmer, Dorsey, & Mustillo, 2004, p. 866).

Case management is particularly indicated in psychotic conditions and in dysregulated patients with complex symptomatology and impaired psychosocial milieus; that is, clinical situations of individuals and families with multiple problems. These patients and their families need the provision and coordination of multiple services and the involvement of multiple agencies. Case management is especially helpful for families that lack initiative, resourcefulness, and the know-how as to how to deal with complicated therapeutic, educational, rehabilitation, and medical services. A related concept to case management is the promising concept of *wraparound.*

Wraparound

Wraparound is a more involved, therapeutically guided coordination of interventions for complex psychiatric conditions in which, to the severity of the child's psychopathology, a significant family dysfunction is an added complication. Wraparound is an approach to treatment that developed as an effort to overcome the fragmented, uncoordinated way in which services traditionally are provided to youths receiving services for multiple problems from multiple child serving agencies. Wraparound puts more attention on the way the service delivery is planned. In this modality, provision of services, access to and coordination of services, is more deliberate and more strategic.

This service is widely used because of its versatility and flexibility. This service is difficult to operationalize and to study, but its unique appeal lies in its relatively simple philosophy, namely, to identify the community services and supports that a family needs and promote and provide those interventions as long as they are needed. The planning process involves the family and is very individualized and flexible, is community based, uses a team approach, and addresses a broad range of life domains including outcomes that are determined and measured (Farmer, Dorsey, & Mustillo, 2004, pp. 867–868).

Intensive Outpatient Therapy (IOT)

Intensive outpatient therapy is indicated when there is evidence of decompensation during a first psychotic break or during a relapse of a primary psychosis. This is the first step in gaining control of the psychotic process or in dealing with an emotional or behavioral breakdown. This approach is also the indicated intervention when the child or the parents refuse to accept the recommendation of hospitalization. The successful implementation of IOT is illustrated in the following vignette:

> An 8-year-old white boy was evaluated because of severe hyperactivity and aggressive behaviors; he had been excluded from the school bus for fighting and disruptive behaviors, and had been suspended from school for severe aggressive and unmanageable behaviors. He had also been involved in a number of fights and was considered a, "classroom clown." Surprisingly, he had no prior psychiatric treatment.
>
> The child's behavioral difficulties went back at least a year, and the difficulties in managing him, at school and at home, had progressively increased. He had reached developmental milestones on time, had no medical or neurological history, and had enjoyed good physical heath. It was felt that he was very bright and had been considered a candidate for the gifted and talented program. He always had difficulties making and keeping friends due to his overbearing and controlling behaviors.
>
> During the psychiatric assessment, the examiner needed to give the child frequent verbal redirection for him to stay seated, to stop roaming the office, to discourage him from getting into office items. To control his hyperactivity the examiner sat him in an armchair and moved the chair against the table, physically corralling him on his chair. He responded to this intervention and was able to engage and to focus on the task of drawing. As he started drawing, he kept on asking to play with the toys present in the office but he was told that he would not be allowed to do so until he completed the drawing task.
>
> The child was likable and quite engaging. The examiner was able to keep him on task, and he was able to complete the assigned drawings; during that task, humor and active engagement were used. The family expressed disbelief that the child was quiet, participating, and "minding" the examiner.
>
> The drawings related to aliens and had a psychotic and paranoid flavor. He drew a number of aliens, including an alien persecuting a scared child. Aliens, destructiveness, and persecution themes in the drawings had an obsessive quality.
>
> The child was able to maintain appropriate eye contact; his affect was unrestricted, but still appropriate; his mood was mildly elated. He endorsed auditory

hallucinations telling him to do bad and mischievous things; he said he did not obey the voices. He also endorsed scary visual hallucinations: he saw frightening monsters. He stated he did not like to hear the voices or see the monsters because they made him scared. He endorsed florid paranoid ideation, feeling that people talked about him and spied on him; he also felt that people followed him and were after him. Furthermore, the child felt controlled by a robot. Along with this, he endorsed transparent grandiose delusions: he felt that he had special powers that he could do things that no other child could do, that he was "unstoppable" and that he was "super-strong." He described these beliefs with a congruent elated mood. The child's sensorium was intact.

The diagnosis of mania with prominent psychotic features was made. The boy's mother was told that the child required hospitalization but she declined the recommendation. She did not accept even a partial hospital treatment option (it appeared that the mother was enmeshed with the child and that she did not want to separate from him). The psychiatrist told the mother that considering her reservations, he was going to initiate treatment on an intense outpatient basis; the mother was told that if treatment did not progress well or that if the child demonstrated further deterioration, the option of hospitalization would be reconsidered.

Because the child had difficulties swallowing pills, he was given samples of Risperidal M-Tabs, 0.5 mg, and was told to take two the first day, and then one BID. He was also prescribed Depakote sprinkles 125 mg capsules, to take two caps BID. He was asked to return for a follow-up visit in three days.

At the scheduled follow-up, the mother reported that there was a slight improvement. He appeared calmer and was minding her more. The child continued displaying sleeping difficulties. He demonstrated more behavioral organization and looked less hyperactive. The elation had decreased and the psychotic features had begun to improve: he was neither hearing command hallucinations nor seeing the monsters he had previously reported; the paranoid feelings were not better, though. He still endorsed ideas of reference and persecutory feelings. The child's mood was euthymic and he continued being very engaging. His medications were adjusted to Risperidone liquid 0.5 mg TID, and Depakote sprinkles, 250 mg q AM and 375 mg q HS. He was asked to return in four days. The child continued progressing; he was able to remain in his home environment and to attend his local school. Although cost effectiveness was not a primary consideration, the stabilization of this child, using IOT, was very cost effective.

Partial Hospital Programs

These interventions are indicated when patients do not respond to less intense interventions (i.e., outpatient or even intense outpatient programs), and the school feels unable to contain the child. The school may consider the child extremely disruptive to the learning environment of other students, or determines that the student poses a safety risk for himself or the other students. With increasing frequency, students who make terrorist threats need, at least, partial hospital evaluation prior to readmission into the school.

Partial hospital treatment is indicated when the family is supportive of treatment, when the family feels able to control the child at home, when there are no issues concerning violence between the child and the family, or when there are no concerns of abuse. Intense and regular communication is expected on a daily basis between the family and the partial program. Since children in partial programs attend therapeutic school programs, broader opportunities for additional assessments of other areas of the child's functioning are available: learning attitude, learning habits, attentional capacity, learning level, interpersonal relations with teachers and other students; these and other evaluations are carried out a daily basis. Children in partial hospital programs attend group therapy on a daily basis and receive age appropriate education regarding nutrition, exercise, safe sex, STDs, illegal drugs, and medication compliance. Furthermore, these patients receive regular individual therapy and the family is expected to participate in family therapy at least weekly, if not more often. Partial hospital treatment allows a more intense adjustment and monitoring of psychopharmacological treatments. If patients improve, they are referred to either intense outpatient treatment or to regular outpatient follow-up. If patients do not improve or if their condition deteriorates, they are referred to an acute hospital program.

Acute Inpatient Care

Acute hospitalization is indicated when there is a considerable decline in the level of adaptive functioning, the patient is either at risk to himself or to others, or is unable to cope with basic daily demands due to the nature of his symptoms. This means that the child is unmanageable at school or at home. Acute hospitalization is also indicated when less intense forms of intervention including outpatient, intensive outpatient, or partial hospitalization are insufficient to contain the impact of a psychotic illness. Acute hospitalization is necessary for containment and control of suicidal and self-destructive behaviors, for containment and control of aggressive, assaultive, and homicidal behaviors, and for control of distressing and incapacitating psychotic symptoms. Due to the limited length of stay, and to maximize utilization of inpatient stay, intense psychopharmacological treatments are frequently implemented, or more correctly, initiated. Upon satisfactory resolution of suicide or homicide risks and either a substantial amelioration of the psychotic symptoms or achievement of mood stabilization, or both, patients are transitioned to partial hospital programs.

Residential Treatment Programs (RTP)

When psychotic patients do not recover completely following acute care treatment, or when the mood stabilization is insufficient to guarantee safe functioning back in the community, either at home or at school, due to enduring problems with aggression/homicidal ideation or suicidal/self-abusive behaviors, residential treatment programming is recommended, for further stabilization. This treatment modality is also indicated for children and adolescents who make significant improvement in mood or in psychotic features but retain marked conflicts with their families, or when the families feel unsafe about the patient's return. Residential treatment is needed when there is prominent alcohol or chemical dependency comorbidity. RTP is also indicated in treatment resistant cases, and in psychotic children with multiple acute hospitalizations without any significant lasting response. Extensive individual and group therapy interventions are deemed necessary; family therapy becomes mandatory to deal with dysfunctional family and interpersonal conflicts. RTP offers the family the opportunity to learn more effective means of illness management. Residential programs offer good opportunities for medication trials, and for medication adjustments, and close psychopharmacological monitoring. Depending on the degree of recovery, the patient may be transitioned to day hospital (that is, the child returns back to his or her family) or if the family nexus is irreparably broken, placement outside of the family is indicated.

Group Home Placement

This nonhospital option is reserved for psychotic patients who do not have families upon successful completion of residential treatment; this is the case with emotionally disturbed children under the care of CPS (these children are wards of the State). Placement is also an option for children who have broken affective links with their families, and for those patients whose families feel insecure or unsafe with their return. A great many number of these children have been victimized either physically, sexually, or both. Many of these patients have a history of violence toward parents or siblings or have a persistent pattern of defiance and disobedience; some have had problems with the law. Some children do not want to return to the family of origin; these children may have been neglected or abused by their progenitors and do not have a positive bonding to them.

Juvenile Detention Center

When the psychotic child displays conduct disorder comorbidity and persists in a pattern of antisocial behavior, he becomes involved with the judicial system. If he is charged with breaking a law, he may end up in a juvenile detention center. Researchers have consistently found that in juvenile populations, mood disorders, neurological disorders (including seizures), and psychotic disorders are very prevalent.

CHAPTER 10

Psychopharmacological Treatment

Considerations in the Clinical Use of Antipsychotic Medications

The following assertions summarize the issues discussed in this chapter:

- Antipsychotic medications are key components in the comprehensive treatment program of severely mood dysregulated children and adolescents with psychotic symptoms, and for children and adolescents with psychotic disorders.
- The second generation antipsychotics (SGA) seem to offer advantages over classical antipsychotics, but they do have their own disadvantages.
- The CATIE report (Lieberman, Stroup, et al., 2005) raises questions regarding the role of the first generation antipsychotics (FGAs) and of perphenazine in particular, in the treatment of adult schizophrenia. Perphenazine performed as well as most of the atypical studied (risperidone, quetiapine, ziprasidone, except for olanzapine which demonstrated a gradient of therapeutic superiority over all the medications tried, including perphenazine); olanzapine was, however, the most adiposogenic and prodyslipidemic antipsychotic.[1]
- For some SGAs, the purported advantages are counterbalanced by deleterious health risks: metabolic, cardiovascular, and others. Cost of medication is an increasing concern.
- The SGAs have important tymoleptic functions: they demonstrate antimanic and antidepressant effects.
- Most of the knowledge base in the conceptualization and treatment of psychotic disorders in children and adolescents is derived from adults. It is encouraging that research of SGA medications in pediatric populations is on the rise.

- By and large, there are no evidence-based data to support the broad and extensive use of antipsychotics in children and adolescents.
- Atypical antipsychotics may pose serious health risks for children and adolescents; these medications can aggravate certain medical conditions or be the cause of new medical complications.

BIOETHICAL ISSUES IN PSYCHOPHARMACOLOGICAL RESEARCH

Fegert (2003) asserts that the present cautionary rules against children's participation in research (Nuremberg Code, the Helsinki Convention, European Bioethical Convention) is actually unethical because the protective regulations may contribute not to the avoidance of risk but to the increase of risk for children and adolescents (p. 5). In usual clinical practice the risks and benefits of treatment are borne individually by patients and doctors, and are usually determined scientifically on the basis of clinical trials. Without the appropriate scientific data being available these risks and benefits cannot be determined appropriately. In the United States, investigative commissions were formed following reports of previous medical abuse. In the Belmont Report, the National Commission for the Protection of Human Subjects (1978) formulated four fundamental principles for medical ethics requirements: freedom from harm, healing (care), justice, and respect for the patient's autonomy. Fegert states that the application of those bioethical principles to the psychopharmacological treatment of psychosis in children and adolescents mean, among other things:

1. Need for effective therapies, free from side effects, as much as possible, in both acute and long-term treatments. This meets the requirement of freedom from harm.
2. Attainable therapeutic goals. This meets the requirement for healing and care.
3. Children, as a group, should receive at least the same degree of protection and same kind of safety and quality of treatment as adults. This meets the requirement for justice.
4. Child and adolescent psychiatrists must facilitate children and adolescents' greatest participation possible in treatment decisions, even in patients suffering from a severe psychosis. This meets the requirement for autonomy. (Fegert, 2003)

In order to increase children and adolescents' benefits from research participation, Fegert advises that:

1. The treatment of children and adolescents with schizophrenic psychoses (and other psychoses) must proceed under the same scientific standards of safety as in adult medicine.
2. Due to legal stipulations, at present, there exists a persistent uncertainty that is frequently passed on as a legally binding question to the person in custody, and to the patient being treated, because the pharmaceutical firms will refuse liability if the substance is used in an off-label context.
3. Precisely in such situations, sufficient consultation with parents is, from both an ethical and medical–legal perspective, the main precondition for responsible action. (p. 9)

Are children able to consent to treatment? Some researchers consider that the construct of informed consent becomes a construct that goes against the best interest of children. During treatment and consultations, parents behave as addressees on behalf of the children although the children are expected to cooperate in the treatment. A distinction is being made between *assent* and *consent*, understanding by *assent* the child or adolescent's willingness to undergo treatment which, though it does not have the status of legal consent, is still an important prerequisite for clinical research (p. 6).

A hopeful and encouraging development in future pharmaceutical research is the expectation that the upcoming new drugs will be required to be tested on sensitive populations: women of childbearing age, children and adolescents, and the elderly.

Clinicians underestimate children's (adolescents, and even late latency children's) capacity for understanding the complexities of risk–benefit assessment and to make decisions on their own behalf. Clinicians take a paternalistic or even a patronizing attitude toward children and adolescents because they suffer from a serious mental disorder, but even under these clinical circumstances, children and adolescents can assent to treatment, and participate in major decisions regarding treatment choices.

INTRODUCTION TO ATYPICAL ANTIPSYCHOTICS

This section deals specifically with the use of atypical antipsychotics currently in use in the United States. In less than a decade, atypical antipsychotics have become the dominant force in the treatment of adult and childhood psychosis. As a result of this rapid change, the typical antipsychotics have been progressively relegated to the sidelines of psychiatry practice (this is particularly true in the United States). The CATIE report (2005) may revive interest in FGAs.

This writer foresees a revival of some FGAs in the field of psychiatry that likely may extend into the field of child and adolescent psychiatry. Because perphenazine was tried in the CATIE study, there is a summary description of FGAs in appendix B, followed by general considerations in the use of FGAs, in the same appendix.

Although conventional antipsychotics have a therapeutic effect on psychotic features as a whole, and on positive schizophrenic symptoms in particular, this action is often achieved at a cost of mood and cognitive impairments. In general, the improvements in positive symptoms are frequently accompanied by an increase in negative symptoms or some cognitive dulling. It is possible that these effects are the result of overdosing of FGAs. In the CATIE study (2005) perphenazine demonstrates as good or better tolerability than the other atypicals (risperidone, ziprasidone, quetiapine, and olanzapine at an average 200 mg of chlorpromazine/day).

The first generation of antipsychotics has as a primary mechanism the DA blockade. The second generation of antipsychotics also blocks the DA receptors, and in addition, has critical modulating effects on other neurotransmitter receptor and modulatory sites, particularly at the serotonin (5-HT) receptors (Tamminga, 2001, p. 987).

Working memory may be impaired by a deficiency of dopamine D2 and D3 receptors and the chronic use of antipsychotic drugs, which block D2 receptors. Since D2 receptor densities are higher in children and adolescents than in adults, these effects may help to explain why children and adolescents are especially sensitive to adverse events affecting the CNS [some degree of cognitive dulling]. Because the absolute number of occupied receptors can be higher in the pediatric population than in adults, the probability of developing EPS may be increased (McConville & Sorter, 2004, p. 21).

A number of theories to explain the "atypicality" of the new neuroleptic medications have been proposed, including a high affinity for 5-HT2 receptors, a high affinity for dopamine D4 receptors, and a fast dissociation from the dopamine D2 receptor (Kapur & Remington, 2001, pp. 505–506). It appears that the fast dissociation theory has a greater heuristic value.

The therapeutic appeal of the atypical antipsychotics seems based on their better tolerability (the CATIE study raises questions in this regard), and in what is described as a broader spectrum of therapeutic action. Atypicals are represented to be effective on positive and negative symptoms, to have a favorable effect on mood, and to have a capacity for sparing or even improving cognitive functioning (these assertions have not been clearly demonstrated). All these effects are proposed to enhance treatment adherence (and this is not necessarily so, either).

Carpenter (2001) expressed reservations about the purported broad-spectrum therapeutic effects of these medications:

> Antipsychotic drugs are effective for psychosis but are not broadly antischizophrenic in therapeutic action. The new generation of drugs is less likely to cause

negative symptoms and cognitive impairments (compared to haloperidol in most studies), but efficacy for primary negative symptoms has not been documented, and controlled-study evidence for pro-cognitive efficacy (rather than reduced adverse effects) is modest. These aspects of schizophrenia mainly account for a reduced quality of life and other functional outcomes. (p. 1772)

It is likely that the purported advantage in cognition and negative symptoms from SGAs results from the high FGAs doses used as comparators. In the CATIE trials, perphenazine, at relatively low dose, 200 mg chlorpromazine/day equivalence, was as effective as quetiapine (up to 600 mg/day), risperidone (up to 6 mg/day), and ziprasidone (up to 120 mg/day). Olanzapine demonstrated some therapeutic superiority but it was used up to 30 mg/day, beyond recommended PDR levels.

Kapur and Remington (2001) reached similar conclusions to Carpenter's cited above:

In summary then, the word atypical should mean an antipsychotic with low EPS and lack of sustained prolactin elevation. Effects on a number of other features of schizophrenia, such as negative symptoms, mood, cognition, and functional outcome, are all very desirable clinical therapeutic goals. However, they are neither consistently realized nor of a substantial magnitude with the current generation of antipsychotics (p. 504).

In the CATIE trials there was no significant difference among the antipsychotics tried (perphenazine, olanzapine, risperidone, ziprasidone, and quetiapine). Although the new generation antipsychotics seem to be more effective and appear to have a broader spectrum of action, they are far from being free of serious side effects (their nature, extent, and severity will be reviewed in chapter 13). Atypical antipsychotic medications have metabolic, endocrinological, cardiovascular, and even neurological side effects. Furthermore, SGAs are very expensive. Atypicals appear to offer a better margin of safety regarding the risk of sudden death or other serious cardiovascular side effects.

From patients' subjective perspective, the major obstacles to treatment, expressed by more than half of the patients interviewed in one study, are medication side effects. The latter not only affects the patient individually but may also have impact on the family: if the patient looks overmedicated or if he or she develops EPS or TD (and here we need to add: if the patient increases weight inordinately or if he or she displays signs of a metabolic syndrome), the family may not support the use of antipsychotics (Bowes, 2002, p. 58). Furthermore, according to Tandom, it is because of the atypicals' EPS advantage that patients get better cognition, less TD, better compliance, and less dysphoria. If the EPS advantage is lost, these benefits vanish (Tandon et al., 1999, p. 60). See commentary above.

There are only a handful of studies that demonstrate superiority of one atypical over others, and in these studies there are questions of methodology. In the Clinical Antipsychotic Trials of Intervention Effectiveness (CATIE) a double-blind, placebo controlled, "head to head" study of chronic schizophrenic adults, was carried out utilizing olanzapine, risperidone, quetiapine, ziprasidone, and perphenazine; olanzapine demonstrated some therapeutic superiority over the other antipsychotics. Olanzapine had a longer staying power, reduced psychopathology to a greater degree, and was most effective in preventing relapse and rehospitalization, in comparison to the other antipsychotics (Lieberman, Stroup et al., 2005).[2] Different atypicals may not work in the same manner or may affect the brain functioning in different ways.[3]

Some published studies are biased to sponsored company products, while other studies suffer from sample size, length of the studies, optimal therapeutic doses, statistical analysis, and/or a comprehensive survey of side effects (Rogers, 2002). The manufacturer's supported studies bias explains amusing paradoxes like the one reflected in the title article by Heres et al. (2006), "Why Olanzapine Beats Risperidone, Risperidone Beats Quetiapine, and Quetiapine Beats Olanzapine: An Exploratory Analysis of Head-to-Head Comparison Studies of Second Generation Antipsychotics." In this study, the authors revealed a clear link between sponsorship and study outcome; in 90% of the abstracts reviewed, results were rated as showing an overall superiority of the sponsor's drug. Even more striking, different comparison of the same two antipsychotics led to contradictory overall conclusions depending on the sponsor of the study (p. 189). It is progressively evident that SGA comparisons to FGAs, like haloperidol, are lopsided in favor of SGAs because haloperidol doses, when used as a comparator, are excessive, thus producing higher side effects rates (particularly, impact on negative symptoms and cognitive performance). These biases make the other antipsychotics appear more beneficial and more benign.

Most of the sparse references so far published, relate to short-term treatments; for a number of psychotic conditions, optimal therapeutic effects only occur after many months of antipsychotic treatment.[4] The CATIE trial is the longest head-to-head, controlled study so far. Studies of long-term treatment outcomes and long-term side effects of atypical medications are lacking, particularly in children and adolescents.

Little is known about the interactions between psychotropic medications and the brain (Critical Breakthroughs, 2001, p. 1). The same maybe said about the long-term effects of atypicals on other organ systems and on the human genome.

There has been a dramatic increase in the prescription of antipsychotic medications in recent years. Approximately 10% of all antipsychotic prescriptions written in the United States are for use in children and adolescents (17 years or younger). The majority of children who receive antipsychotic medications are in the 7 to 12 and 13 to 17 age groups, 43 and 47% respectively; 10% of those receiving these medications are under 7 years of age (McDougle, 2003, p. 4).

There are limited literature references available to guide the child and adolescent psychiatric clinicians in the use of antipsychotic medications, and atypical antipsychotic medications in particular: "In many ways, physicians treating these patients (children and adolescents) are becoming the pioneers of this emergent field" (Critical Breakthroughs, 2001, p. 1).

Since knowledge of the mechanism of the therapeutic action and long-term side effects of atypical antipsychotics is lacking, we should look with concern at the rapid expansion of the use of these medications in children's nonpsychotic conditions. At the present time the atypical medications are being used in a vast array of nonpsychotic disorders. It has been estimated that more than 75 to 85% of the atypicals are currently being used outside of the psychosis categories (off-off label). There are growing concerns with overprescription of medications in children, and with overprescription of antipsychotics, in particular: "Although close scrutiny suggests that most medications were prescribed appropriately, roughly two-thirds of all antipsychotics were prescribed for no psychotic conditions" (Clinical Breakthroughs, 2001, p. 1). Atypical antipsychotic costs are enormous when compared with those of FGAs. From a public health perspective, questions are being raised regarding the cost–benefit ratio. The CATIE report justifies a reconsideration of the role of FGAs.

The increase in the prescription of antipsychotic medications for children and adolescents in the Texas Medicaid program from 1996 to 2000, has been unprecedented: "[T]here was a sizable increase of 494% in the prevalence rate of children and adolescents receiving atypical antipsychotics—a fact that reflects the growing acceptance of these medications by clinicians" (Patel, Sanchez, Johnsrud, & Crismon, 2002, p. 225), even though the safety and efficacy of these products have not been demonstrated in pediatric populations. "It is difficult to evaluate the long-term effects of atypical antipsychotics in children and adolescents, as these agents are relatively new to the market and few long-term studies have been performed… effects on learning and cognition as well as growth and development have yet to be determined" (p. 226). There is reason to believe that the Texas experience is not an isolated one and that the broad use of atypical antipsychotics is widespread across the nation, and beyond.

Although, experiences in the use of antipsychotics in institutional settings are hardly generalizable to broader settings, it is still illustrative that in the "real world," the adherence to preferred practices for the administration and monitoring of these medications is infrequently adhered to (Pappadopulos, Jensen et al., 2002). These authors note, that among children and adolescent inpatients, atypical antipsychotics are mainly prescribed for aggression rather than psychosis (p. 111), and that, for the treatment of aggression, antipsychotics are the most commonly prescribed agents across most inpatient settings (p. 112). Only 9.7% of all diagnoses in the sample were psychotic in nature (p. 119). Preferred practices are not followed in the use of antipsychotics and there was a lack of systematic monitoring of side effects and questionable polypharmacy (p. 117), as well as a systematic lack of targeting of therapeutic effects (p. 118). There is a dearth of evidence to support the current practices involving the use of antipsychotic medications to treat aggression in youth (Pappadopulos, MacIntyre II, et al., 2003, p. 145). A major concern related to the fact that neuroleptic treatment that begins in childhood may last a lifetime and may thus have incalculable neurological and functional impact (Labellarte & Riddle, 2002, p. 12). To these concerns we need to add the potentially detrimental effect that these medications have on weight gain and other metabolic effects, with implications for shortening the life span. Because of gaps in our knowledge regarding long-term safety and efficacy of atypical antipsychotics, controlled trials [particularly in children and adolescents] are urgently needed in this area (Schur et al., 2003, p. 141).

As reported by Gelenberg (2002),

> [T]he Expert Consensus Guidelines for the Treatment of Schizophrenia recommended the new generation of antipsychotics as the treatment of choice in almost all cases of schizophrenia. Nonetheless, an estimated 20% to 25% of patients in United States, who take antipsychotics, still use first-generation agents. The consensus guidelines recommended "typical neuroleptics" in only three groups of patients: (1) stable patients who tolerate the older agents and have had a good clinical response; (2) patients requiring long-acting injectable preparations (although now, there are effective parenteral atypical alternatives, i.e., Consta, IM risperidone and Geodon IM); and (3) patients for whom only conventional antipsychotics sufficiently control aggression and violence. (p. 17)

To these, we add (4), patients who, for lack of health resources, cannot afford the more expensive atypical prescriptions. It is far better for some patients to receive medications with some added risks, than to receive no medications at all. See previous commentaries on the CATIE report, above. Questions regarding efficacy and safety of atypical antipsychotics, in children and adolescents, are still largely unanswered.

NONANTIPSYCHOTIC EFFECTS OF ATYPICAL ANTIPSYCHOTICS

The new group of neuroleptic medications has mood modulating functions and antiaggressive activities besides their represented antipsychotic effects; because of that, an appropriate nomenclature for these medications would be welcome. Because of the multiple receptor affinities (which explain their broad therapeutic effects), atypicals have received the colorful label of "promiscuous drugs." In this regard, Swartz (2003) argues that atypicals are nonspecific antischizophrenic drugs: they have demonstrated effectiveness for most of the established psychiatric Axis I and II diagnoses, regardless of the presence of psychosis in those conditions (pp. 12–13).[4] Atypical antipsychotic medications also have demonstrated some efficacy in the treatment of cognitive deficits of schizophrenia (see chapter 14).

Some atypicals may decrease the life span due to long-term metabolic, endocrinological, or cardiovascular side effects, including the risk of sudden death (see chapter 13). In addition, "atypical antipsychotics as a group were found to have significantly higher frequencies of EEG abnormalities than typical neuroleptics at each step of the four-level EEG abnormality rating scores" (Centorrino, Price, Tuttle, et al., 2002, p. 112). Each atypical antipsychotic has its own side effect profile risk; clinicians need to familiarize themselves with the health risks of each atypical antipsychotic.

ARE ATYPICAL ANTIPSYCHOTICS BETTER THAN CONVENTIONAL ANTIPSYCHOTICS?

Food and Drug Administration regulatory procedures assure that drugs approved for the treatment of schizophrenia have documentation of efficacy. What follows is complicated. The physician must decide which drug, at what dose, in what combination, for what period of time, for which aspect of illness, whether to use off-label and at what risk and cost. This decision is case specific, is modified over time, and must weigh patient wishes and alternative approaches. The empirical data is [sic] inadequate. (Carpenter, 2001, p. 1771)

In a sophisticated meta-analysis, Chakos et al. (2001) found that, of 10 comparisons of second generation versus typical antipsychotics, six found significant differences that favored the second-generation antipsychotics on measures of treatment efficacy; four found no significant difference between treatments (p. 520). This means that in 40% of the analyzed studies there was no evidence of therapeutic efficacy difference between the atypicals and the typicals. Even in areas where atypicals are purported to be superior to typicals, such as in effects on tardive dyskinesia, only two of five studies reported reduction in tardive dyskinesia prevalence; the remaining three studies showed no difference in tardive dyskinesia rates. The CATIE report (2005) substantiates the latter analysis.

As has been pointed out, above, in the CATIE report perphenazine performed equally as well or better than other atypical antipsychotics (ziprasidone, risperidone, quetiapine) but not as well as olanzapine; perphenazine was used at 200 mg chlorpromazine equivalent dose/day, that is, at a low dose, whereas olanzapine was used up to 30 mg/day, that is, above 800 mg chlorpromazine equivalency/day. Moreover, perphenazine demonstrated less toxicity and a better tolerability than olanzapine.

There are an increasing number of publications which indicate that the therapeutic effectiveness difference between conventional and atypical medications is modest at best: no significant statistical differences in treatment response were found in the last observation carried-forward analysis between haloperidol and olanzapine in first psychotic episode treatment groups at 12 weeks. In acutely ill and severely symptomatic patients, relatively low doses of haloperidol or olanzapine were both effective in reducing symptom severity by the end of the 12-week period (Lieberman, Tollefson, et al., 2003). When compared with patients given a low dose of haloperidol, risperidone-treated patients experienced similar improvements in positive and negative symptoms and similar risks in psychotic exacerbations (Marder, Glynn, et al., 2003). Even the gold standard treatment for schizophrenia, clozapine, does not always live up to its expected superiority: in a double blind, 52-week trial, Lieberman, Tollefson, et al. (2003) studied 164 patients in China who had experienced their first psychotic episode. The investigators found a 71% cumulative response rate at 12 weeks for clozapine-treated patients compared with 62% for the chlorpromazine patients, but no difference between the drugs at 1 year, with a cumulative response rate of 81% for clozapine and 79% for chlorpromazine (Woerner, Robinson, et al., 2003, p. 1515). To reiterate, in the CATIE study, olanzapine demonstrated therapeutic superiority over the other studied medications (risperidone, quetiapine, ziprasidone, and perphenazine) at higher than recommended doses. There was no significant difference in therapeutic effectiveness among risperidone, quetiapine, ziprasidone, or perphenazine. For all the atypicals, in about 75% of patients, the initial medication was discontinued during the 18 months of the study for lack of effectiveness or tolerance problems (Lieberman, Stroup et al., 2005). These results are comparable to the CAFÉ study (Lieberman, McEvoy, Perkins, & Hamer, 2005). The apparent superiority of olanzapine other the other SGAs, except for clozapine, was corroborated in the CATIE II results (McEvoy, Lieberman, Stroup, et al., 2006, p. 608).

A meta-analysis of the relapse prevention role of antipsychotics shows that the magnitude of the advantage of the atypicals over conventionals is modest. Despite the proposed superiority of the new antipsychotics, the number of treatment failures in both groups was high. The available data do not allow for any conclusions about whether this modest superiority for the new antipsychotics (measured in relapse prevention) is related to enhanced efficacy, better adherence, or a combination of these factors (Leucht et al., 2003, p. 1219).

The meta-analysis conducted by Davis, Chen, and Glick (2003) reached different conclusions to that of Chakos et al. (2001), cited above. According to the new analysis, clozapine produced a better response than first generation antipsychotics (FGA), in the treatment of schizophrenia, with an effect size of d = 0.49, whereas amisulpride, risperidone, and olanzapine clustered around an effect size of d = 0.25 units. The effect of amisulpride, risperidone, and olanzapine over FGAs is somewhat less than half the effect of FGAs over placebo or clozapine over FGAs. Large risperidone and olanzapine studies found consistent differences versus FGAs (p. 555). The authors disagree with prior assertions that the second generation antipsychotics (SGAs) are equally efficacious as a homogeneous group; according to their analysis, aripiprazole, quetiapine, remoxipride, sertindole, and ziprasidone show similar efficacy to FGAs (p. 556). See the CATIE I and CATIE II reports commentaries above. Jibson (2003) disagrees with Davis, Chen, and Glick's (2003) conclusions: He asserts that there are aspects of the meta-analysis that preclude their being taken as the last word on the subject.

> Most conspicuous was the decision to limit studies to those involving risperidone doses > 4 mg/day and olanzapine > 11 mg/day, but allow studies with quetiapine doses as low as 150 mg/day and ziprasidone and aripiprazole studies without any minimum dose. Clearly, these conditions are not equivalent, since appropriate clinical doses of risperidone and olanzapine were compared to potentially sub-therapeutic doses of quetiapine, ziprasidone, and aripiprazole. This bias would affect the outcome in precisely the direction noted. (p.)

Jibson added that recent clinical trials have a trend toward higher drop-out rates and smaller effect sizes even for comparator medications, such as haloperidol, that are known to be effective. Newer drugs show smaller effect sizes than the older ones, reflecting a probable artifact of the increasingly treatment-resistant population that self-selects for these studies (p. 14). It is unclear what the implications of this meta-analysis are for the field of child and adolescent psychiatry.

INDICATIONS FOR ANTIPSYCHOTIC TREATMENT

This section discusses some rational principles for the use of atypical antipsychotics in psychotic disorders of children and adolescents. The main tenets of this section include:

- There are no FDA approved antipsychotic medication indications for use on children and adolescents.
- There is limited evidence-based support for the use of antipsychotics in children and adolescents.
- Most of the antipsychotic medication use in children and adolescents is off label.
- There is increasing concern that antipsychotic and other psychotropic medications are overused in children and adolescents.
- Antipsychotic medications have serious potential side effects.

There are no accurate or reliable tests for the diagnosis of psychotic and behavioral disorders in children and adolescents. At the present time, there is no way of proving that a patient suffers from schizophrenia or a bipolar disorder.

The diagnoses of schizophrenia and bipolar disorders are based, preferentially, on expertise and clinical judgment. As a result, clinicians' psychopharmacological approach is empirical and seldom based on treatment protocols. This is particularly true for the treatment of psychosis in children and adolescents. The symptoms of greatest concern, for which antipsychotics are used, include: severe tantrums, aggression, self-injury, severe irritability, affective lability, hallucinations, and delusions (McDougle, 2003, p. 4).[5]

Not all the psychotic symptoms require psychopharmacological treatment, and not all the psychotic features respond to psychopharmacological treatment.. There are a number of psychotic symptoms that may be considered part of the human condition, or that emerge under stressful situations; if symptoms are situational and transitory, and do not interfere with the adaptive capacity, they do not merit pharmacological treatment. Thus, hallucinations during the bereavement period are normative as much as are the presence of a paranoid attitude after trauma, tragedies, and unforeseeable events. Hallucinations that are supportive in nature (i.e., hearing God telling the child to behave, hearing an angel telling the child not to worry, or to be good, etc.) are not experiences that need to be targeted for treatment. Cultural and religious beliefs condoned by a group, that may not have consensual validation by nonadherents to this group, are not the purview of the field of clinical psychiatry. The psychiatrist needs to be familiar with the patient and family's religious and cultural backgrounds to recognize beliefs accepted within the patient's cultural milieu.

When the psychotic symptoms motivate the patient to act on distorted perceptions or abnormal beliefs they need to be treated. The distortions and abnormal sense of reality alter the patient's judgment and sense of behavior propriety. Special attention is recommended for the following clinical circumstances:

1. The psychotic symptoms overwhelm the child's ego (executive system) and the child becomes unable to carry out basic responsibilities of daily living such as eating, hygiene, sleep, personal care, school attendance, and learning.
2. The child displays bizarre behavior, induced by psychosis, behaves at odds with his family, school, social, cultural, or religious milieus.
3. The child displays profound withdrawal and interpersonal isolation that interferes with adaptation at the school and other social environments.
4. The child experiences command hallucinations that place other people or the child's safety at risk.
5. Hallucinations or delusions promote demoralization in the child and, as a result, the child considers suicidal or self-abusive behaviors.
6. The child experiences auditory hallucinations that erode the patient's sense of self and undermine his or her self-esteem and interest in life.

7. Hallucinations interfere with concentration and motivation for school-work.
8. Hallucinations terrify the child and make him feel a continual sense of danger.
9. Paranoid beliefs activate the child to act against the perceived attacker or persecutor.
10. The child has an intense sense of reliving a past traumatic experience.
11. The child's psychosis distorts the child's body image and the child attempts to change his distorted sense of self by means that are either detrimental to health or which put the child's physical health at risk.
12. Grandiose delusions impair the child's sense of propriety and judgment pertaining to social, sexual, or lawful behavior.
13. The child is agitated and aggressive and neither the aggression nor the agitation responds to the specific treatment of the primary disorder(s). Atypical antipsychotics are preferentially used in the treatment of agitation and aggressive behaviors (see the TRAAY recommendations below).
14. The child is in a premorbid or "prodromal" condition (see the Pace program, chapter 6).

In general, hallucinations respond to antipsychotics faster than delusions; at times, hallucinations respond while the delusions do not. Occasionally, neither the hallucinations nor the delusions respond to antipsychotics. The optimal treatment of mania with prominent delusions, hallucinations, or thought disorder has not been determined in any age group. Specifically, whether antipsychotic medication is essential for treating of mania with psychotic features, and if so, for what duration, remains unknown (Kafantaris, Coletti, et al., 2001, p. 1448).

USE OF ATYPICAL ANTIPSYCHOTICS IN AGGRESSIVE BEHAVIOR

Maladaptive aggression accompanies different forms of psychopathology. Affective disorders (depression, bipolar disorders), PPD, mental retardation, psychosis, PTSD, ADHD, and others can produce maladaptive aggression (Steiner, Saxena, & Chang, 2004, p. 3).[6] The Treatment Recommendations for the use of Antipsychotics for Aggressive Youth (TRAAY) developed by the Center for the Advancement of Children's Mental Heath and the New York State Office of Mental Health, offers specific guidelines for the use of antipsychotic medications in patients with violent and destructive behaviors. The recommendations were developed from a review of actual prescribing practices, consensus derived from focus groups, consensus of clinical and research experts, and a review of the current pertinent literature (Pappadopulos, MacIntyre II, et al.,

2003). Although, the recommendations have specific relevance for the use of atypical antipsychotics in aggressive behaviors, the principles delineated have broader applicability for the general use of atypical antipsychotic medications. Fourteen recommendations were issued.

TABLE 10.1 Treatment Recommendations for the Use of Antipsychotics in Aggressive Youth (TRAAY)

1. Conduct a comprehensive psychiatric evaluation before starting pharmacological treatment.
2. Determine target symptoms and treatment outcomes.
3. Start treatment with psychosocial and educational interventions.
4. Use appropriate treatments for primary disorders:
    - For aggressive youth with verifiable history of ADHD, consider stimulants before antipsychotics;
    - For aggressive youth with current depressive or anxious symptoms consider SSRI or dual mechanism antidepressants before using antipsychotics;
    - For aggressive youth with mania or verifiable history of bipolar disorders consider mood stabilizers before using antipsychotics;
    - For aggressive youth with psychotic symptoms, consider antipsychotic medications at appropriated doses before targeting the treatment of aggression.
5. Consider atypical antipsychotic first rather than conventional antipsychotics.
6. Use a conservative dosing strategy: "Start slow, go slow, taper slow strategy."
7. Use psychosocial crisis management interventions before medications for acute or emergency treatment of aggression.
8. Avoid frequent use of Stat or P.R.N. medications to control behavior.
9. Assess side effects routinely and systematically
10. Ensure an adequate trial (enough dose and appropriate length of treatment) before changing medications.
11. Use a different atypical after a failure to respond to an adequate trial of the initial first-line atypical.
12. Consider adding a mood stabilizer after a partial response to an initial first-line atypical.
13. If the patient does not respond to multiple medications consider tapering one or more medications.
Candidates for discontinuation:
    - Medications with the highest potential for side effects;
    - Medications with the highest potential for drug interactions;
    - Medications or combinations of medications whose side effects may be misinterpreted as treatable symptoms;
    - Medications with limited empirical evidence to support their efficacy (use);
    - Optimal tapering and discontinuation are completed in small increments over 2- to 4-week period.
14. Consider discontinuing medications in patients who show remission of aggressive symptoms for six months or longer.
To the above recommendations we add:
15. Atypical medications with supportive empirical evidence should be used before others lacking that literature support.
16. Atypical antipsychotics with the safest side effect profile should be used before considering others with more serious side effects.
17. Psychiatrists need to be aware of provider's medication formulary and family's financial resources when considering the best psychopharmacological alternatives for each patient.
18. The CATIE results (Lieberman, Stroup et al., 2005), suggest the FGAs, like perphenazine, may be considered as an effective and a cost effective alternative.

Source: Modified from Pappadopulos, MacIntyre II et al. (2003, pp. 147–157).

The child psychiatrist needs to know that even though he or she attends to the above principles, there is a growing public apprehension over the overuse of these medications in children; especially, there is increasing criticism over the use of antipsychotic medications for behavioral control. Furthermore, there is a growing concern about the serious health risks that antipsychotic medications pose to the safety of children when they are combined with physical interventions; for example, restraint/hold, four-point restraint, or seclusion (see chapter 13). These interventions are progressively perceived as coercive and traumatic (Allen, Currier, et al, 2003, p. 17). Consumers favor benzodiazepines and atypical antipsychotics over restraint or seclusion (p. 24). In the experts' opinion, even in psychiatric emergency settings, injectables [intramuscular injections (IM)], are only needed in 10% of the cases (p. 28). It is likely that consumers' perceptions are more favorable with the parental antipsychotics olanzapine, and particular with ziprasidone that produces tranquilization without neuroleptization.[7]

Meta-analytic studies showed rather conclusively that ADHD treatment with stimulants and related compounds reduces aggression significantly. The antiaggressive effects are more pronounced in overt aggression that tends to be more impulsive and affectively charged. There is abundant evidence that treatment of childhood onset psychosis, PDD, and mental retardation with antipsychotics results in reduction of overt aggression. Divalproex reduces overt aggression in bipolar offspring and also decreases the affectively charged PTSD-related aggression (Steiner, Saxena, & Chang, 2004, pp. 3–4).

Patel, Crismon, et al. (2005) highlighted that there is no empirical support for the extensive used of atypical antipsychotics for the treatment of aggressive behavior in children and adolescents. Risperidone is the only atypical that has persuasive evidence for efficacy against aggressive behavior across different psychiatric conditions in children and adolescent (p. 272); however, the supporting data come mostly from short-term studies There are recent long-term studies that support chronic risperidone use in developmentally impaired populations. Although, the use of atypicals for aggressive behavior is off-label, the evidence from randomized control studies represents an evidence-based treatment approach (p. 274). Underutilization of nonpsychopharmacological treatments and other psychosocial approaches is a major concern. Psychotherapeutic approaches for treatment of aggression of children and adolescents show significant efficacy, and parent management techniques (PMT), and multisystemic therapy (MST), have shown efficacy in the treatment of aggressive youth (p. 276). In spite of this, the effect size of psychopharmacological treatment is greater than the psychosocial intervention(s) one(s) (p. 277).

There is also a growing concern regarding the psychiatric hospital and residential treatment programs' physical restraining practices, which are responsible for most of the untimely deaths while the patients are in custody. Children account for up to 26% of the reported deaths in psychiatric facilities (Currier, 2003, p. 62).

TABLE 10.2 Issues that Need to be Considered in the Selection of Antipsychotic Medications

- Nature of the therapeutic alliance
- Nature of the psychiatric condition
- Specific target signs and symptoms
- History of family medication response
- Past history of medication response (therapeutic and adverse events)
- Patient preference
- History of treatment adherence
- History of medication effectiveness
- Presence of medical and psychiatric comorbidity
- Nature of concomitant medications
- Availability of appropriate formulations (vehicles or medication presentation), e.g., fast-dissolving oral, short- and long-acting intramuscular
- Medication costs
- Access to and availability of medications
- Risk of obesity, diabetes and dyslipedimias.

Source: Modified from Consensus Development Conference (2004, p. 598).

CHOOSING ANTIPSYCHOTIC MEDICATIONS

A number of issues need to be taken into account in the selection of antipsychotic medications (see table 10.2).

Despite the lack of controlled studies, the American Academy of Child and Adolescent Psychiatry practice parameters and recent pediatric psychopharmacological review articles favor atypical antipsychotics agents as the "Standard of Care" for children and adolescents with psychotic conditions (Pappadopulos, Guelzow, et al, 2004, p. 830). Prevailing clinical thinking and psychiatric practice recommend the second generation agents over the first generation ones. However, greater experience with atypical antipsychotics (strengths and limitations) make the Patient Outcomes Research Team (PORT) recommendations from 1998 still valid: "We do not recommend preferential use of second generation agents over first generation ones but rather focus on the wider options now available to clinicians and patients in selecting the best treatment for the individual" (Bender, 2005, p. 36).

IS THERE AN APPROPRIATE TIME TO INITIATE ANTIPSYCHOTIC MEDICATIONS?

There would be limited controversy regarding the use of antipsychotic medications according to the parameters described in indications for antipsychotic medication, cited above. These indications for treatment make the use of antipsychotics mandatory. However, could the expression of a florid syndrome be aborted? Should the subthreshold syndromes receive earlier attention and intervention? Should the psychiatrist wait for the unfolding of the clinical syndrome to intervene or should he or she take steps to prevent the development of more severe symptoms? There are a number of concepts related to risk factors and vulnerability issues related to the development of serious psychoses (see table 10.3).

Research indicates that, preceding the development of psychosis in schizophrenia, up to 80 to 90% of patients report a number of symptoms including changes of perception, beliefs, cognition, mood, affect, and behavior, and that about 10 to 20% of schizophrenics develop psychotic symptoms abruptly without any apparent prodromal symptoms (Addington, 2004, pp. 588–589). In other studies, up to 73% of first-episode patients experience a prodromal phase that starts with nonspecific prodromal signs (e.g., depression, anxiety, low self-esteem) or negative symptoms (such as, poor concentration, lack of energy, worsening work performance); 20% of first-episode patients present with positive symptoms (such as suspiciousness, perceptual abnormalities, disorganized symptoms), and negative or nonspecific symptoms; and 7%, with positive symptoms only (Knowles & Sharma, 2004, p. 597). For the prodromal aspects of bipolar disorders see chapter 8. In relation to studies correlating

TABLE 10.3 Risk, Vulnerability, and Related Concepts

Risk factor is a characteristic associated with heightened probability of a later onset of a disorder.

Precursor is any characteristic that occurs prior to the event or clinical outcome; a forerunner of a disorder or the one that precedes or indicates the approach or presence of another.

Precursors are best understood as *risk indicators*, or as manifestations of other *risk modifying precursors* (maternal exposure to influenza and perinatal brain insults are proposed as risk modifying precursors; minor physical anomalies and skin abnormalities are considered risk indicators). Risk indicators may become *risk modifiers* (anxiety in social situations, and overreactive behavior in boys and underreactive or withdrawn behavior in girls); these behaviors may expose these children to added risks.

Risk factors that cannot be changed are described as *fixed markers*. The ones that can be changed are called *variable risk factors*. These are dubbed *causal risk factors* if the manipulation of the factor changes the outcome. When it does not change the outcome, they are called *variable markers*.

Vulnerability markers are the equivalent of risk indicators or fixed markers. Some vulnerability factors are called *endophenotypes*, or *endophenotypic markers* (abnormalities in attention, cognition, and information processing, and psychophysiologic abnormalities such as eye tracking disorders).

Prodrome refers to early symptoms and signs that a person experiences before the full-blown syndrome of an illness becomes evident. A problem with the concept of prodrome is that it is determined retrospectively.

Risk mental state indicates a mental state that confers increased risk for the affected person for the development of a severe psychotic disorder.

Source: Yung & McGorry (2004, pp. 67–68).

prodromal symptoms and schizophrenia outcomes, the following caveats are relevant:

1. Not all individuals with schizophrenia present with precursors, risk factors, or known vulnerabilities.
2. Risk factors are only helpful as heuristic etiological factors to some subgroups of schizophrenic patients.
3. Not all the individuals with identifiable risk factors will develop schizophrenia; actually, the majority will not.
4. It is not possible to use the precursors as predictors for use in identifying individuals at high risk of schizophrenia.
5. These concepts cannot be used in targeted interventions to prevent the onset of schizophrenia (p. 69). The same caveats are applicable for prodromal bipolar features.

The PACE Clinic in Melbourne, Australia (Phillips, Leicester, et al., 2002), is pioneering an early intervention program in what they defined as an ultra high risk population for psychotic disorders (subjects are between 14 and 30 years of age). A number of assessment scales were developed for subjects to participate in this research project.[8] The enthusiasm for early intervention should be tempered by a number of reservations:

1. To this day, it is impossible to separate false positives from so called schizophrenic prodromal syndromes (Davidson & Weiser, 2004, p. 578).
2. Antidepressants, anxiolytics, and mood stabilizers may be as helpful in dealing with prominent prodromal symptoms as atypical neuroleptics (Remington & Shammi, 2004, p. 581).
3. Some atypicals like olanzapine failed to demonstrate superiority over placebo in prodromal syndrome interventions (p. 584).
4. Atypical antipsychotics are not innocuous pharmaceuticals; most SGAs may elicit potentially serious adverse events. The same reservations are applicable to prodromal bipolar features.

DOES THE TIMING OF INITIATION OF TREATMENT OF PSYCHOSIS INFLUENCE PROGNOSIS?

Some investigators have expressed concerns that if treatment of schizophrenia is not started early and promptly, the therapeutic response is decreased and the prognosis is compromised. Ho, Alicata, et al. (2003) do not find support for these concerns. In their view, "On the basis of our findings as well as [those of] other investigators...the pattern of mostly small correlation coefficient and the paucity of significant differences between patients with long and short duration of untreated initial psychosis do not support the frequently expressed belief that long periods of untreated psychosis have a pronounced impact on neurocognitive functioning or on brain morphology in schizophrenia" (p. 146). These authors argue that structural brain abnormalities and cognitive deficits are evident by the time patients first come to treatment, that the neurodevelopmental theory of schizophrenia posits that abnormal or genetic factors interfere with early brain development (neurulation, cellular proliferation, migration, differentiation, and synaptogenesis), and that later brain development processes (e.g., apoptosis and synaptic pruning) or neurodevelopmental events (e.g., stress, illicit drugs, head trauma) interact with the already aberrant neuropathology to produce the symptoms and signs of schizophrenia. Thus, the structural brain abnormalities and cognitive deficits found in schizophrenic patients may be primarily neurodevelopmental in origin. Several studies have shown that schizophrenic patients with poor outcome exhibit greater ventricular enlargement over time, suggesting that additional pathogenic processes may contribute to further deteriorative progression in these deficits. If such pathogenic processes are also present around the onset of clinical symptoms, it appears that untreated psychosis is not a contributing factor (pp. 142–148). The authors substantiated their proposition on a later neuroimaging study (Ho, Alicata, et al., 2005). The authors concluded, again, that there were no significant associations between hippocampal volumes and duration of untreated initial psychosis (p. 1527).

A Scandinavian study conducted by Rund et al. (2004) corroborated Ho, Alicata, et al.'s (2003) findings (cited above). This was a large study group: the number of patients participating in the study was larger than in any prior studies of its kind. Also, the neuropsychological test batteries included tests of a wider range of cognitive functions compared to former studies. The Scandinavian authors found no association between duration of untreated psychosis and any of the cognitive measures. Strong associations were demonstrated between poorer premorbid school functioning and neurocognitive deficits, especially in verbal learning and working memory. No relationship was found between neurocognitive functions and clinical measures except for an inverse correlation of positive and negative syndrome scale and working memory, and a positive correlation between positive symptom and motor control. The authors did not find any correlation between medication types (FGAs vs. SGAs) or dose and neuropsychological results, either (pp. 470–471).

CLINICAL APPLICATIONS OF ATYPICAL NEUROLEPTICS

In general, atypical antipsychotics have broad antischizophrenic effects (for both positive and negative symptoms) and positive mood modulating effects. Some atypicals appear to have positive effects on cognitive functioning. There is a growing application of atypical medications to a broad variety of psychotic and mood disorders (mostly bipolar disorders), aggressive behaviors, movement disorders, and in many other psychiatric conditions. Gracious and Findling (2001) suggest the following indications (see Table 10.4).

There is no research evidence indicating that either first or second generation antipsychotics were effective for primary negative symptoms of schizophrenia, although they are useful for negative symptoms secondary to positive psychotic symptoms (Bender, 2005, p. 60). Lamotrigene has shown positive results on negative symptoms on both bipolar disorders and schizophrenia. Because of the broad-spectrum therapeutic effects, the atypicals act as a "pharmacological

TABLE 10.4 Common Uses of Atypical Antipsychotics in Children and Adolescents

- Psychosis
  Schizophrenia
  Brief psychotic disorder
  Schizoaffective disorder
  Psychotic disorder NOS
- Mood disorders
  Treatment resistant bipolar disorder
  Bipolar disorder with psychotic features
  Major depression with psychotic features
- Movement disorders
  Tic disorders or Tourette's syndrome
  Stereotypic movement disorder
- Autism and pervasive developmental disorders
- Intermittent explosive disorder

Common uses in pediatric medicine"

- Sedation; paradoxical response to benzodiazepines
- Drug-induced (e. g., steroids) psychosis
- Delirium (e. g., meningitis or ketoacidosis)
- Chorea
- Organic personality disorder
- Agitation (hospitalization or immobilization)
- Self-injurious behavior (e. g., biting)
- Anorexia nervosa

Potential uses in child psychiatry:

- Disruptive behavior disorders
  Conduct disorder
  Severe or treatment resistant ADHD
- Schizoid or schizotypal personality traits
- Borderline personality traits
- Severe stuttering

Sources: Gracious & Finding (2001); Critical Breakthroughs (2001); Bogetto, Bellino, Vaschetto, and Ziero (2000).

shotgun" treatment on a variety of aspects of the disease (schizophrenia) in all patients (Kapur & Remington, 2001, p. 503). Many clinicians are using the broad unspecific therapeutic effects to deal with a multitude of clinical issues in their practice. A more rational and more sophisticated and perhaps more effective approach to schizophrenia (and other psychotic conditions) may lie in independently targeting the pathophysiological mechanisms of each clinical dimension (i.e., positive, negative, cognitive, and affective) with more selective drugs that can be combined and individually titrated to the needs of each patient (Kapur & Remington, 2001, p. 503).

STRENGTH OF ATYPICAL ANTIPSYCHOTIC RESEARCH DATA

Based on the strength of the research evidence, Jobson and Potter (1995) categorized available data at the following levels:

Level A: Data is supported by two or more randomized control trails. There is good research-based evidence supporting a clinical recommendation.

Level B: Data is supported by at least one randomized trial. There is fair research-based evidence supporting a clinical recommendation.

Level C: Data is supported by opinion, case reports, and studies that do not meet randomized, controlled-trial criteria. Data is primarily based on group opinion, with minimal research-based evidence to support a clinical recommendation. Lack of evidence does not mean lack of efficacy. (Jobson & Potter, 1995, pp. 458–459)

A related guideline, developed by Ghaeme (2002) will be discussed in chapter 12.

ISSUES REGARDING TREATMENT WITH ANTIPSYCHOTIC MEDICATIONS IN CHILDREN AND ADOLESCENTS

No psychopharmacological treatment should be initiated without a comprehensive assessment including, developmental and family history, previous response to medications (including family members' response), review of systems, and a physical and neurological examination. Blood tests, EKG, and baseline laboratory tests are indicated; other studies may be necessary dependent on the patient's individual and medical circumstances.

The physician should anticipate adverse event effects and will request pertinent tests to monitor the potential side effects of the prescribed antipsychotic. Physicians will remind families and patients that all antipsychotic and mood stabilizing medications with FDA indication(s) for adults, do not have FDA indication for use in childhood and that children, as a group, have more frequent and more severe adverse event reactions than adults.

There is a growing concern with the expanding practice of polypharmacy in childhood. This is one of the most critical issues that must be studied (Zonfrillo, Penn, & Leonard, 2005, p. 16). Child psychiatrists seem to be progressively complaisant about the practice of polypharmacy. It seems that the psychiatry field is becoming less concerned and probably less attentive to polypharmacy increased risks.

BASELINE STUDIES FOR ANTIPSYCHOTICS WORKUP

Current standards of practice demand a comprehensive physical and neurological examination plus a variety of laboratory examinations prior to the initiation of antipsychotic medication. Child and adolescent psychiatrists need to pay attention to a number of issues prior to, and during the prescription of antipsychotics as suggested, with modifications by Bryden, Coletti, Dicker, et al. (2001; for baseline assessments before initiation of treatment of antipsychotic medications see table 10.5).

RECOMMENDATIONS FOR THE USE AND SELECTION OF ANTIPSYCHOTICS

1. Only one antipsychotic medication should be used at a time. Combinations of antipsychotics should not be tried until monotherapy with different available agents, including conventional antipsychotics, has been used for an extended period of time, for at least six weeks, at therapeutic doses

TABLE 10.5 Baseline Assessments for Antipsychotic Treatment

Physical examination (pulse, blood pressure)
Weight and height (BMI, measurements of waist and hip circumference)
Neurological evaluation
AIMS, EPS, Barnes, Simpson-Angus assessment scales
CBC, hepatic, renal and thyroid function
Insulin level, hemoglobin A1c
Urine drug screen
Glucose and lipid profile
K+, Mg++
Prolactin level
Lactate, pyruvate, and ketone levels to rule out mitochondrial disorders
EEG
EKG: QTc Interval.
CSF studies to rule out occult CNS infections.

Source: Modified from Bryden, Carrey, & Kutcher (2001).

(for each medication), or when single medications at therapeutic levels bring forth unacceptable side effects or increased health risks. There is no evidence-based data to support the use of antipsychotic combinations.

2. Given the patient's health status, an antipsychotic medication with a better-known effectiveness and a more benign side effect profile should be tried first.

3. Atypical antipsychotic medications with supportive literature should take priority over the ones without published evidence.

4. The CATIE report (2005) stimulates the thinking that perphenazine (and probably other FGAs) could be considered alternative treatment options for children and adolescents.

5. Psychiatrists should inform parents or guardians that although antipsychotic medications are extensively used in current psychiatric practice, these medications are not Federal Drug Administration (FDA) approved for use in pediatric populations. Child and adolescent psychiatrists need to appreciate that they carry a higher legal liability for prescribing medications off label.

Table 10.6 lists a number of considerations for using antipsychotic medications with higher health risks.

1. In patients with overweight/obesity (BMI > 30), the clinician should select medications that are least likely to aggravate the patient's risks of obesity as well of those of hyperglycemia or diabetes, hypercholesterolemia or hyperlipedemia, or other metabolic syndrome features, sleep apnea, or gall bladder disease.

2. "Counteractive polypharmacy," the concomitant use of a medication to counteract side effects of another drug, should only be used when the

TABLE 10.6 Considerations in the Selection of Antipsychotic Medications for Patients with Higher Health Risks

1. The patient's psychiatric condition
2. Target symptoms
3. Target deficits
4. Prior history of antipsychotic use
5. The patient's health history including:
   (a) Cardiovascular history
   (b) History of:
       Overweight or obesity
       Diabetes and lipidemia history
       History of endocrinological problems:
           Menstrual problems, polycystic ovarian disease, gynecomastia
       Sexual dysfunction
       Sleep apnea

patient responds specifically only to a given drug and that medication brings on undesirable health risks. The clinician needs to try alternative medications prior to exposing the patient to long-term detrimental side effects. It is not a sound practice to use polypharmacy from the very beginning with the goal of preventing a potential antipsychotic side effect (i.e., risperidone plus cabergoline to avoid hyperprolactinemia).

On the other hand, the concomitant use of weight attenuating agents (i.e., amantadine, nizatidine, or sibutramine, and others) has been proposed to decrease the rate of weight gain and other metabolic complications promoted by some atypical antipsychotics.

3. When the patient has gynecomastia, menstrual or other endocrine difficulties, neuroleptics with low prolactin elevation induction risk should be used.

4. If the patient has prior exposure to neuroleptics and subsequently developed undesirable metabolic or neurological side effects, antipsychotics with a lower likelihood of reproducing these complications should be selected.

5. The nature of the comorbidity and possible interactions with concomitant medications will also have a bearing in the antipsychotic selection.

6. When there is no response to atypicals, FGAs and other medications should be considered. A number of psychotic children do not respond to atypical antipsychotic medications. If patients do not show benefits in their psychotic symptoms, after a meaningful time and at a high enough dose, the antipsychotic should be discontinued. The caveat is that even though the atypical medication may not be effective against psychotic symptoms, it may have produced beneficial effects in mood, anger control, sleep, or other symptoms. These beneficial effects are frequently not appreciated until the medications are discontinued. Patients who do not respond to atypical antipsychotics may respond to conventional ones. Nonantipsychotic medications and alternative nonpsychopharmacological approaches (psychosocial interventions) should be tried when there is no response to antipsychotic medications.

7. Occasionally, psychotic symptoms do not respond to antipsychotic medications but respond to mood stabilizers, SSRIs, or other medications. In patients whose psychosis is unresponsive to antipsychotics, psychosocial interventions need to be intensified, and techniques of symptom management (blocking of hallucinations, cognitive behavioral therapy, and others) will assist the child and family to handle the symptoms more effectively. PTSD-related psychoses have limited response to antipsychotic medications; psychosocial interventions should be used preferentially instead, or they should be combined with psychotropics.

The above principles are in line with Tandon and Jibson's (2005) guide to major principles of pharmacotherapy for schizophrenia (see table 10.7).

TABLE 10.7 Guide to the Major Principles of Pharmacotherapy for Schizophrenia

1. Agent Selection. Select antipsychotic agents based on patient factors and physician factors. Input from the child and family is very desirable.
2. Initiation of Therapy.
   (a) Allow adequate duration of antipsychotic therapy (4 to 6 weeks at optimal dose).
   (b) If no response or inadequate response, change antipsychotic within 8 to 12 weeks. Obviously, antipsychotic will need to be changed sooner if problems with tolerability develop.
   (c) Use continuous antipsychotic treatment (not targeted or intermittent).
3. Dose Adjustments and Switching Strategies
   (a) If patient display cognitive deficits, avoid anticholinergic medications.
   (b) If patient experiences side effects, consider a dose adjustment or change of agent.
   (c) If the patient has been on a typical medication consider switching to an atypical. If the patient does not respond to atypicals, some typical antipsychotics may be considered.
4. Adjunctive Treatments
   (a) Adjunctive treatments should be used for the treatment of nonpsychotic associated symptoms such as depression or anxiety, particularly if psychotic symptoms have abated.
5. Noncompliance, No Response to Therapy
   (a) Insure patient is taking medication. Check medication levels if pertinent.
   (b) When there are objective indicators that the child or adolescent is not taking the medications as prescribed, parents will be made aware of this, and they will be expected to increase surveillance over medication intake.
   (c) If parents cannot insure regular medication intake consider a child's referral to CPS.
   (d) If an adolescent does not comply with medications in spite of parents' best efforts, consider sublingual preparations or depot antipsychotics. All along, psychiatrists and therapists will make efforts to understand the motivational sources that promote a lack of compliance and the depth of patient's denial.
6. These principles should be respected with regard to continuing use.

Source: Modified from Tandom & Jibson (2005, p. 92).

MEDICATION MONITORING

Vinks and Walson's (2003) indications for therapeutic drug monitoring are listed in table 10.8.

TABLE 10.8 Factors to Attend to in Medication Monitoring

Inadequate response
        Higher than standard dose required
        Serious and persistent side effects
        Suspected toxicity
        Suspected noncompliance
        Suspected drug–drug interactions
        New preparations, changing brands
        Emerging illnesses
        Presence of other illnesses such as hepatic, renal, inflammatory diseases, and others

Source: Modified from Vinks and Walson (2003).

ANNOTATIONS TO THE TIMA ALGORITHM (2003)
FROM A CHILD AND ADOLESCENT PSYCHIATRIC PERSPECTIVE

Choice of antipsychotic (AP) should be guided by considering the clinical characteristics of the patient and the efficacy and side effect profiles of the madication.

Any stage(s) can be skipped depending on the clinical picture or history of antipsychotic failures.

First episode or never before treated with a NGA

Stage 1
Trial of a single NGA
(ARIPIPRAZOLE, OLANZAPINE, QUETIAPINE, RISPERIDONE, or ZIPRASIDONE)

Partial or Non-Response

Stage 2
Trial of a single NGA
(not NGA tried in Stage 1)

Partial or Non-Response   Partial or Non-Response

Stage 2A
Trial of a single agent
FGA or NGA
(not NGA tried in Stage 1 or 2)

Partial or Non-Response

Stage 3
CLOZAPINE

Partial or Non-Response

Stage 4
CLOZAPINE
+
(FGA, NGA or ECT)

Clozapine Refusal

FGA = First Generation AP
NGA = Newer Generation AP
ECT = Electro-Convulsive Therapy

Non-Response

Value in cozapine failures not established

Stage 5
Trial of a single agent
FGA or NGA
(not NGA tried in Stages 1, 2, or 2A)

No controlled studies

Stage 6
Combination Therapy
E.g. NGA + FGA, combination of NGAs, (FGA or NGA) + ECT, (FGA or NGA) + other agent (e.g. mood stabilizer)

Notes to the Algorithm

1. Since the research data-based for constructing algorithms on children and adolescents is limited, by necessity the algorithms for the use of atypical antipsychotics for children and adolescents are preliminary or tentative and largely borrowed from the ones constructed for adults. The algorithm under discussion is based on the TIMA Antipsychotic Algorithm (2003).

2. Every new onset psychotic episode in children and adolescents necessitates a comprehensive psychiatric evaluation complemented with pertinent medical, neurological, laboratory and imaging studies. See "Aids in the Diagnosis of Psychosis," chapter 5, and chapters 6 and 7 for the differential diagnosis of psychotic disorders in children and adolescents. Parallel considerations will be applied to situations of relapse or deterioration of clinical condition. Attributing deterioration to the illness clinical course may be erroneous.

3. There are no pediatric algorithms for the treatment of schizophrenic disorders in childhood. Child and adolescent psychiatrists, and adult psychiatrists who treat child and adolescent psychosis seek guidance from the adult algorithm. The CATIE results (Lieberman, Stroup et al., 2005) are likely to promote a change in the schizophrenia algorithm. This writer believes that a reconsideration of some first generation antipsychotics will be in order, based on perphenazine therapeutic effectiveness, tolerability, and cost-effectiveness when compared with SGA comparators (olanzapine, risperidone, ziprasidone, and quetiapine). In this writer's opinion the "big winner" in the CATIE trial was perphenazine: it performed as well as the other atypicals at a low dose (about 200 mg of chlorpromazine equivalence/day), had good tolerability, and cost far less than the competitor atypicals. The initial CATIE results raise serious questions about the present schizophrenia algorithm. It appears that the SGAs' effectiveness and tolerability is not equal; it seems that there are gradients of therapeutic superiority of some atypicals over others, and that some atypicals have serious issues with tolerability. Changes in the current algorithm are likely in the near future.

4. This writer recommends the use of antipsychotic medications that have significant data-base, level 1 evidence (as first-line medication for treatment of psychotic disorders in children and adolescents. See Table 12.

5. This writer objects to the present TIMA antipsychotic algorithm as a clinical guide for the psychopharmacological treatment of severe psychosis of childhood:

    (a) There is no evidence base to support the use of aripiprazole, olanzapine, ziprasidone, or quetiapine as first-line medication in childhood for the treatment of primary psychosis in childhood. There is supportive controlled data for the use of risperidone as a first-line agent for psychotic disorders in children and adolescents.

    (b) The CATIE study would suggest that perphenazine should be considered, at least at the same level, than risperidone, ziprasidone, or quetiapine.

    (c) If other studies confirm the therapeutic superiority of olanzapine, this medication will need to be considered as a first-line medication against severe psychosis of childhood. The CATIE II results (McEvoy, Lieberman, Stroup, et al., 2006), adds support for this consideration. Since this medication is associated with frequent metabolic toxicity, the initiation of this medication will necessitate the compulsory implementation of protective measures to decrease the metabolic risks; these include: dietary counseling, promotion of regular exercising and fitness, and the concomitant use of weight attenuating medications (see chapter 13).

    (d) For noncompliant psychotic adolescents, risperidone IM extended form (Consta) is a new alternative to haloperidol decanoate or fluphenazine decanoate traditional options.

    (e) This writer considers the use of perphenazine and mood stabilizer early in the nonresponsive downward track rather than using these drugs as the last resort choices prior to consideration of clozapine or ECT.

    (f) It is unclear what will be the role of emerging electrical and magnetic brain stimulating technologies and how proven psychosocial paradigms will need to be implemented to enhance the pharmacological interventions. Alternative treatments for the treatment of mood disorders are discussed in chapter 11.

(g) Psychopharmacologic treatment needs to be complemented by ongoing psychosocial interventions. Appropriate psychoeducational programming is fundamental (see chapter 9). Other interventions (i.e., speech and language therapy, occupational therapy, physical therapy) will be implemented as pertinent; medical and other ancillary services will be accessed as necessary.

6. Since the long-term consequences of extended use of atypical medications in children and adolescents is unknown, systematic medication side effect risk monitoring, including pertinent laboratory monitoring, is mandatory. The psychiatrist will be attentive to learning interferences created by medication side effects or the presence of comorbid disorders. Attention to the learning processes and to concentration difficulties, in particular, are central concerns for pediatric patients. Stimulant medication or alternative treatments to deal with comorbid ADHD may be necessary.

7. Because chronic psychotic youth have a higher risk for suicide or even homicidal behaviors, these risks will need to be monitored on a regular basis. Psychiatrists will be equally attentive to the use or abuse of alcohol or other illegal drugs, common complications of chronically psychotic patients.

8. The psychiatrist will also be attentive to the issues of medication compliance and to adherence to other psychosocial treatments. Early changes to alternative medications are in order if tolerability is compromised or there is a lack of therapeutic effectiveness. Sensitive use of antidepressant, antianxiety medications or others are indicated when there is significant depressive, anxiety or additional comorbidity. A mood stabilizer may be indicated if there is indication of mood instability or if the psychiatrist is seeking augmentation effects.

9. Psychosocial interventions, including appropriate psychoeducational programming, and ongoing individual and family interventions, are essential components of the comprehensive treatment plan for chronically psychotic children. The psychiatrist will monitor compliance to these interventions in each follow-up appointment.

   Li = Lithium
   DVP = Divalproex   *Depakote*
   AAP = Atypical Antipsychotics
       Olanzapine, Quetiapine, Risperidone, Clozapine, Aripiprazol, ziprasidone.
   AC = Anticonvulsants
       Divalproex, Carbamazepine, Oxcarbazepine, Lamotrigene
   CONT = Continue Therapy
   ETC = Electroconvulsive Therapy

Source: Miller, Hall, Buchanan, et al. (2004, p. 501).

Following the recommendations for monitoring weight, diabetes, and dyslipidemias related to SGAs, the Consensus Development Conference guidelines could be modified for children and adolescents in the following manner: A modification of the Consensus Development Conference (2004, p. 599) is presented in table 10. 9.

For patients with a higher risk for diabetes and those treated with other medications that may increase this risk (e.g., valproate, lithium, depoprovera), it may be preferable to initiate treatment with an SGA that appears to have a lower propensity to induce weight gain or glucose dysregulation (p. 599).

DRUG CHOICE AND DOSAGE

Except for the CATIE I study (Lieberman, Stroup, et al., 2005) there is no definitive study that demonstrates superiority of one atypical antipsychotic over

TABLE 10.9 Monitoring Recommendations for Weight, Diabetes, and Dyslipidemias

	Baseline	1st month	2nd month	3rd month	6th month	1 year
Personal and family history	X					X
Medical history	X				X	(1)
Weight/BMI	X	X	X	X	X	(2)
Height	X			X	X	Yearly
Waist circumf.	X	X			X	Yearly (3)
Blood pressure	X	X		X	X	Yearly (4)
Fasting glucose	X		X	X	X	(5)
Lipid profile	X		X	X	X	Yearly (6)
Insulin, Cortisol	X			X	X	Yearly (7)
EKG	X			X	X	(8)

1. or more often if an illness emerges
2. or more frequently if there is a rapid increase of weight or BMI
3. or more frequently if there is a rapid increase of weight or BMI
4. or more frequently it there is emergence of dizziness or related symptoms
5. or more often if diabetes related symptoms (polydypsia, polyphagia, polyuria, or others) unfold.
6. or more frequently if there is a rapid increase of weight or BMI
7. or more often if the person has Acanthosis Nigricans, history of diabetes, or if the patient has gained weight or BMI rapidly
8. or more often if the patient has a cardiovascular history, or if dizziness, fainting, chest pain, or related symptoms develop

Source: Modified from the Consensus Development Conference (2003).

another one. "Despite the publication of several treatment guidelines, there is significant variation in pharmacological treatment practice that cannot be explained away by 'patient heterogeneity.' Efforts to promote evidence-based 'best possible' pharmacotherapy of schizophrenia have hitherto been unsuccessful" (Tandon & Jibson, 2001, p. 982). Obviously these concerns are even more important in regard to the use of antipsychotics in children. The CATIE study showed that olanzapine has a gradient of therapeutic effectiveness superiority over the other comparator antipsychotics (perphenazine, quetiapine, ziprasidone, risperidone).[9] The CATIE II (McEvoy et al., 2006) results substantiated the therapeutic superiority of clozapine and corroborated the gradient of superiority of olanzapine over risperidone and quetiapine in the treatment of chronic adult schizophrenics.

Treatment of bipolar disorders in childhood is empirical; there are no established norms for the treatment of pediatric bipolar disorder. Although SGAs are demonstrating antimanic efficacy in adults, there are no rigorous controlled studies demonstrating similar effects in childhood. Furthermore, most of the evidence-based studies in adults are short-term. The reader will be reminded that the current accepted view is that bipolar pediatric disorders are chronic conditions.

Bryden, Coletti, Kutcher, et al. (2001) recommend a very conservative optimal dose for atypicals, 300 mg chlorpromazine equivalents/day and, (1) attention to clinical status, physical heath, and prior medication response; (2) monitoring for clinical response; (3) change of the antipsychotic if no response in six weeks or earlier, or if side effects become intolerable (pp.123–124). Bryden, Coletti, et al.'s conservative dose recommendations are applicable to children and adolescents with moderate psychopathology. For children with severe psychosis, clinicians use more often than not, doses that are akin to levels used in adult patients, that is, 600 to 800 mg of chlorpromazine equivalence dose/day, or even higher. There are multiple issues related to the use of antipsychotic medications at doses above the recommended levels (see table 10.10).

PHASES OF TREATMENT

In the use of antipsychotic medications, Tandom, as reported by Bowes (2002), identifies three distinct treatment phases, each with its own characteristics and

TABLE 10.10 Caveats in the Prescription of High Dose Antipsychotics

Patient may not be responding for lack of adherence.
1. Attend to psychosocial stressors and to adherence to psychosocial interventions.
2. Change on medications may not be needed.
3. Attend to GADE (Genetic variation, Age, Disease, Environmental factors).
4. There is no evidence-based support for the use of high dose antipsychotics. Unpublished cases in which high dose therapy was ineffective may outnumber published positive reports.
5. Current dose concentration may be too high and the resulting adverse effects may resemble worsening of the disease being treated.
6. Rapid medication clearance should be considered.
7. Higher doses may not help. Higher doses may decrease effectiveness.
8. Higher doses increase adverse events and costs, adding pressure for noncompliance.
9. Most of the reports on higher doses are anecdotical and uncontrolled.
10. Antipsychotics work in 6 to 8 weeks. Increases above the recommended doses are not advised during the initial 6 to 8 weeks.
11. Polypharmacy may cloud attributions of clinical response.
12. Oversedation does not equal improvement.
13. If higher doses are tried, increase monitoring and attend to added potential risks.

Sources: Pierre, Wirshing, & Wirshing (2004, p. 35); Preskorn (2004, pp. 39–43).

treatment goals: acute, symptom resolution phase, and long-term maintenance phase. This scheme is also applicable for considerations of pediatric bipolar treatment. In the treatment of children and adolescents with severe psychotic disorders, we propose parallel treatment chronology goals to Tandom's scheme:

First Phase

Promoting a therapeutic alliance for the initiation of treatment. Oftentimes, families are in shock, and it is hard for them to accept that the child has a serious psychotic illness. Efforts are directed toward breaking the individual and family denials, and to promoting the child and family's alliance for the initiation of multimodal treatments. Since antipsychotic medication is one of the pillars for improvement or resolution of the psychotic process, it is imperative to educate the family on the nature of the psychotic illness, and to discuss at length the antipsychotic target symptoms and the nature of medication side effects. Both child and family should be given ample opportunity for discussing benefits and potential medication risks. A parallel consideration will be given to the use of a mood stabilizer in childhood. Psychiatrists will propose target symptoms and will educate patients and families about potential side effects, including a full explanation of each medication's "black boxes" or serious warnings, when pertinent.

Second Phase

The psychiatrist monitors medication compliance and adherence to other psychosocial interventions. The clinician needs to methodically monitor adaptational stressors at school, at home, in the social milieu (parental discipline and consequences), and also becomes vigilant for signs of alcohol or drugs abuse.

Third Phase

This is the maintenance phase in which the psychiatrist continues monitoring for early evidence of psychotic or mood disorder relapse, and for medication and psychosocial interventions adherence. If the child maintains stability for an extended period, the psychiatrist will attempt to use lower therapeutic doses. The psychiatrist will also pay attention to the patient's health and other aspects of the patient's development, and will monitor his or her response to the comprehensive rehabilitation program. The psychiatrist monitors and promotes optimal child functioning at the school, within the family, and in the social milieu. All along, the psychiatrist will keep in mind that medication side effects are a major hindrance to treatment compliance; thus, detailed exploration of medication side effects should be done systematically in each therapeutic contact. Long-term side effects such as tardive dyskinesia, weight gain, diabetes, dyslipedimias, cardiovascular, and others require attentive monitoring. Females are particularly sensitive to side effects that may affect their perceived attractiveness and gender role functioning: weight gain, hair loss, acne, polycystic ovarian disease, and others.

Clinicians need to be attentive to any source of developmental interference and, if found, it should be addressed appropriately and without delay. Developmental interference refers to any detrimental influence from the psychosocial milieu that interferes with normal child and adolescent development (Nagera, 1966).

COMPLIANCE AND THERAPEUTIC ADHERENCE

Frequently the concepts of therapeutic compliance and adherence are used interchangeably; there is a difference between these two concepts, though. *Compliance* refers to a passive acceptance of the physician's recommendations, often without recognition of the presence of a problem, or without a clear understanding of the nature of the therapeutic goals. *Adherence* refers to the patient's deliberate efforts to follow the physician's recommendations, accepting the presence of a problem, and actively pursuing the agreed on therapeutic goals. Kane (2004), states that the belief that the prescribed therapy will be effective is one of the most important factors affecting treatment adherence; that is, that therapy will reduce symptoms and prevent relapse. Kane also highlights the role of the family and the therapeutic alliance in sustaining adherence: other factors affecting adherence include family or social support (family agreement with the intervention and the commitment to carry them out); presence of comorbid substance abuse; and the quality of the therapeutic alliance. Since the adherence is multifactorial, an individualized treatment approach within the context of the therapeutic alliance is necessary (p. 34).

The Treatment Outcomes Research Team (TORT; 1998) recommendations for adult schizophrenic patients, which have relevance for the child psychiatric field, emphasize that maintenance dosage was preferred over targeted, intermittent medication maintenance strategies which increase risk of symptom worsening or relapse (Bender, 2005, p. 36), and even compliance difficulties.

In the treatment of children and adolescents, understanding of the parents' theory of the illness and the underlying belief system is fundamental. If the treatment plan disagrees with the parents' theory of illness, it is unlikely that they will comply with the treatment recommendations.

Gabbard and Kay (2001) quote Basco and Rush (1966), who suggest that psychiatrists should always assume that obstacles to compliance exist and discuss potential problems and their solutions before they even arise. The authors emphasize the need for the establishment of a long-term therapeutic relationship based on trust. Within this context, common obstacles to treatment adherence can be identified; these include cognitive variables, treatment variables, social system variables, and variables involving intrapersonal and interpersonal factors (pp. 1959–1960).

It was thought that because SGAs have better tolerability than FGAs, that the adherence to those medications would be better. That is not necessarily so. Emergent data regarding comparison of adherence between patients taking typicals versus atypical antipsychotic medications is of concern. In a VA adult outpatient population, "patients receiving typical agents were without medications for approximately 7 days per month, while those receiving atypicals were without medication for approximately 4 days per month" (Dolder et al., 2002, p. 105). Dolder et al. concluded that, "The refill rates observed in this study highlight the pervasive, problematic degree of antipsychotics non-adherence in patients with psychotic disorders, including those who have prescriptions for atypical agents" (p. 106).

Psychiatrists are not good at judging the degree of compliance of their patients. When clinicians were asked to rate the degree of compliance of their patients using rating scales and interviews, on a threshold of 70% compliance, they rated the lack of compliance at 6% whereas data obtained from the use of microelectronic devices showed the rate of nonadherence as high as 62% (Kane & Turner, 2003, p. 3).

Compliance has significant implications for the frequency of relapse and rehospitalization, both psychiatric and medical. The costs of hospitalization for nonadherent patients were three times higher than the hospitalization costs for adherent patients. There is not a significant difference in adherence between patients taking typical or atypical antipsychotics (Gilmer et al., 2004, p. 695). Patients who were partially adherent (16%) were 2½ times more likely to be psychiatrically hospitalized that adherent patients, and patients who were nonadherent (24%) were three times more likely than adherents to get hospitalized; excess fillers (19%), had two times the risk of being hospitalized. Medical hospitalization was also correlated with adherence. Of relevance for the field of child psychiatry are the findings that patients living with their families or in supervised environments have higher levels of compliance; that compliance is lower in African-American and Hispanic populations (p. 697).

In adult schizophrenics, 40% of patients stop the antipsychotic within the first year, and 75% within two years (Brecher et al., 2002, p. 287). It is well known that bipolar disorder patients are poor compliers, even though they may experience positive medication effects. Parents need to redouble their efforts to insure that children adhere to the recommended dose, frequency, and intake details (i.e., to consume the medication after meals).

Regardless of the mediating intervention (individual, group, family, or community oriented approach) compliance will not improve unless compliance per se is made a very specific goal of those interventions (Zygmunt, Olfson, Boyer, & Mechanic, 2002). Attention needs to be given to contextual cues and reinforcements that are more amenable to intervention within the treatment programs. Besides individual variables, the psychiatrist needs to consider contextual factors that may impede or encourage a higher rate of adherence (p. 1654). Psychoeducational interventions without medication adherence as a key treatment element were generally less likely to improve adherence (p. 1661). There is a caveat with the psychoeducational approaches: "For some patients, increasing knowledge about their illness and about medication and its side effects may actually be disturbing. In other contexts, interventions that impart information associated with a high level of fear have been shown to reduce adherence and activate defensive avoidance" (Zygmunt et al., 2002, p. 1661).

Lacro, Dunn, Dolder, et al. (2002) found a very high incidence of nonadherence in a meta-analysis of an adult schizophrenic population. Nonadherence increases the risk of relapse, emergency visits, and rehospitalization (p. 892). The literature reviewed showed a broad a range on nonadherence, between 4% and 72%, with a median 40% of nonadherence (p. 894). The authors identified a number of factors that make nonadherence more likely (see table 10.11). Pediatric clinicians know very well that children psychoses and manic symptoms are poor compliers. Parents need to intesify their efforts to insure that pediatric bipolar patients adhere to their medications.

TABLE 10.11 Factors Associated with Lack of Adherence

Poor insight
Negative attitude or subjective medication response
   (family's apprehension to medications)
Short duration of illness
History of substance abuse
Nature of symptoms
       Severity of psychosis
       Presence of mood symptoms
       Inpatient status
       Previous history of nonadherence
Medication related factors
       High antipsychotic dose
       Limited intake supervision
       Severity of medication side effects
Environmental factors
       Poor therapy alliance
       Infrequent physician/ clinician contact
       Inadequate discharge planning
       Poor aftercare environment

Source: Lacro et al. (2002).

For adults, other factors thought to be related to poor adherence were not confirmed in the literature review: age, gender, ethnicity, marital status, education level, neurocognitive impairment, severity of psychotic symptoms, severity of medication side effects, route of administration, and family involvement (Lacro et al., 2002, pp. 991–905).

A Finnish study did not find evidence for a statistically significant superiority in acceptability of novel atypical drugs when compared to conventional antipsychotics (Wahlback, Tuunainen, Ahokas, & Leucht, 2001, p. 230). It is interesting that Scott and Pope (2002), propose that it was not the actual experience of side effects but the fear of side effects that increases the risk of nonadherence (Scott & Pope, 2002, p. 389).

Velligan (2003) reported that of a group of schizophrenic adults, whose compliance was followed three months after hospital discharge, 55% endorsed by self-report, compliance with medication and doses prescribed; however, compliance was 40% according to pill counts, and only 23% when the medication was monitored by blood levels (p. 3). There is no reason to believe that compliance in chronically psychotic children and adolescents is any better.

According to Velligan, partial compliance creates significant problems for clinicians. Partial compliance makes it difficult to determine whether medications are working adequately, whether dosing is appropriate, and whether concomitant medications are required. Medication changes and addition of medications are more likely to occur in patients who are not fully compliant with the prescribed medications (p. 14). It is optimistic if not naïve to think that adherence to treatment recommendations is better in the field of child and adolescent psychiatry. For relevant factors related to adherence difficulties in children and adolescents see table 10.12.

Compliance in children and adolescents is more complex than it is in adults. Children rarely seek treatment on their own, and seldom like to take medications. Adolescents abhor acknowledging that they have problems; thinking about things that they need to do to get better is the farthest thing from their minds. Adolescents hate to admit that they need to see a psychiatrist or a therapist. Taking medications goes against the developmental strivings of autonomy. For many adolescents, going to therapy or taking medications at certain scheduled times are "unbearable inconveniences." It takes a dedicated parent to set priorities in the child's life and to overcome the child's denials and avoidances; adolescents like to enjoy the illusion that they do not have any problems or that they can do everything on their own. In other words, the alliance with the child's parent(s) regarding the need for medications is fundamental; if the parent is in agreement with medication intake, it is likely that the medication compliance will be enforced. If the parent has reservations about the medication or, worse, if the parent is against medication intake, the chances of medication compliance are minimal.

TABLE 10.12 Factors Associated with Adherence Problems in Children and Adolescents

Children Issues

Denial of illness[1]
Developmental issues
Autonomy and control needs
Conflict with other interests[2]
Peer pressure
Drug abuse[3]

Parental issues

Reservations about psychotropics
Poor supervision
Parent–child conflict[4]
Lack of parental alliance[5]
Parental Illness (medical or psychiatric)

Financial matters:

Medications are not covered by insurance
Copayments may be high
Families may have more pressing financial needs than paying for medications, no matter how important they may be

1. Adolescents seldom feel they need to be on medications. Older preadolescents and adolescents frequently think that they can control emotions and behavior on their own. Above everything else, adolescents abhor to "depend on a medication," to achieve well-being, except for those with drug-dependence.
2. It is quite common for adolescents to avoid taking sedative medications at night because they induce sleep and interfere with late-night online, phone, or other social activities.
3. The preadolescent or adolescent may not want to give up drug of abuse, and prefers to continue abusing drugs than taking prescribed medications.
4. It is more likely that a parent will have a persuading influence on the child if the relationship is positive; if not, the child may behave oppositionally against medication intake.
5. If the parental figures disagree about medications, it is likely that the child seeks support in medication avoidance from the parent who objects to its use.

Many parents suffer from moderate to severe psychiatric pathology themselves, and lack the dedication and deliverance needed to attend to the diverse facets of their children's treatment plan. Many parents forget to take children to the psychiatric and psychotherapy appointments; they frequently forget to give the medications or supervise their intake. It takes a parent with a real conviction and willingness to make a persistent effort to stay on top of the implementation of the child's treatment plan. If the psychiatrist recognizes psychopathology in the parent(s) she should make efforts to refer the parents for appropriate assessment and treatment. The psychiatrist will also be attentive to parents' abuse of alcohol or illegal drugs and to neglectful or abusive parenting, and will take the appropriate steps to deal with these pathologies and developmental interferences.

Clinicians need to acknowledge that attending psychiatric and psychotherapeutic appointments creates work conflicts for many parents; many employers lack understanding for the employee's individual or family circumstances, and frown at the idea of the employee's need to leave the workplace on a regular basis. The therapeutic alliance is a very important factor in insuring therapeutic adherence; nonetheless, the psychiatrist should not assume that because the child and family attend scheduled appointments on a regular basis that this means that the medication or other aspects of the treatment plan are being followed as prescribed. Parents and children want to please their psychiatrist or therapist, and dislike revealing anything that would compromise the psychiatrist or psychotherapist's regard. In the same vein, parents do not like to share lapses in the care or supervision of their children, fearing the psychiatrist or psychotherapist's criticism.

When inquiring about treatment compliance and medication adherence in particular, the psychiatrist should ask nonleading questions like: How often do you forget to take the medications? This is a far better and more revealing question than asking, are you taking the medications? The psychiatrist needs to remember that the patient wants to please his physician and may avoid bringing issues he or she knows would displease the treating psychiatrist. Furthermore, the psychiatrist will ask the patient, what medications are you taking? Similarly, the psychiatrist will ask, how are you taking the medication? The physician will explore how the patient takes each one of the prescribed medications. This is more informative than fostering a leading inquiry by mentioning the medications that the patient is supposed to be taking rather than allowing the patient to disclose what medications he or she is taking, the way the patient takes them, the schedule, and the like. All along, the psychiatrist will compare the medications and dosage schedule declared by the patients with the ones he or she had recommended. Any discrepancies will be explored. Of equal importance is knowledge of the patient's medication rituals. If the patient does not have one, the psychiatrist could encourage the patient to develop one.

SIDE EFFECTS MONITORING

Broad questions regarding the presence of side effects are not effective in introducing and exploring the topic of side effects and the problems of compliance. A good start is to ask the patient what problems have arisen with the medications, and then, to explore systematically the presence of GI, sedative (Is the child sleeping in class?), cognitive/learning (Is the child keeping up with her grades?), memory, concentration (Are medications interfering with attention and learning?), or language interference (Is the child experiencing difficulties in word finding? Is the child having problems making or completing sentences?). Are there balance or coordination problems? How is the appetite? (Is the patient gaining weight? Is the child eating more than before?). Any sleep problems? Does the child complain of difficulties falling sleep or of waking up in the middle of the night? Any neuromuscular side effects (tremor, EPS?), any sexual side effects? Male adolescents may complain about erectile or ejaculatory difficulties. Sexual side effects need to be inquired about in sexually active adolescents. Only when the psychiatrist takes into account the patient's point of view, may issues related to noncompliance, and other treatment adherence obstacles be revealed, understood, and worked through.

Parents are very apprehensive regarding side effects that produce sedation (more so if the child sleeps in class), constriction of affect (parents miss the sense of liveliness of the child), and overweight (because of teasing, or because of personal complaints from the child). Any of these side effects render compliance very difficult.

Adherence is likely when the physician listens to the patient's concerns regarding medication side effects. Taking the complaints related to medication side effects seriously is a powerful intervention in itself. When patients feel understood they are better able to trust their psychiatrists and to follow the treatment recommendations and be open about nonadherence and the emergence of side effects. Actually, the patients should be encouraged to report side effects; this increases the therapeutic alliance (Weiden, 2002, p. 392).

The key to medication education is to translate our notion of symptoms into something the patient considers being a problem, which can be helped with the medication. When emphasizing adherence to avoid relapse and rehospitalization it is probably a better strategy for the physician to inquire about life and future goals. In this manner, the clinician may hear about the patient's desire to go back to school, to work, or to have a romantic involvement. The psychiatrist may articulate to the child and the family how adherence to treatment recommendations may help the child to achieve those goals.

The literature shows a strong correlation between therapeutic alliance, medication adherence, and outcomes in chronic psychosis, and probably, in chronic psychiatric illness. Although medications are important, medications alone are not enough. Patients who have a good relationship with their doctors are more likely to stay on medications, less likely to relapse, and generally will do better in other aspects of their lives (p. 391). Doctors need to strive to create a therapeutic alliance and to strengthen the alliance in every contact with the patient. A good alliance helps to foster supportive relationships outside of the family and to strengthen the therapeutic relationship with the family and other supportive persons or systems, in the child's life.

DISCONTINUATION OF ANTIPSYCHOTICS AND SWITCHING OF ANTIPSYCHOTICS

The staying power of atypical antipsychotics is poor. In the CAFÉ and CATIE reports three out of four patients discontinued the initial medications during

12 months and 18 months, respectively, because of lack of effectiveness or tolerability problems (Lieberman, McEvoy, et al., 2005; Lieberman, Stroup, et al., 2005). Winnas (2003) asserts that the two most compelling reasons to switch antipsychotics in the treatment of adults are a need for an enhanced clinical response and to improve tolerability. Four steps to ease the transition are suggested: (1) Assess response and side effects with the existing medication. (2) Weigh the pros and cons of switching, with input from the patient and caregivers. (3) Select a replacement with characteristics that could improve the patient's functioning. (4) Choose a switching strategy while considering safety and efficacy data. The greatest risk in a relatively stable patient is the reemergence of psychosis. The author stressed care when switching patients who: (1) Might harm themselves or others if the psychosis reemerges during the switch. (2) Patients who were recently stabilized after an acute psychotic episode and have been maintained on the medication that controlled the symptoms for less than six months. (3) Patients who cannot adhere to oral medications and are being maintained on long acting depot formulations.

Other factors that need to be considered during a switching transition are: need for more frequent psychiatric visits, the patient's willingness to change, the influence of external stressors such as bereavement, emerging illnesses, aspects of the workplace or living environment, medication costs, and coverage by third party payers (pp. 53–54). Many of these concepts and concerns are also applicable to antipsychotic switching in children and adolescents.

If an antipsychotic is ineffective in relieving target symptoms after many weeks of treatment at therapeutic dose levels, or if intolerable side effects develop, a new antipsychotic needs to be tried. There are three strategies for changing one antipsychotic medication to another: (1) abrupt discontinuation and immediate start of the new antipsychotic; (2) tapering of the ineffective or intolerable medication and starting of the new medication at full dosage; and, (3) the cross-over strategy in which tapering of the old drug is concomitant with a progressive titration of the new medication (p. 61). In adults, research has not demonstrated any clinical difference among the mentioned strategies, and there are no clear or specific guidelines as to what are the best switching strategies. The Consensus Development Conference (2004) recommends cross-titration as the safest approach for medication switching; they also advise against abrupt discontinuation of antipsychotics (p. 599).

In children and adolescents, abrupt discontinuation and immediate start of antipsychotic medications has two clinical drawbacks: (1) risk of medication withdrawal symptoms that may be misidentified as side effects of the new medication; (2) risk of withdrawal dyskinesia of the first drug that may be misattributed as a side effect of the new medication. Many parents are apprehensive about the abrupt discontinuation strategy, and are more accepting and comfortable with the other medication switching approaches. Complications with the first strategy of switching are illustrated in the following vignette:

Greg, an 8-year-old white boy, with severe psychosis and aggressive behavior, received treatment with quetiapine up to 600 mg/day for eight weeks without any significant therapeutic benefit; actually, his enuresis had worsened. A rapid tapering of quetiapine over three days and initiation of a small dose of aripiprazole, 5 mg/day, was implemented. About the third day of this regime, the patient began to display severe balancing problems and involuntary movements of the mouth and neck; gross tremor was observed and gait became very unstable. The patient had been receiving valproic acid and consideration was given to a high level of that medication. However, valproic acid level was 86, within the therapeutic range. Withdrawal dyskinesia to quetiapine was considered, and increasing quetiapine to previous levels caused the movements to disappear. Quetiapine taper was accomplished at a slower pace without any problems.

Particular care is recommended when switching from clozapine to other antipsychotics, and when changing patients from depot formulations to oral antipsychotics. How long should a patient need to continue on medications? Gitlin et al. (2001) consider that the decision to continue an antipsychotic is entirely based on clinical judgment and that the therapeutic alliance has a very important bearing upon it.

The vast majority of clinically stable individuals [adults] with recent-onset schizophrenia will experience an exacerbation or relapse after antipsychotic discontinuation, even after more than a year of maintenance medication. However, clinical monitoring and a low threshold for reinstating medications can prevent hospitalizations for the majority of these patients.... Current consensus suggests approximately 1 year of antipsychotic treatment for a first episode of schizophrenia followed by consideration of medication discontinuation for stable patients.... In essence, this study may be viewed as an attempt to apply targeted medication approach to a recent-onset schizophrenia cohort; patients were followed regularly when not receiving medications and treatment was re-started as soon as symptom exacerbation occurred. (p. 1836).[10]

CHAPTER 11

Mood Stabilizing Medications in the Treatment of Psychotic Disorders of Children and Adolescents, Other Treatments, and Alternative Treatments

For a variety of reasons, other medications are added frequently to the psychopharmacological treatment of chronic psychotic conditions in children and adolescents. Among these, mood stabilizers (valproate, lithium, lamotrigene, and others) play a significant role in the treatment of chronic psychotic disorders, more so if the conditions are mood related or if the disorders have a prominent mood component.

As with many other psychotropic medications used in child and adolescent psychiatry, use of mood stabilizers except Lithium is off label, that is, they are not FDA approved for use in this population or for these treatment objectives. As with many other psychotropic medications used in child and adolescent psychiatry, there are limited evidence-based data to support the use of mood stabilizers in childhood. Psychiatrists need to be alert and wary about polypharmacy in child and adolescent psychiatric patients and its added risks, which include tolerance problems, drug interactions, compliance, and additional costs.

This chapter provides a brief overview of clinical applications of the use of mood stabilizers in childhood. Currently the designation of mood stabilizers covers three groups of medications: lithium, anticonvulsants, and atypical antipsychotics. This chapter deals with clinical use of lithium and anticonvulsants in child and adolescent psychiatric patients. Atypical antipsychotics are covered in chapter 12.

The use of antidepressants in the treatment of bipolar depression is a highly debated issue among adult and child and adolescent psychiatrists. Gijsman,

Geddes, Rendell, et al. (2005) defend the use of antidepressants in the short-term phase treatment of bipolar depression (p. 1548). This proposition is in disagreement with the American Psychiatric Association guidelines for the treatment of bipolar disorders. Use of antidepressants in bipolar disorder I patients should be accompanied by a mood stabilizer.[1]

ANNOTATIONS TO THE ALGORITHM FOR TREATMENT OF ACUTE HYPOMANIC/MANIC/MIXED EPISODES IN PATIENTS WITH BIPOLAR DISORDERS

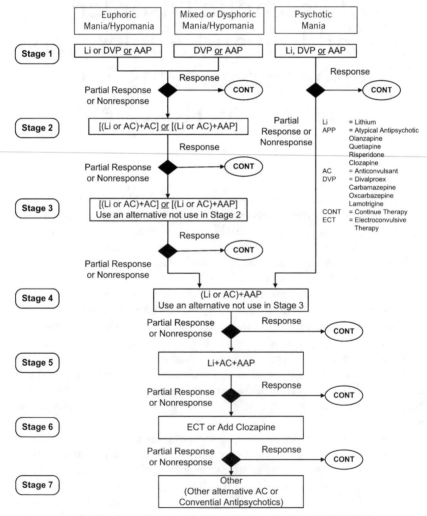

Consider decreasing or tapering/discontinuation of antidepressant medications.

Source: Suppes et al., 2005, pp. 873–876.

Notes

For symptom threshold use the frequency, intensity, number, and duration guidelines (FIND; Kowatch, Fristad, et al. (2005, p. 215). The threshold for the diagnosis needs to take into account the FIND guidelines and (1) the context of symptoms; (2) the impairment of adaptive functioning, and; (3) the presence of concurrent symptoms (p. 215). In addition, a timeline of onset, offset, and duration of symptoms is very helpful as well as an inquiry into comorbid conditions, including all the behavior, anxiety, mood, and other symptoms (BAMO, p. 218). Since suicide risk in BPD is very high, this risk needs to be assessed systematically (p. 217). The comprehensive evaluation should include collateral information (school, relatives, friends, etc.), a comprehensive medical exploration, substance abuse inquiry, and reactions or response to previous medication trials. A cross-sectional inquiry should be complemented with a longitudinal one. A three-generation genogram detailing history of psychiatric illness and emphasizing mood disorders: depression, manic–depressive illness, and family history of suicide should be included. (p. 218).

The medication algorithms were developed for the acute phase treatment of children and adolescents (ages 6 to 17) who met diagnostic DSM-IV criteria for BPD-1 manic or mixed episode (Kowatch, Fristad, et al., 2005, p. 219). The strongest database for the construction of the pediatric bipolar algorithm was taken from controlled studies in children and adolescents (level of evidence A) with complementary data from controlled adult (level of evidence B), supplemented by weaker database: open and retrospective studies (evidence C), and the least generalizable data (evidence D), case reports and panel consensus (p. 219).

1. The pharmacotherapeutic plan for mood stabilization according to Pavuluri and Naylor (2005), includes: (1) comprehensive history; (2) rapid wean-off of all the ineffective medications; (3) discontinuation of SSRIs; and (4) discontinuation of stimulants (p. 24). Pavuluri and Naylor, 2005, recommend the implementation of the acronym RAINBOW therapy as a key component of a comprehensive approach to the treatment of pediatric bipolar disorders:

   *R*outine. To establish strict daily routines, including consistent sleep time.

   *A*ffect regulation/anger control. Implement techniques of mood self-monitoring.

   I can do it. Help the child to develop a positive self-story.

   *N*o negative thoughts. Restructure negative thinking. "Live in the now."

   *B*e a good friend/balanced lifestyle. Organize play dates and build positive ties; foster a balanced lifestyle and a good self-care.

   *O*h. how can we solve it? Encourage problem solving.

   *W*ays to ask and get support. Develop a supportive network (p. 25).

2. For stage 1: Monotherapy, Kowatch, Fristad, et al. (2000), advised monotherapy with mood stabilizers or atypical antipsychotics. Li, Val, CBZ, OLZ, QUE, RISP are placed on an equal footing (pp. 220–221).

   The first medication choice for nonpsychotic mania is either lithium or divalproex (pp. 220–221). Pavuluri and Naylor (2005) also considered that the first treatment of choice is either lithium or divalproex; these medications have an established track record (mainly based on adult BPD studies) (p. 25). The SGAs alone may be more effective when irritability is prominent and demands a faster response not possible with mood stabilizers. SGAs plus a mood stabilizer (Li or Val) is an effective first-line strategy for severe cases, especially those with psychotic features (p. 25). It is questionable if medications that have A and B level of evidence should be placed at the same level of recommendation as medications which do not have controlled studies in children and adolescents. Findling, McNamara, Stansbrey et al. (2006) reported that pediatric patients with bipolar disorder who initially stabilized on combination Li/DVPX and who subsequently experienced recurrence of symptoms while receiving Li or DVPX monotherapy can be effectively re-treated with the reinitiation of combined Li/DVPX treatment (p. 1460).

3. For stage II, augmentation is recommended when there has been minimal or moderate response to monotherapy (Kowatch, Fristad, et al., 2005, p. 220). A switch to a different agent among the monotherapy alternatives is recommended if there has not been any response or the agent has not been tolerated. If there has been a partial response, an addition of the other monotherapy

alternatives is advised (Li + Val, Li + OLZ, Li + QUE, etc.). If atypical antipsychotics produce partial response, Li, Val, or CBZ could be added (p. 223). Adult bipolar I patients who responded to olanzapine for a manic or mixed episode were randomized to olanzapine or placebo. Olanzapine significantly prolonged the time to symptomatic relapse in all three types of mood disorders (manic, mixed episodes, depressed, including rapid cycling). Olanzapine appears to be more effective in preventing manic and mixed episodes than depressive episodes (p. 254).

4. For stage III, a third monotherapy alternative not tried in previous stages is an acceptable alternative. A lack of response to two monotherapy agents does not predict failure of an agent of a different class (p. 254).

5. For stage IV, for children who have not responded to previous monotherapy trials, a combination of mood stabilizers is considered a choice (Kowatch, Fristad et al., 2005, p. 223). As the clinician confronts progressive nonresponse, the need and risks of polypharmacy increase but the supportive evidence data for use of such drug combinations is wanting.

6. Stage V, therapeutic trials with ziprasidone, aripiprazole, or oxcarbazepine, could be implemented as less desirable alternatives, when there has been no response to more tried alternatives or tolerability has become a problem.

7. If patients have been recalcitrant to previous therapeutic efforts, clozapine is an alternative for children and adolescents; ECT remains an alternative for refractory adolescents (p. 224).

8. For BPD-I, manic or mixed, acute with psychosis, the database is limited (mostly level D). See, Findling et al. (2006) above. Kowatch, Fristad, et al. (2005) recommend a combination of traditional mood stabilizers (Li, Val, or CBZ) plus an atypical antipsychotic (p. 224). Adult data show a counterintuitive response to valproate or olanzapine: valproate being more effective than olanzapine in psychotic mania, and olanzapine being better than valproate in nonpsychotic mania (Tohen, Baker, et al., 2002, p. 1016). Similar observations have been made with lithium; see below.

9. There is insufficient data to develop a treatment algorithm for BPD-I depressed (Kowatch, Fristad, et al., 2005, p. 225). Antidepressants may be used if preceded by a mood stabilizer. Lamotrigine is a promising alternative in these circumstances. Quetiapine appears to be a very promising agent for the treatment of bipolar depression in adults (Calabrese et al, 2005). In a randomized equipoise adult trial (NIMH, Systematic Treatment Enhancement Program for Bipolar Disorder –STEP-BP) on bipolar resistant depression, there were no differences in primary pairwise comparison analyses of open label augmentation with lamotrigine, inositol, and risperidone. Post hoc secondary analysis suggests that lamotrigine, may be superior to inositol and risperidone in improving treatment resistant bipolar depression (pp. 213–214).

Psychosocial interventions may help in reducing the frequency and intensity of depressive episodes. ECT remains an alternative for severe, treatment-refractory bipolar depression (pp. 213–214).

For breakthrough depression, Pavuluri and Naylor (2005), recommend lithium or lamotrigine as the first choice, and lithium plus lamotrigine as their second choice (p. 25).

For breakthrough aggression, these authors recommend a switch to SGA monotherapy, when the aggression is mild, or to a mood stabilizer plus a SGA for moderate to severe aggressive presentations. Clonidine is an alternative to subdue rage attacks (p. 25).

For breakthrough anxiety, cognitive behavior therapy (CBT) remains the first choice of treatment. SSRIs may be used with caution. Benzodiazepines or buspirone are alternative choices. Propanolol may be used for performance anxiety (p. 25).

10. Stabilization of BPD should precede treatment of comorbid disorders when such conditions negatively affect the child's psychosocial or academic functioning. When indicated, proven psychosocial intervention should be tried (Kowatch, Fristad, et al., 2005, p. 226). It is better to treat each comorbid condition sequentially (p. 227).

11. Suicide risk demands consistent and systematic monitoring. Data regarding the long-term use of lithium are compelling. In adults with BPD Li treatment is associated with an eightfold reduction of suicidal behavior (p. 229).

12. Treatment maintenance goals include prevention of relapse and recurrences; reduction of sub-threshold symptoms, suicide risks, affective cycling, and mood instability; reduction of vocational and social morbidity, and promotion of wellness (diet, sleep hygiene, fitness, dental and medical care, abstention from tobacco and alcohol, birth control, protection against STDs, etc.). There are limited randomized, controlled maintenance studies in children and adolescents. It is not known how long a child or adolescent will need to be maintained in treatment. Current guidelines recommend a minimum of 18 months. A consideration for tapering or discontinuation of medications should be given in cases where children have achieved steady remission for 12 to 24 months (p. 229).

13. Medication side effects should be an ongoing concern and systematic monitoring of potential side effects should be the rule. Cognitive side effects should be kept in mind and will be monitored regularly (p. 230).

14. The recent CATIE (Lieberman, Stroup, McEvoy, et al., 2005) results stimulate a reconsideration of the role of first generation antipsychotics based on therapeutic effectiveness, tolerability, and cost-effective considerations when compared with SGA. A comparable study to CATIE's, in mood disorders, is needed.

15. It is unclear what will be the role of emerging electrical and magnetic brain stimulating technologies in the treatment of primary affective psychoses of childhood or how proven psychosocial paradigms will need to be implemented to enhance the pharmacological interventions. See below.

16. Substance abuse comorbidity will require the concomitant implementation of alcohol/chemically dependency treatments.

17. In an adult prospective cohort study, 58% of the participants achieved recovery during up to two years of follow-up; 48.5% of participants experienced recurrence during up to two years of follow-up (the majority of the recurrences, 70%, were to the depressive pole). Results demonstrated that mood episodes, and particularly depressive episodes, are prevalent and likely to recur in spite of guideline treatments (Perlis, Ostacher, et al., 2006, p. 221). Predictors of recurrence include: residual mood symptoms (residual manic symptoms appear to confer risk for both manic and depressive recurrence), and significant anxiety in the year prior to the study, which confers risk for depressive recurrence (p. 222).

LITHIUM

Lithium has a double-blind, placebo-controlled, prospective study (Geller et al., 1998). In this study lithium demonstrated therapeutic superiority over placebo in the treatment of bipolar disorders. First introduced into psychiatry by Cade in Australia in 1949, lithium received FDA approval for the treatment of mania in 1970, and for prophylaxis of bipolar disorder in 1974. Lithium has stood the test of time, and remains an efficacious and a cost-effective treatment for bipolar disorder (Freeman, Wiegand, & Galenberg, 2004, p. 547). Currently, lithium is the only FDA-approved psychotropic for acute mania and maintenance treatment for children and adolescents.

Lithium is a monovalent cation and the lightest alkali metal. Substitution of other cations (sodium, potassium, calcium) may contribute to its therapeutic effects. Lithium is minimally protein-bound, does not undergo biotransformation, and is excreted by the kidney. Brain levels, measured by in vivo nuclear magnetic resonance, peak 0 to 2 hours after maximum blood serum levels (pp. 457–458). Lithium's mood stabilizing mechanism of action is unknown.

Lithium provides short- and long-term effects. Ultimately, it is believed that lithium causes changes in gene expression. The following short-term effects are being considered:

1. *Depletion of inositol.* Lithium is a noncompetitive inhibitor of inositol and promotes inositol depletion. This explains lithium's profound impact on mood in bipolar and depressed disorders, and its minor effects in control subjects. Depletion causes effects on neurotransmitters and second messenger systems (adrenergic, serotonergic, and cholinergic receptors that are coupled to the inositol cycle via G proteins); this cycle in turn, regulates protein kinase C action, leading to a reduction of protein kinase C isoenzymes in the frontal cortex and hippocampus, areas known to be involved in the pathophysiology of mood disorders.

2. *Glycogen synthase kinase-3 (GSK-3) inhibition.* This effect has an impact on a number of neurotransmitter systems. GSK-3 is an inhibitor of the Wnt protein-signaling pathway, which affects neuronal transduction. It appears that lithium mimics Wnt signaling, and because of this effect, it inhibits a stimulating cascade of events that causes stimulation of the protein kinase C activity. Lithium stabilizes the cytoskeleton structures by inhibiting the GSK-3 activity on the catenins that produce changes in the cytoskeleton.

3. *Affects major neurotransmitter systems.* Lithium has an effect in most of the major neurotransmitter systems. It is proposed that lithium increases glutamate uptake, normalizes low gamma-amino-butyric acid in the CSF, and enhances norepinephrine and serotonin functions. Lithium has proven antagonist effects on 5HT1A and 5HT1B autoreceptors, producing an increase of serotonin at the synaptic cleft.

4. *Resynchronization of hypothalamic oscillators.* Lithium administration causes a resynchronization of the hypothalamic oscillators (major and minor), altered in bipolar disorders (pp. 548–549).

5. *Increases neuronal viability and function.* Chronic lithium use increases neuronal viability and function in human brains. It is likely that the long-term lithium beneficial effects are mediated by neurotrophic and neuroprotective actions (Bachmann, Schloesser, et al., 2005, p. 51).

Clinical Indications

Acute Mania

Lithium has clinical effects on acute mania irrespective of the presence of psychotic symptomatology. In general, manic psychotic patients respond better to lithium than manic patients without psychosis. Lithium is less effective in patients with mixed or dysphoric mania, rapid cycling, a greater number of previous episodes, mood incongruent delusions, or in manic patients with concurrent substance abuse (Ketter, Wang, & Post, 2004, p. 582).

Bipolar Depresion

Patel et al. (2006) demonstrated that lithium may be effective in decreasing depressive symptoms in adolescents with bipolar depression. About half (48%) of the patients achieved a response but only 30% reached remission (p. 294).

VALPROATE

There are no published double-blind, placebo-controlled studies of the use of valproic acid in children and adolescents for the treatment of bipolar disorders. Valproate was the first alternative mood stabilizer to be studied. First introduced as an antiepileptic in France in 1967, it was first introduced into the United States in 1978, and received approval for the treatment of mania in 1995. Valpromide, a primary amide of valproic acid, is reported to be twice as potent as the parent compound. Vaproate has antiepileptic activity against a variety of seizure disorders and has also antikindling properties (Bowden, 2004, p. 567). Divalproex obtained FDA approval for mania in 1995. Valproate increases the concentration of GABA by activating its synthesis and inhibiting its catabolism (p. 568). Divalproex causes a reduction of the GABA plasma levels, which correlate with the improvement of manic symptomatology (p. 568).

Sodium valproate and valproic acid attain peak concentration within two hours and divalproex within three to eight hours. Valproex, the extended release form, is absorbed faster. Absorption is delayed if the drug is taken with food (p. 568). Valproate is highly protein bound. The binding is increased by a low-fat diet and decreased by high-fat diets. Only the unbound form of the drug crosses the brain–blood barrier (BBB). Valproate is metabolized primarily in the liver by glucoronidation. Oxidative pathways produce a number of metabolites some with antiepileptic, others with toxic effects. Less that 3% of the drug is excreted unchanged by urine and feces (pp. 568–569). Valproate is the only major antiepileptic that does not induce hepatic chromosomal enzymes (p. 576).

Wassef et al. (2005) report lower effectiveness of divalproex versus valproic acid in a large sample (N = 9,260) of patients resulting in a longer inpatient length of stay for subjects on divalproex in comparison to patients on valproic acid. The length of stay difference is maintained even if the patients on valproic acid are switched to divalproex. Valproic acid's higher peak serum concentration might account for its association with a shorter length of stay. Extended release divalproex (Depakote ER) has an even lower peak serum concentration.

The authors now switch patients who cannot tolerate valproic acid to delayed release, not to extended release, divalproex (p. 336). Allen, Hirschfeld, Wozniak, Baker, and Bowden (2006) demonstrated a linear relationship of valproic serum concentration to response and optimal serum levels for the treatment of acute mania (p. 272). Evidence from their study indicates that higher valproate levels are associated with greater efficacy (as measured by effect sizes) across the groups defined in the study (p. 274).

Valproate antiepileptic and mood-stabilizing mechanisms are unknown. Valproate inhibits the catabolism of GABA, increases its release, decreases GABA turnover, increases GABA-Beta receptor density, and may also increase neuronal responsiveness to GABA (p. 570). Valproate increases GABA levels in the brain and enhances neuronal responsiveness to GABA. Other theories as to how valproate works are discussed in an endnote.[2]

As far back as 1996, Bowden et al. determined that the therapeutic range of valproate was between 45 and 125 mcg/ml. Although, a linear relationship regarding therapeutic effectiveness and valproex level has been demonstrated in the treatment of acute mania, see above, in cyclothymia and bipolar II disorders, patients may respond to therapeutic levels below 50 mcg/mL. Levels above 100 mcg/mL increase the risk of hematologic side effects (decrease white blood and platelet count), sedation, and appetite increase. More over, levels above 100 mcg/mL are less efficacious than levels between 75 and 100 mcg/mL (p. 569).

Only the unbound drug crossed the blood-brain barrier and is bioactive. Thus when valproic is displaced from protein binding sites through drug interactions, the total drug concentration may not change [the relationship between dose and total valproate concentration is nonlinear], however the pharmacological active unbound drugs does increase and may produce signs and symptoms of toxicity (Idem).

Clinical Applications

Valproate has FDA approval for mania in adults, sole or adjunctive treatment of simple and complex absence seizures, for adjunctive treatment of a variety of absence seizure, and other seizure disorders, and for prophylaxis of migraine.

Acute Mania

Seven controlled trials (four placebo-controlled, one haloperidol-controlled, one lithium-controlled, and one placebo- and lithium-controlled) have demonstrated valproate effectiveness in acute mania. Antimanic effects could be augmented by the coadministration of lithium, carbamazepine, or antipsychotics (PDR, 2005, p. 570). Valproate may also be effective in the treatment of secondary manias (p. 572). Valproate is more effective than lithium in manic patients with rapid cycling and in bipolar patients with substance abuse, and is less effective with schizoaffective disorder, bipolar type (p. 574).

Prophylactic Treatment Effects

Valproate reduces the intensity and frequency of episodes (mania and depression) in adults and extends the time to new episodes, including patients with rapid cycling, mixed bipolar disorder, bipolar II disorder, and schizoaffective disorder (p. 572).

Impulsive Aggression

Valproate reduces impulsive aggression in patients with personality disorders.

Cotherapy in Schizophrenia

Coadministration of antipsychotics and valproate produces a significant improvement of the Positive and Negative Syndrome scale (PANSS) scores. It is proposed that antipsychotics should be limited to breakthrough manias in patients treated with valproate (p. 573).

Catatonia

GABAergic drugs like valproate may be beneficial in the treatment of catatonia. Benzodiazepines have an established role in the management of catatonia (Ginsberg, 2005, pp. 29–30).

Drug Interactions

Valproate increases the levels of phenobarbital, phenytoin, and TCAs. Carbamazepine decreases the levels of valproate and fluoxetine may boost valproate concentrations. Coadministration of valproate and lamotrigine should be done with extreme caution. The risk of Steven–Johnson's syndrome increases with this combination. Children are particularly vulnerable to this potentially fatal outcome.

CARBAMAZEPINE (CBZ)

There are no published double-blind, placebo-controlled studies on the use of carbamazepine in children and adolescents for the treatment of bipolar disorders. CBZ increases limbic gamma amino butyric acid (GABA) type B receptors, decrease GABA and dopamine turnover, inhibits inositol transport, and weakly inhibits calcium influx by a NMDA mediated effects in preclinical trials. Chronic Li, CBZ, VPA use increases hippocampal GABA-B and decreases GABA turnover, suggesting that hippocampal GABA-B receptor mechanisms and a decrease of GABA turnover could be effects involved in medications that stabilize mood (Ketter, Wang, & Post, 2004, p. 585). A list of some of the complex CBZ functions appears in an endnote.[3]

The active CBZ-E metabolite can yield therapeutic and adverse effects similar to CBZ but is not detected in conventional CBZ assays. Thus, the unwary clinician may misinterpret the significance of therapeutic or adverse effects associated with low or moderate CBZ serum concentrations. The CSF and serum levels of CBZ-E (or CBZ-E/CBZ), but not of CBZ, are associated with improvement of mood disorders and clinical improvement of depression, respectively (Ketter et al., 2004, p. 585).

CBZ in blood is 76% protein bound, and is more rapidly metabolized to CBZ-10,11-epoxide (a metabolite with equipotency to CBZ as an anticonvulsant in animal screens) in younger age groups than adults (PDR, 2006, p. 2279). If there is no hint of therapeutic response at moderate doses, it is unlikely that pushing the medication to very high doses will be beneficial (Ketter et al., 2004, p. 585). Carbamazepine alters the concentration and metabolism of many medications.[4]

Carbamazepine is available as chewable 100 mg tablets, tablets of 200 mg, XR tablets of 100, 200, 400 mg, and as a suspension of 100mg/5ml (PDR, 2006, p. 2281). CBZ suspension should not be administered concomitantly with other medication suspensions because of the risk of precipitation (p. 2379).

Clinical Indications

CBZ should not be used in patients with history of bone marrow depression, porphyria, hypersensitivity to the medication, or sensitivity to TCAs, or con-comitantly with MAO inhibitors (PDR, 2005, p. 2378). CBZ is indicated in the following neurological (seizure disorders and trigeminal neuralgia, migraines, and others) and psychiatric conditions.

Treatment of Acute Mania

Carbamazepine and valproate are more effective than lithium in producing remissions in patients with bipolar disorders with comorbid substance abuse (Bowden, 2004, p. 574). CBZ antimanic response is considered to be comparable to lithium or neuroleptics, or in other studies, to valproate (Ketter et al., 2004, p. 588). The overall aggregated antimanic efficacy reported in mixed studies (16 with CBZ, 4 with OXC) in 179 patients was 59%; the one for lithium was

61%; for adjunctive neuroleptic, 56%; and adjunctive placebo, 33% (p. 587). These results should be read with caution; the number of patients is small and the aggregation of CBZ and OXC is not justified. Actually, it is misleading, because it gives OXC a legitimacy that needs to demonstrated; OXC needs to prove its efficacy and tolerability on its own and should not do so by riding on the coattails of the parent compound.

Prophylaxis

CBZ may have an equal prophylactic antimanic and antidepressant efficacy in contrast to its less potent acute antidepressant efficacy compared to the antimanic effects (p. 588). CBZ efficacy in rapid cycling patients is mixed (p. 590).

In maintenance treatment, CBZ seems to be more effective than lithium in patients with nonclassical manias (bipolar II, bipolar NOS, bipolar disorder with mood incongruent delusions or comorbidity). CBZ may be effective in VPA resistant illness, and a CBZ plus VPA combination may be effective in patients with little or no response to either agent alone (p. 589). It is proposed that the left insula hypermetabolism is a marker for CBZ response (p. 590).

The overall rate of prophylaxis efficacy in mixed studies in 242 patients was reported as 54%. There were 13 studies with CBZ and 2 studies with OXC (one study has 8 and the other 4 patients). The response rates for lithium were 63%, and for placebo 22% (p 589). The reservations expressed about the antimanic efficacy are also applicable for the ones on prophylaxis. Regarding long-term treatment safety, there are only data related to six-month treatment in epileptic children (PDR, 2006, p. 2280).

OXCARBAZEPINE

At the joint Annual Meeting of the American Academy of Child and Adolescent Psychiatry, in Toronto, Canada, Wagner et al. (2005) presented a poster to report the results of a double-blind, placebo-controlled trial of 116 outpatients (aged 7 to 18 years, mean 11.1 +/– 2.99) with bipolar disorder (manic or mixed), treated with oxcarbazepine or placebo. In this study, oxcarbazepine did not show any therapeutic superiority over placebo. These findings were published in *The Brown University Child and Adolescent Psychopharmacology Update* (2005, pp. 6–7).

This anticonvulsant has limited evidenced-based studies for applications in psychiatry. It is purported to have CBZ clinical effects and to have a more favorable side effect profile. OXC does not cause autoinduction and yields less heteroinduction than does CBZ (Ketter et al., 2004, p. 585). Drug–drug interactions are less problematic with OXC than with CBZ (p. 585). OXC is available in film-coated tablets of 150, 300, and 600 mg, and in suspension (300 mg/5 ml) (PDR, 2006, p. 2286). OXC may render oral hormonal contraceptives ineffective (p. 2382).

LAMOTRIGENE

There are no published double-blind, placebo-controlled studies of the use of lamotrigene in children and adolescents for the treatment of bipolar disorders. Lamotrigene inhibits the reduction of dihydrofolate to tetrahydrofolate by inhibiting the enzyme dihydrofolate reductase. This may result in inhibition of nucleic acid and protein synthesis, secondary disruption of neural structure and functions, and tertiary disruption of mood (Shelton & Calabrese, 2004, p. 615). Lamotrigene inhibits use-dependent Na+ channels, allowing continued normal depolarization but suppressing paroxysmal firing. Lamotrigene inhibits glutamate release secondary to ischemia (neuroprotection) and also inhibits excitotoxic epileptic discharges (p. 616). Oral lamotrigene is absorbed rapidly and readily crosses the BBB, reaching peak brain concentrations in two to three hours. The t1/2 is approximately 27 hours and only about half of the concentration is protein bound. It is believed that lamotrigene psychotropic mechanisms are associated with its antiepileptic activity.

Research data supports the notion that lamotrigene–induced inhibition of Na+ flux at presynaptic use-dependent and voltage-sensitive Na+ channels. The inhibition is greatest in paroxysmal depolarized, rapidly firing neurons. Thus, preferential attenuation of paroxysmal wave trains while sparing the initial stimulus could permit normal neuronal activity to continue unimpeded, while suppressing seizure activity and affective instability (p. 617). The presynaptic inhibitory effects of lamotrigene results in the decreased release of the excitatory amino acid glutamate. This may explain lamotrigene's mood stabilization. Lamotrigene is 55% protein bound (PDR, 2006, p. 1450). Lamotrigene (Lamictal) is available for oral administration in 25, 100, 150, and 200 mg scored tablets. It is also available in chewable dispersible tablets of 2, 5, and 25 mg (PDR, 2006, p. 1457).

Clinical Indications

Adjunct Antiepileptic

Adjunct therapy for adults with partial seizures, and for children and adult patients with generalized seizures secondary to Lennox-Gastaut syndrome.

Bipolar Depression

Lamotrigene monotherapy is an efficacious and well-tolerated treatment for bipolar depression. No increase in the rate of switch to mania was observed with lamotrigene treatment (p. 618).

Chang et al. (2006) using monotherapy in the majority of 31 enrolled adolescents, reported that no subject developed mania during the 8 weeks of the study. Lamotrigene was well tolerated with not rashes considered medication related. The authors stated that they obtained robust results, an 84% and 63% response based on primary and secondary criteria, respectively, and a remission rate of 58%. This remission rate is higher than the remission rates published for lithium and valproate (p. 302).

Bipolar Disorder Maintenance

Lamotrigene was superior to placebo at prolonging the time to a mood disorder (manic, hypomanic, mixed episode, and rapid cycling bipolar disorders, particularly bipolar II, with predominant depressive symptoms). Lamotrigene has a better cognitive profile than phenytoin, diazepam, carbamazepine, and even valproate. It is believed that lamotrigene produces a general activation of brainstem arousal and vigilance systems (p. 619).

USE OF ANTIDEPRESSANT MEDICATIONS

Silva, Gabbay, et al. (2005) made a comprehensive review of the use of antidepressant medication in children and adolescents. Antidepressants are used effectively in a broad array of adult psychiatric conditions. In children and adolescents, studies and indications lag behind the adult counterparts. Antidepressants are FDA approved for use in children and adolescents for treatment of OCD and MDD. For OCD, sertraline is FDA approved for children 6 years of age and older, fluoxetine for children 7 years of age and older, fluvoxamine for children 8 years and older, and clomipramine for children 10 years and older. Among all the antidepressants considered useful for MDD, only fluoxetine has FDA indications for children 8 and older (pp. 44–45). The authors reviewed the use of antidepressants in anxiety disorders, ADHD, MDD, OCD, PTSD, and selective mutism. The latest antidepressant warning regarding increased suicidal ideation is stated in the review; however, the review overlooks cautioning psychiatrists about these agents' risk for mania induction. This is a serious concern in the treatment of serious depressions in children and adolescents, since differentiating unipolar from bipolar depression is not an easy endeavor.

Clinicians will strive to ascertain the accuracy of the depressive syndrome by making a detailed inquiry into the epigenesis of the mood disturbance, a comprehensive assessment of concurrent comorbidities, and a meticulous exploration of family history and of previous responses to psychopharmacological and psychosocial treatments; additionally, diagnosticians will gather information regarding developmental achievements including cognitive levels, learning capacities, and social skills. The clinician will also strive to ascertain history of mania or hypomania in the patient's past.

Antidepressant medication in the treatment of bipolar disorder is controversial; it may be used with caution in the treatment of children and adolescents with bipolar depression if preceded by mood stabilizers. Because antidepressants carry the risk of increased suicidal ideation and mania induction, the use of antidepressant medication for the treatment of bipolar depression should monitored very closely. Goodwin and Ghaemi (2005) express strong reservations about antidepressant use in adult bipolar depressed patients. They state that there is evidence indicating that antidepressants worsen mixed states and are associated with a faster relapse rate (p. 2077). In spite of the later warning, Tohen, Zarate, et al. (2003) reported the use of antidepressants in 9% of a mostly manic adult follow-up cohort (p. 2101). Apparently the manic switch risk with the use of antidepressants is increased with the presence of substance abuse comorbidity (Lieberman, 2005a, p. 11).[5]

ELECTROCONVULSIVE THERAPY (ECT) AND OTHER BRAIN STIMULATING TECHNOLOGIES (REPETITIVE TRANSCRANIAL MAGNETIC STIMULATION- RTMS)

ECT is a established electrical stimulating technique employed in the treatment of severe mood disorders. An electrical current, applied to the skull, simulates a seizure, believed to bring about ECT therapeutic effects. The use of ECT in children and adolescents is controversial, and in certain states in the Union, this treatment intervention has been politicized and proscribed. This technique may be a life saving intervention for patients with profound melancholia, or unresponsive mania, for those that refused to eat, for those with stupurous or agitated catatonia, or for patients with unremitting suicidal ideation. Although there is an ongoing reappraisal of ECT, still remains a therapeutic modality of last resort because of the belief that electroshock treatments injures the brain.

There has been some interest in new developed, non-convulsive interventions, purported to have therapeutic effects akin ECT. TMS shows some promise as a novel antidepressant therapy. Gelenberg (2003, July) reports two separate negative findings in the use of TMS for bipolar depression and mania. This technique remains an experimental treatment (p. 25).

TABLE 11.1 Suggested Doses for Mood Stabilizers in Children and Adolescents

Medication	Initial dose preschoolers in mg/day	Maximal dose mg/day	Initial dose preadolescents in mg/day	Maximal dose mg/day	Initial Dose adolescents in mg/day	Maximal dose mg/day
Lithium carbonate[1]	150 BID	300–450	300 BID	900–1200	300 TID	1200–1800
Lithium citrate	150 BID	300–450	300 BID	—	—	—
Lithobid	300/day	300–600	300 BID	600–900	300 BID	900–1500
Eskalith-CR	122.5 mg BID	450 mg	225 BID	900–1350	450 BID	1350–1800
Valproate[2]	125 BID	375–500	250 BID	750–1000	500–1000	1500–2000
Depakene	75 BID	100–150 BID-TID	200 BID-TID	600–800	—	
Depakote sprinkles	125 BID	375–500	250 BID	750–1000	—	
Depakote ER	250 q HS	250–500	250–500 q HS	750–1000	500–1000 q HS	1500–2000
Carbamazepine[3]	50 BID	150–200	100 BID	200–400	200 BID	800–1200
Tegretol XR	100 mg q HS	200	200 BID	300–400	200 BID	800-1600
Oxcarbazepine[4]	150 BID	450–600	150–300 BID	900–1200	300 BID	900–1800
Lamotrigene[5]	Not indicated		12.5 BID	200–250	12.5 BID	200–400

[1]The 2006 edition of the PDR indicates that lithium (Lithobid) is not recommended for children under 12 years of age (p. 1671). Lithium is titrated according to tolerance, clinical response, and blood levels. Children tolerate higher blood levels than adults: in preadolescents a level, up to 1.5 mEq/l, is acceptable in acute titration; in adolescents, a level up to 1.2 mEq/l is permissible in acute titration. Therapeutic levels are usually lower for maintenance. Thyroid function tests and renal function require periodic evaluations.

[2]Valproate is titrated according to tolerance, clinical response, and blood levels. Liver functions tests need close monitoring at the initiation of treatment and then at regular intervals. Early preschoolers are more prone to toxicity than older children. Therapeutic level: 50–100 mcg/ml; up to 100–125 mcg/ml could be permissible, if there is satisfactory tolerance.

[3]Carbamazepine is titrated according to tolerance, clinical response, blood levels, and the degree of autoinduction or heteroinduction. Therapeutic levels: 8–12 mcg/ml.

[4]Oxcarbazepine is titrated according to tolerance and clinical response. OXC does not required blood level monitoring.

[5]Lamotrigene requires a very slow induction in children and adolescents. In general, an initial dose of 12.5 BID is recommended. Dose is increased, tolerance permitting, 12.5 mg every week to every other week. When the upward titration reaches 50 mg BID, the increase of the dose can be done by increments of up to 25 mg every week. Afterwards, it is safe to increase dose by increments of up to 50 mg/week, if patient is tolerating medication well and efficacy has not achieved. In children and adolescents coadministration of valproate and lamotrigene is not recommended.

ALTERNATIVE TREATMENTS

Placebo controlled, double-blind studies and metanalysis of controlled studies consistently show that S-adenosyl-L-methionine (SAMe) in doses of 400 to 1600 mg/day produces antidepressant effects comparable to conventional antidepressants (Lake, 2005, p. 91). Folate and vitamin B_{12} are essential cofactors for the synthesis of SAMe and should be recommended to patients using SAMe or conventional antidepressants (p. 91). Eicosapantaenoic acid (EPA), an omega-3 fatty acid, has demonstrated effectiveness against moderate depressive mood. Rare cases of hypomania have been described in depressed patients with BD taking EPA (p. 91). According to Stoll (2005), pure DHA did not show any effects in bipolar disorder and there is mounting evidence that EPA is the active component of fish oil (p. 24). There are anecdotal reports of bleeding with omega-3 fatty acids use because these agents can block platelet aggregation (p. 25).

St. John's Wort (SJW) has been used for the treatment of moderate to severe depressions; results are contradictory; it seems that SJW is as effective as conventional antidepressants (CAs) in moderate depression, but it is not as effective as CAs in the treatment of severe depressions (Lake, 2005, p. 91); 5-hydroxitryptophan (5-HTP), is also as good as CAs for the treatment of moderate depression. It has also been used for augmentation in a combination of CAs. Acetyl-L-carnitine (ALC) has not been studied in comparison to CAs but has been investigated in controlled, double-blind studies in severely depressed patients; ALC seems to ameliorate symptoms of cognitive impairment when depression is related to age related-cognitive decline. Folate and vitamin B_{12} improve mood by themselves and enhance the antidepressant effects of SAMe. (p. 92).

According to Stoll (2005), folic acid partially worked in men. On the other hand, it converted women from an approximate 50% response rate to fluoxetine to a 90% response rate (p. 26). Stoll recommends Metanx and Folgard brands because they are helpful to the heart and are also very effective as an augmentation strategy in bipolar and depression treatment (p. 26).

Patients on SAMe or EPA need to be monitored for signs of hypomania, and patients on a combination of CAs plus 5-HTP need to be monitored for the emergence of serotonin syndrome (Lake, 2005, p. 95). Somatic, mind–body, and energy information treatments of depressed mood include exercise, total or partial sleep deprivation, yoga, tai chi, and qigong, as well as treatments without empirical validation based on energy or information such as bright light exposure and electroencephalogram feedback (p. 95). For instance, regular exercise at least 30 minutes three times a week may be as effective as CAs, SJW, or cognitive therapy for moderate depressive mood (p. 95). People who exercise are less depressed than people who do not exercise, and score 7.3 point less on the Beck Depression Inventory. Most studies conclude that resistance training and aerobic exercises are effective in reducing symptoms of mild to moderate depression, and in one study there was a dose–response relationship between exercise and reduction of depressive symptoms (Leard-Hansson & Guttmacher, 2006, p. 29). Patients who exercise in a bright-lit (2500 lux–4000 lux) indoor environment experience more significant improvement in mood and greater sense of vitality than individuals with depression who exercise indoors in ordinary room light (400 lux–600 lux) (p. 93). Also, regular exposure to dim red or blue light is probably as effective as CAs, and exposure to dim green light two hours before exposure to natural light may accelerate the response to CAs. Partial sleep deprivation improves moderate depressed mood. One night of total sleep deprivation followed by sleep phase advance improves severe depressed mood, and partial sleep deprivation combined with maintenance lithium therapy and morning bright light exposure may be more effective than either approach in bipolar depression (p. 94).

Mindfulness training is probably as effective as cognitive therapy in moderate depressed mood. If has been suggested that the mechanism of action of yogic breathing might be similar to vagal nerve stimulation (VNS) in that both approaches involve modulation of the balance of sympathetic and parasympathetic autonomous tone. Regular yoga practice, including specialized breathing techniques and postures may be as effective as CAs (p. 93). Biofeedback, acupuncture, and electro-acupuncture may also have an ameliorating effect in some forms of depression (p. 94).

CHAPTER 12

Overview of Atypical Antipsychotics

The clinical objective of this chapter entails a review of the evidence-based literature for each atypical antipsychotic in the areas of very early schizophrenia, early schizophrenia (VEOS-EOS), and schizoaffective disorders, other psychotic disorders (OPD), mania/bipolar disorders, autism/pervasive developmental disorder (PDD), disruptive behaviors (DD), Tourette's disorder (TD), and other conditions (aggressive behaviors, and others), specifically for children and adolescents. Each medication will have a summary table indicating the highest available scientific evidence for the category of these disorders in children and adolescents. Each medication review begins with a summary of its clinical experience followed by the evidence-based summaries of each medication; each review ends with a table of suggested doses for preschoolers, preadolescents, and adolescents. The suggested doses are tentative and preliminary.

Biederman, Spencer, and Wilens (2004) state that pharmacotherapy should be part of a comprehensive treatment plan and that it should not be used to the exclusion of other interventions or after other interventions fail. The ingredients of a successful psychopharmacological intervention are realistic expectations and a clear definition of target symptoms. They add that, pharmacotherapy should be started early, before the onset of complications, chronicity, or social incapacitation. Furthermore, they advise that before initiation of psychotropic treatment, the child and the family need to be made familiar with the risk and benefits of the medications, the available alternative treatments, and the likely side effects, including short-term, long-term, and withdrawal side effects (p. 931). Risks associated with no treatment should also be discussed.

It needs to be reiterated that there is no FDA approval for the use of these medications in children and adolescents, and that the current use of these drugs in these populations is off label. No atypical medications, currently in use in the United States, have been demonstrated to be either effective or safe in children or adolescents. Most of the sparse literature on the use of atypicals in children and adolescents relates to uncontrolled short-term efficacy and tolerability reports. There are limited long-term studies related to the safety or effectiveness of these medications. The limited available literature is skewed to favorable therapeutic effects and benign side effects results; negative research outcomes or data reflecting frequent or severe side effects are rarely reported. It is imperative for physicians to represent this to parents when discussing medication options. Parents need to know that by consenting to atypical medications for their children, to a certain extent they will be participating in a clinical experiment.

In regard to atypical antipsychotics, an English language MEDLINE search from 1974 to 2003 identified 176 reports, including 15 double-blind, controlled trials, 58 open-label trials, 18 retrospective chart reviews, and 85 case reports or series. Of this literature, 43% corresponded to risperidone, 21% to olanzapine, 14% to clozapine, 11% to quetiapine, 6% to ziprasidone, 2% to aripiprazole, 3% were miscellaneous (Cheng-Shannon, McGough, Pataki, & McCracken, 2004, p. 373). Particulars of the highest evidence base of this body of publications will be mentioned in the corresponding sections.

In attending to issues related to medication side effects, clinicians will keep in mind that the U.S. Food and Drug Administration (FDA) is a conservative agency under significant pressure from political entities and pharmaceutical manufacturers. The FDA is slow to respond to emerging concerns regarding medication safety. For instance, the FDA only took action on Abucal and Redux after the dangerous nature of these medications far surpassed the threshold of medical concern. More pertinent, issues with atypicals' induction of obesity or metabolic dysregulation elicited only a belated response.

Clinicians need to attend to emerging publications on side effects, reflect on standards of practice, and attend to evidence-base guidelines in the use of atypical antipsychotics. They also should rely on their own observations and experience when evaluating the safety of a given atypical drug prior to prescribing it for children and adolescents. It is important to remember that children and adolescents display side effects patterns that are different from those described for adults (see chapter 13).

In a recent antipsychotic survey in adults, Atypical Antipsychotic Therapy and Metabolic Issues (AtAMI), a number of psychiatric practices raised concerns: psychiatrists rarely monitor hypertension or ask laboratories to detect hyperglycemia or hyperlipedemia. Efforts to address metabolic disturbance were inadequate because 29% of the respondents indicated they would not alter therapy or refer a patient who gained weight. Of more serious concern, more than 40% of psychiatrists expressed a willingness to risk diabetes (43%) or weight gain (48%) in their patients with schizophrenia by deciding to continue treatment with high risk antipsychotics such as olanzapine (Nasrallah & Newcomer, 2004, S12–S13). This survey raises concerns about the bland if not lackadaisical attitude of a number of practicing psychiatrists in regard to side effects from emerging atypical medications.

Psychiatrists and other physicians need to remember their own liability risk when they prescribe off label medications for children and adolescents. It is likely that the ongoing safety concerns regarding stimulants and antidepressant medications will have a ripple effect on most of the other psychotropics prescribed for children, and mood stabilizers and atypical antipsychotics, in particular.

Following Ghaemi's (2002) *Evidence-Based Medicine: Levels of Evidence*, the purported research support for each atypical antipsychotic indication will be labeled as follows:

Level 1: Double-blind, randomized studies
Level 2: Open, randomized, prospective, outcome studies
Level 3: Large naturalistic studies (n > 100), case control studies
Level 4: Small naturalistic (n = 10–100) studies
Level 5: Retrospective chart reviews
Level 6: Case reports clinical observations on one or a few cases
Level 7: Uncontrolled case studies
Level 8: Anecdotal reports (modified from Ghaemi, 2002, p. 20)

Level 1 represents the best research evidence, and Level 8, the least valuable one. Only level 1 evidence will be discussed or annotated in the present text. Table 12.1 summarizes the highest evidence base for the SGAs currently in use in the United States.

For an overview of receptor affinity of the atypical antipsychotics currently in use in the United States see table 12.2.

TABLE 12.1 Highest Level of Evidence-Based Support for Atypical Antipsychotics Currently in Use in United States for the Treatment of Children and Adolescents

	VEOS/EOS	OPD	BP	PDD	DD	TD	Other
Clozapine	1	—	4	6	—	—	
Risperidone	1	3	4	1	1	1	1
Olanzapine	3		4	4	—	6	
Quetiapine	3	3	2	5	—	6	
Ziprasidone	—	—	—	—	—	1	
Aripiprazole	—	—	—	—	—	—	

VEOS/EOS: Very early onset schizophrenia, early onset schizophrenia, schizoaffective disorder; OPD: other psychotic disorders; BP: bipolar disorders, including mania; PDD: pervasive developmental disorder, including autism; DD: disruptive disorders; TD: Tourette's disorder.

TABLE 12.2 Receptor Affinity of Atypical Antipsychotics

Receptor binding profile	Clozapine	Risperidone	Olanzapine	Quetiapine	Ziprasidone	Aripiprazol
D1	++	-/+	+++	+	-/+	-
D2	++	+++	++	++	+++	++/+++
D3		++/+++	+/++		+++	++/+++
D4		++	+		+	+/++
5-HT2A		++++	++/+++		++++	++/+++
5-HT1A		+	-		+++	+/++
5-HT2C		+/++	++		+++	
5-HT1D		+	-/+		+++	
5-HT2	++++	++++	++++	+++	+++	+/++
α1	+++	++++	++	++++	++	
α2	+++	++++	-	+	-	
H1	++++	+	++++	++++	+	+/++
μ1	++++	-	++++	+++	-	-
5-HT reuptake		1,400	>15,000		53	
NE reuptake		28,000	2,000		48	

Source: Modified from Kapur & Remington (2001, p. 507); Daniel et al. (1999, p. 492).
D=Dopamine; 5-HT=Serotonin; α=Adrenergic; H=Histamine; μM=Acetylcholine (muscarinic).

CLOZAPINE

Clozapine is unique in its clinical effectiveness and side effect profile; clinical applications and side effects, and its use in treatment will be covered in this review. For the other atypicals, a broad discussion of side effects is covered in chapter 13.

Clinical Implications of the Use of Clozapine

Clozapine is considered the most effective atypical antipsychotic available. It has a broad-spectrum therapeutic action and is considered superior to the other SGAs in therapeutic effectiveness. The side effect risks are potentially very serious and for that reason clozapine is not a first line medication. It is reserved for refractory cases. Clozapine is an option for severe psychotic and mood disorders, which have not responded to other second generation medications.

Clozapine should also be considered in cases of protracted suicidality and in patients with persistent aggressiveness and impulsivity, when these dimensions of psychopathology have not responded to alternative treatments. So far, clozapine is only FDA approved for resistant schizophrenia in adults. See endnote for information regarding clozapine receptor affinity and cytochrome activity.[1]

In December 2005, Novartis announced some changes related to parameters of clozapine monitoring. During the first six months, WBC and ANC will be monitored weekly; after six months, tolerance permitting, blood monitoring will be biweekly. After one year, other things being equal, blood monitoring may be done monthly. For patients who are rechallenged on clozapine, weekly blood monitoring for the first 12 months is recommended (Bess & Cunningham, 2005, p. 1).

Clinical Applications

Clozapine has demonstrated superior effectiveness on positive and negative symptoms and is still the golden standard against which all the other atypical antipsychotics medications are measured. Clozapine has been demonstrated to be:

1. Effective in at least some patients for whom the typical neuroleptics have failed;
2. Preferentially effective with so-called negative symptoms (apathy, amotivation, etc.);
3. Beneficial for symptoms related to mood and cognition (Kapur & Remington, 2001, p. 504).

Clozapine appears to have a decisive advantage in decreasing aggression in comparison to the other atypicals (Citrome, Bilder, & Volavka, 2002, p. 210). Clozapine may be of particular benefit to patients with treatment refractory schizophrenic spectrum illness who demonstrate hostile and aggressive behaviors (Marder & Wirshing, 2004, p. 446). Clozapine shows superiority over olanzapine and risperidone in the reduction of levels of hostility; this effect is independent of its antipsychotic activity and is also independent of clozapine's sedative effect (Citrome, Bilder, & Volavka, 2002, p. 210).

Clozapine also may be the preferred agent for patients with schizophrenia who are at a higher risk of suicide. Large epidemiological studies have found that mortality from suicide is reduced in patients taking clozapine (Marder & Wirshing, 2004, p. 446). The most convincing study demonstrating antisuicidal benefits in adults was based on a comparison of clozapine and olanzapine in 980 patients with schizophrenia, considered at risk for suicide. In that study, clozapine was more effective in reducing suicidal risk than olanzapine (Meltzer, 2002).[2] Unfortunately, the lives saved by clozapine's antisuicidal activity may essentially be offset by the deaths associated with weight gain and its complications (Marder & Wirshing, 2004, pp. 451–452). Patients should not be considered treatment refractory or partial responders until they have had an adequate trial of clozapine (p. 453). Clozapine may also have advantages for patients with polydipsia–hyponatremia syndrome (p. 446). Clozapine also reduces impulsivity (Meltzer, 2002, p. 281).

The acid test of therapeutic superiority of atypical antipsychotics over conventional antipsychotics is their impact on chronic resistant schizophrenia. The effectiveness of second generation antipsychotics (risperidone, olanzapine, and newer atypicals), other than clozapine, in the reduction of symptoms in treatment resistant schizophrenia has not been established (Chakos, Lieberman, Hoffman, Bradford, & Sheitman, 2001, p. 523). Patients who are more severely symptomatic at baseline are the most likely to benefit from clozapine treatment (p. 524). The CATIE II report substantiated the therapeutic superiority of clozapine over other second generation antipsychotics, mainly, olanzapine, risperidone and quetiapine (McEvoy, Lieberman, Stroup, et al., 2006).

Clozapine might be more effective than other antipsychotics because of its additional effects, which include mood stabilization, and catatonia prophylactic effects, similar to lithium. Its mood-stabilizing effects differ from the decrease in mania severity produced by antipsychotics. Clozapine also shows narcotic analgesia effects that are blocked by naloxone (Swartz, 2003, p. 13). Accumulating evidence suggests that clozapine is particularly effective for manic symptoms that are nor responsive to other agents (Marder & Wirshing, 2004, p. 447). Clozapine has a very low risk of TD; actually, this medication has antidyskinetic activity. In clinical practice, the more the dyskinetic symptomatology, the better the antipsychotic results.

Reports suggest that Clozapine decreases the frequency of smoking among schizophrenic patients (Procyshyn, Ihsan, & Thompson, 2001, pp. 292–293) and that it may also be effective for adult patients with borderline personality disorder (Parker, 2002, pp. 348–349; Swinton, 2001, pp. 580–591).

Blood levels are correlated with therapeutic effectiveness; levels around 450 mcg/ml are considered therapeutic. Plasma level studies show that patients with higher clozapine plasma levels had an excellent response, whereas those with lower levels had a poor response (Davis, Chen, & Glick, 2003, p. 556). A typical daily dose of 300 to 400 mg/day (about 5 mg/kg) is associated with plasma levels ranging from 200 to 400 mg/ml (Marder & Wirshing, 2004, p. 445).

A Summary of Evidence-Based Support for the Use of Clozapine
in Children and Adolescents

Disorders	VEOS/EOS	OPD	BP	PDD	DD	TD
Evidence	1	—	4	6	—	—

VEOS/EOS: Very early onset schizophrenia, early onset schizophrenia, schizoaffective disorders; OPD: other psychotic disorders; BP: bipolar disorders, including mania; PDD: pervasive developmental disorder, including autism; DD: disruptive disorders; TD: Tourette's disorder. For rating details on this table, see above.

Side Effects

Black Boxes—Serious Warnings, *Physicians Desk Reference* (PDR, 2006, pp. 2176–2178): Clozapine has a Black Box for the following serious potential adverse events for children and adolescents: (1) agranulocytosis, (2) seizures, (3) myocarditis, (4) other adverse cardiovascular and respiratory effects.

1. Agranulocytosis occurs in 1 to 2% of patients in the first six months of treatment, but its incidence decreases thereafter. Clozapine-induced agranulocytosis is reversible if clozapine is discontinued before patients develop infections; because of this, clozapine can be used safely (Marder & Wirshing, 2004, p. 443). With mandatory weekly white blood cell monitoring in the first six months of treatment and biweekly monitoring thereafter, the risk of death due to this side effect is 1 in 10,000 (Jibson & Tandon, 2003, p. 62).
2. Myocarditis is a fatal risk; this complication is most frequent during the first months of treatment; 85% of the myocarditis occurred at normal doses within the first two months of therapy. Myocarditis is often associated with eosinophilia (Marder & Wirshing, 2004, p. 449).
3. Other cardiovascular and respiratory adverse effects: Tachycardia appears to be related to clozapine anticholinergic activity. Hypotension is caused by alpha-adrenergic blockade (Marder & Wirshing, 2004, p. 449).
4. Obesity, diabetes, and dyslipidemia risk. According to the Consensus Developing Conference (2004), clozapine and olanzapine carry the highest risk in this regard (p. 597).

Clozapine should not be stopped abruptly; there is a risk of psychosis reactivation or of cholinergic rebound.

Adverse Events

Common Side Effects
The most common side effects are sedation, sialorrhea, orthostatic hypotension (OH), tachycardia, and weight increase.

Serious Side Effects
Granulocytopenia, agranulocytosis (neutropenia). During premarketing testing the cumulative incidence of hematological side effects, including agranulocytosis, at one year was reported as 1.3%. Revised reports put the incidence at one year at about 0.8%. Agranulocytosis increases with age and may be higher in women. Presence of HLA-B38 may predispose to clozapine related agranulocytosis. Granulocytopenia and agranulocytosis are a major burden for compliance with clozapine because of the need for weekly monitoring of white blood cells (WBC). It appears that the risk of agranulocytosis drops significantly after the first six months of treatment. Even with the new U.S. parameters of WBC monitoring, two countries have less stringent requirements for the prescription of clozapine: in the United Kingdom, the WBC is monitored weekly for the first

18 weeks, followed by biweekly monitoring till the 52nd week, and monthly thereafter. In Australia, there is a weekly monitoring for the first 18 weeks followed by monthly monitoring thereafter (Mechcathie, 2003, p. 8).

Seizures. Up to 1.3 to 3.5% of patients on clozapine develop seizures. Clozapine lowers the seizure threshold in a dose dependent fashion.

Cardiomyopathy. It is a rather common adverse event, and is not limited to the first month of therapy. Twenty-eight cases of myocarditis (including 18 deaths) and 41 cases of cardiomyopathy (including 10 deaths) have been reported. It is likely that many more cases go on unreported.

Respiratory arrest. Clozapine may aggravate the respiratory status of patients with respiratory insufficiency.

Excessive weight gain. Clozapine tends to promote the most weight gain among all the atypical antipsychotics. The ranking from the greatest weight inducer to the least is: clozapine > olanzapine > risperidone > quetiapine > aripiprazole ≥ ziprasidone.

Elevation of liver enzymes. Transient asymptomatic elevation of liver function tests has been reported in as many as 50% of patients treated with clozapine. Fatal, acute fulminating hepatitis is rare, with an incidence of 0.001% (Marder & Wirshing, 2004, p. 453).

CPK elevation. Greater than 20,000 CPK units in the absence of other NMS features have been reported (Rosebush & Mazurek, 2001, p. 3).

Fatal constipation. Constipation occurs in 14 to 60% of patients taking clozapine; serious constipation could become lethal.

Glucose and lipid metabolism disturbances. Caution should be exercised in the use of clozapine when the patient is overweight, when there is history of diabetes mellitus, or if the patient has history of serum lipid elevation (hypercholesterolemia, hypertriglyceridemia) (Domon & Webber, 2001). Clozapine is strongly associated with hyperglycemia, diabetes mellitus, and diabetic ketoacidosis. The latter, although infrequent, may cause death. Patients with these disorders, or who are at risk for development of these disorders, should only be treated with clozapine or olanzapine as medications of last resort. If the use of clozapine is mandatory, the clinical monitoring of these conditions should be particularly close. Domon and Webber estimate a 10-fold increase of hyperglycemia risk in adolescents treated with clozapine. Since underreporting is the norm, the true incidence and risk with this drug could be higher.

Dyslipidemias. Whereas patients taking clozapine or olanzapine increased the level of triglycerides more than 30%, the increase was only 19% in those taking risperidone. Levels of triglycerides decreased in patients taking haloperidol or fluphenazine (Marder & Wirshing, 2004, p. 451).

Physicians need to periodically monitor glycemia and lipidemia; weight and BMI also need to be monitored on a regular basis. The blood glucose and lipid panel should be monitored at least every six months and measurements of weight and blood pressure at every visit in patients on maintenance treatment with clozapine (Gelenberg, 2002, p. 5–6).

Orthostatic hypotension. This side effect is dose dependent, and tachycardia may be associated with syncope or, rarely, with cardiovascular collapse. These adverse events are more common at the beginning of therapy or when the medication is prescribed at high doses.

Pancreatitis. There have been reports of pancreatitis associated with clozapine treatment (Gelenberg, 2002, p. 5).

Fever. Clozapine induced fever probably occurs in 20 to 25% of patients, usually within the first month of treatment. Acetaminophen is a reasonable antidote. Of course, fever can signal infection, the possibility of which should be explored. Worse still, it could indicate agranulocytosis or a neuroleptic malignant syndrome that requires an urgent differential diagnosis and urgent medical management. If these more serious concerns are ruled out, fever per se is not a reason to discontinue clozapine (Gelenberg, 2002, Vol. 25, p. 15).

Eosinophilia requires temporary or permanent interruption of clozapine.

Venous tromboembolic complications. Clozapine has also been associated with this condition (Gelenberg, 2003b, Vol. 26. p. 27).

Managing of Clozapine Side Effects

Neutropenia. Monitor WBC and the absolute neutrophil count (ANC) according to new monitoring parameters, see above. Patients are to be warned about unexplained fever, flulike symptoms, or sore throats; consider using granulocyte colony stimulating factor (GCSF).

Sedation. Titrate up slowly and give as much medication as possible in early evening or nighttime; use the lowest effective dose, get a blood level.

Enuresis. For nocturnal enuresis, treat with DDAVP or terazacin (Hytrin); for urinary urgency, treat with oxybutynin, for refractory cases consider imipramine.

Seizures. To decrease seizure risk, obtain a preclozapine EEG, titrate up slowly, using the lowest effective dose; get regular blood levels, and repeat EEG if clozapine dose is 600 mg/day or greater, or if the blood level is above 600 mcg/ml; treat with divalproex sodium, and continue clozapine at lower or same dose if effective (beware of any potential synergistic effects on bone marrow).

Constipation. Consider exercise, high fiber diet, or increase fluid intake; consider stool softeners.

Sialorrhea. Attempt to lower the dosage; treat with pirenzepine, clonidine, or guanfacine; as a last resort, treat with benztropine. Intranasal ipratropium bromide may also be tried (Marder & Wirshing, 2004, p. 453).

Tachycardia. Titrate up slowly or reduce dose; considered beta-blockers.
Orthostatic hypotension. Titrate up slowly or reduce dose; use divided doses, and if possible, increase salt intake (modified from *Child and Adolescent Psychopharmacology Update*, 2003, p. 4).

Clozapine Suggested Initiating Dosing

< 6 years of age	6–9 years of age	10–13 years of age	14 years of age and older
NR	NR	12.5–25 mg/day	25 mg/day

NR: not recommended.

Clozapine Suggested Therapeutic Maintenance Dosing

< 6 years of age	6–9 years of age	10–13 years of age	14 years of age and older
NR	NR	200–400 mg/day	200–600 mg/day

NR: not recommended.

RISPERIDONE

Clinical Summary of Risperidone Use with Children and Adolescents

Except for clozapine, risperidone is the oldest second-generation antipsychotic available in the United States. Risperidone, in comparison to its competitors, is the most studied antipsychotic in children and adolescent psychiatric populations. It has the most published data to support its use in a number of conditions of childhood and adolescence, including controlled studies in the treatment of schizophrenia spectrum disorders, Tourette's disorder, conduct and disruptive disorders in children with subaverage IQ, autistic disorder, mentally retarded children, and others. Double-blind studies have demonstrated risperidone effectiveness in most of the areas of severe psychopathology in children and adolescents with a satisfactory tolerability. In comparison, clozapine has one controlled study on childhood onset schizophrenia, quetiapine has two controlled studies, one as an adjunctive medication for adolescent mania, and the other for the treatment of mania and mixed disorders. There are very few published studies on the use of the new atypical aripiprazol with children or adolescents..

Risperidone is one of the most commonly used antipsychotics in clinical practice. Studies of children and adolescents have demonstrated that risperidone is safe, convenient to use, fairly well tolerated, and that it has a rather benign side effect profile. Risperidone has many presentation forms (concentrated, rapid absorption, intramuscular, and depot form) making this antipsychotic a versatile medication for emergencies, acute conditions, stabilization, maintenance, relapse prevention, and for patients with compliance difficulties. Furthermore, due to the availability of risperidone in very small oral dosing, it can be used in safe amounts in very small children.

Weight gain, EPS, hyperprolactinemia, proarrythmic risks, limited antidepressant effects, and anticholinergic side effects represent a limitation. Risperidone has a moderate risk for obesity, diabetes, and dyslipidemias. The concerns regarding the health implications of hyperprolatinemia are under active scientific discussion.

It had been expected that risperidone would be granted an indication for use in children and adolescents. If this had happened, risperidone would have been the first second-generation antipsychotic with FDA approved indications for children. In mid-2005, however, the FDA denied the application for risperidone indication for children and adolescents with developmental disorders.

Risperidone should be considered a first line antipsychotic medication for use in children and adolescents based in the above considerations. This proposition buttressed by the Expert Consensus Guidelines Series (Optimizing Pharmacologic Treatment of Psychotic Disorders, 2003) in adults. Risperidone was considered the first line antipsychotic for first psychotic breaks, for relapse, for patients who need to be switched from other antipsychotics, and was also considered the first choice if clozapine failed (Kane, Leucht, Carpenter, & Docherty, 2003), and as has been stated, risperidone is the most broadly researched atypical antipsychotic among children and adolescents.

Clinical Activity

Risperidone demonstrated a significant superiority on relapse prevention over haloperidol. It appears that in the treatment of a general population with chronic schizophrenia clozapine and risperidone may be equally effective. Risperidone in combination with mood stabilizers was associated with more rapid and significant improvement of manic symptoms. Risperidone plus a mood stabilizer was equally effective in patients with or without psychosis, suggesting that risperidone like olanzapine has antimanic properties independent of its antipsychotic effects (Yatham, Grossman, Augustyns, Vieta, & Ravindran, 2003, p. 146). At the end of 2003, risperidone received FDA approval for the treatment of mania in adults.

Several studies have indicated that risperidone may significantly enhance cognitive functioning, particularly verbal working memory, when compared with haloperidol (Goff, 2004, p. 500). In a meta-analysis by Davis, Chen, and Glick (2003), olanzapine vs. clozapine and risperidone vs. clozapine showed no significant differences. Six olanzapine vs. risperidone studies yielded no significant differences in the effectiveness of these medications (p. 556).

In the CATIE report, risperidone was less effective than olanzapine and was as effective as perphenazine, quetiapine, or ziprasidone (Lieberman, Stroup, et al., 2005, p. 1218). It needs to be stated, however, that olanzapine was used at higher than recommended doses, and that risperidone dosing was at a modal average dosing. A long-acting, injectable risperidone is now available. Data shows that depot formulations lower relapse rates by 15% compared with oral antipsychotics, largely because of poor compliance with the oral regimes.

An epidemiological study raised concerns that women who used antipsychotic and antiemetics dopamine antagonists, that elevate prolactin levels, have a modest but significant increase in the development of breast cancer; this risk increases in a monotonic, dose dependent fashion with exposure to larger cumulative dosages (Wang et al., 2002, p. 1152). Long lag periods are generally thought to be required between tumor initiation and the diagnosis of breast cancer (p. 1153). When the study was controlled for parity and age of first delivery, the concerns regarding hyperprolactinemia and cancer did not hold (see chapter 13).

Representative Studies

Risperidone in the Treatment of VEOS/EOS and Schizoaffective Disorders
Level 1 evidence. Sikich, Hamer, Malekpour, Sheitman, and Lieberman (2001) conducted a randomized, double-blind study comparing risperidone (N = 19; dose range 1–6 mg/day), olanzapine (N = 16; dose range 5–20 mg/day), and haloperidol (N = 15; dose range 2–8 mg/day) in 50 children and adolescents between the ages of 8 and 19 years (mean age 14.8 years) with moderate psychotic symptoms occurring in patients with schizophrenia spectrum disorders.

Comment: This was a small randomized study. There were no significant differences between risperidone and olanzapine in therapeutic effectiveness, and both medications had a better therapeutic effect than haloperidol.

Level 1 evidence. Csernansky, Mahmoud, and Brenner (2002) reported on a double-blind, randomized study in which 177 patients received risperidone, and 188 received haloperidol. The Kaplan-Meier estimate for relapse risk was 34% in the risperidone group and 60% in the haloperidol one ($p < 0.001$). This represented a 48% risk reduction for patients assigned to risperidone in comparison to patients assigned to haloperidol. Patients on risperidone showed improvements from baseline in total scores, and in positive and negative symptoms, disorganized thoughts, and in anxiety and depression (pp. 18–19).

Risperidone in the Treatment of Conduct Disorder
Level 1 evidence. Aman et al. (2002) conducted a randomized, double-blind, placebo-controlled study comparing risperidone and a placebo in the outpatient treatment of severe conduct problems in 118 children, 5 to 12 years of age, with subaverage intelligence. Patients were diagnosed with conduct disorder, oppositional defiant disorder, or disruptive behavior disorder NOS, with or without ADHD. The authors concluded that risperidone 0.02 to 0.06 mg/kg/

day is effective and well tolerated in the treatment of children with subaverage intelligence and severe behavioral problems.

Comment: This is a valuable short-term study demonstrating a significant effect of risperidone on behavior disturbances in children with subaverage intelligence; adverse events are in accordance with previously described risperidone side effects. Long-term studies are necessary to corroborate long-term effectiveness and medication safety.

Another large level 1 evidence study, with a similar design, was conducted by R. Snyder et al. (2002) on 110 children between 5 and 12, with a range of IQ between 36 and 84, or a Vineland score of 84 or less. The authors concluded that risperidone appears to be an adequately tolerated and effective treatment for children with subaverage IQs and severe disruptive disorders such as aggressive and destructive behaviors.

Comment: Statements regarding the previous study are pertinent for this study as well.

Risperidone in the Treatment of Autism/PPD

Level 1 evidence. McCraken, McGough, Bhavik, et al. and the Research Units on Pediatric Psychopharmacology Autism Network (2002) conducted a double-blind, placebo-controlled, eight-week clinical trial of risperidone in children with autistic disorders and behavioral problems.

Adding to extensive literature of the effectiveness and safety of risperidone in the treatment of autism and neurodevelopmental disorders, the article by the Research Units of Pediatric Psychopharmacology Autism Networks (2005) expands on issues of efficacy and safety of risperidone in long-term treatment of autistic features (aggression, temper outbursts, and self-injurious behavior).

Comment: This randomized study demonstrates a decrease of maladaptive behavior in autistic/PDD children. Since this group of children has lifelong psychopathology, long-term studies of effectiveness and safety are necessary to justify risk–benefit decisions.

Risperidone for the Treatment of Autism

Level 1 evidence. McDougle et al. (2005) from the Autism Network of the Research Units of Pediatric Psychopharmacology, conducted an eight-week, double-blind, placebo-control trial (N = 101) and a 16-week, open-label continuation study (N = 63) for children and adolescents with autism. Risperidone was effective in decreasing repetitive and stereotyped patterns of behavior, interests, and activities.

Risperidone in the Treatment of Tourette's Disorder

Level 1 evidence. Gaffney et al. (2002) compared the efficacy and tolerability of risperidone and clonidine in a randomized, double-blind study involving 21 patients (7–17 years) with Tourette's disorder. The authors concluded that the study established that risperidone efficacy was equal to clonidine in the treatment of tic symptoms in children and adolescents. The child psychiatric field will benefit from publications like this in which the agent under investigation does not show advantages or superiority over the comparator, and by publications of studies with negative outcomes.

Risperidone Treatment of Other Psychiatric Conditions

Treatment of Aggression
Level 1 evidence. Buitelaar, van der Gaag, Cohen-Tettenis, and Melman (2001) conducted a six-week, double-blind, randomized trial study of the safety and efficacy of risperidone in the treatment of aggression in 38 hospitalized adolescents (33 boys) with a primary diagnosis of DSM-IV disruptive behavior disorders and subaverage intelligence.

Mental Retardation
Level 1 evidence. Zarcone et al. (2001) conducted a placebo controlled, double-blind study of the efficacy of risperidone on aberrant behavior (e.g., aggression and self-injurious behavior) in 20 patients with developmental disabilities, including five children (6–12 years), six adolescents (13–18 years), and nine adults. The authors conclude that risperidone was effective in reducing aberrant behavior for most patients.

Level 1 evidence. Van Bellinghen and De Troch (2001) conducted a four-week double-blind, placebo-controlled study to evaluate the efficacy of risperidone in the treatment of behavioral disturbances in 13 children and adolescents (6–14 years) with borderline IQ.

Summary of the Evidence-Based Support for the Use of Risperidone in Children and Adolescents

VEOS/EOS	OPD	BP	PDD	DD	TD	Other
1	3	4	1	1	1	1

VEOS/EOS: Very early onset schizophrenia, early onset schizophrenia and schizoaffective disorder; OPD: other psychotic disorders; BP: bipolar disorders, including mania; PDD, pervasive developmental disorder, including autism; DD: disruptive disorders; TD: Tourette's disorder. For rating details on above table, see above.

Risperidone Suggested Initiating Dosing

< 6 years of age	6–9 years of age	10–13 years of age	14 years of age and older
0.125 mg/day	0.25–0.5 mg/day	0.5–1 mg/day	1 mg/day

Risperidone Suggested Therapeutic Dosing

< 6 years of age	6–9 years of age	10–13 years of age	14 years of age and older
0.25–0.75 mg/day	0.5–2 mg/day	1–3 mg/day	2–4 mg/day

OLANZAPINE   *Zyprexa*

Summary of Clinical Use of Olanzapine in Children and Adolescents

Olanzapine does not have significant double-blind controlled studies in child and adolescent populations. In adults, olanzapine has demonstrated a broad spectrum of therapeutic action including antipsychotic effects and strong antimanic and mood regulating properties. Olanzapine is deceptively easy to use (once/day dosing), and it is fairly well tolerated. It is very sedative and has significant anticholinergic side effects. In small children, olanzapine produces severe aberrations of the appetite.

Except for clozapine, olanzapine poses the greatest health risks among SGAs. Olanzapine has a relative contraindication for patients suffering from obesity, diabetes mellitus, or dyslipidemias, and for those with family history of diabetes mellitus or dyslipidemias. Because olanzapine causes such a severe weight increase in children and adolescents and may induce a metabolic syndrome, this medication should not be considered a first line antipsychotic in youth. This medication should be reserved for children or adolescents who do not respond to more benign weight inducing, and less metabolic disturbing antipsychotics. The CATIE study (see below) clearly highlighted the serious weight promoting and metabolic risks of this antipsychotic (Lieberman, Stroup, et al., 2005, p. 1215). Now concerns are being raised about olanzapine intramuscular formulation safety and about Lilly's variable standards as to how to alert the medical community to olanzapine emerging risks.

A study of eight children and adolescents between 10 and 18 years of age found similar pharmacokinetic parameters as those reported in nonsmoking adults. The metabolism of olanzapine is increased by cigarette smoking, and results in a 30% reduction in serum levels (Jibson & Tandon, 2003, p. 61). Olanzapine is readily oxidized in air when the protective coating is removed, which occurs when the tablet is cut or crushed. In these circumstances the portion of the medication, not consumed immediately, must be discarded (Jibson & Tandon, 1998, p. 219). The manufacturer does not recommend splitting tablets (for drug interactions see appendix A).

Clinical Activity

Studies demonstrate olanzapine has strong effects on positive and negative symptoms, and a positive impact on cognitive functioning. Olanzapine can increase frontal lobe dopamine. Phase I of the Clinical Antipsychotic Trials of Intervention Effectiveness (CATIE I) showed that olanzapine was the most effective antipsychotic among the medications tried (perphenazine, olanzapine,

Zyprexa

risperidone, quetiapine, and ziprasidone). Olanzapine had the lowest rate of discontinuation, produced a greater reduction in psychopathology, had a longer staying power, and a lower rate of hospitalizations due to exacerbations of schizophrenia (Lieberman, Stroup et al., 2005, p. 1218). These results need to take into account that olanzapine was used at higher than recommended doses in relation to its competitors: 20.1, 20.8, 543.4, 3.9, 112.8, mean modal dosing in mg/day, for olanzapine, perphenazine, quetiapine, risperidone, and ziprasidone, respectively (Nasrallah, 2006, p. 55). The CATIE II report (McEvoy, Lieberman, Stroup, et al., 2006) corroborated the CATIE I findings regarding olanzapine better effectiveness than risperidone, quetiapine or ziprasidone.

Olanzapine is currently approved as an antimanic monotherapy medication. It has demonstrated antimanic properties comparable to lithium (Schulz, Olson, & Kotlyar, 2004, p. 464), and was superior to divalproex in therapeutic effectiveness and remission rates irrespective of the presence of psychosis; however, it displayed more toxicity than divalproex. The olanzapine group also showed improvement in motor activity, sleep, and language–thought disorder items of the YMRS (Tohen, Baker, et al., 2002, p. 1016). The results of the comparison of antimanic effects of olanzapine and divalproex were counterintuitive: divalproex did better than olanzapine in mania with psychotic features, and olanzapine did better than divalproex in mania without psychotic features (Tohen, Baker, et al., 2002, p. 1016). This pattern of action is similar to lithium. See lithium, chapter 11. Another comparison of olanzapine and divalproex confirmed no difference in treatment outcome but did note more sedation and weight gain in the olanzapine group (Schulz, Olson, & Kotlyar, 2004, p. 464). Olanzapine also appears to have antidepressant, antisuicidal (less so than clozapine), and prophylactic effects. In a path analysis to control for negative symptoms and EPS, a statistically significant greater effect of olanzapine on depression compared with placebo was observed, and at medium (10 ± –2.5 mg/day) and at high doses, reductions in BPRS Anxiety/Depression scale scores were similar to those seen with haloperidol (p. 464).

The augmentation study by Sheldon et al. (2001), already a classic in the treatment of depression, demonstrated that the combination of olanzapine with fluoxetine was far superior than the outcome for either olanzapine or fluoxetine alone. This study broke new ground on the treatment of refractory depressive disorders. Olanzapine may have a role in the treatment of anorexia nervosa (Schulz, Olson, & Kotlyar, 2004, pp. 465–466).

By mid-2004, olanzapine was the only atypical FDA approved for the treatment of acute mania and bipolar maintenance in adults, and in combination with fluoxetine (Symbiax), for the treatment of bipolar depression in adults.

An injectable, rapid acting preparation of olanzapine has been developed and is superior to placebo in doses of 10 mg; this vehicle is as effective as haloperidol with significant lower untoward side effects (Schulz, Olson, &

Kotlyar, 2004, p. 464). Parenteral olanzapine is contraindicated in patients whose agitation or disinhibition is caused by benzodiazepines. Combination of olanzapine with divalproex should only be used with added caution. However, adult patients treated with a combination of Depakote and olanzapine experienced significantly smaller increases in cholesterol than patients treated with olanzapine monotherapy, and patients treated with a combination of valproate and risperidone experienced a decrease in cholesterol levels (Casey et al., 2003, p. 190). It must be recognized that olanzapine is more hepatotoxic than divalproex.

Olanzapine has positive antidyskinetic functions. Prior to conducting their prospective study of the putative therapeutic effects of olanzapine on TD, Kinon, Basson, Stauffer, and Tollefson (1999) undertook a retrospective analysis of three large clinical trials that included 129 patients with presumptive TD at baseline prior to receiving olanzapine. The authors found the patients' baseline AIMS total scores were reduced in the first week of olanzapine treatment and remained significantly lower throughout weekly ratings. Retrospective mean reductions of 55 and 71% were found at weeks 6 and 30 respectively (p. 2).

Kinon's group designed a double-blind study in which patients with preexisting TD received olanzapine for eight months in one of four treatment arms with up to two, two-week periods of 75% dosage reduction. Full discontinuation of medication was thought to be unethical. Seventy percent of subjects no longer met restricted TD criteria after up to eight months of treatment. Furthermore, there was no statistically significant rebound worsening of TD during the blinded dose reduction periods (p. 3).

A comparison of olanzapine to risperidone showed a slightly lower level of EPS with olanzapine, but there were comparable rates of akathisia and acute dyskinesia with the two drugs (Tran et al., 1997b). When compared to risperidone and haloperidol, olanzapine had superior cognitive effects. The general cognitive index derived from six domain scores (motor skills, attention, verbal fluency and reasoning, nonverbal fluency and construction, executive skills, and immediate recall, measured at 6, 30, and 54 weeks of treatment) revealed a significantly greater benefit from olanzapine treatment relative to risperidone. The study also showed that there were no significant differences between risperidone and haloperidol. After conservative Bonferroni adjustment, only immediate recall revealed a significant improvement over the other comparators. On the 17 tests measured, only the Hooper Visual Organization Test showed a significant improvement. The medication doses used in this study were olanzapine 5 to 20 mg/day, risperidone 4 to 10 mg/day, and haloperidol 5 to 20 mg/day (Purdon et al., 2000, p. 249). The doses of risperidone and haloperidol were clearly excessive and place olanzapine in an advantageous position in relations than the comparators.

Representative Studies

The MEDLINE search from 1974 to 2003 on atypical antipsychotics identified 37 studies with olanzapine: eight for psychosis, four for mania, three for tic disorders, five for PDD, three for eating disorders, four for other indications, and 10 small case reports. There were no pediatric double-blind, controlled studies (Cheng-Shannon et al., 2004, p. 385). Information regarding the therapeutic use of olanzapine in children and adolescents is limited. Literature is limited to open label studies in a number of areas as indicated above. In addition, there are small pharmacokinetic studies and data of toxicity in overdose in children (Lilly, 2004).

Summary of Evidence-Based Support for the Use of Olanzapine in Children and Adolescents

VEOS/EOS	OPD	BD	PDD	TD	Other
3		4	4	6	

VEOS/EOS: Very early onset schizophrenia, early onset schizophrenia, schizoaffective disorder; OPD: other psychotic disorders; BP: bipolar disorders, including mania; PDD: pervasive developmental disorder, including autism; DD: disruptive disorders; TD: Tourette's disorder. For rating details on above table, see above.

Olanzapine Suggested Initiating Dosing

< 6 years of age	6–9 years of age	10–13 years of age	14 years of age and older
NR	2.5–5 mg/day	5 mg/day	5 mg/day

Olanzapine Suggested Maintenance Therapeutic Dosing

< 6 years of age	6–9 years of age	10–13 years of age	14 years of age and older
NR	5–10 mg/day	5–15 mg/day	5–20 mg/day

NR: not recommended.

QUETIAPINE   Seroquel

Summary of the Clinical Experience with Quetiapine

There is limited research support for the use of quetiapine in children. Quetiapine, except for clozapine, displays the most benign EPS profile among the second-generation antipsychotics; it also has moderate weight and metabolic side effects profiles and does not increase prolactin secretion. Quetiapine is a very safe medication, although it is very sedative; due to its short half-life, it is recommended for twice a day dosing. Single night dosing is on the rise; single dosing schedule will greatly increase tolerability since BID dose titration is frequently problematic. For BID dosing, increasing experience demonstrates that assertive rapid titration creates rapid tolerance to sedative side effects. In the author's experience, if the child or adolescent reaches tolerance to 100 mg of quetiapine in the morning, without sedation, the patient will be able to tolerate any further dose increases without experiencing drowsiness. Quetiapine carries a moderate risk for obesity, diabetes, and dyslipidemias. Quetiapine appears to have favorable neurocognitive effects. Since the ratio of dose initiation to therapeutic dose is large, and there is a small available oral dosing, quetiapine can be safely prescribed to very small children in appropriate amounts. Because of its strong sedative properties at lower doses, quetiapine is commonly used as a sleeping medication.

A recent report alerts clinicians to the potential for intranasal quetiapine abuse (Pierre, Shnayder, Wirshing, et al., 2004, p. 1718). There was also a report of intravenous quetiapine abuse (Hussain, Waheed, & Hussain, 2005, pp. 1755–1756) (for drug interactions, see appendix A).

Clinical Activity

This atypical antipsychotic has demonstrable impact on positive symptoms, negative symptoms, affective disturbance, and cognitive deficits commonly found in schizophrenia (Kasper & Muller-Spahn, 2000). A number of studies provide evidence that quetiapine is effective at improving global symptoms of schizophrenia, as well as positive and negative symptoms associated with the illness, particularly at higher doses (Lieberman, 2004b, p. 479).

Regarding quetiapine effect on mood, treatment with this atypical resulted in significant improvement in BPRS factor I (somatic concerns, anxiety, guilt feelings, depressive mood) and Kay's depressive factor (sum of PANNS items: anxiety, guilt feelings, depression, somatic concern and preoccupation) compared to treatment with haloperidol (Lieberman, 2004, p. 480). Quetiapine was superior to haloperidol in reducing depressive symptoms. This result was a direct effect of quetiapine on depressive symptoms and was not related to quetiapine impact on positive or negative symptoms or on EPS (p. 480). A report on quetiapine in bipolar depression appears below.

Cognitive deficits (in executive function, attention, and verbal memory) improved to greater extent in doses of 300 to 600 mg/day compared to haloperidol at 12 mg/day dose after 24 weeks of treatment (Lieberman, 2004, p. 479). Furthermore, Velligan et al. (2002) reported cognitive improvement in patients on quetiapine 600 mg/day ($p < 0.02$) in comparison to patients on haloperidol $\leq$ 30 mg/day. There were specific differences in executive function (Verbal Fluency Test, $p < 0.04$), attention (Stroop Color Word T, $p < 0.03$), and verbal memory (Paragraph Recall Test, $p < 0.02$). (However, the doses of haloperidol are excessive and put haloperidol in disadvantage to quetiapine). The authors stated that the group differences were not solely due to the benztropine use, medication side effects, or changes in symptomatology. The improvement in cognitive performance (attention, memory, and executive function) is predictive of role functioning and community outcome (including global functioning, occupational functioning and social skills) in patients with schizophrenia (pp. 239–240). The comparison haloperidol dosing was excessive.

Quetiapine appears to be a strong alternative for the treatment of bipolar depression. Calabrese et al. (2005) concluded that quetiapine monotherapy has significant antidepressant efficacy in a group of patients with bipolar I and II depressive disorders. The magnitude of the clinical improvement was substantial (p. 1358). The effect size is considered low if it is less than 0.4, moderate if the effect size is 0.40 to 0.79, and large if the effect size is larger than 0.80. The effect size for quetiapine, 600 mg QHS, for bipolar I depression, was estimated at 1.09, compared to published size effects for olanzapine 0.32 alone and 0.68 for olanzapine-fluoxetine combination (p. 1359).

In the CATIE report, quetiapine had the highest discontinuation rate (see below) among the antipsychotics studied (quetiapine, olanzapine, risperidone, ziprasidone, and perphenazine). Olanzapine was superior in therapeutic effectiveness to all the compared medications, and there was no significant therapeutic effectiveness difference among quetiapine, risperidone, ziprasidone, and perphenazine (Lieberman, Stroup, et al., 2005, pp. 1209, 1218). See CATIE commentaries above. In the CATIE II report, olanzapine showed, again, better effectiveness than quetiapine, risperidone and ziprasidone (McEvoy, Lieberman, Stroup, et al., 2006).

Quetiapine has a very low EPS prevalence, and produces no elevation of prolactin; quetiapine has no hematologic or cardiologic side effects. Contrary to olanzapine and risperidone, EPS rate with quetiapine does not increase with higher doses. Of all the antipsychotic medications, quetiapine may have the least potential for inducing EPS and is currently the preferred medication for treatment of behavioral toxicity in patients with Parkinson's disease (Lieberman, 2004, p. 480). Quetiapine should be the choice alternative for patients who have displayed neurological side effects to alternative antipsychotics.

Regardless of the length of treatment (up to 52 weeks) prolactin levels were consistently below baseline in quetiapine-treated patients, and there was a low incidence of reproductive system or hormonal adverse side effects such as impotence, decreased libido, or vaginal dryness (0.3%); abnormal ejaculation (0.2%); and of amenorrhea, galactorrhea, and gynecomastia (0.1%) (p. 480). The above effects appear to be related to quetiapine and clozapine transient adhesiveness to the D2 receptors, or "transient occupation theory." The transitory high occupancy of the D2 receptors is sufficient to relieve psychotic symptoms without causing EPS or prolactinemia (Bowes, 2002, p. 57). FDA approval for quetiapine in mania for adults was granted in January 2004.

Quetiapine has a very low risk of inducing EEG abnormalities (Centorrino et al., 2002, p. 113) and it may be helpful in reducing tardive dyskinesia (*Schizophrenia Research*, 2001, pp. 309–310).

In a long-term maintenance, open-label study of quetiapine in the treatment of schizophrenia, Kasper, Brecher, Fitton, and Jones (2004) reported a 91.5% drop-out rate in a cohort of 674 patients followed up for up to 208 weeks or more; 46.7% discontinued treatment due to lack of efficacy. According to Kutcher (2004), the high percentage of lack of efficacy is troubling and raises questions about the medicine, or the trials or both. The good news is that patients who responded to this medication during the initial weeks were able to maintain the efficacy up to 208 weeks or longer from the time of initiation, with relatively low incidence of side effects (p. 10). Since the data on long-term "staying maintenance" is unknown, this high drop-out rate cannot be compared with that of other atypicals. There is a great deal of switching of atypical medications, in children and adolescents, at the initiation of treatment either for tolerance factors or for lack of efficacy. The highest discontinuation rate of quetiapine, 82%, in the CATIE I study, mentioned above, among the antipsychotics studied, is in line with Kasper et al. (2004) study discussed previously.

Representative Studies

The MEDLINE search from 1974 to 2003 identified 19 published studies of quetiapine use in children and adolescents. There were no pediatric double-blind, controlled studies of quetiapine monotherapy (Cheng-Shannon et al., 2004, p. 385).

Quetiapine for the Treatment of Bipolar Disorders

Level 1. Quetiapine appears to have mood modulating functions as demonstrated in a double-blind, randomized, placebo control study of this atypical as an adjunct in the treatment of adolescent mania. The results of this study indicate that quetiapine in combination with divalproex is more effective at reducing manic symptoms associated with bipolar disorder than divalproex alone. Quetiapine was well tolerated and the percentage of patients completing the study (73%), was greater on quetiapine plus divalproex (93%) than the ones on DVP + placebo (53%) (DelBello, Schwiers, Rosenberg, & Strakowski, 2002, pp. 1220–1221).

Comment: This randomized study, with only a small number of cases, demonstrates the impact of quetiapine as an adjunct in the treatment of adolescent bipolar disorder.

Level 1. DelBello, Kowatch, Adler, et al. (2006) reported on the first published double-blind controlled study of a mood stabilizer versus an atypical antipsychotic for the treatment of mania or mixed states in adolescents with bipolar disorder. The study demonstrated that both quetiapine and divalproex were associated with significant improvement of changes in the YMRS from baseline to end point. Although the therapeutic effectiveness between the two medications was not statistically significant, the YMRS scores improvement was better for quetiapine than for divalproex. Adolescents who received quetiapine had a more rapid reduction in manic symptoms than those receiving divalproex. Based on secondary measures, the response and emission rates in patients treated with quetiapine were greater that those treated with divalproex. Both medications were well tolerated and an equal number of subject on each medication completed the study (pp. 310–311).

Summary of Evidence-Based Support for the Use of Quetiapine in Children and Adolescents

VEOS/EOS	OPD	BP	PDD	DD	TD
3	3	2	5	—	6

VEOS/EOS: Very early onset schizophrenia, early onset schizophrenia, schizoaffective disorder; OPD: other psychotic disorders; BP: bipolar disorders, including mania; PDD: pervasive developmental disorder, including autism; DD: disruptive disorders; TD: Tourette's disorder. For details regarding ratings on above scale, see above.

Quetiapine Suggested Initiating Dosing

< 6 years of age	6–9 years of age	10–13 years of age	14 years of age and older
12.5 mg BID	12.5–25 BID	25 mg q AM &	25–50*mg q AM &
	50 mg q HS	50–100 mg q HS	

Quetiapine Suggested Therapeutic Maintenance Dosing

< 6 years of age	6–9 years of age	10–13 years of age	14 years of age and older
25–50 mg BID*	100 mg BID*	100–200mg BID*	100–300mg BID*

* Due to sedative side effects, physicians adjust the dose at AM, and tend to prescribe about 25% of the dose at AM, and the rest, 75% of the dose, at bedtime. As discussed in the text, single night dosing is becoming more common in clinical practice. Single-dosing increases tolerability.

ZIPRASIDONE

Summary of Clinical Experience with Ziprasidone

A pharmaceutical competitor of ziprasidone created an aura of apprehension about this medication's cardiological side effects long before this medication had obtained FDA approval. The orchestrated campaign against this product was very successful in creating physicians' apprehension about ziprasidone. These fears are unjustified; the alarming purported side effects of ziprasidone never materialized, and were dispelled by the Clinical Antipsychotic Trials of Intervention Effectiveness (CATIE I) trial (Lieberman, Stroup, McEvoy, et al., 2005). Ziprasidone is an eminently safe and effective second-generation antipsychotic in adults. There is limited literature to substantiate safety and effectiveness in childhood. So far, ziprasidone has not been associated with torsades des pointes (TdP), and has demonstrated no lethality in overdose (see chapter 10, note 7).

Its weight neutrality, its favorable metabolic side effects and prolactin profiles, render ziprasidone an attractive therapeutic option. Ziprasidone is an optimal antipsychotic medication for overweight and obese children and adolescents. Ziprasidone also appears to have significant antidepressive effects and a favorable neurocognitive effect. A minor disadvantage is that it is a twice a day medication, and that it requires food in the stomach for optimal absorption. There is an ongoing empirical experimentation with single nightly dosing.

The CATIE Phase I (2005) report indicated that there is no difference in cardiological risk among the antipsychotics tried (perphenazine, olanzapine, risperidone, quetiapine, and ziprasidone). However, ziprasidone should not be used with persons who suffer from Long QTc syndrome or concomitantly with medications that prolong the QTc.

Regarding the pediatric use of ziprasidone, Blair, Scahill, State, and Martin (2005) raised some concerns regarding the safety of this antipsychotic in children, based on an uncontrolled study of 20 children with a variety of diagnosis: Tourette's, OCD, or PDD. In the June 2006 issue of the *Journal of the American Academy of Child and Adolescent Psychiatry*, there is a lively point-counter-point debate on the issue of safety of ziprasidone in pediatric populations. Loebel, Miceli, Chappel (Pfizer employees), and Siu (Pfizer consultant) (2006, June) pinpoint a number of methodological problems in the Blair et al. (2005) article: measurements were random and uncontrolled, and suffer from other shortcomings, not in line with the International Conference in the Harmonization of Technical Requirements for Registration of Pharmaceuticals (ICH) E14 guidelines on the clinical evaluation of QT/QTc intervals. There are issues with the Bazett's correction norms (the Fridericia method is more accurate, QtcF), lack of placebo or other controls and a number of issues with the data interpretation. These authors also mention that the publication by DelBello et al. (2005) based on the study of 63 children and adolescents with bipolar mania or schizophrenia suggests that ziprasidone is safe and well tolerated in the children and adolescent population. The DelBello et al. study, using standardized ECG conditions, showed no subject with QTc increase exceeding 60 ms. The authors concluded the Blair et al. conclusions are potentially misleading (pp. 636–637).

Martin, Blair, State, Leckman, and Scahill (2006, June) replied to the Loebel et al. critique. The authors recognized that their findings were based on a prematurely terminated study (because the dead of the only adult subject in the study. These authors assert that the adult death was not related to ziprasidone treatment) and an incomplete dataset. The authors stand by the previous recommendations of requiring close ECG monitoring when using ziprasidone in children. They also state that Ziprasidone should be considered a second line option in pediatric populations, and that manual reading of QTc measurements, ideally by a pediatric cardiologist, will improve reliability [and accuracy] (pp. 638–639). It could be concluded that Martin et al. (2006) concede to the criticisms and reservations of Loebel et al. (2006) regarding issues on methodology and data interpretation of Blair et al. (2005) article.

Ziprasidone has antimanic properties, and has obtained the FDA antimanic indication for treatment of bipolar disorders (see below).

The CATIE Phase I (2005) report indicated that 79% of patients placed on ziprasidone discontinued the medication during the 18 months of the study (Lieberman, Stroup et al., 2005, p. 1209). The anticipated concerns regarding QTc interval prolongation and TdP did not materialized (p. 1218). The result of other SGAs (except for olanzapine, which appears to demonstrate effectiveness superiority) including ziprasidone, were similar to perphenazine, a conventional antipsychotic (p. 1218). In this study ziprasidone was the only medication associated with improvement of the metabolic variables (p. 1215).

Ziprasidone has probably both agonist and antagonist activity (Sallee et al., 2003, p. 905). Ziprasidone is an antagonist at dopamine D2 and serotonin 5-HT2A receptors, and an agonist at 5-HT1A receptors, mostly located in neocortex in the pyramidal glutaminergic neurons where their action is inhibitory. Dopamine agonists appear to increase intracortical inhibition (p. 905).

A twice a day dose with ziprasidone will produce adequate steady state occupancies at the 5-HT2 and D2 receptors (p. 905). The bioavailability of ziprasidone is enhanced by the administration of food. Ziprasidone bioavailability is 60% when taken with food, and only 30% when taken on an empty stomach, so patients should be informed of the importance of taken ziprasidone with food (Jibson & Tandom, 2003, p. 62). Maalox does not affect ziprasidone bioavailability but slows its Tmax for about 3 hours. Ziprasidone is more than 99% protein bound—primarily albumin and alpha-1-acid glycoprotein (p. 510).

Because of concerns with the cardiovascular side effects, the initial recommended doses were subtherapeutic and probably activating. Clinical experience has shown that the titration and therapeutic doses need to be adjusted upward. Consensus is developing that ziprasidone doses below 120 mg/day, in adults, are mainly antidepressant, and that true antipsychotic effects are demonstrable with ziprasidone in doses above 120 mg/day. This is also true for many children and adolescents.

The upper therapeutic recommended dose is 160 mg/day. There are incipient clinical experiences indicating that ziprasidone doses above 160 mg/day increase its therapeutic effectiveness without increasing the cardiovascular risks.

Clinical Activity

Ziprasidone is indicated for the treatment of schizophrenia; its efficacy in the treatment of recently hospitalized schizophrenic or schizoaffective patients was demonstrated at daily doses, ranging from 40 to 200 mg/day, for a broad range of schizophrenic symptoms in four to six weeks placebo control trials (Daniel, Copeland, & Tamminga, 2004, p. 511). Ziprasidone's therapeutic effects are comparable to those of olanzapine and risperidone (p. 511).

In a study reported by Weiden, Simpson, Potkin, and O'Sullivan (2003), Ziprasidone efficacy and tolerability were evaluated in patients with schizophrenia and schizoaffective disorder who were switched from conventional or atypical antipsychotics to ziprasidone in multicenter, parallel group trials. Stable outpatients with persistent symptoms or troublesome side effects on a conventional antipsychotic (N = 108), olanzapine (N = 104), or risperidone (N = 58), were switched to an open-label, six-week flexible dose trial of ziprasidone (40–160 mg/day). The authors concluded that when stable but symptomatic outpatients were switched from their previous antipsychotic medication to ziprasidone, the change was well tolerated, in general, and was associated with symptom improvement six weeks later. Improvement occurred for patients who had been on atypicals or conventional antipsychotics (p. 580).

There is now a parenteral, intramuscular preparation that uses sulfobutyl ether beta-cyclodextrin to solubilize the drug by complexation. This preparation is useful in dealing with patients in acute states of agitation associated with psychosis. The bioavailability of ziprasidone is 100% when used intramuscularly, with peak concentration postdose of 60 minutes or earlier (Daniel, Copeland, & Tamminga, 2004, p. 510). Improvement of agitation was seen as early as 15 to 30 minutes, and was sustained for up to two to four hours with ziprasidone, at either 10 or 20 mg IM. The subjective experience of ziprasidone IM has been reported as a more comfortable tranquilization than previous experiences with previous antipsychotics (pp. 511–512). An interval of two hours for additional doses is recommended for patients receiving 10 mg IM, and a four-hour interval for those receiving 20 mg. Patients should not receive more than 40 mg of parenteral ziprasidone in 24 hours (p. 515). Contrary to other parenteral medications (haloperidol, haloperidol plus lorazepam, lorazepam, risperidone, olanzapine, and others) ziprasidone IM induces tranquilization without sedation. It is common for patients to return to therapeutic activities shortly after receiving parenteral ziprasidone; that is rarely the case with the other parenteral medications.

Harvey et al. (2004) studied the neurocognitive effects of the patients switched to ziprasidone described above (Weiden et al., 2003). They concluded that switching schizophrenic patients from other antipsychotics to ziprasidone was associated with improvements across a wide range of cognitive domains, including learning and memory, attention and vigilance, and executive functions. The effect was greater for those switched from conventional antipsychotics and risperidone than from those switched from olanzapine to ziprasidone (pp. 110–111).

Ziprasidone and Mania

Ziprasidone demonstrated efficacy and tolerability as an antimanic agent in acute bipolar mania on a three-week, placebo control trial. Ziprasidone produced rapid, sustained improvements, relative to baseline and placebo, in all primary and secondary efficacy measures at endpoint. Significant improvements were observed within two days of treatment initiation and were maintained throughout the three weeks (Keck, Versiani, et al., 2003).

Representative Studies

The MEDLINE search from 1974 to 2003 identified 11 studies on pediatric use of ziprasidone; there was one double-blind, controlled study for the treatment of Tourette's disorder (Cheng-Shannon et al., 2004, p. 386).

Summary of the Evidence-Based Support for the Use of Ziprasidone in Children and Adolescents

VEOS/EOS	OPD	BD	PDD	DD	TD
—	—	—	—	—	1

VEOS/EOS: Very early onset schizophrenia, early onset schizophrenia, schizoaffective disorder; OPD: other psychotic disorders; BP: bipolar disorders, including mania; PDD: pervasive developmental disorder, including autism; DD: disruptive disorders; TD: Tourette's disorder. For details regarding ratings on above table, see above.

Ziprasidone Suggested Initiating Dosing

< 6 years of age	6–9 years of age	10–13 years of age	14 years of age and older
NR	20 mg BID	20 mg BID	20–40 mg BID*

Ziprasidone Suggested Therapeutic-Maintenance Dosing

< 6 years of age	6–9 years of age	10–13 years of age	14 years of age and older
NR	20–40 mg BID*	20–60 mg BID*	40–80 mg BID*

*Due to sedative side effects, physicians tend to adjust the dose at AM, and tend to prescribe about 25% of the dose at AM, and the rest, 75% of the dose, at bedtime once a day dosing, PM single dosing is on the rise.

ARIPIPRAZOLE   Ability

Summary of the Clinical Experience with Aripiprazole

Aripiprazole is the newest second generation antipsychotic on the U.S. market and, so far, has no evidence-based literature to support its use in children. Aripiprazole is rapidly attracting the attention of child and adolescents psychiatrists for its benign side effect profile. Aripiprazole is minimally sedative, has negligible anticholinergic side effects, and has shown no metabolic complications; it also has no prolactin elevating properties and displays no cardiovascular side effects.

Difficulties with agitation (akathisia) at the beginning of treatment probably represent a response to a high initial dosing. Children under 10 years of age are more susceptible to acute dyskinesias and other EPS adverse events than adolescents, or adults. It also appears that aripiprazole has a favorable impact on neurocognitive functioning. The preliminary positive impressions with this novel antipsychotic need to be corroborated by rigorous research to establish safety and effectiveness of aripiprazole in the treatment of children and adolescents.

It has been proposed that aripiprazole is a weight neutral medication. However, according to the 2006 PDR, aripiprazole increases weight equal or greater that 7% of body weight in 30% of patients with a baseline BMI < 23, in 19% of patients with a baseline BMI between 23 and 27, and in 8% of patients with a baseline BMI > 27 (p. 920). This indicates that aripiprazole will tend to increase the most weight in patients who are below ideal BMI and in those within the ideal BMI range. This pattern of weight increase is not unique to aripiprazole.

Even though aripiprazole is the newest atypical in the U.S. psychiatric field, it has rapidly gained an important place within the adult antipsychotic armamentarium. For instance, in adults, psychiatric experts gave risperidone and aripiprazole first line rating for first episode (schizophrenia) with predominant negative symptoms. Aripiprazole also received strong recommendations for first episodes with predominant positive and negative symptoms, for a multiepisode patient with predominant positive symptoms, for a multiepisode patient with predominant negative symptoms, and for a multiepisode patient with both prominent positive and negative symptoms (Kane et al., 2003, p. 9). It is likely that early uncritical warm reception for aripiprazole may be tempered by the results of the CATIE I (Lieberman, Stroup, McEvoy, et al., 2005) and CATIE II (McEvoy, Lieberman, Stroup, et al., 2006) reports. In the first report, ziprasidone showed less effectiveness than olanzapine and a similar effectiveness as risperidone, quetiapine, or perphenazine. In the second report, olanzapine again, demonstrated therapeutic superiority over risperidone, quetiapine or ziprasidone.

Aripiprazole has antimanic effects and obtained FDA antimanic monotherapy indication for adults in late summer 2004. Aripiprazole had significantly greater efficacy than placebo for the treatment of bipolar disorder patients in acute mania or mixed episodes, and was well tolerated in a randomized controlled trial (Keck, Marcus, et al., 2003). Aripiprazole is effective for motor tics in Tourette's disorder (Ginsberg, 2005b, pp. 21–22).

Although preliminary observations appear to indicate that arpiprazole is a safe medication, it is too early to say what its extended and long-term side effect profile will be, particularly in children and adolescents. Also, will aripiprazole be as effective as older atypical antipsychotics? The CATIE trial (2005) raises some questions in this regard. Time, research, and extended clinical use of this medication will tell. Ginsberg (2005e) states that aripiprazole appears to precipitate or worsen psychosis in a subset of vulnerable patients (p. 30) (for drug interactions, see appendix A).

Clinical Activity

Kane et al. (2002) reported on a four-week, double-blind clinical trial in which patients with schizophrenia and schizoaffective disorder received aripiprazole 15 and 30 mg/day, and haloperidol 10 mg/day; there was also a placebo control group. For both doses of aripiprazole, mean change in PANSS total score from baseline separated from placebo by week two (p. 769). These improvements were comparable to the ones produced by haloperidol (p. 770).

Saha et al. (2001) reported at the 7th World Congress of Biological Psychiatry held in Berlin in 2001, on the results of a phase III study including 404 hospitalized patients with a DSM-IV diagnosis of schizophrenia or schizoaffective disorder with acute relapse. Aripiprazole's side effects and tolerability are appealing: a favorable EPS profile, no increase in plasma prolactin, minimal somnolence, nor significant cardiac QTc prolongation, minimal orthostatic hypotension or tachycardia, minimal change in weight, no effect on plasma glucose levels, and no significant elevation of cholesterol or triglycerides (Gelenberg, 2003, p. 10). Aripiprazole induces a normalization of hyperprolactinemia related to risperidone (Shores, 2005, pp. 42–45).

Representative Studies

The MEDLINE search from 1974 to 2003 identified three pediatric studies of aripiprazole. There were no published controlled studies in childhood or adolescent patients (Cheng-Shannon et al., 2004, p. 286).

Summary of the Evidence-Based Support for the Use of Aripiprazole in Children and Adolescents

VEOS/EOS	OPD	BP	PDD	DD	TD
—	—	—	—	4	—

VEOS/EOS: Very early onset schizophrenia, early onset schizophrenia; OPD: other psychotic disorders; BP: bipolar disorders, including mania; PDD: pervasive developmental disorder, including autism; DD: disruptive disorders; TD: Tourette's disorder. For details regarding ratings on above table, see above.

Aripiprazole Suggested Initiating Dosing

< 6 years of age	6–9 years of age	10–13 years of age	14 years of age and older
NR	2.5 mg/day	2.5–5 mg/day	5 mg/day

Aripiprazole Suggested Therapeutic Dosing

< 6 years of age	6–9 years of age	10–13 years of age	14 years of age and older
NR	5–7.5 mg/day	5–15 mg/day	5–20 mg/day

NR: not recommended.

CHAPTER 13

Side Effects of Mood Stabilizers and Atypical Antipsychotics

This chapter provides an overview of developmental issues related to side effects, and then reviews the most common adverse events and concerns related to mood stabilizers and atypical antipsychotics. There are clear developmental differences in adverse event expression or side effects risks when mood stabilizers and antipsychotics are used in children and adolescents. All the mood stabilizers and antipsychotic medications produce adverse events. Each mood stabilizer and each atypical antipsychotic medication has its own adverse events profile. Prescribing physicians need to be familiar with the spectrum of risks for each of these medications.

Currently, concerns with cardiovascular and metabolic complications take center stage in current mood stabilizing and antipsychotic treatments. Children and adolescents are more vulnerable to these risks. Sudden-death risk with the use of atypical antipsychotics is due to cardiovascular and metabolic risks, or the result of pancreatitis or liver failure. Females have an increased risk for these complications. Polypharmacy increases the risk of side effects. Increase in pediatric psychotropic polypharmacy is on the rise. Caution must be exercised when initiating these practices (Zonfrillo, Penn, & Leonard, 2005, p 19). It is alarming the lack of safety and efficacy data for the combined use of psychotropics in children (Berrettini, 2005, p. 5).

UNRESOLVED ISSUES RELATED TO SIDE EFFECTS

Research on side effects, short- and long term, in children and adolescents, needs to take the preeminence that effectiveness has been given in clinical pharmacological studies. In general, there are no systematic studies of side effects reactions even for pharmacutical products approved by the FDA for use in children and adolescents. Most of the pharmaceutical products currently on the market lack comprehensive profile studies of long-term side effects; there are no gender sensitive studies or developmentally sensitive side effects research regarding specific side effects in preschool, preadolescent, or adolescent populations. Two systems have been developed for the systematic study of adverse events:

The most common protocols for the investigation of side effects are the *Coding Symbols for Thesaurus of Adverse Reaction Terms* (COSTART), and the *Medical Dictionary for Regulatory Activities*). Researchers do not use these protocols consistently (Greenhill, Vitiello, Riddle, et al., 2003, p. 637).

The Med Watch and World Health Organization databases collect Adverse Events (AE) practitioners' spontaneous reports. The sensitivity and validity of postmarketing surveillance needs to be improved, and passive surveillance based on spontaneous reporting should be supplemented by active surveillance, based on prospective studies and systematic studies of cohorts of patients (p. 638).

There is not an accepted dictionary of AE definitions. Although there is a standard definition for serious side effects, there is no corresponding one for mild, moderate, or severe AEs. The definition of severe AEs, used in some psychopharmacology studies, mixes issues that do not have the same dimension of concern: "AE prevented functioning in at least one important area (e.g., unable to sleep for more than 1.5 hours; no food at breakfast, lunch or dinner, even if had snack later at night) or posed a major threat to the child's health (e.g., seizures, loss of consciousness, hallucinations)" (p. 640). It is hard to understand how insomnia or appetite loss is placed on the same dimension of severity as a seizure episode or loss of consciousness.

TYPES OF STUDIES ON DRUG INDUCED TOXICITY

The term *adverse events* (AE) refers to any negative occurrence in mental or physical functioning that occurs during a psychopharmacological treatment. AE may be "unrelated," "likely related," or "definitely related" to the drug being taken. The occurrence may be judged "frequent" if occurring in more than 5% of the patients taking that medication, "infrequent" when more than 2% but less than 5% of the patients are affected, and "rare" if less than 1% is affected. The severity of the AE is considered "mild," "moderate," or "serious." Serious is an AE that is life threatening or fatal, one that requires or prolongs inpatient hospitalization, or that results in congenital malformations, or in a persistent significant disability (Greenhill, Vitiello, Riddle, et al., 2003, p. 629).

In the study and research of side effects, a number of variables (factors) need to be taken into account. The following are descriptors for the categories of side effects that are listed below: (T): toxicity refers to the temporal presentation of side effect(s) after initiation of a drug (D): definition describes the nature of the emerging side effect; (E): example describes specific side effects events; (PADM): Possible Ascertainment Design and Methods relates to research strategies needed to ascertain the causal attribution of the side effect.

(T) Acute: (D) Emerging after brief drug exposure. (E): rash. PADM: Controlled clinical trial.

(T) Chronic: (D) Emerging after a long-term drug exposure. (E): tardive dyskinesia. PADM: Naturalistic extended follow up.

(T) Proximal: (D) Emerging during drug exposure and disappearing after discontinuation. (E): Lithium-induced tremor. PADM: Controlled clinical trial, naturalistic follow up, ABA intrasubject design.

(T) Distal: (D) Emerging after considerable time since drug exposure ended. (E): DES-induced vaginal adenocarcenoma. PADM: Naturalistic follow-up, spontaneous reporting and epidemiologic tracking.

(T) Anticipated: (D) Already known to be associated with drug use or suspected based on previous reports or preclinical data. (E): Stimulant-induced anorexia, valproic-associated polycystic ovary disease. PADM: Targeted, drug-specific adverse event scale.

(T) Unanticipated: (D) No previous concerns. (E): Fenfluramine-induced cardiotoxicity. PADM: Systematic, open, broad-range scales (Vitiello, Riddle, Greenhill, et al., 2003, p. 635).

ISSUES AND ADVERSE EVENTS IN CLINICAL RESEARCH WITH CHILDREN

Psychopharmacologic research in children and adolescents is making steady progress but it is still limited. There is a great disparity between the extent of psychotropic medication use in children and adolescents and the research data supporting its use.

To a great extent, assumptions about pediatric psychopharmacology have been borrowed from adult patients. Although some extrapolations from adults to children are valid, a number of issues pertaining to pediatric pharmacodynamics, pharmacokinesis, and developmental psychopharmacology are specific to childhood and adolescence; these particulars need further elucidation through systematic short- and long-term studies. Pertinent studies with large numbers of patients for extended periods of time are needed. Of late, we have been made aware that data related to negative outcomes and serious side effects are seldom published, which has caused a disproportionate bias toward the purported positive effects of medications.

Erroneous pharmacological generalizations from adults to children have been made. Examples of a developmental differential response in children include: (1) anticholinergic desipramine side effects (constipation and dry mouth) are less pronounced in children under 18 years of age than in adults (Galanter & Walsh, 2002), and (2) contrary to report in adult patients, olanzapine increases the levels of prolactin in children and adolescents (Alfaro et al., 2002).

The NIMH Collaborative Multisite Multimodal Treatment Study of Children with ADHD (MTI) demonstrated that the largest source of variance in the AE data, when a drug specific checklist was used, came from the type of informant (p. 629). This is pertinent to the study of antipsychotic side effects. Lethal adverse reactions may reflect developmental susceptibility of children for catastrophic side effect responses. Since the mid-1990s, there have been at least five serious, though rare, adverse events associated with psychotropic medications in children and adolescents. These include sudden deaths related to desipramine for ADHD (3 children), four deaths in children taking methylphenidate, clonidine, and other drugs; 25 deaths related to hepatotoxicity, plus four deaths secondary to hemorrhagic pancreatitis in pediatric patients taking valproic acid, and 11 cases of extreme hepatotoxicity, which resulted in death or liver transplant in individuals being treated with pemoline for ADHD (Greenhill et al., 2003, p. 628). At the present time it is unknown how many children had fatal outcomes with atypical drugs (ketoacidosis, cardiovascular events, etc.). Of course, it is likely that the number of actual fatalities is larger due to underreporting.

DEVELOPMENTAL ASPECTS OF PSYCHOTROPIC SIDE EFFECTS

Adverse events (AE) are developmentally sensitive. Substantial AE data are available for adults, but it is unknown whether AE risks or patterns of risk are similar in children and adolescents. Age and developmental stage can play an important role in determining AE patterns to pharmacological interventions. Thus, Reye's syndrome (secondary to aspirin) and "gray baby syndrome" (due to chloranfenicol) are examples of unique medication reactions in childhood that are not observed in adults. The same is true for fatal arrhythmias secondary to use of desipramine in childhood and the exfoliating dermatitis reaction to lamotrigene in childhood. The polycystic ovarian syndrome risk described with valproate should be included in this category. AE risks may be similar across development for some complaints; however, some risks may be significantly more common in children or adolescents than in adults (Woods, Martin, Spector, & McGlashan, 2002, pp. 1439–1441). Sometimes, it takes many years to recognize the deleterious side effects of a medication. Pemoline was in use for more that 20 years before a rare, unexpected, and serious AE hepatic failure, was discovered (Greenhill et al., 2003, p. 629).

Although data are preliminary, children and adolescents treated with atypical medications have been shown to be especially sensitive to a number of potential AEs. Some evidence suggests that the incidence or severity of EPS, TD, hyperprolactinemia, weight gain, sedation, hypotension, seizures, hepatotoxicity, tachycardia, and hypersalivation maybe greater in pediatric subjects than in adults. Nevertheless, significant variability in AE profiles exists among these medications and, based on the accumulated evidence so far, treatment recommendations must take into account individual patient factors, including family medical history (Labellarte & Riddle, 2002, p. 100). The greater vulnerability to adverse events in children and adolescents in comparison to adults is summarized in table 13.1.

Similarly represented AEs included EPS (except for an apparent higher frequency of akathisia for aripiprazole which seems higher than the EPS data reported in adults). Overrepresented adverse effects included sedation, weight gain, and liver function abnormalities (Woods et al., 2002, p. 1442). These authors cite a number of examples of differential developmental AEs using olanzapine as the prototypical antipsychotic (see table 13.2).

TABLE 13.1 Developmental Sensitivity to Antipsychotic Medications Side Effects in Children in Comparison to Adults

Symptom	< 10 years of age	11 to 18 years of age
EPS		
Acute dystonia	>>>	>>
Akathisia	>>>	>
Parkinsonism	>>>	>
Sialorrhea	>>>	>/=
Galactorrhea	-	>>
Tardive dyskinesia	>>/>>>	>>
Sedation	>>	>>
Insomnia	>/>>	>/>>
Enuresis	>>>	>
Encopresis	>>	=
Constipation	>>	>
Seizures	>>	>
Weight gain	>>>	>>/>>>
Hepatotoxicity	>>	>
Orthostasis	>>	>
Rhinitis (noisy breathing)	>>>	>>
Behavioral toxicity		
Suicide	>>	>
Hostility	>>	>
Dysphoria	>>	>

>>>   Particularly sensitive to this side effect in comparison to adults
>>   More sensitive to this side effect than adults
>   Somewhat more sensitive than adults
=   Equally sensitive to this side effect than adults
Source: Labellarte & Riddle (2002); Woods et al. (2002).

TABLE 13.2 Developmental Differences in Atypical Medications Side Effects

	Children	Adolescents	Adults
Extrapyramidal side effects	=	=	=
Tardive dyskinesia	>>	>/>>	
Agitation	>>	>	
Hostility	>>>	>	
Sedation	>>	>	
Weight gain, appetite increase	>>>	>>>	
Diabetes	<<<	<<	
Suicide and suicidal attempts	>	>	
Prolactin increase	>>	>>	
Neuroleptic malignant syndrome	=	=	=
Seizures	>>	>	
Liver abnormalities	>>	>	
Anticholinergic Side effects	<	</=	

=   Equal for children, adolescents and adults.
>>>   A great deal more common than in adults
>>   Much more common than in adults
>   More common than in adults
<<<   A great deal less common than in adults
<<   Much less common than in adults
</=   Less or equal than in adults
Source: Based on Woods et al. (2002, pp. 1442–1444).

The developmental observations on children and adolescents side effects support the following propositions:

1. Development is likely to modify the expression of medications side effects of mood stabilizers and of antipsychotic medications..
2. Mood components developed during treatment with antipsychotics may represent neuroleptic dysphoria (see below); this may be a common antipsychotic side effect in childhood and adolescence.
3. Close monitoring of mood stabilizing and antipsychotic side effects is mandatory; this includes a pertinent inquiry and testing for the presence of side effects for which children and adolescents seem to be particularly vulnerable.

Gender Differences

The volume of distribution of lipophilic drugs is greater in women than in men; although the blood volume is smaller, the lipid compartments are larger (the proportion of adipose tissues is 33% in postpubertal younger women and 48% in the elderly, in contrast to the proportion of 18% in young men and 36% in elderly men). Increased adiposity prolongs the half-life of antipsychotics in women, leading to accumulation over time. After steady state, dosing intervals for women should be longer than for men. Aging brings a decrease in intracellular water, a decrease in protein binding, and a decrease in tissue mass; this increases the proportion of body fat resulting in increased concentration of antipsychotics in the brain, and their accumulation in lipid compartments. Drug metabolism decreases because of relative enzymatic inactivity, decreased blood flow to the liver, and a decrease of liver mass. Renal excretion is progressively impaired with age. A greater amount of adipose tissue in women indicates lower doses to prevent unnecessary side effects (Seeman, 2004, p. 1327).

Gender Related Side Effects

A meta-analysis of 332 patients exposed to cardiovascular medications suggested that women are at a higher risk of developing torsades des pointes (TdP) than males in response to drugs that prolong cardiac repolarization (Ito, 2005, p. 41). QTc interval in women was significantly higher than in men among people with cardiovascular comorbidity (p. 42). Thus, female patients with mental disorders with QTc prolongation seem to be at a higher risk of cardiovascular diseases (p. 86). Table 13.3 indicates factors that are associated with prolongation of QTc and risk of TdP.

Also, antipsychotic adverse events tend to be more severe in women than in men.

1. Acute dystonia, contrary to previous beliefs, is more common in women than in men.
2. Pulmonary embolism seems to be more common in women.
3. QTc side effects may be more common in women than in men because women have longer QT intervals than men on average. The QT interval is genotype dependent.

TABLE 13.3 Factors Associated with Increased Risk of QT Prolongation and Torsades de Pointes

Prolonged QTc
Female sex
Advanced age
Bradycardia
Hypokalemia
Hypomagnesemia
Congestive heart failure (low EF)
Cardiac arrythmias
Combination of drugs (ion channel blockers, cytochrome P450 enzymes inhibitors)
Genetic polymorphisms of gene coding cardiac ion channels or enzymes in liver
    metabolising drugs

Source: Zareba & Lin (2003, p. 298).

4. Antipsychotics' increase of body mass index is more prevalent in women than in men. Obesity is particularly stigmatizing for women. Women appear to be at a higher risk than men for obesity related side effects (diabetes mellitus, hypertension, cardiovascular disease, and hyperlipidemia).
5. Women are more susceptible to hyperprolactinemia, and as a result, are more prone to amenorrhea and galactorrhea. Individuals with schizophrenia are at increased risk for osteoporosis and bone fractures due to low estrogen levels, inactivity, cigarette smoking, and polydipsia. Even benign side effects like sedation, similar in both sexes, may have devastating consequences for women, such as the loss of child custody (Seeman, 2004, pp. 1327–1328).
6. Newer antipsychotics may increase pregnancy risk. If a woman has been treated with a prolactin-raising antipsychotic, and she is switched to one that does not elevate prolactin, her chances of becoming pregnant increase (Gelenberg, 2002, Vol. 25, p. 17)

When considering adverse medication side effects, the clinician will keep in mind that the patient may be reacting to the medication constituents rather than to the principal compound. All the atypicals contain animal-derived lactose; risperidone and quetiapine contain bovine-derived magnesium stearate. There are also hypothetical risks of Creutzfeldt-Jacob disease (mad cow disease) when using materials derived from contaminated animals, as well as issues related to lactose intolerance, which is estimated to be present in 50 million Americans. Use of animal-derived constituents may also have a number of ethnic, religious, and dietary implications (Sauer & Howard, 2002, p. 1249).

ELICITATION OF SIDE EFFECTS

Unlike tests for efficacy, which can pose a single specific research question and then test it, safety monitoring has to use a broad, flexible vigilance method for detecting any safety issues, expected or unexpected, from mild to serious (Greenhill et al., 2003, p. 632). In determining AE, a sound clinical practice would recommend the following:

- Children and adolescents themselves should become a primary source of information.
- More than one source of information (parents, teachers, and others) is more accurate for detecting and reporting AE.
- Spontaneous, passive reporting or a general unspecific inquiry is unsatisfactory, since patients may either fail to report important AEs or the psychiatrist may fail to make pertinent inquiry of AEs related to the medication in question.

- Monitoring of side effects needs to be systematic and standardized; specific checklists may be useful for this objective (p. 633).

The extent and severity of AEs in children and adolescents have not received enough attention in the investigation of psychotropic medications. Most of the published studies on psychotropic pediatric use do not collect or report data on AE in a systematic fashion. The FDA ought to demand AE studies in pediatric populations and develop new systems of vigilance and monitoring of the psychotropics in current use to insure detection of AE trends and to alert practitioners of emerging concerns.

MOOD STABILIZERS: SIDE EFFECTS

Weller, Kloos, Hitchcock, and Weller (2005) question whether lithium and antiepileptic agents are safe for use in children. They also remind physicians that except for lithium, which is only approved for use in children over 12 years of age, none of the other anticonvulsants are approved for use in childhood. The authors stress that the evidence base for the use of mood stabilizers for the treatment of bipolar disorders in children and adolescents is sparse. According to these authors, valproate or lithium should be tried first for the treatment of nonpsychotic pediatric mania, and they consider olanzapine, quetiapine, or risperidone as alternative first-line treatments. The authors think that other anticonvulsants may be justified, when the first-line treatments are unsuccessful or tolerance problems emerge (pp. 31–32). The most significant concern with polypharmacy is the increased risk of medication related AEs (Zonfrillo et al., 2005, p. 18).

Lithium

The 2006 PDR contains no Black Boxes for lithium carbonate or its controlled-release forms, Eskalith-CR (pp. 1406–1408) or Lithobid. Short-term side effects include gastric irritability, nausea and vomiting, polyuria, and tremor. Small children are prone to reactivate enuresis, or become enuretic for the first time. Gastric irritability is one of the most common causes for lithium discontinuation in children.

Teratogenicity

Uncommon, Predictable, Potentially Serious
Lithium's teratogenic effects are no greater than those in placebo-controlled studies, and lithium is the medication of choice for pregnant bipolar manic patients.

Seizure Potential

Uncommon, Predictable, Potentially Serious

EEG abnormalities were found in nearly two thirds of patients treated with lithium, including background slowing with high-voltage anterior delta activity and a 17% risk of spike discharge. Recent use of lithium may contribute to the association found between EEG abnormalities and bipolar disorder (Centorrino et al., 2002, p. 114). Among commonly prescribed psychotropics for children and adolescents, lithium and bupropion are the most epileptogenic drugs.

Neurotoxicity

Uncommon, Predictable, Potentially Serious

Neurotoxicity, delirium, and encephalopathy have been described with lithium; concomitant ECT and neuroleptic medications increase this risk. Neurotoxicity is not necessarily associated with elevated lithium blood levels. It is suggested that patients with high levels of psychosis and anxiety are at a greater risk for neurotoxic reactions. Such reactions may be irreversible and neurological deficits (ataxia, movement disorders, memory problems, and fine motor deficits—slowing in performance rate) have been reported after lithium intoxication (Freeman, Wiegand, & Gelenberg, 2004, p. 555).

Tremor affects between 4% and 65% of patients receiving lithium. Tremor may decrease overtime. Severe tremor may indicate toxicity. Interestingly, elimination of caffeine makes the tremor worse because caffeine stimulates renal lithium clearance (p. 555).

Thyroid Problems

Common, Predictable, Remediable

Female patients and persons over 50 years of age are more likely to develop hypothyroidism with lithium treatment. In some studies, the rate of hypothyroidism is about 3.5% for males and about 15% for female, a fourfold gender difference. If the there is history of family hypothyroidism the risk of lithium-induced hypothyroidism is increased. Clinical practice mandates thyroid hormone supplementation if thyrotropin is increased (pp. 555–556).

Renal Dysfunction

Rare, Unpredictable, Feared, and Potentially Very Serious

Renal morbidity in lithium treated patients is rare; however, lithium may cause renal tubular damage. Renal concentration ability may get compromised with lithium use, and as a result patients may experience polyuria. No significant histopathological changes are observed in patients on long-term lithium therapy, except in those who had experienced acute lithium intoxication. Patients on therapeutic lithium levels, in long-term treatment, maintain glomerular function and renal clearance without significant impairment. Diabetes insipidus, caused by kidney lack of response to antidiuretic hormone, may develop in about 10% of patients in long-term lithium treatment. This complication may respond to thiazides or amiloride (p. 556). Creatinine should be measured every two to three months at therapy initiation, and thereafter, annually or semiannually in stable patients.

Cardiac Problems

Rare, Unpredictable, Potentially Serious

Sinus node dysfuction is more prevalent in patients who have taken lithium for at least a year. A-V block, T-wave abnormalities, and ventricular irritability have been reported. For further issues related to lithium side effects and drug interactions.[1]

Valproate Side Effects

Valproate has been associated with better tolerability than lithium in the treatment of bipolar disorders. Valproate is less likely than other anticonvulsants to cause cognitive impairment. Valproate does not cause renal disease, extrapyramidal side effects, thyroid, cardiac, dermatological, or allergic effects (Bowden, 2004, p. 574). Cognitive dulling may be dose related and is less frequent than with lithium (p. 575).

The 2006 PDR contains identical Black Box warnings for the following valproate brands: Depacon (valproate sodium injection, p. 412), Depakene (valproic acid, p. 417), Depakote sprinkle capsules (p. 422), Depakote tablets (divalproex sodium, p. 427), and Depakote-ER (divalproex sodium extended release tablets, pp. 433).

Hepatotoxicity

Uncommon, Unpredictable, Potentially Serious

Hepatic failure resulting in fatalities has been reported with valproate. Children under the age of 2 are at considerable risk, more so if they are on multiple anticonvulsants. Liver function tests should be performed prior to the initiation of treatment and at frequent intervals thereafter. The prevalence of hepatic failure is about 1 in 50,000 cases. No hepatic fatalities have been reported on persons over 10 years of age. Valproate induces a hepatocellular liver injury with predominant elevation of alanine aminotransferase (ALT); in cholestatic liver injury, the alkaline phosphatase (ALP) is predominantly elevated, and in mixed liver injury, both ALT and ALP are elevated. Liver injury is defined as ALT level of three times or more of the upper normal range, and ALP of more than twice the upper normal range, or total bilirubin (TBL) of more that twice the upper normal range if associated with elevations of ALT and ALP (Navarro & Senior, 2006, p. 731).

Teratogenicity

Uncommon, Predictable, Potentially Serious
Valproate has been associated with neural-tube defects (e.g., spina bifida). Prevalence is estimated at about 1 to 1.5% in childbearing women. Multivitamins with trace elements and folic acid are recommended in childbearing women on valproate.

Pancreatitis

Rare, Unpredictable, Potentially Fatal
Rapid, progressive, hemorrhagic pancreatitis in children and adults has been associated with valproate, and it is contraindicated in urea cycle disorders (UCD). Valproate may produce hyperamonemia (despite normal liver function tests), and thrombocytopenia (levels above 100 mcg/ml increase this risk) (PDR, 2006, pp. 418, 423, 429, 435). Valproate may be lethal when taken in overdose.

Common Side Effects

Gastrointestinal irritation: nausea, dyspepsia, vomiting, diarrhea. Valproate is better tolerated that lithium carbonate and is easier on the upper GI tract than the less irritating extended-release lithium salts: Lithobid, and Eskalith–CR.

Tiredness and drowsiness. The new presentation, the extended-release form, Depakote ER, given once a day, at bedtime, bypasses this problem

Benign elevations of hepatic transaminases are reported.

Weight gain. About 57% of adult patients on valproate gain weight. In children, about 40% of patients in valproate gain weight (Benbadis & Wilner, 2005, p. 89). Patients with low BMIs gain more weight than patients with normal or greater BMIs. The weight increase may be greater with certain combinations of medications: lithium, atypical antipsychotics, and others.

Reduction of platelets and low WBC count may represent a response to high levels of valproate. Reduction of the dose may increase the platelets and the WBC count (p. 89).

Hair loss may be temporary and greater in women than in men. Multivitamins containing selenium may be helpful. See endnote for other issues related to valproate side effects.[2]

Carbamazepine Side Effects

The 2006 PDR contains the same Black Box warnings for all the carbamazepine brands, Tegretol and Tegretol-XR (pp. 2278–2279).

Aplastic Anemia, Agranulocytosis

Rare, Unpredictable, Feared, and Potentially Fatal
The risk of this complication is five to eight times greater than in the general population. Risk in the untreated general population is about six cases per million per year for aplastic anemia. The vast majority of cases with leucopenia do not progress to the more serious condition of aplastic anemia or agranulocytosis. Because of the very low incidence of agranulocytosis and aplastic anemia, the vast majority of minor hematologic changes observed in patients on Tegretol, are unlikely to signal the occurrence of either abnormality. Discontinuation of the drug should be considered if there is any significant evidence of bone marrow suppression. CBZ side effects are the reason for medication discontinuation in more than 22% of patients. In this regard, CBZ fares worse than lithium in some studies (Ketter, Wang, & Post, 2004, p. 590). Early in therapy and before autoinduction, at high doses, CBZ produces neurotoxicity (sedation, ataxia, diplopia, and nystagmus). Dizziness, ataxia, and diplopia emerging one to two hours after a CBZ dose, is an indication that the adverse effect threshold has been crossed and that a change in the schedule or a reduction of medication is required (p. 591).

Common Side Effects

Dermatologic: Common, Unpredictable, Nonserious with Discontinuation
Rash. A morbiliform rash may evolve in 1 of 10 patients. The rash tends to reappear promptly after the medication is rechallenged. Between 25 and 30% of patients who develop a rash with CBZ, will also develop the rash when switched to OXC. Rarely this rash is the prelude of Stevens-Johnson syndrome. A rash presenting with systemic illness or with involvement of the eyes, mouth, or bladder constitutes a medical emergency and mandates immediate CBZ discontinuation (p. 591).

Hematologic: Rare, Unpredictable, Potentially Fatal
A benign leucopenia is common. CBZ should be discontinued if the WBC falls below 3000 and the absolute neutrophil count falls below 1000 to 1500/mm3. Agranulocytosis and aplastic anemia have been reported at a frequency of 1 in 10,000 to 1 in 100,000 patients. Adding lithium may improve the WBC indices. Patients should be alerted to development of fever, sore throat, oral ulcers, petechiae, and easy bruising or bleeding. Most of the serious hematological reactions occur in the first three months of therapy. Blood and hepatic indices

should be monitored at two, four, six, and eight weeks of CBZ initiation, and every three months, thereafter.

Hepatotoxicity: Rare, Unpredictable, Potentially Serious
Patients should be medically evaluated if they develop malaise, abdominal pain, or other serious gastrointestinal symptoms. CBZ should be discontinued if liver enzymes reach threefold the upper limit of the normal range.

Cardiovascular: Rare, Unpredictable, Potentially Serious
CBZ may affect heart conduction.

Endocrinologic and Other Effects: Rare, Unpredictable, Potentially Serious
CBZ is less likely than lithium to promote weight gain. It may induce hyponatremia. CBZ increases HDL and total cholesterol, and also decreases T4, free T4 index, and less consistently, T3, but rarely induces hypothyroidism. CBZ is teratogenic. Mothers on CBZ treatment should be discouraged from breastfeeding. Carbamazepine may render oral contraceptives ineffective. For further issues related to CBZ side effects and cytochrome induction.[3]

Oxcarbazepine Side Effects

The 2006 PDR contains no Black Box warnings for Trileptal (oxcarbazepine, pp. 2281–2286). However, a letter from the manufacturer, Novartis, dated April 18, 2005, alerts the medical community to an important drug warning regarding Trileptal. The updated warning calls physicians' attention to serious dermatological reactions, including Stevens-Johnson syndrome (SJS) and toxic epidermal necrolysis (TEN) reported in children and adults in association with Trileptal use. The potential for dermatological reactions has been added to the warning section of the prescribing information. The manufacturer indicates that the frequency of these serious skin reactions exceeds the estimated rates in general population by a factor of 3 to 10. The background incidence in the general population is in the range of 0.5 to 6 cases per million person years. Also, in the section of precautions, a new heading, "Multi-Organ Hypersensitivity," was added. OXC has yielded comparable anticonvulsant efficacy as CBZ and VPA; its side effect profile is comparable to VPA and more favorable than CBZ. OXC's side effect profile in bipolar patients is less known. OXC appears to yield less neurotoxicity and rash than CBZ. OXC has not been associated with blood dyscrasias (Ketter et al., 2004, p. 592). OXC may induce untoward GI effects and may increase hepatic transaminases, but seems to have less effect on lipids. Weight increase with OXC is less than with VPA.

Hyponatremia is more common with OXC than with CBZ. It is likely that OXC has effects on the thyroid indices. OXC above 900 mg/day, increased testosterone and gonadotropin levels in normal male volunteers. OXC may decrease the effectiveness of hormonal contraceptives. It is considered that OXC is less teratogenic (p. 593).

There are three major areas of difference between CBZ and OXC:

1. OXC is a modest enzymatic inducer but may also reduce serum concentrations of certain medications, diminishing their clinical effects. OXC induces heteroinduction, not autoinduction. Most of the metabolic induction effects are not clinically significant except for effects on hormonal contraceptives (p. 598).
2. OXC is rarely affected by enzyme inhibitors (OXC is primarily metabolized by arylketone reductase).
3. OXC metabolite, MHD is not inhibited by VPA, contrary to VPA inhibition of CBZ-E, which may render that metabolite toxic. OXC does not induce VPA metabolism (pp. 598–599).

Lamotrigine Side Effects

The 2006 PDR contains a bold Black Box warning for Lamictal (lamotrigene; p. 1449). Serious rashes, including Stevens-Johnson syndrome (SJS), have been reported in association with lamotrigene treatment. Incidence of SJS is approximately 8 cases per 1,000 (0.8%) in pediatric patients (below 16 years of age). In a prospectively followed cohort of 1,983 pediatric patients with epilepsy, there was one rash-related death in worldwide post marketing experience; underreporting is likely.

Other than age, there are as yet no factors identified that are known to predict the risk of severe rashes. It has been suggested that coadministration of lamotrigene with valproate, exceeding initial recommended doses, or exceeding the recommended dose escalation, may increase the risk. Nearly all life-threatening rashes occur during the initial two to eight weeks of treatment. Lamotrigene may also be associated with benign rashes; currently, it is impossible to distinguish a benign rash from a malignant one; as such, discontinuation of medication is advised at the first evidence of rash. Discontinuation of the drug does not stop the rash from becoming life threatening or avoid the development of a permanent and disfiguring condition.

In controlled monotherapy treatments of lamotrigene in patients for mood disorders, lamotrigene was associated with headaches, sleep disturbances, nausea, and vomiting. Although rash prevalence with lamotrigene did not exceed the prevalence seen with placebo, rash is considered as the side effect that is most likely to complicate the drug's clinical use. In more than 3,500 patients, rash was observed in 10% of patients on lamotrigene and 5% in patients on placebo. Lamotrigene caused drug discontinuation in 3.8% of patients and hospitalization in 0.3% of treated patients due to Stevens-Johnson syndrome and toxic epidermal necrolysis. Apparently, the rate of serious rashes has decreased over the years, mostly due to a decrease of the initial dose (Shelton & Calabrese, 2004, p. 619).

The serious lamotrigene rash is confluent, with predominant face and neck involvement; the rash may be tender, purpuric, or even hemorrhagic, and is accompanied or preceded by fever, malaise, pharyngitis, anorexia, or lymphadenopathy. Any rash with features suggestive of a serious reaction necessitates an immediate drug cessation and close monitoring of hepatic, renal, and hematologic involvement (p. 622). The rash may be prevented by a very slow titration schedule and by avoiding coadministration with valproate, which increases lamotrigene t1/2 from 25.4 hours to 69.6 hours (p. 624).

ATYPICAL ANTIPSYCHOTICS: SIDE EFFECTS

A number of typical and atypical antipsychotics increase the QTc interval and augment the risk for torsade de pointes (TdP) and ventricular arrhythmias.

Cardiovascular Risk

QT relates to the time lapse from the beginning of the QRS until the end of the T-wave; this corresponds to the ventricular systole. The QT is a good indicator of repolarization and involves sodium, calcium, and potassium channels. It is potassium channels that are considered the most relevant in drug-induced arrhythmias. The QT measurements are corrected for the heart rate; this is the so-called QTc. Computer generated QTc values may be inaccurate (Stubbe & Scahill, 2002, p. 7). See issues with OTc measurements in the Ziprasidone section of chapter 12.

QTc Prolongation

Rare, Unpredictable, Potentially Fatal
The upper limits of normal (ULN) of QTc duration for children and adolescents have been reformulated, and currently are described as 450 msec for males, and 460 msec for females. A QTc equal or greater than 500 msec, or a prolongation greater than 60 msec, both predict risk for TdP. When the medication-induced prolongation is equal or greater than 10% of the QTc baseline duration, further studies are needed. The computerized reading failed to classify QTc prolongation in 6 of 10 subjects with QTc duration equal or greater than 460 msc (Labellarte, Crosson, & Riddle, 2003, p. 643).[4]

Stubbe and Scahill (2002) recommend that the EKGs should be read by clinicians well trained in QTc calculations. They also advise pediatric cardiological consultation if the baseline EKG is abnormal, if there is history of syncope or dizzy spells, or when there is a family history of sudden death (p. 12).[5] Some antipsychotics impact heart conduction and increase the risk of arrhythmias and sudden death; more so if there is coprescription of other drugs that prolong the QTc.[6]

The QT interval changes with the time of the day (nighttime intervals are about 20 msec longer than daytime ones). In addition, QTc is about 20 msec shorter for male adolescents than for females (Vieweg & McDaniel, 2003a, p. 5); patients with a history of cardiovascular disease have longer intervals than those without this history (p. 6).

Stressors and the heart rate also prolong the QTc. If the QTc is prolonged beyond a certain threshold, repolarization may occur simultaneously with depolarization, causing ventricular arrhythmias (TdP) that can degenerate into ventricular tachycardia, fibrillation, and death (Wirshing, Danovitch, Erhart, Pierre, & Wirshing, 2003, p. 54).

A prolonged QT interval may be congenital or acquired. Ventricular arrhythmia is the most frequent cause of syncope and sudden death related to prolonged QTc associated with medications. The QTc prolongation is due to a blockade of the potassium channels preventing potassium from flowing out of the cells (Stubbe & Scahill, 2002, p. 7). The acquired prolonged QT interval may be caused by a number of factors, including electrolytic abnormalities (hypokalemia, hypocalcemia, or hypomagnesemia), metabolic or endocrine disturbances, or be induced by a number of medications; females are at a higher risk for this complication (p. 7). Other factors that increase this risk include potassium depletion, reduced cardiac ejection fraction, toxins, and CNS insult. Currently, the QTc is the best available predictor for assessing risk for potentially fatal arrhythmias (Stubbe & Scahill, 2002, p. 10).

Long QT syndrome (LQTS) is a congenital condition that should be suspected in all patients who present with a history of syncope, particularly if it is recurrent or associated with exercise or pain. Often these episodes are precipitated by intense emotion, loud noises, or vigorous exercise. Hereditary LQTS should be investigated in children with seizures of unknown origin, near drowning, congenital deafness, or bradycardia, and in those with affected family members or a family history of SIDS, syncope, seizures, or sudden death (Friedman, Mull, Sharieff, & Tsarouhas, 2003) (see related sudden death syndromes).[7]

Thus, congenital LQTS is an important cause of morbidity and mortality among youth (Vieweg & McDaniel, 2003c, p. 3). Beta-blockers are the recommended first-line therapy for this condition; additional treatments may include ablative surgery or implantation of a pacemaker or cardiac defibrillator. Patients with LQTS should be restricted from competitive sports, encouraged to drink electrolyte-enriched fluids during exercise, and advised to avoid loud noises and emotional stress (Friedman et al., 2003). Nine percent of pediatric LQTS patients present with sudden cardiac death. More than 70% of these patients will die within 15 years if not treated (Vieweg & McDaniels, 2003a, p. 7).

Pimozide and droperidol also have a considerable TdP risk. Because of prior extensive use, haloperidol has the most literature reports of association with TdP (Vieweg & McDaniel, 2003d, pp. 2–3). There are no reports of clozapine-associated TdP, but this product has a box warning regarding myocarditis. There are a number of reports related to risperidone-associated TdP and sudden death (p. 3). Olanzapine does not appear to be associated with TdP. Quetiapine is associated with TdP reports. Medications that inhibit CyP450 3A4 are particularly problematic when coprescribed with quetiapine. To date, there have been no reports of ziprasidone-associated TdP. In spite of this, a rigorous compliance with the package insert is recommended (pp. 3–4).

The ranking of propensity for QTc prolongation is as follows: ziprasidone, clozapine > quetiapine > risperidone > olanzapine > aripiprazole (Strakowski, 2003b, p. 57).

A number of medications become deadly when given in combination. For example, pimozide, which increases the QTc in a dose dependent manner, is a 3A4 substrate; when combined with clarithromycin or other macrolide antibiotics or other 3A4 inhibitors like nefazodone, a strong 3A4 inhibitor, TdP may ensue due to the increasing blood levels of pimozide caused by the 3A4 metabolic inhibition. Other contributions to this fatal combination stems from the fact that clarithromycin also prolongs the QTc, thus causing an additive QTc interval prolongation (Sandson, 2003, p. 38). Even the innocuous grapefruit (which inhibits 3A4 and 1A2 systems, among others) may bring about disastrous consequences when interacting with medication that prolongs the QTc interval (p. 52). The propensity to develop TdP, and the accompanying patient morbidity and mortality, were the primary reasons that the antihistamines terfenadine and astemizol (Hismanal) and the promotility agent cisapride (Propulsid) were removed from the U.S. market in recent years. Thioridazine (Melleril), mesoridazine (Serentil), and pimozide (Orap) may well follow the same fate in future years (p. 92). The risk of QTc prolongation is increased when there is drug interaction among the medications prescribed. For instance, clomipramine (CMI) uses the 3A4 metabolic pathway; erythromycin, a broad-spectrum antibiotic, is a potent blocker of the 3A4 system. The addition of erythromycin to a person being treated with CMI may result in a dramatic increase in the levels of clomipramine, with potentially toxic side effects. Persons with genetic deficits in a particular metabolic pathway are at a higher risk of reaching potential toxic levels due to the lack of enzymatic capacity (7 to 10% of Caucasians, and 1 to 3% of Asians have a genetic deficiency of the cytocrome 2D6 enzyme). On the other hand, there is group of people with overactive enzymatic systems that require higher medication doses (Wirshing, Danovitch, Erhart, Pierre, & Wirshing, 2003, p. 54).

TABLE 13.4 Elements in the Evaluation of QTc Prolongation

- 12-lead EKG
- Measurement of K, Mg, Ca, and thyroid hormone
- Cardiac history
- Personal/family history of syncope or sudden death
- Palpitations, presyncope plus QTc prolongation are grounds for an immediate referral to a cardiologist.

Source: Vieweg & McDaniel (2003c, p. 3).

Elements included in the valuation of QTc prolongation are listed in table 13.4.

For the new generation of antipsychotic medications (risperidone, olanzapine, quetiapine, ziprasidone, and aripiprazole) administered to children, a baseline EKG is recommended. Accepted threshold parameters are:

- PR interval of less than 200 msc
- QRS interval of less than 120 msc
- QTc interval of less than 450 msc.[8]

When the steady-state antipsychotic drug dose is reached, the EKG should be repeated, and interval measurements obtained to insure that they have not significantly changed (Vieweg & McDaniel, 2003c, p. 2). Zareba and Lin (2003) advise a more conservative approach for patients with QTc baseline interval equal or greater than 450 ms:

- Patients with QTc equal or greater than 450 ms are likely to develop pro-arrhythmias.
- These patients need repeated EKG after a first dose of antipsychotic medication and then at steady state. In the case of QTc > 0.50 sec on a drug or a combination of drugs, the drug needs to be replaced with another one (or other ones) without QTc prolongation effects, confirmed by the same type of EKG testing.
- If there is a likelihood of drug–drug interaction, additional EKG monitoring will be required (if another drug affecting an ion channel or acting through the same hepatic metabolic pathway is added or a currently introduced antipsychotic drug is added on top of such a drug).
- These patients should have careful monitoring of magnesium and potassium since hypokalemia and hypomagenesemia (caused by vomiting or diarrhea) may aggravate QTc prolongation (p. 303).

To reiterate, QT prolongation syndrome commonly has a history of syncope, dizzy spells, and sudden death (p. 303). Of greater concern is the recently recognized Brugada syndrome, characterized by an EKG pattern of right bundle branch block and ST segment elevation in the right precordials with normal QTc duration. This congenital syndrome is more than three times more common than the LQTS and is associated with sudden death due to ventricular tachycardia (including TdP). Typically, this syndrome is present in Caucasians and Asian men. Ventricular fibrillation is the most commonly documented terminal arrhythmia. The mortality rate for this syndrome may be as high as 6.7%. Antipsychotics, as well as TCAs, may induce the Brugada syndrome. The syndrome may be sufficiently incapacitating to warrant heart transplantation as a last treatment resort (Vieweg & McDaniel, 2003b, p. 4).

Medications of all classes may affect cardiac conduction (cisapride, terfenidine). Tricyclic antidepressants (desipramine and imipramine) are clearly associated with cardiac conduction delays, and at least seven deaths in young patients have been linked to their use (p. 4). Thioridazine and other typical and atypical antipsychotics also increase the QTc interval and are known to have caused sudden death.[9]

There are other medications seldom considered as potential inducers of TdP. Among these are flextime, the R isomere of citalopram (R citalopram), and methadone, which have the potential for increasing the QTc interval in persons with other cardiovascular risks (Vieweg & McDaniel, 2003b, pp. 4, 5).

All atypicals prolong the QT interval to some degree by reducing the flow of repolarizing K+ currents, making the myocardium more excitable. There is a very low risk of arrhythmia development with QTc intervals below 450 ms. In fact, atypicals behave like type III antiarrhythmics and overdrive the ventricle, and suppress other emerging ventricular arrhythmias (Wirshing et al., 2003, p. 54).

Physicians are not careful enough to avoid coprescriptions that may increase the risk for catastrophic arrhythmias in person already receiving medications with proarrythmic potential.[10] See endnote for medications likely to increase the QTc interval.[11] Families should be warned of potential medication side effects and of the medications that need to be avoided (macrolide antibiotics, antidepressants, antifungal, and others), as well as being informed of the risks of herbals and over-the-counter products that may inhibit the P450 system. Psychiatrists need to collaborate closely with family practitioners, pediatricians and other specialists to avoid combination of medications with potential toxic side effects.

In summary, it is difficult to choose an antipsychotic drug in common use that does not have adverse cardiac side effects. Treatment resistance and extrapyramidal side effects have led to increased use of atypical antipsychotics despite the fact that their nonneuropsychiatric adverse effect profile (e.g., body weight gain, cardiovascular and anticholinergic effects) is not better and often worse than the conventional antipsychotic drugs (Buckley & Sanders, 2000, p. 225).

Unfortunately, thioridazine is not the only medicine with potential lethality. The literature suggests that all currently available antipsychotics have electro-physiological properties that are likely to increase the risk of sudden death. There are case reports of TdP and sudden death for most of the antipsychotic drugs. Thus, until there is substantially more evidence, it would be prudent to assume that all the available antipsychotics have the potential to increase the risk of serious ventricular arrhythmias and, thus, sudden cardiac deaths (Ray & Meador, 2002, p. 483).[12]

Although, not germane to the child and adolescent psychiatric populations, recent concerns with increased stroke and mortality with the use of atypicals in demented elderly, highlight the added cardiovascular risks associated with SGAs.

SUDDEN DEATH: RARE, POTENTIALLY PREDICTABLE

Epidemiological studies indicate that exposure to antipsychotic medications is associated with sudden death. The association is valid for current use, not for past use. Sudden cardiac risk was the highest among patients receiving butyrophenone antipsychotics, mainly pipamperone and haloperidol, even at low doses (Straus et al., 2004, 1295). Sudden cardiac death is associated with antipsychotic use rather than with schizophrenia itself. This risk is fourfold and remains high throughout long-term use (p. 1297). Sudden death commonly occurs in patients between 10 and 35 years of age, particularly during exercise even in patients with only mild obstruction hypertrophic obstructive cardiomyopathy (HOC). The incidence of sudden death is 4 to 6% a year in children and adolescents and 2 to 4% a year in adults. Even brief episodes of asymptomatic ventricular tachycardia on ambulatory EKG may be a risk factor (Park, 2002, p. 272).[13]

Cardiovascular factors are not the sole cause of sudden death risk; metabolic complications, diabetic ketoacetotic crisis (DKA; even in persons who are not hyperglycemic), acute pancreatitis, and other acute illnesses (hematologic, hepatic, and others) may promote a fulminating death. Nasrallah and Newcomer (2004), assert that the best means for prevention and early detection of DKA and pancreatitis are regular laboratory screenings and being on alert for signs and symptoms of polyuria, polydipsia, mental status changes, and acute abdominal symptoms (like pain, nausea, vomiting, and others) (p. S11).

Regarding sudden death, Koller, Cross, Doraiswamy, et al. (2003) alert physicians about the incidence of pancreatitis associated with atypical antipsychotics. This pharmacovigilance study, based on spontaneously reported adverse events, and likely to suffer from underreporting, uncovered 192 cases of pancreatitis associated with antipsychotic use: 22 patients died. Most of the cases of pancreatitis occurred within six months of antipsychotic initiation. The association was of 40, 33, 16, and 12% for clozapine, olanzapine, risperidone, and haloperidol treatments, respectively (p. 1123). Only 23% of the patients had received valproate concomitantly; some had received valproate for extended periods of time without experiencing difficulties (p. 1129).[14]

Of pertinent relevance for child psychiatrists, 10 pediatric patients (less than 18 years of age) were affected; 4 patients were treated with olanzapine, 3 with risperidone, 1 with clozapine, 1 with haloperidol, and 1 with a combination of clozapine and haloperidol (p. 1126). A 15-year-old died because of direct complications of pancreatitis (p. 1127).

Sudden Death and Physical Restraint

Extreme care should be exercised in restraining patients with underlying cardiac pathology. Persons, who ultimately experience sudden death, display a state of "excited delirium or an endogenous acute psychotic episode" preceding the restraint (Dimaio & Dimaio, 2001). Deaths usually occur after the restraint hold has been applied. "Immediately after the struggle ends, the individual becomes unresponsive, develops cardiopulmonary arrest and does not respond to cardiopulmonary resuscitation...[sudden death] invariably occurs after the struggle (physical restraint) has ended" (pp. 500, 502). During correctly applied restraint techniques, respiratory related deaths (asphyxiation) rarely occur. This is in agreement with Dimaio and Dimaio: "While virtually all deaths in manic delirium are probably caused by the physiological reactions to a violent struggle (with or without the interaction of illegal drugs), in occasional cases positional asphyxia may play a role in a death" (p. 504). Persons who die after the struggle of a restraint have "an underlying physiological lesion of the conduction system of the heart (Wolf-Parkinson-White syndrome, prolonged QT syndrome, or others) [that] predisposes them to develop an arrythmia" (p. 503). Fatal arrythmias are precipitated by a catecholamine release and the prolonged hypokalemia (lasting 90 minutes or more) that ensues from the physical struggle during the restraint. "This period has been referred [to]...as the time of post-exercise peril, in that there is a risk of cardiac arrythmias during this period" (p. 501). Patients who are under the influence of illegal drugs (e.g., cocaine or amphetamines), are at an increased risk of developing arrythmogenic effects during a restraint-related struggle. The psychiatrist and the restraining team need to exercise judgment and maximal care during these high-risk situations. Atypical antipsychotics may also contribute to the fatal event since these medications may have been used before as primary treatments, and are commonly added as prn drugs in cases of agitation and are administered before or concomitantly with the physical intervention.

Sudden death has been associated with both conventional antipsychotics and with clozapine. The etiology of the cause of death in these contexts is not clear; it is probably secondary to ventricular arrythmia. It may be associated with sudden increase of clozapine dose; clozapine increase should not exceed more than 50 mg every two days (Marder & Wirshing, 2004, p. 449). Also, it is safe to assume that every severely obese patient may have an underlying cardiomyopathy and that they may develop cardiac arrhythmias during a physical restraint.

WEIGHT GAIN: COMMON, PREDICTABLE, POTENTIALLY SERIOUS

Antipsychotics may act on the hypothalamic feeding center and stimulate the appetite directly. Antagonism of serotonin (5-HT2C) or histamine (H1) and other receptors and neurotransmitters may play a role in antipsychotic-related weight gain (Nguyen, Yu, & Maguire, 2003, p. 59).

Agents that stimulate the 5-HT2C receptors such as fenfluramine and M-chlorophenyl-piperazine have been associated with weight loss; agents that antagonize these receptors are thought to increase appetite and to cause weight gain. Agents that antagonize the histamine receptor induce weight gain, and there is an exponential relationship between the antipsychotics' H1 affinity and the potential for inducing weight gain. Clozapine and olanzapine have strong affinity for 5-HT2C and H1 receptors; these atypicals are the greatest promoters of weight gain among antipsychotics (Nguyen et al., 2003, p. 59). Clinical trials have shown convincingly that atypical antipsychotics pose a greater risk of weight gain and central adiposity than do most of the older typical antipsychotics (Wirshing et al, 2003, p. 49).

Peripheral antagonism of H1 receptors appears to interfere with satiety signals; affinity to histamine H1 receptors is strongly correlated with weight gain potential (Wirshing et al., 2003, p. 50). Weight gain is associated with increased morbidity and mortality in a wide range of conditions, including hypertension, coronary heart disease, cerebrovascular disease, type 2 diabetes mellitus, various cancers, sleep apnea, and respiratory problems (Brecher, Rak, Melvin, & Jones, 2000, p. 288). Weight gain causes negative psychosocial stress and may compromise compliance.

The higher the BMI, the greater the risk of sudden death, cerebrovascular accident, and congestive heart failure in both sexes (Amatruda & Linemeyer, 2001, p. 952). The ratio of waist girth to hip girth is significantly associated with diabetes, hypertension, and gallbladder disease in women 40 to 59 and with menstrual abnormalities in women 30 to 39 years old, even in women with comparable total body fat.

Obese individuals with high waist–hip ratios show decreased hepatic extraction of insulin, higher posthepatic insulin levels, and more insulin resistance (p. 953). Clozapine and olanzapine are associated with the greatest weight gain, followed by risperidone, ziprasidone (and aripiprazole); reports on quetiapine have been inconsistent. Weight gain associated with quetiapine, risperidone, and ziprasidone tends to plateau within the first few months, whereas patients on clozapine or olanzapine may tend to continue gaining weight for 9 months or more (p. 50). In the CATIE report (Lieberman, Stroup, et al., 2005), cited above, patients on quetiapine gained more weight than patients on risperidone (p. 1220).

There is considerable evidence, particularly in patients with schizophrenia, that treatment with SGAs can cause a rapid increase in body weight in the first few months of therapy and that it may not reach a plateau even after one year of treatment (Consensus Development Conference, 2004, p. 597). Adolescents and young adults are particularly susceptible to antipsychotic induced weight gain. Adolescents are particularly susceptible to metabolic dysregulation; extreme weight gain (> 7% baseline body mass) for olanzapine and risperidone was observed in adolescent inpatients, and extreme weight gain was seen in 78% of patients of an adolescent group (for 6 months the weight gain averaged 1.2 kg/month without leveling off). Risperidone's apparent metabolic advantage for adults does not seem to be present for children and adolescents. Risperidone's effect on prolactin may explain this metabolic disturbance. Children and adolescents have an exquisite end-organ sensitivity related to prolactin levels (Wirshing et al, 2003, p. 50).

The extent of weight gain reported is indeed worrisome, if not alarming. During 12 weeks of follow-up, 19 of the 21 (90.5%) patients treated with olanzapine, and 9 of the 21 (42.9%) patients treated with risperidone showed a 7% increase of weight, which is considered extreme weight gain. The relative average increase of weight was 11.1% in the olanzapine group and 6.6% in the risperidone group. The average absolute weight gain for olanzapine and risperidone was 7.2 kg and 3.9 kg, respectively. The rates were 1.5 (olanzapine) and 1.9 (risperidone) times higher than the rates reported in adults. Olanzapine may have caused more robust weight gain because of its combined 5-HT2C and histamine-1 antagonistic effects. Risperidone exerts mostly 5-HT2C inhibitory and a weak H1 antagonistic effect. Male gender was a prominent risk factor, with significantly more males (67.7%) than females (42.1%) showing extreme weight gain. Concerns about weight gain were particularly higher for those subjects with lower baseline weight; they gained more weight during treatment with atypical antipsychotics than did patients with a higher BMI. Neither efficacy of the neuroleptic treatment (change in PANSS) nor its dosages was associated with the proportional weight gain (Ratzoni et al., 2002, pp. 341–342). The CATIE study, in adults, confirmed that olanzapine poses serious heath risks; olanzapine was the most weight promoting and, in this regard, the most toxic of the SGAs studied, and was associated with a greater increase in glycosylated hemoglobin, total cholesterol, and triglycerides (Lieberman, Stroup, et al, 2005, p. 1215).

The ranking of atypicals regarding weight gain induction in children and adolescents is: clozapine > olanzapine > risperidone > quetiapine > aripiprazole ≥ ziprasidone.[15] Loss of weight is very difficult, even in highly motivated persons.[16] Obesity is related to multiple health risks and to a higher prevalence of psychiatric disorders in children and adolescents (Mustillo et al., 2003). The American Academy of Pediatrics has advised the membership to take a more active role in stemming the increasing prevalence of obesity in childhood and adolescence. Child psychiatrists can contribute to identification and management of this complex and vexing problem. Obesity is a major source of multiple heath risks, and a major factor in self-esteem difficulties. Obesity is clearly associated with an increased incidence of depression and anxiety disorders, school and vocational difficulties. Obese children have a higher risk of suicide. The importance of taking detailed family and medical histories and of identifying risk factors for obesity and diabetes mellitus should not be underemphasized (detecting acanthosis nigricans, as a marker for DM, etc). Barnhill proposes an aggressive treatment of obesity (2001). For an overview of the treatment of obesity, see chapter 14.

METABOLIC SIDE EFFECTS: UNCOMMON, PREDICTABLE, POTENTIALLY SERIOUS

The combination of obesity, hyperinsulinemia, insulin resistance, hypertension, and a predisposition to noninsulin dependent diabetes mellitus is postulated to be part of a common metabolic abnormality caused by a combination of hyperinsulinemia and insulin resistance (Amatruda & Linemeyer, 2001, p. 953). Paradoxically, "in circumstances of chronic hyperinsulinemia such as obesity, relatively less insulin can be available to the CNS as an adiposity signal" (Figlewicz, 2003, p. 83). Waist measurements of 102 cm (> 40 inches) in men and 88 cm (> 35 inches) in women are indicative of a component of the metabolic syndrome and are strong predictors of diabetes and other medical complications, including heart disease and sleep apnea (Marder & Wirshing, 2004, p. 449). The higher the BMI at age 18, the greater the risk for the development of diabetes with any additional weight gain. As expected, weight gain also increases the risk if there is a family history of type 2 diabetes (Amatruda & Linemeyer, 2001, p. 954).

DIABETES MELLITUS (DM): UNCOMMON, PREDICTABLE, POTENTIALLY SERIOUS

Numerous case reports have documented the onset and exacerbation of diabetes, including the occurrence of hyperglycemic crisis, following initiation

TABLE 13.5 Risk Factors for Type 2 Diabetes

- Family history of diabetes
- High-risk ethnicity:
  American Indian, African American, Hispanic American, Asian, or South Pacific Islander
- Insulin resistance or conditions associated with insulin resistance:
  Acanthosis nigricans, hypertension, dyslipidemia, or polycystic ovarian syndrome

Source: Carlson, Sowell & Cavazzoni (2003, p. 6).

of treatment with SGAs. Several of these events occurred within a few weeks of initiation of SGA treatment (Consensus Development Conference, 2004, p. 598). The risk of type 2 diabetes increases with weight gain; it is not a surprise then, that diabetes is more prevalent among patients taking atypicals (Wirshing et al., 2003, p. 50). All atypicals were associated with a significant increase in diabetes risk in patients younger than 40. It is likely that, besides the effects on weight, atypicals may alter insulin and glucose metabolism (p. 51). Table 13.5 indicates risk factors for the development of DM.

Chronic psychiatric illness is by itself a significant risk for DM. More than 15% of medication naïve patients with schizophrenia had impaired fasting glucose tolerance, compared to none in a matched healthy comparison group. Patients with higher fasting plasma levels of glucose, insulin, and cortisol were more insulin resistant than the healthy matched subjects (Ryan, Collins, & Thakore, 2003, p. 286). Furthermore, in patients with schizophrenia, fasting concentration of plasma glucose correlated positively with the waist–hip ratio, waist circumference, BMI, plasma triglyceride level, and age (p. 286). This study and others suggest that the illness of schizophrenia (and probably others) is associated with aspects of the metabolic syndrome; this explains why patients with this illness die prematurely (p. 288). Table 13.6 contains a list of factors that increase the risk for the development of DM.

TABLE 13.6 Factors that Increase the Risk for the Development of Diabetes Mellitus

1. Family history of diabetes mellitus
2. Recent weight changes, polyuria, and polydipsia
3. Habitual inactivity
4. Ethnicity
   African American
   Asian American
   Hispanic American
   Native American (Pimia Indians)
   Pacific Islanders
5. BMI > 25, waist circumference > 35 inches for women, and > 40 Inches for men.
6. Having delivered a baby of more than 9 pounds and/or history of gestational diabetes.
7. History of hypertension
8. HDL cholesterol that is ≤ 35 mg/dl, and/or a triglyceride level of 250 (or more) mg/dl
9. Fasting glucose > 126 mg/dl, random glucose > 200 mg/dl or an abnormal findings in the glucose tolerance test, or hemoglobin A1c > 6.1 %

Clozapine and haloperidol were associated with significant elevation of mean glucose levels after eight weeks of treatment; olanzapine was associated with significant elevation with glucose levels after 14 weeks of treatment. Risperidone was not associated with glucose level changes. Fourteen percent of patients (6 given clozapine, 4 given olanzapine, 3 given risperidone, and 1 given haloperidol), developed abnormally high levels of glucose (>125 mg/dl) during the course of treatment. Changes in glucose levels were independent of weight increase: the highest association was present in olanzapine treated patients followed by clozapine and risperidone. In a small number of patients (7) with preexisting diabetes, antipsychotic treatment did not have a deleterious effect on glucose metabolism. There was a rate of 14% of diabetes in this study. This corresponds to double the rate in the U.S. population (Lindenmayer et al., 2003, p. 294). The overall annual diabetes mellitus incidence rate of 4.4%, in patients with schizophrenia on a stable regime of antipsychotic monotherapy, was considerably higher (about eightfold) than the estimated rate of 0.63% in the general U.S. population (Leslie & Rosenheck, 2004, p, 1710).

Differences in diabetes mellitus risk across antipsychotic medications did not become apparent until 14 months after the end of the stable period. Hence, the additional diabetes mellitus risk associated with clozapine and olanzapine took more than a year to develop. This interval should offer ample time for clinicians to identify weight gain and/or elevated diabetes mellitus risk and perhaps to change the antipsychotic regime accordingly (p. 1710).

The mechanism underlying the metabolic disturbance is unclear. Some reports indicate that from 2 to 36% of patients receiving atypical antipsychotics experience metabolic disturbances. It is possible that decreases in serotonergic 5-HT2A and 5-HT2C signaling, which influence appetite and caloric intake, physical activity, pancreatic functioning, and metabolic rate may be the pathophysiological factors (Nasrallah & Newcomer, 2004, p. S9).

Olanzapine and clozapine are also associated with a significant increase of the levels of cholesterol and triglycerides (p. S9). Clozapine, olanzapine, and quetiapine are associated with higher prevalence of diabetes than conventional antipsychotics for all the age ranges; risperidone was not (Marder & Wirshing, 2004, p. 450). Olanzapine's role in the causation of diabetes is one of the most actively debated topics in the contemporary use of atypical antipsychotics. There is a preponderance of clinical observations and data culled from multiple sources that demonstrate a strong association between olanzapine and diabetes mellitus (DM). The pharmaceutical company, Lilly, has persistently claimed that olanzapine has no causative role in the onset of DM. See above for comments about the CATIE report.

Case reports indicate that the mean time for onset of glucose dysregulation is three months after the beginning of olanzapine treatment (Koro et al., 2002, p. 244). These British authors conducted an epidemiological study using different referent groups to compare the risk of diabetes development among users of different antipsychotics, in a cohort of 19,637 schizophrenic patients. The study was supported by Bristol-Myers-Squibb, a Lilly pharmaceutical competitor.

The prevalence of diabetes and obesity among individuals with schizophrenia and affective disorders was approximately 1.5 to 2.0 times higher than in the general population. Epidemiological data suggest an increased prevalence of obesity, impaired glucose tolerance, and type 2 diabetes in people with psychiatric illness (Consensus Development Conference, 2004, p. 597). The incidence of diabetes among all the patients with schizophrenia treated with antipsychotics was 4.4/1000 person years. Women exhibited a higher incidence rate than men (5.3 vs. 3.5/1000 person years). The incidence rate within three months of a prescription was 10.0/1000 person years for olanzapine (95% confidence interval 5.2–19.2), 5.4/1000 person years for risperidone (3.0–9.8), and 5.1/1000 person years for conventional antipsychotics (4.5–5.8) (Koro et al., 2002, p. 245).

Particularly alarming because of the relevance for the field of child and adolescent psychiatry was the report of diabetes in 12 patients (N = 131 patients) younger than 19 years of age, and the report of one patient with acidosis (N = 6 patients) below 19 years of age (Koller et al., 2003, p. 737). Patients had been treated for disorders other than schizophrenia, including aggression, agitation, anxiety, autism, conduct disorder, bipolar disorder, and Tourette's disorder (p. 737). The time for the emergence of hyperglycemia ranged from one day to 48 months; however, 67% of patients experienced the problem within six months or less from risperidone initiation (p. 739). For patients with previously diagnoses of hyperglycemia, deterioration of glycemic control was noted in 71% of those patients on risperidone monotherapy (p. 739). Four patients on risperidone monotherapy died (p. 740). The following issues raise serious concern regarding the use of olanzapine in children and adolescents:

Olanzapine induces marked weight increases in children and adolescents.
Olanzapine induces a voracious appetite and aberrations in feeding behavior; scavenging behavior has been observed in small children.
Olanzapine use may be associated with hyperglycemia and other disorders of glucose metabolism, diabetes mellitus, and hyperlipedimias. (Psychiatric Drug Alerts, 2002, p. 12). See CATIE reports, 2005, 2006.

Epidemiological studies demonstrate a high degree of concurrence between diabetes and depression; a meta-analysis concludes that diabetes doubles the odds for depression. Also, schizophrenic patients have been reported to manifest a higher incidence and severity of diabetes than the general population (Figlewicz, 2003, p. 89). Diabetes seems to increase the severity of tardive dyskinesia (p. 89).

A number of factors may explain the association of diabetes with atypical use, such as weight gain and the disruption of glucose metabolism. Diabetes is strongly and consistently associated with obesity and weight gain. Antagonism of histamine receptors is also known to cause weight gain. It is possible that serotonin antagonism may also play a role. Weight gain may be due to an increase of leptin secretion that in turn leads to a disturbance of insulin secretion and diabetes mellitus. Lastly, dopamine has been shown to stimulate insulin secretion by a beta-mediated mechanism (Koro et al., 2002, pp. 245–246). Gupta, in an article sponsored by Lilly (2003), advises caution regarding rushing into attributing a major role in the causation of diabetes to antipsychotics.

> There is a well-established increased risk of diabetes among mentally ill, particularly patients with schizophrenia or bipolar disorders. However, the data in the field to date are equivocal regarding a potential causative relationship between antipsychotic use and diabetes. While epidemiological studies uniformly report increased risk with antipsychotic use, the various influences of the underlying disease and medication therapy have not been separated….Epidemiological studies…suffer from several limitations, including their retrospective and nonrandomized structure….To date, however, no clear pattern has emerged in the literature regarding differential risk between agents in the atypical class. (p. 6)

The CATIE report clearly demonstrated that olanzapine produces glycemic and dyslipidemic effects far above the other medications studied (risperidone, quetiapine, ziprasidone, and perphenazine) (Lieberman, Stroup et al., 2005).[17]

There are converging trends indicating that some atypicals such as clozapine and olanzapine may pose a significant risk for the elicitation of diabetes or for leading to complications of this illness. The Consensus Developing Conference (2004), corroborated these observations: "Despite the limitations in study design, the data consistently show an increased risk for diabetes in patients treated with clozapine or olanzapine compared to patients not receiving treatment with FGAs or with others SGAs" (p. 598).

The ranking of association of diabetes with SGAs is as follows: Clozapine=olanzapine>quetiapine=risperidone>ziprasidone=aripiprazole. In the CATIE report, olanzapine was associated with an increase in glycosylated hemoglobin and with an increase in total cholesterol and triglycerides (Lieberman, Stroup, et al., 2005, p. 1215).[18,19]

DYSLIPIDEMIAS: UNCOMMON, PREDICTABLE, POTENTIALLY SERIOUS

Atypicals have been associated with hyperlipidemia. Although, the cause of this association is unknown, there are concerns regarding elevations in triglycerides because that represents an independent heart disease risk. Severe hypertriglyceridemia has been reported with clozapine and olanzapine (Wirshing et al., 2003, p, 53).

Clozapine and olanzapine which produce the greatest weight gain are associated with the greatest increase in total cholesterol, LDL cholesterol, and triglycerides, and with a decrease in HDL cholesterol. Aripiprazole and ziprasidone do not seem to be associated with a worsening of serum lipids, and risperidone and quetiapine have intermediate effects on lipids (Consensus Developmental Conference, 2004, p. 598). In the CATIE report (Lieberman, Stroup, et al., 2005), only ziprasidone promoted weight loss and a decrease of cholesterol and triglycerides. Weight and blood pressure should be checked at every visit; fasting glucose, triglycerides, and cholesterol should be monitored every three months. For some patients, achieving antipsychotic effects is extremely difficult, and an effective treatment should not be discontinued because of some side effects without seriously considering the consequences (Wirshing et al., 2003, p. 54). Ranking of the association of dyslipidemias and SGAs is as follows: Clozapine = olanzapine > quetiapine > risperidone > aripiprazole ≥ ziprasidone.

In the CATIE report, olanzapine was associated with an increase in total cholesterol and triglycerides (Lieberman, Stroup, et al., 2005, p. 1215). In the CATIE study, ziprasidone was the only antipsychotic that improved a number of metabolic syndrome factors. Despres, Golay, Sjöström, and the Rimonabant in Obesity–Lipids Study Group (2005), described that rimonabant (a cannabinoid-1 receptor [CB1] blocker) offers a pharmacological approach to improve the unfavorable cardiovascular risk profile in high-risk obese or overweight patients with hyperlipidemia (p. 2133).

ENDOCRINOLOGICAL SIDE EFFECTS

Aina, Nandagopol, and Nasrallah (2004) state that, prior to the initiation of treatment, multiple endocrinological abnormalities have been demonstrated in schizophrenic patients; these abnormalities include: anomalies in growth hormone, the hypothalamic-pituitary-adrenal axis, the hypothalamic-pituitary-thyroid axis, the hypothalamic-pituitary-gonadal axis, diabetes, vasopressin, oxytocin, renin/angiotensin, melatonin, neurotensin, cholycystokinin, neuropeptide Y, somatostatin, neurosteroids, substance P, and leptin. Prolactin is a major stress-induced hormone like cortisol and growth hormone, but is not as widely studied as these (p. 78).

Polycyst Ovarian Disease (POD)

Common, Predictable, Potentially Serious
Polycystic ovary syndrome consists of oligoovulation or anovulation (manifested by oligomenorrhea or amenorrhea), hyperandrogenemia, and polycystic ovarian disease as demonstrated by ultrasonography. The diagnosis is functional: the presence of polycystic ovaries is not necessary to make the diagnosis, and polycystic ovaries by themselves do not make the diagnosis of POD (Ehrmann, 2005, p. 1223). In POD the level of luteinizing hormone is elevated or the ratio of LH/FSH is increased. LH promotes androgen production in the theca cells and insulin acts synergistically with LH to enhance androgen production of the thecal cells (p. 1225).

POD remains one of the most common hormonal disorders in women with an estimated prevalence between 5 and 10%. It is understood that the syndrome is a complex multigenic disorder. POD and the metabolic syndrome share insulin resistance as a central pathogenic feature, and POD might be viewed as a sex-specific form of the metabolic syndrome (Ehrmann, 2005, p. 1227). Many psychotropic medications promote weight gain; some psychotropics such as valproic acid have also been associated with polycystic ovarian disease. Obesity is present in about 30 to 40% of POD cases and the greater the BMI the greater the risk of anovulatory infertility.

The risks for obesity and polycystic ovarian disease may be aggravated by atypical antipsychotics. Abdominal obesity is associated with menstrual abnormalities; these abnormalities subside when the patients lose weight. Hyperandrogenism is also associated with menstrual irregularities. Compared with hyperandrogenized women of similar body weight, patients with acanthosis nigricans were more hyperinsulinemic and insulin resistant (Amatruda & Linemeyer, 2001, p. 956).

It is likely that hyperinsulinemia is the cause of the polycystic ovarian syndrome rather than the result of it. Hirsute women with polycystic ovary disease have higher insulin levels than those without hirsutism; there is a significant correlation between plasma insulin and plasma testosterone or androstenedione (Amatruda & Linemeyer, 2001, p. 956).

Hyperprolactinemia

Predictable, Rather Common, Potentially Serious
Prolactin is secreted episodically (with peak levels at night and through levels at noon). Prolactin release is inhibited by dopamine released from the hypothalamus. Stress, exercise, and hypoglycemia may increase the prolactin levels. Estrogens decrease prolactin response to dopamine and increase the response

to TSH. Insulin induces prolactin secretion. Prolactin is the only anterior pituitary hormone that is produced by the tuberoinfundibular neurons governed by dopamine (Vieweg & Fernandez, 2003, p. 58). Prolactin is released in response to stress and to nipple stimulation. Endogenous substances like estrogen, opioids, substance P, growth hormone-releasing hormone, gonadotropin-releasing hormone, oxytocin, vasopressin, histamine, bradykinin, and others stimulate prolactin release; GABA, somatostatin, acetylcholine, glucocorticosteroids, and gonadotropin-associated peptide, decrease prolactin levels (Aina et al., 2004, p. 78).

Elevated prolactin levels do not necessarily lead to clinical symptoms and have not been demonstrated to be intrinsically harmful. They do cause hypogonadism via negative feedback by inhibition of gonadotropin-releasing hormone leading to inadequate levels of follicle stimulating hormone (FSH) and luteinizing hormone (LH) (Wirshing et al., 2003, p. 55). Atypical antipsychotics are less likely to cause hyperprolactinemia than conventional antipsychotics. Most of the newer agents, except risperidone, produce minimal D2 blockade in the tuberoinfundibular area (Vieweg & Fernandez, 2003, p. 57).

Children and adolescents in long-term treatment (for up to 1 year) with risperidone show a transient elevation in serum prolactin during the initial three to four weeks; these levels begin to drop after the fourth to seventh week and return to within normal limits by weeks 40 to 48 in a majority of cases. Only 2.2% of children (13/592) developed symptoms hypothetically attributable to prolactin; 9 of the 13 children showed resolution of symptoms by the end of the study. No correlation was demonstrated between prolactin levels and attributable symptoms, even when male gynecomastia was included. These findings are in agreement with other studies in adults that show no association between prolactin levels and attributable symptoms (Findling, Kusumakar, et al., 2003, 1368).

Seventy-one percent of children and adolescents on risperidone, developed hyperprolactenimia, and 25% of the subjects experienced sexual side effects at the end point (Saito, Correll, Gallelli, et al., 2004, pp. 355–356). The tendency of risperidone to normalize over time may not apply to older children or to girls (p. 356). Atypicals do cause transitory elevations of prolactin levels, but they do it to a lower level than conventional antipsychotics.

Clinical Effects Of Hyperprolactinemia

Behavior

Direct effects: Hostility, depression, and anxiety were more frequently reported in women with hyperprolactinemia than in women with normal prolactin levels or in women with regular menstrual cycles (Halbreich & Kahn, 2003, p. 350). Cognitive impairment due to hypogonadism is possible.

Bones

Decreases in bone mineral density due to testosterone or estrogen deficits. Trabecular bone mass has been found to be reduced in young women with amenorrhea secondary to hyperprolactinemia.

Breast

Engorgement, galactorrhea, gynecomastia. A major concern regarding hyper-prolactinemia is its potential role in the development of breast cancer. Wang et al. (2002) raised the question whether dopamine antagonists might act as modest initiators or promoters of breast malignancies (p. 1153). They found that women who used antidopaminergic medications, antipsychotics, and antiemetics (that elevate the levels of prolactin), have a modest but significant increased risk for the development of breast cancer; this effect appears to be dose dependent and cumulative (p. 1152).

Halbreich and Kahn (2003) also argued that hyperprolactinemia is associated with breast cancer. The incidence of breast cancer was 3.5 times higher among psychiatric patients than among patients in the specialized radiology clinic, and 9.5 times higher than the reported incidence in the general population. Prospective data suggest that high plasma levels of prolactin are associated with an increase of breast cancer in postmenopausal women (pp. 347–348). Bowden (2003) indicated that Wallaschofski et al., (2003), proposed that a marker of platelet stimulation (ADP-stimulated P-selectin expression) was higher in hyperprolactinemic patients on antipsychotic medications than in nonprolactinemic controls; this may increase the risk of idiopathic venous thromboembolism (VTE) in patients receiving antipsychotics (p, 55). More research is needed to elucidate this serious concern.

Seeman (2004) argued that studies addressing the relationship of hyperpro-lactinemia and breast cancer concerns have not been controlled for two potent breast cancer risks: age at first giving birth and parity status. The younger a woman is at the time of her first pregnancy and more children she has, the less likely she is to develop breast cancer. When this is taken into account, the risk of breast cancer is not increased in women with schizophrenia treated with antidopaminergic agents (pp. 1327–1328).

Cardiovascuardiovascular: Effects Due to Low Levels of Estrogen or Testosterone

Menstrual function: Anovulation, amenorrhea.
Sexual function: Reduced libido and arousal; orgasmic dysfunction; in males, gonadal dysfunction. For the causes of hyperprolactinemia, see table 13.7.

The most common medications causing hyperprolactinemia are antipsy-chotics, dopamine receptor blockers, methyldopa, antidepressants, antihy-pertensives (reserpine), estrogens, opiates, cimetidine, and metoclopramide. Prolactin levels were studied in patients receiving atypical antipsychotics (Saito,

TABLE 13.7 Causes of Hyperprolactinemia

- Hypothalamic diseases
- Pituitary diseases (lactotroph adenomas)
- Medications
- Other causes of hyperprolactinemia include: primary hypothyroidism, chronic renal failure, cirrhosis, neurogenic, and idiopathic causes (p. 60).
- Pregnancy produces a physiological hyperprolactinemia (values up to 200 ng/ml to 600 ng/ml have been described). Nipple stimulation and stress (physiological or psychological) are other factors that cause prolactin elevation.

Source: Snyder (2001, p. 194).

Correll, & Kafantaris, 2003). Thirty-nine patients (18 females, 21 males, mean age = 13.44, SD = 2.66, range 5–18) were the study subjects. 21 patients were on risperidone, 12 on olanzapine, and 6 on quetiapine. Mean duration of treatment was 11.78 weeks (SD = 0.94; range, 6–15 weeks). Hyperprolactinemia, defined as a prolactin level > 25.4 ng/ml, was present in 53.8%. Seventy-one percent of risperidone treated patients showed hyperprolactinemia vs. 29% of those treated with olanzapine or quetiapine (chi-square $p = 0.017$). The risperidone treated patients had higher end point levels, 46.08 ng/ml (SD = 30.2), compared with the olanzapine or quetiapine-treated groups, 22.86 ng/ml (SD = 16.8, $p = 0.013$) (pp. 413–414). Galactorrhea occurs in about 10 to 15% women with hyperprolactinemia. A minority of women who have galactorrhea have hyperprolactinemia and abnormal menses (P. J. Snyder, 2001, p. 195).

Hummer et al. (2005) stated that, "We were not able to confirm the hypothesis that treatment with prolactin-increasing antipsychotics enhances the risk of osteoporosis" (p. 165). They add that a number of schizophrenic patients suffered from osteopenia or osteoporosis despite the fact that they had never received treatment with prolactin-increasing neuroleptics (p. 165). The authors commented on the well-known positive association of osteoporosis with BMI and level of psychopathology (p. 166). The authors conclude that schizophrenic patients suffer from low bone density, and that male patients were more affected than females; these patients also have a number of additional risk factors that may contribute to this problem (cigarette smoking, alcohol consumption, vitamin D deficiency, immobility, poor nutrition, and low level of gonadal hormones (p. 166).

In men hyperprolactinemia causes hypogonadism resulting in decreased libido, including impotence, and infertility. Galactorrhea in males is infrequent (p. 166). Hyperprolactinemia reduces the testosterone levels in men which may lead to decrease libido, impotence, infertility, gynecomastia, and, rarely, to galactorrhea (Wirshing et al., 2003, p. 55). Hyperprolactinemia resulting in androgen deficiency may cause gynecomastia. Marijuana and digioxin ingestion results in breast enlargement by interacting with the estrogen receptor (p.

55). Increase of peripheral aromatase activity and conversion of androgens into estrogens in adipose tissue may be involved in the gynecomastia observed in obese men (p. 664).

The diagnosis of gynecomastia is not easy; it is difficult to differentiate between true gynecomastia and an increase of adipose tissue in obese boys or men. A careful physical examination is needed. Gynecomastia is usually bilateral but can be unilateral. Gynecomastia needs to be distinguished from chest wall tumors (lipomas, neurofibromas, lymphomas) and, most importantly, from male breast cancer (Matsumoto, 2001, p. 663). Malignancies of the adrenal gland, tumors of the testis, and other systemic diseases need to be considered in the differential diagnosis of gynecomastia. In persistent pubertal macromastia, the breast enlargement reaches adult female size; his condition is idiopathic (p. 665).

Quetiapine causes thyroid function side effects. A decrease of up to 20% of total and free thyroxine (T4) has been observed at the higher end of quetiapine dose range; this finding has been detected during the first 2 to 4 weeks of therapy with quetiapine. These changes have no clinical significance. Increase in TSH was observed in about 0.4% of patients (Lieberman, 2004b, p. 482).

NEUROLOGICAL SIDE EFFECTS

Sedation

Very Common, Predictable, Usually Transitory and Nonserious
Most of the atypical antipsychotics are sedative at treatment initiation; in general, patients develop tolerance to these medications' sedative effects. Not all the atypicals induce the same degree of sedation. Sedative effects interfere with alertness and learning. Sleeping in the classroom might indicate antipsychotic medication sedative side effects. Rarely is it necessary to dose medications like risperidone and olanzapine BID. The coadministered medications may cause sedation or increase the atypicals' sedative effects. Clonidine is a very sedative medication; guanfacine is less so. Anticonvulsants are frequently sedative; that is the case with valproic acid, carbamazepine, and oxcarbazepine, among others. The ranking of atypicals regarding sedative side effects is as follows: aripiprazole (+/-)=ziprasidone (+/-)<risperidone (+)<olanzapine (++)=quetiapine (++)<clozapine (+++) (Measure Minutes, Nasrallah, 2004, p. 1).

Extrapyramidal Side Effects (EPS)

Common, Predictable, Rarely Serious
EPS refers to untoward neurological manifestations of neuroleptic treatment (other nonneuroleptic medications may also elicit these symptoms). EPS

includes a constellation of symptoms such as tremor (Parkinsonian tremor), dystonias (acute dystonias, athetosis, muscular rigidity, gait disturbance, and others), oculogyric crisis, and akathisia. Sialorrhea frequently accompanies other EPS symptoms. These symptoms may be acute or chronic. Acute symptoms are commonly distressing, dramatic, and even painful, but rarely serious, except for the picture of laryngeal spasm that constitutes a true medical emergency, and the worrisome neuroleptic malignant syndrome (see below); in general, acute symptoms resolve promptly with appropriate treatment. Chronic symptoms (tardive dyskinesia, tardive akathisia, tardive Tourette's, and others) may be incapacitating and socially stigmatizing; these conditions are less responsive to treatment than acute symptoms.

Stimulant medications induce EPS symptoms occasionally; in general, the EPS-stimulant related symptoms are most commonly orobuccal dyskinesia (OBD). Symptoms are worst at the peak of the medication blood level; symptoms start waning as the blood levels decrease. When the symptoms are due to stimulant alone, children are symptomless in early morning before receiving the stimulant medication and after the medication wanes.

When patients receive stimulants and antipsychotics, concomitantly, diagnosis of the EPS is more complex. Children with a history of neurological damage or those who had developed prior EPS reactions to antipsychotics are vulnerable to the EPS side effect from neuroleptics. Even for those patients with low EPS potential, stimulants and related medications (like atomaxetine, see below), may induce involuntary movements. Sometimes, a medication that by itself does not produce EPS may unleash this side effect when it interacts with other medications.

Atypical antipsychotics differ in the potential for eliciting neurological side effects. Risperidone is the closest to a typical antipsychotic in this regard, and as such, it is not uncommon for risperidone to induce acute dyskinesias and other EPS symptoms. It is difficult to say if the other SGA are more benign than resperidone in this regard. Risperidone is somewhat unpredictable in this regard. For children and adolescents on risperidone, as the dose ascends over 3 to 4 mg/day there is a linear increase in the risks of dyskinesia. Children and adolescents are more susceptible to EPS AE than adults (see above). All the atypical antipsychotics (including, although rarely, clozapine) produce EPS AE in children and adolescents. In the CATIE I report there was no difference in EPS rates among the studied antipsychotics (olanzapine, risperidone, quetiapine, ziprasidone, and perphenazine) (Lieberman, Stroup, et al., 2005, p. 1215).

Dyskinesias do not always present with bilateral, symmetrical signs; occasionally, dyskinesias are more prominent on one side of the body or limited to only a sector of the body, such as a part of the face; this is also true for cogwheeling. Children may also display isolated, episodic, oculogyric crises, which create diagnostic confusion, mainly, considerations of a seizure disorder.

The complexities of diagnosing a neuroleptic related movement disorder is exemplified in the following vignette:

> A 9-year-old white girl was referred for psychiatric evaluation by a child psychiatrist, for increased aggression and irritability. She had displayed extreme temper tantrums at home and school. The family was concerned with the child's frequent "meltdowns," lasting for up two hours. She was described as being mean to her siblings, irritable, and displayed "mood swings" and poor anger control.
>
> The child had a prior acute psychiatric hospitalization at age 7, for six days, after she attempted to jump from a second floor window. The family reported that she had received the diagnosis of Asperger's by a developmental pediatrician. Two years before, a psychological testing indicated the presence of a thought disorder; psychometric testing showed a VIQ: 84, PIQ: 83, and a FSIQ: 83.
>
> The child had been under the care of her maternal grandmother since 7 months of age. Her biological mother was psychiatrically incapacitated, and the biological father was described as a violent man who suffered from drug abuse. Even though the natural mother was around, the patient was not attached to her; she was bonded preferentially to her grandmother, whom she considered the most important person in her life.
>
> There was no history of developmental delays but there had been difficulties with learning in areas of math, reading, and comprehension. The family denied a history of seizures, head trauma, fractures, or surgeries. The child had been sexually molested at age 6 by a babysitter's uncle who killed himself after he was accused of sexual perpetration. She had received treatment with sertraline, risperidone (up to 8 mg); she had also been tried on Adderall but this product activated her. At the time of the assessment the child had been receiving quetiapine 50 mg at bedtime.
>
> *Mental status examination*: the child was small for her age and had difficulties warming up to the examiner; she was not spontaneous but she was cooperative and forthright in her answers. Her affect was constricted but appropriate. She endorsed paranoid ideation, feeling that people talked about her, watched her, and followed her. She denied any other perceptual disturbances as well as suicidal or homicidal ideation.
>
> Neurological evaluation: she was fully oriented to day, date, month, and year. She had solid right and left orientation and performed contralateral limb commands without difficulties. There were no cerebellar signs or difficulties with finger sequencing. Fundoscopy was unremarkable. Right planter response: toes fanned up, except for the big toe; the left plantar response was flexor.
>
> During the examination, she displayed intermittent rolling of the eyes up and to the right. There was mild cogwheeling at the neck and elbows. There was no tremor, no choreathetosis. The diagnosis of an unusual EPS reaction was made.
>
> Because the neurological features were unusual and an immediate neurological consultation was requested. The consultant neurologist reported presence of ocular dystonia. He also performed an EEG and found bilateral spiking. Imaging was ordered. The MRI was unremarkable.
>
> This patient had an uncommon form of EPS, to a neuroleptic rarely causing

this reaction. It is likely the patient had been sensitized to EPS by her exposure to large doses of risperidone. The patient also had complex partial seizures.

Although, the most common cause of oculogyric crisis is neuroleptic medication or other antidopaminergic treatment, carbamazepine, lithium, and pentazocine have also been reported to evoke this side effect (Ayd, 2000, p. 714). A very bothersome and deceptive side effect is akathisia. Usually the patient or the patient's parents complain that the child is restless, hyperactive, and uneasy, or that the child displays agitation, dysphoria, inability to sit still, insomnia, and the like. These symptoms may be misjudged to be psychotic agitation or uncontrolled mania, resulting in treatments that are inappropriate or that aggravate the condition (i.e., when the psychiatrist increases the antipsychotic dose). Homicidal and suicidal behavior, severe impulsive behaviors, and sudden attempts to run away have been reported. Akathisia promotes medication noncompliance. For an overview of treatment of akathisia, see chapter 14. Haan, Lavalaye, Booiij, et al. (2005) report that negative subjective experiences (akathisia) are related to D2 receptor occupancy by antipsychotics and that monitoring for feelings of comfort, self-confidence, and safety may guide clinicians and researchers in finding the optimal D2 occupancy. All 38 items of the Subjective Well-Being Under Neuroleptic scale were negatively correlated with D2 receptor occupancy as measured in SPECT imaging studies (p. 1544).

Drug induced Parkinsonism is another EPS AE that occurs during the initiation of antipsychotics. In Parkinsonism, patients may look medicated. Negative symptoms related to a psychotic illness or depressive features related to a mood disorder are part of the differential diagnosis of antipsychotic-related Parkinsonism. Perioral tremor (rabbit syndrome) is an uncommon late form of EPS (Findling, McNamara, & Gracious, 2003, p. 334). EPS side effects are mainly due to the high affinity of atypicals for the D2 receptor. It is also likely that for the same reason, risperidone is associated with increased incidence of tardive dyskinesia and other tardive disorders (tardive akathisia, tardive dystonia, and even tardive Tourette's). EPS, in children and adolescents, has also been observed with ziprasidone and aripripazole, and to a less extent with olanzapine. Quetiapine rarely induces EPS, but quetiapine-related TD has been reported.[20]

It is important to remember that stimulants and other psychotropic medications (i.e., SSRIs, and others) may either cause involuntary movement disorders by themselves or may aggravate preexistent or coexistent movement disorders. The author witnessed an acute orofacial dyskinesia after the smallest extended long-released methylphenidate 10 mg, on a 5-year-old girl. This case is similar to the 6-year-old girl who developed oraofacial dyskinesia after taking the first dose of methylphenidate (a 10 mg tablet). Facial contortions persisted the following day after the patient received only 5 mg. The movements were predominant in the lower face, mostly around the mouth including chewing and puckering movements, writhing, and slight protrusion of the tongue. The patient also made soft clucking sounds. The episodes occurred 30 minutes after the ingestion of 5 mg of methylphenidate and lasted for five hours (Senecky, Lobel Diamond, et al., 2002, pp. 224–226). Orobuccal dyskinesias (OBD) need to be differentiated from oral apraxias; in the latter, there are no spontaneous involuntary movements, but the child labors with the production of speech, often making gestures as he or she makes efforts to articulate, resembling OBD.

Connor (1998) mentions that withdrawal dyskinesia may not improve until the stimulants are discontinued. "Continued stimulant treatment in the face of neuroleptic withdrawal may initiate, exacerbate, or prolong the duration of the neuroleptic withdrawal dyskinesia in certain children. Children with pre-existing basal ganglia pathology may be particularly vulnerable to this possible neuroleptic withdrawal-stimulant interaction" (Connor, 1998, pp. 247–248). Surprisingly, there are not too many reports on stimulants. A case of orofacial dyskinesia after a peak dose of methylphenidate (5 mg) was reported in another 6-year-old girl (*The Brown University Child and Adolescent Psychopharmacology Update*, 2003, p. 8; see case described above). It is not uncommon for children who receive higher doses of stimulants to display apparently involuntary movements including perioral and tongue movements simulating neuroleptic side effects (EPS). On the other hand, EPS-like movements are also described after stimulants are withdrawn.

Many cases of adverse side effects of SSRIs—EPS—have been described. Pies (1997) wrote an editorial on the subject: "Must We Consider SSRIs Neuroleptics?" Fluoxetine is the biggest offender in the literature on adults, and acute dystonia is the most common EPS symptom reported. The authors reported on a 15-year-old female who developed torticollis, bradykinesia, and cogwheel rigidity on fluoxetine (Diler, Yolga, Avci, & Scahill, 2003, pp. 125–126). Akathisia is a commonly reported EPS reaction with SSRIs treatment. Other EPS symptoms, such as oculogyric crisis, sustained upward eye gaze, and other EPS symptoms have also been reported. It is well established that children with neurodevelopmental problems, including mental retardation, have increased vulnerability for the development of EPS (Lindsey, Kaplan, Koliatsos, Walter, & Sandson, 2003, p. 1269).

EPS Monitoring

Extrapyramidal side effects encompass a range of deleterious side effects. Jibson and Tandom (1998) describe the clinical costs of EPS secondary to antipsychotics:

1. Increased motor side effects (Parkinsonian symptoms, dyskinesias, etc.).
2. An increase of negative symptoms (secondary negative symptoms).

3. An increase of cognitive symptoms (problems with attention, learning, memory, slowing of neuropsychological functioning).
4. An increase of akathisia (neuroleptic dysphoria, see below).
5. A higher likelihood of noncompliance (secondary to all the above), and,
6. A greater risk of tardive dyskinesia (pp. 224–225).

EPS also may offset gains in negative symptoms associated with the resolution of active psychosis (p. 221).

The psychiatrist should systematically monitor all patients on antipsychotics for the development of extrapyramidal side effects (EPS). In every follow-up appointment, children and adolescents should be examined for the presence of choreathetotic movements, cogwheel rigidity, and the presence of orofacial dyskinesia. Simple component tests of the AIMS examination such as, (1) asking the child to extend his or her arms in front, with spread fingers, and with the eyes closed will readily reveal choreathetosis, and the degree of Parkinsonian tremor; (2) asking the child to close the eyes and open the mouth leaving the tongue inside and still, readily reveals involuntary movements of the tongue, mouth, face, and jaw in children with orobuccal-facial dyskinesia; hypersalivation when present is obvious; (3) as the psychiatrist assesses for involuntary movements of mouth and face, she or he will observe for associated involuntary movements of hands and forearms, feet and legs; (4) the psychiatrist needs to examine for the presence of cogwheel rigidity. It is difficult to identify these movement disorders without examination unless the dyskinesias are advanced and severe.

When evaluating EPS, the psychiatrist will be mindful of a number of medications that ordinarily are not considered offending agents for these side effects. Dystonic movements may develop with the ingestion of many drugs including phenytoin, carbamazepine, TCAs, antihistamines (i.e., diphenhydramine—Benadryl), Ketamine, lithium, and others (Menkes, 2006, p. 171).

Withdrawal Dyskinesia

Common, Usually Benign, and Transitory
This dramatic and often alarming movement disorder appears shortly after antipsychotic medications are discontinued. The child begins to display increased hyperactivitiy and severe orobuccal-lingual dyskinesia. The most concerning aspects of this syndrome are the tongue darting, the persistent tongue protrusion and lip licking, and the intense involuntary movements of the mouth, lips, and face. The onset of the syndrome is rather abrupt; the fading of this syndrome, on the other hand, is rather slow. Fortunately, this syndrome fades away in the majority of the cases. The author has seen multiple and severe withdrawal dyskinetic cases but has only seen one case that remained symptomatic for a prolonged time. This child will be described below.

Frequently, the symptoms begin to recede during the first or second week or so, after the onset of symptoms. Reassurance should be given to the parents, to the child, and to other significant others, including teachers and clinical staff; this is imperative since there are no known treatments for this condition. Most of the time, the condition resolves spontaneously.

The darting of the tongue and the gross mouth and jaw dyskinetic movements may take some weeks to fade away; the choreathetotic movements slowly disappear in a few months. Children with neurological background (brain lesions/injuries, cerebral palsy, static encephalopathy, etc.) are particularly sensitive to antipsychotic extrapyramidal side effects; caution and closer monitoring should be exercised when using antipsychotic medications in this population. Baseline neurological evaluations and AIMS assessments are mandatory prior to antipsychotic initiation for these children.

Akinesia, an extrapyramidal side effect that may be confused with agitated catatonia, could also be confused with the syndrome of postpsychotic depression. Postpsychotic depression may respond to antidepressant medications whereas akinesia needs to be treated with anti-Parkinsonians (Biederman, Spencer, & Wilens, 2004, p. 962), or beta-adrenergic blocking agents.

Neuroleptic Dysphoria/Akathisia

Common, Unpredictable, Potentially Serious
Akathisia is one of the most common neuroleptic side effects; it has been associated with suicide and violent behavior. The subjective unpleasant mood, an important aspect of the akathisia syndrome, is often unrecognized. Therefore, patients who are irritable or complain of tension or panic can be given excessive treatment rather than a dose reduction. Dysphoria can occur in the absence of objective signs of akathisia (King, Burke, & Lucas, 1995). These effects have also been observed in child and adolescent populations. Clinical examples will be illustrated below. The subjective side effects of neuroleptic antipsychotic medications have not received the attention and importance that they deserve. Neuroleptics are frequently, if not invariably, associated with a number of side effects of which the extrapyramidal, autonomic and subjective (feelings of dysphoria) symptoms are the most troublesome. Although the previous statement is particularly true for the classical neuroleptics, it is also true for some second-generation antipsychotics. The subjective feelings are difficult to evaluate, and complaints of this type have often been dismissed as exaggerated or delusional. These side effects should not be underestimated; they may affect the patient's compliance, social autonomy, and quality of life (Lader & Lewander, 1994, p. 5). There is controversy regarding the meaning of mood and affective symptoms in chronic psychotic patients. Some consider them part of the illness, while others feel they are part of the extrapyramidal side effect syndrome. The affective changes induced by neuroleptics are of particular

concern; mood swings, crying, sadness, anxiety, agitation, panic attacks, and phobic states, among others, have been described (p. 7).

The affective, cognitive, and social impairment side effects induced by neuroleptics have been labeled the neuroleptic induced deficit syndrome (NIDS) (p. 7). These adverse reactions have also received the denominations of dyscognitive syndrome, neuroleptic dysphoria, akinetic depression, and subjective aspects of akathisia (p. 10). These reactions need to be differentiated from negative symptoms that are part of the primary illness, postpsychotic depression (neuroleptic treatment may contribute to the post psychotic depression syndrome in susceptible individuals), personality disorders, and in children, neurodevelopmental deficits (nonverbal disabilities, affective aprosody, etc.).

It is assumed that these side effects are mediated via antagonism of central dopamine D2 receptors (p. 9). These side effects may also adversely affect the success of other treatment modalities such as psychotherapy and behavioral and cognitive therapies, and may impede the rehabilitation process (p. 10). In children and adolescents, interferences with neurocognitive development and interferences with attention and learning (encoding and retrieval) are major concerns. There might be a developmental coloring to the syndromes described in adults. As described above, the dysphoric or mood disordered features of akathisia may be present in the absence of restlessness or pacing.

> Margie, a 5½-year-old white girl, with a diagnosis of very early onset schizophrenia, had been receiving psychiatric treatment since she was 2 years old. On many occasions, Margie had displayed homicidal behavior toward her 2½-year-old sister.
>
> Although, Margie was a somewhat attractive brunette girl, she was strange looking, lacked warmth, and was distant. She was unpredictable in her relatedness; at times, she was remote, other times she sought body contact, violating interpersonal boundaries. With some frequency, she attempted to befriend strangers. Margie had history of multiple acute psychiatric hospitalizations and a history of multiple residential treatment program placements.
>
> On one occasion, symptoms of aggression and psychotic behavior were under fair control with 2.5 mg of risperidone/day. After about four weeks on that medication, the parents began to report that Margie looked very depressed, that she cried for long periods of time, that she was irritable, that she appeared very sad, and even self-abusive. Sleep was also disrupted. When she was examined, she appeared dysphoric, and withdrawn; she endorsed hearing commanding voices and seeing monsters; there was no evidence of hypertonia, orobuccal-facial movements, or cogwheeling. The psychiatrist suspected neuroleptic side effects and ordered a decrease of the risperidone dose; parents reported improvement of the dysphoria, irritability, and crying.

Here is an adolescent example:

> Liz, a petite, 15-year-old white female, had a long history of mood difficulties and progressive deterioration of behavior at home and school. Liz's parents had

been divorced for many years but they still carried on a bitter relationship. Father, a nurse, lived in another state. He did not support psychiatric treatment for his daughter, and disapproved of the use of psychotropic medications. Liz had a history of poor compliance with her psychotropic medications. Liz's father frequently sided with his daughter's misperceptions, distortions, and misbehavior, and blamed Liz's unhappiness and difficulties on her mother. Liz was extremely hostile toward her biological mother and frequently abused her, both physically and verbally. Liz voiced a profound spite toward her mother, and her father seemed to contribute to the child's hatred and negativity toward mother. Liz was convinced that her natural father agreed with her, in more than one way, and felt supported in her attitude that she did not need to take psychotropics. The situation came to a serious crisis when Liz began to display overt paranoid symptoms at school, blaming others for disliking her and accusing peers and teachers of spying on her. She also voiced fears of being poisoned and became very agitated and suspicious. Her sleep became compromised, and hostility and aggression toward her mother escalated. Liz was hospitalized after revealing suicidal ideation, and as expected, had been refusing to take medications.

Because of the agitation, hostility, paranoia, and sleep difficulties, she was given progressive doses of olanzapine. She was started at 10 mg q HS, which was increased progressively to 20, 30, and finally 40 mg/day, seeking a satisfactory response. On this higher dose the paranoia began to recede. However, at this dose she began to complain of a great deal of anxiety; she became very hypochondriacal, fearing that something was wrong with her heart, wondering if she had AIDS, worrying that she had liver cancer, and so on. No amount of reassurance helped. Use of benzodiazepines was of limited use, but decrease of olanzapine to 30 mg, and later to 20 mg, noticeably reduced the dysphoria and anxiety. Because of concerns with weight increase, olanzapine was discontinued later on.

In the two previous examples, the atypical antipsychotic side effects had strong mood components and, in Liz's case, there were prominent anxiety symptoms, too. The mood and anxiety side effects could become a source of diagnostic confusion and the basis for inappropriate polypharmacy. The clinician might mistakenly assume that the patient is now developing a mood/anxiety disorder and would feel inclined to add antidepressants or anxiolytics to the medication regime. The importance of close monitoring of antipsychotic side effects is illustrated in the next preadolescent example.

Phil, a 6-year-old Hispanic adopted male, had been previously followed for homicidal and suicidal behaviors and a history of chronic psychosis. He had been adopted by his Caucasian mother at age 3, after suffering from severe neglect and physical abuse. Phil was a handsome, intelligent, and appealing child. However, he had a peculiar dysprosody: he would talk in a pedantic, monotonous, songlike way, and in a baby-talk fashion. He claimed he heard Osama Bin Laden telling him to kill himself and to kill his mother; he also heard the Scream commanding him to do bad deeds.

Because of prior difficulties with zyprasidone, risperidone, and quetiapine

Phil was prescribed aripiprazol, 7.5 mg/day. Since hallucinations did not respond to this dose, medication was increased to 15 mg. On this dose he reported that he did not hear Bin Laden or the Scream anymore. His mother complained, however, that the child looked depressed and withdrawn and that his speech defect was more pronounced. Phil's affect became very constricted and he appeared moderately depressed; he missed his mother a lot. He was also mildly drowsy and complained of being tired. A physical examination revealed no tremor or orobuccal-facial movements; however, marked cogwheeling was evidenced, as well as severe neck hypertonia. Sensitive decrease of the medication improved his mood and progressively decreased the EPS side effects. The psychiatrist had not suspected EPS till she examined the child and the cogwheeling was detected.

The syndrome of akathisia may be induced by a number of medications other than antipsychotics: SSRIs, theophylline, stimulants, and others. The conjoint use of these medications with antipsychotics may complicate the diagnosis of the problem. The differential diagnosis of akathisia includes: pharmacological induced akathisia (by antipsychotics, and other medications), delirium, severe ADHD, manic behavior, and excited catatonia. Akathisia may present suddenly and dramatically as illustrated in the following example:

Jennifer, a petite 14-year-old white girl, required acute care admission for prominent suicidal behavior. The day prior to the admission she had run away from home with a grown-up male and apparently had become sexually involved. She reported no prior psychiatric history but stated that she had contemplated suicide a number of times, and that she had tried to kill herself three times before. Jennifer endorsed symptoms of depression for the previous three years, and also admitted to a history of severe anxiety including panic attacks with occasional agoraphobia. At the time of admission she had difficulties falling sleep and had lost weight. She had been doing well at school.

The Mental Status Examination disclosed the presence of a very depressed adolescent, very avoidant, unable to make eye contact. She spoke with a very low tone and displayed overt anxiety during the interview. She acknowledged suicidal ideation but disclosed no plans. She endorsed moderated paranoid ideation, believing that people talked about her, watched her, and followed her. The sensorium was intact.

It was considered that Jennifer's prominent psychopathology was mostly an admixture of severe depression and anxiety disorder. Since she had been insomniac and lacking of appetite, mirtazapine was chosen as the only psychotropic agent. Mirtazapine was titrated up to 30 mg/night. Jennifer received no other psychotropics. By the seventh day she was doing so well (mood had brightened, anxiety had dissipated and she was no longer suicidal or paranoid), she was scheduled for discharged the following day.

In the morning of the discharge day the treating psychiatrist was called to the unit. Jennifer was extremely hyperactive and had become very fidgety and restless; she had also started pacing. The child psychiatrist corroborated the cited symptoms and also noticed that Jennifer had difficulties staying seated, that when she sat down she couldn't keep her feet still, and that when she stood up she still kept moving her feet, as if she were marching. She had a mild dysphoria; however, she endorsed no depressive symptoms and reported no anxiety feelings. She negated the presence of suicidal or paranoid ideation. A neurological examination revealed no other evidence of EPS.

Since the only psychotropic on board was mirtazapine, it was felt that this acute akathisia symptomatology was secondary to this antidepressant. The patient was given 10 mg of propanolol stat, and in the lapse of 30 minutes she reported with some degree of surprise that her feet had stopped moving! She became more outgoing and engaging. Jennifer was discharged on the scheduled day on mirtazapine 15 mg/night, propanolol 10 mg BID and was seen three days later. She was not akathisic then.

This was a dramatic development of akathisia in the lapse of less that 24 hours since the psychiatrist had last "rounded" his patient. The response of propanolol was equally dramatic. It is considered that acute akathisia is frequently misdiagnosed and erroneously treated. This vignette is also extraordinary because mirtazapine has been proposed as an agent to treat akathisia (Ginsberg, 2005c, p. 27).

TARDIVE DYSKINESIA: UNCOMMON, PREDICTABLE, POTENTIALLY SERIOUS

Correll, Leutch, and Kane (2004) conducted a meta-analytic review of 11 long-term studies of SGAs; their study supports the expectation that atypical antipsychotics have a reduced risk for tardive dyskinesia compared to FGAs. This finding was true for children, adults, and particularly, for the vulnerable population of the elderly (p. 419). In this review no aripiprazole data was included in the analysis.

Based on pooled data from 12 open-label studies and 15 double-blind studies with risperidone (9 lasting 3 months or more, and 7 lasting one year or more), the incidence of tardive dyskinesia was observed to be 0.2% in 878 adults who completed at least three months of treatment, and was only slightly higher (0.3%) when the study was restricted to the seven one-year studies. A shortcoming of this conclusion is that the incidence was extrapolated only from spontaneous reports of adverse events; this most likely represents significant underreporting (p. 419).

According to Jibson and Tandon (2003), the prevalence of tardive dyskinesia is 0.5% to 1% per year of treatment, for the first line antipsychotic medications, excluding clozapine (p. 60). That means that the risk for the development of this serious side effect increases with the duration of treatment (increased exposure) to atypicals. To complicate matters, there is not a standard definition of TD and it has not been studied systematically. There are no systematic studies of TD in children. Moreover, the incidence of TD varies according to the nature of the cohort; the incidence is smaller in an antipsychotic naïve cohort than in a cohort involving resistant schizophrenics; it is likely that the incidence is less in homogeneous populations by age and diagnostic categories than in heterogeneous populations for diagnoses and age.

In many studies the impact of withdrawal dyskinesia is not discriminated from the unfolding true dyskinesias. This explains why some studies report up to 35.8% of dyskinesia incidence in the placebo group (pp. 420–421). When olanzapine and clozapine were compared (90 patients in each group), olanzapine had an incidence of TD of 2.2%, which was significantly higher than clozapine in which no cases were ascertained ($p < 0.03$) (p. 420). The SGAs' benefits of lower TD risk are decreased when the doses are increased. This is consistent with the observation that higher doses of SGAs are associated with higher incidence of EPS. Furthermore, acute EPS and a higher utilization of anticholinergic medications have been associated with an increase risk for TD (p. 421).

In adult and elderly patients the incidence of SGAs appears to be about one fifth of the risk observed for FGAs (p. 423). It is likely that children and adolescents, who have a higher susceptibility for EPS, and who potentially have a longer time exposure to these medications, may reveal a higher incidence of TD. Although the above study indicates that SGAs have a lower risk for TD than FGAs, the case is mostly made for risperidone; the data for olanzapine is limited and for the other atypicals is either limited or nonexistent. There is limited data on the long-term quetiapine TD risk and, of course, it is unknown what will be the impact of the newest atypicals (ziprasidone and aripiprazole) in this regard.

The following vignette illustrates the vicissitudes of a very severe withdrawal dyskinesia that seemed to continue into a tardive dyskinesia syndrome:

Jittery was an 11-year-old Hispanic male with a long history of psychiatric disturbance. He had multiple psychiatric admissions to local psychiatric hospitals. The author first saw him when he was 9 years old. The hospital psychiatric admissions had been precipitated by suicidal and aggressive behaviors. He frequently talked about killing himself, and frequently got involved in fights with his brother. He also had held a knife to his sister's neck. He used to argue with mother a great deal and had problems minding her. He had a history of multiple suicidal attempts and self-abusive behaviors. There was a long history of impulsivity and hyperactivity. There was an allegation of sexual abuse by a 13-year-old cousin in the past; when Jittery was 9 he reportedly fondled his 5-year-old sister. There was no history of seizures, and a prior EEG had been unremarkable.

Jittery had severe behavioral difficulties at school; he was severely learning impaired and had an obvious speech disorder. Actually, he suffered from a severe mixed language disorder. The presence of aphasia was inferred.

Prior to the first hospitalization and first contact with the author, he was receiving risperidone 8 mg/day and methylphenidate 40 mg q AM, and 20 mg q Noon & q 4 PM. He had been on the high risperidone dose for close to six months. He had also been receiving Neurontin 400 mg BID. At the time of the first psychiatric admission, a history of occasional involuntary movements of the limbs and the tongue was reported.

Risperidone was progressively withdrawn; at about 4 mg/day Jittery displayed conspicuous sniffing and throat clearing, and his hyperactivity and involuntary movements progressively increased. Further tapering of risperidone continued; the hyperactivity remained unchanged, however.

Prior to a subsequent admission he was on Tenex 1mg q AM and Noon and 2 mg q HS, risperdal 2mg q HS, and dexedrine 15 mg q AM and Noon. After the readmission, risperidone was discontinued. Involuntary movements became conspicuously worse, then; Jittery displayed severe oral (buccolingual) dyskinetic movements as well as observable facial muscle contractions (blinking, facial gesturing), and gross choreathetotic movements in the upper limbs with associated involuntary movements of the feet. Furthermore, frequent neck and trunk contractions were noticed. The buccolingual movements consisted of frequent tongue darting and licking, and an ongoing movement of the lips and jaw.

This dramatic picture began to fade by the second week; by the third week most of the buccolingual aspects had receded. The choreathetotic movements took a number of months to dissipate. By the sixth month, evidence of an involuntary movement disorder was no longer present. By that time the patient was on high doses of quetiapine, and it was considered that this neuroleptic was camouflaging or silencing the involuntary movement syndrome. It is important to point out that the stimulants tended to increase or make the involuntary movements more noticeable. However, atomaxetine was more benign in this particular regard.

The diagnosis of withdrawal dyskinesia had been initially made, but later the diagnosis of TD was entertained. Since the involuntary movements reappeared every time attempts were made to decrease the neuroleptic (even quetiapine) we considered that the most correct diagnosis was chronic dyskinesia, most likely tardive dyskinesia.

On 600 mg of quetiapine/day, Jittery did not display evidence of oro-buccolingual movements; he was quite fidgety, however. On quetiapine, there was no observable choreathetotic movement of the hands, and no involuntary movement of the feet. Limited trunk and neck movements were still present. His mood was pleasant but continued displaying difficulties with impulsivity and hyperactivity. As stated, stimulant medications were somewhat helpful for the hyperactivity and impulsivity, but tended to increase the involuntary movements. Jittery continued displaying serious impairments in language and in learning, and impulsivity remained particularly problematic.

Further medication changes were implemented: Jittery began to receive atomaxetin 25 mg q AM and aripiprazole 10 mg q AM. On these medications, the child developed a maculo-papular eruption, mainly in the face and in the trunk, with a limited rash in the limbs. Because of the rash all the medications were discontinued for about five days. Since there was a major behavioral deterioration after the medications were discontinued, he was restarted on atomaxetin, 25 mg, for his severe impulsivity and hyperactivity, and ziprasidone 40 mg BID for aggressive behavior and agitation. Due to sedation, ziprasidone was changed to aripiprazole 10 mg BID, later adjusted to 7.5 mg BID. On these medications the impulsivity and hyperactivity came under satisfactory control and Jittery displayed no orobuccal movements, choreathetosis, or any other evidence of a movement disorder. No evidence of involuntary movement disorder was detectable in this child in subsequent follow-ups. After another inpatient admission for violence toward the family, he was involuntarily committed and observed without psychotropic medication for about a month; he did not show any evidence of EPS then. This clinical example puts into question either the concept of irreversibility of TD in children, or the timetable of reversibility of the withdrawal dyskinesia.

It is likely that the child's neurodevelopmental background and the prolonged exposure to high doses of risperidone may have contributed to this complication. At a later time, when neuroleptics were discontinued for more than two moths, Jittery showed no evidence of orobuccal dyskinesia or other movement disorders. Unexpectedly, one day, he began to show some involuntary movements again. The psychiatrist was puzzled because Jittery was only supposed to be on atomaxetine, 80 mg/day. The psychiatrist reviewed the record carefully and learned that the child was also receiving propanolol 10 mg BID. This medication was discontinued and the movement disorders subsided. In other words, the metabolic interference of atomaxetine brought on by propanolol induced a movement disorder in this child with a diathesis for involuntary movements. Two years later, Jittery remained free from involuntary movement disorders.

A related but different movement disorder is represented by Superman:

This 8-year-old white boy had a long history of aggressive behavior at home and at school. As a result of his violent and psychotic behavior he had undergone multiple psychiatric admissions in the past. His mother reported that he had severe neurodevelopmental difficulties since birth. Actually, the child was "blue and unresponsive at birth." Superman had delays in the development of milestones and a history of severe expressive language difficulties. He also had difficulties progressing in learning, and from the very beginning of elementary school, he had been provided with special education services. He had received speech therapy and occupational therapy for gross and fine motor deficits. There was no history of seizures. Mother began to notice involuntary movements of the mouth and face of her son by the second year of age, long before he started receiving psychotropic medications.

Superman was an engaging and at times endearing blond child who was markedly hyperactive and impulsive. During one of his hospitalizations, he hit peers indiscriminately and even elbowed his psychiatrist in the genital area; he also hit a number of peers in the "privates" (no history of physical or sexual abuse was ever elicited).

One aspect of his behavior was somewhat perplexing: with some frequency, he would go to his room and stay there for long periods of time, and even though he was encouraged to participate in group or other therapeutic activities, he kept to himself. In his room, he stayed quiet, appeared rather placid, and remained isolated and calmed for extended periods of time. At those times, he would respond and would engage when prompted.

On one occasion, during a psychiatric hospitalization, when a physician was nearby, Superman displayed seizure activity: he rolled his eyes backward and became unresponsive for a short while. After a number of EEGs, one tracing was conclusive for the presence of bilateral spiking in the temporal and frontal areas. In retrospect, the very short-lived episodes of eye rolling lasting for a few seconds were most likely seizure episodes, with a frontal lobe focus. The described behaviors, however, remained unabated in spite of treatment with valproate, carbamazepine, and oxicarbamazepine.

The mental status revealed an exuberant hyperactive and impulsive child who required ongoing structuring; he was very oppositional and rarely sat down on the designated chair. He displayed overt expressive language and articulation deficits; he had limited vocabulary, and displayed disturbance in the melodic aspects of language, dysprosody.

The child was very psychotic: he believed he was Superman and felt he could "burn things with the lava that come from my eyes." He had tried to fly from high places before. The child adhered to the conviction that he was Superman even when challenged. Every time the examiner expressed disbelief that he was Superman, he would start enacting contortions in the air, and would throw himself to the ground enacting fights, all this to prove to the examiner he was Superman. The child never lost his delusion that he was the man of steel. Not surprisingly, he used a Superman costume for Halloween.

Superman revealed that he heard voices telling him to kill people; he claimed that the voices told him "to hit people in the nuts." He reported that the voices told him to kill his mother, too. Although, the child was somewhat engaging, his affect was frequently bland and inappropriate. His affect brightened every time he enacted his Superman beliefs. On close observation, he displayed involuntary movements of the mouth, lips, and jaw, and his tongue was very restless. These movements extended to the face, mainly to the lower eyelids and nose. When he was asked to extend the hands with the fingers spread, obvious choreathetotic movements were observed. The examiner also noticed involuntary movements of the neck and trunk. All along, the child displayed generalized fidgeting.

When the psychiatrist called mother's attention to the involuntary movements, she indicated that the child had problems with these movements from a very early age, and reiterated that the movements had been present before he started receiving psychiatric medications.

Treatment of this child posed challenges on many fronts. Psychopharmacologically, the child needed stimulant medications, but these worsened the movement disorder (even atomaxetine made the movement disorder worse). This child also needed antipsychotic medications, but those medications also worsened the movement disorder. The seizure disorder did not respond to three antiepileptic medications.

The history indicated that the oro-buccal-lingual and facial movements preceded the exposure to antipsychotic medications. Technically, this child suffered from a chronic dyskinesia, secondary to cerebral palsy. This was not a case of neuroleptic induced tardive dyskinesia.

Tardive Psychopathology

Rare, Unpredictable, Potentially Serious

Tardive psychopathology is postulated to be more frequent than tardive dyskinesia. Tardive psychopathology includes psychosis, obsessive–compulsive disorders, or depression. It has been proposed that clozapine's ability to treat neuroleptic-resistant schizophrenia is due to this medication's purported ability to specifically treat tardive psychopathology, in a fashion similar to lithium (Swartz, 2003, p. 13).

Neuroleptic Malignant Syndrome (NMS)

Rare, Unpredictable, Serious, Feared, and Potentially Fatal

NMS is a serious, life-threatening side effect of medications that reduce dopaminergic neurotransmission. In its most lethal presentation, NMS is characterized by a fulminating onset of delirium, rigidity, immobility, mutism, staring, and tremulousness. Autonomic disturbances are prominent and are manifested by high fever, diaphoresis, tachycardia, and labile or elevated blood pressure. Mental status changes indicated the presence of an encephalopathy that can be demonstrated by diffused EEG slowing. The most common causative agents are antipsychotic drugs, including most of the newer atypical antipsychotics. Cases of NMS have also been reported with metoclopramide, a dopamine D2 blocking agent used for gastrointestinal symptoms, and with the sudden withdrawal of drugs used to enhance dopaminergic functions, such as levodopa and amantadine (Rosebush & Mazurek, 2001, p. 1). The incidence range of NMS has been estimated to be between 0.02% to 1.8%. However, there is evidence to support the view that NMS frequently goes unrecognized and underdiagnosed, especially for those treated with non-anti-psychotic medications (Christensen, 2004, p. 20).

Haloperidol, for a long time the medication of choice for treating agitation and delirium, was the most common trigger of NMS. Frequently overlooked, antiemetics and sedatives with neuroleptic properties such as prochlorperazine, metoclopramide, and promethazine can also trigger NMS (Caroff, 2003, p. 38).

Factors that increase patients' risk for NMS include dehydration, agitation, low serum iron, underlying brain damage, catatonia, and history of prior NMS episodes (p. 39). In addition, high room temperature and the diagnosis of affective disorder have been implicated as contributory factors (Rosebush & Mazurek, 2001, p. 3).

The typical case scenario is that of an undernourished, inadequately hydrated, catatonic or agitated patient on multiple medications who receives a rapid dose increase of a high potency antipsychotic drug. NMS was common in the era of rapid neuroleptization and in patients with very high doses of potent antipsychotic drugs. However, NMS can occur in patients on low doses or in stable antipsychotic regimes, particularly in those receiving polypharmacy. Lithium is often implicated in these reactions; SSRIs may also lower the NMS threshold (Rosebush & Mazurek, 2001, pp. 2–3).

Contemporary experts stress the importance of early detection of NMS to undertake effective treatment. Although, identifying early signs is difficult, if not impossible in fulminating cases, patients with incipient NMS show the following symptoms: unexpected mental status changes, new onset catatonia, refractory EPS, and bulbar signs such as rigidity, dysphagia, or dysarthria (Caroff, 2003, p. 39). Other researchers have corroborated that mental status changes (especially confusion) and extrapyramidal symptoms usually precede other signs of NMS, and that temperature elevation may represent a late sign of a potentially fulminating course (Christensen, 2004, p. 21)

It appears that the neuroleptic malignant syndrome (NMS) is more frequent with conventional than with atypical antipsychotics. All currently marketed atypicals, except for ziprasidone, have been linked to at least one case of NMS in adults. Reports in pediatric patients are limited to two adolescent cases treated with risperidone (Labellarte & Riddle, 2002, p. 99). Probably, there is considerable underreporting of this potentially lethal complication.

In the NMS clinical course, it is postulated that an acute phase reaction (APR), an immunological reaction, initiates NMS. APR causes a cascade of events that can be precipitated by infections, muscle injuries, strenuous exercise, burns, surgery, and, perhaps psychological stress. Fever, leukocytosis, muscle breakdown, and low iron serum level are seen in APR and are all found in NMS (p. 99). The most common immediate causes of death associated with NMS are cardiac and respiratory arrest, pulmonary emboli, disseminated intravascular coagulation, and myoglobinuric renal failure (Christensen, 2004, p. 22).

NMS is a poorly understood syndrome that usually occurs within hours or days of initiating antipsychotic medications (Wilkaitis et al. 2004, p. 437). Besides the risks described above, NMS is more frequent in men than in women and occurs more often during the summer months. The NMS risk is also increased by rapid titration, physical restraint, and intramuscular use (p. 438).

In a review of the pertinent literature, Silva, Munoz, Alpert, Perlmutter, and Diaz (1999) reported that, with few exceptions, the NMS clinical presentation in children and adolescents was similar to the one described in adults. The triad of *fever*, *tachycardia*, and *rigidity* characterizes the presentation in children and adults; alteration of consciousness was seen in 72%, including coma in 19.4%. Boys are affected twice as often as girls. Children show a higher rate of dystonia (40.8 vs. 29% for all the ages), and a lower rate of tremor (32.7 vs. 48% for all ages). The course could be fulminating or could last up to 18 days.

There are no pathognomonic tests for NMS but a laboratory profile supports the diagnosis: leukocytosis in the absence of infection, elevated levels of muscle enzymes creatine phosphokinase (CPK), serum alanine aminotransferase (ALT), aspartate aminotransferase (AST), and lactate dehydrogenase (LDH), and low levels of serum iron. Calcium is usually low; BUN and creatinine will increase if renal function is compromised by myoglobinuria. Urine myoglobine is increased (Rosebush & Mazurek, 2001, pp. 1–2).

Silva, Munoz, et al. (1999), report that fatality outcomes have dropped sharply, but underreporting is a concern. Prior to 1986 the mortality rate was 21%; the mortality risk being higher early in the NMS onset. The authors were unable to locate any NMS fatalities in children from 1986 until the publication of their article in 1999.

The decrease of NMS frequency and its apparent better prognosis may be related to the clinician's growing awareness of early antipsychotic discontinuation and the need for a more aggressive medical treatment approach. Children who had been receiving anticholinergics along with the antipsychotics, and had those medications discontinued at the time of the NMS onset, had a better outcome than those kept on them (pp. 190–193). The differential diagnosis of NMS includes infection plus EPS, anticholinergic toxicity, serotonin syndrome, heat stroke, retarded catatonia, and malignant hyperthermia (Rosebush & Mazurek, 2001, p. 3).

The neuroleptic malignant syndrome cannot be differentiated from malignant catatonia (MC; previously called lethal catatonia), either clinically or by laboratory testing. The hallmarks of malignant catatonia are acute onset of excitement, delirium, fever, autonomic instability, and catalepsy. Until the advent of ECT most of the patients died. Those clinical features are similar if not identical with the features observed in the neuroleptic malignant syndrome. Both clinical syndromes respond to benzodiazepines and ECT (Taylor & Fink, 2003, p. 1236). ECT should be considered early in the course of MC. Other conditions commonly associated with catatonic features include delirious mania, benign stupor, and malignant hyperthermia (p. 1235).

It is proposed that simple catatonia, malignant catatonia, and NMS share a common pathophysiology; this involves a reduction of dopaminergic neurotransmission within the basal ganglia-thalamocortical circuits. Hypodopaminergia may underlie muscle rigidity (Mann, Caroff, Campbell, Cabrina, & Greenstein, 2003, p. 7). MC appears to be a nonspecific syndrome that may occur in association with diverse neurological, medical drug-induced, and psychiatric illnesses (p. 9). ECT is the preferred treatment for MC and its effectiveness and survival rates are better when the treatment is initiated during the first five days of the onset of symptoms. Even severely debilitated patients have tolerated ECT without incident (p. 12).

Although, the serotonergic or serotonin syndrome shares many clinical features with NMS, the etiologies of the syndromes are different. The serotonergic syndrome is caused by agents that stimulate specific central and peripheral serotonin receptors, mainly, 5-HT1A and 5-HT2; probably 5-HT3 and 5-HT4 are also involved in causing GI symptoms and affecting dopaminergic transmission (Sternbach, 2003, p. 16). Serotonin syndrome has been reported as a result of interactions between MAOIs, including selegiline and reversible MAOIs inhibitors (RIMAs), and various serotonergic compounds (p. 16).

LeDoux, Braslow, and Brown (2004) argued about the role of C-reactive protein (CRP) in the pathogenesis of the serotonin syndrome (SS). SS occurs when there is an acute increase in extracellular serotonin in the presence of an impaired serotonin metabolism. Vascular disease and depression are linked to elevated CRP. CRP activates platelets, promoting the release of serotonin, and inhibiting the endothelial nitric oxide synthase, which is an "off" signal for the release and action of the platelet-derived serotonin. Thus, CRP may contribute to the SS by perpetuating the release of serotonin and inhibiting the nitric oxide synthase. They postulate that CRP may help to predict patients at risk for SS (p. 1499). The serotonin syndrome may be differentiated from the NMS clinically as outlined below (see table 13.8).

Boyer and Shannon (2005) emphasize that no laboratory tests confirm the diagnosis of serotonin syndrome (SS). However, the presence of tremor, clonus, or akathisia, in the absence of additional extrapyramidal signs should lead clinicians to consider this diagnosis. A history of prescriptions and OTC drugs, use of illicit substances, and dietary supplements may be informative. The physical examination should focus on the assessment of deep-tendon reflexes, clonus, muscle rigidity, ascertaining mydriasis, dryness of oral mucosa, the intensity of bowel sounds, skin color, and the presence or absence of diaphoresis (p. 1115). The evolution of this syndrome is revealing: SS onset is usually rapid, often occurring minutes after ingestion of the injurious agent or of the poisoning substance (p. 1114). Hyperthermia and muscular hypertonia appear late in the syndrome development (p. 1113).

Originally, the serotonin syndrome excluded the addition or increase of antipsychotics prior to the onset of the syndrome. However, serotonin syndrome has been reported with combinations of risperidone and paroxetine; olanzap-

TABLE 13.8 Differential Diagnosis Between the Serotonin Syndrome and the Neuromalignant Syndrome

Serotonin syndrome	NMS
• Psychomotor agitation	• Immobility
• Clonus, mioclonic jerking, hyperreflexia, fasciculations	• These findings rare in NMS
• GI disturbances: nausea, vomiting, diarrhea	• Constipation and paralytic ileus
• Antecedent ataxia	• No history of ataxia
• Seizures, severe hypotension, ventricular tachycardia, and disseminated intravascular coagulation (DIC)	• Rarely present in NMS

Source: Rosebush & Mazurek (2001, p. 4).

ine, mirtazapine and tramadol, and olanzapine with lithium and citalopram. The 5-HT2 antagonism effect of these antipsychotics may have led indirectly to an overactivation of 5-HT1A receptors resulting in the serotonin syndrome (Mann et al., 2003, p. 19).

NMS cases treated with bromocriptine (a D2 receptor agonist) and dantroline (a peripheral relaxant that interferes with the release of calcium from the sarcoplasmic reticulum) showed no significant benefit over supportive care. When these drugs are used, there is a tendency for a recrudescence of autonomic abnormalities and of elevation of the CPK when these agents are withdrawn.

> In our experience with over 50 patients with NMS, the natural course of the syndrome—even in the most severe cases—has been for the autonomic disturbances, as well as the laboratory abnormalities, to peak in the first 48 hours. They begin to improve significantly within 72 hours solely with cessation of the putative offending agents, administration of antipyretics, application of cooling blankets and replacement of intravenous fluids. (Rosebush & Mazurek, 2001, p. 5).

There are anecdotal reports that benzodiazepines are helpful; ASA or acetominophen are important therapeutic agents.

> Fever, EEG abnormalities, and alteration of consciousness appear to be related to a poor prognosis. Complications or NMS include respiratory failure, deep vein thrombosis with risk of pulmonary embolism, contractures if immobility is prolonged, entrapment neuropathies, renal failure, muscle weakness, and infections such as pneumonia and urinary tract infections. (p. 6)

NMS residual symptoms included residual rigidity, brachial plexus palsy, residual dysarthria, liver function abnormalities, atelectasis, increase of prolactin levels, and the development of other abnormal movements. Rare sequelae include seizures, DIC, and cerebellar degeneration. Following a NMS episode patients are at a higher risk of suffering a recurrence if antipsychotic medications are reintroduced within the first two weeks of the full syndrome resolution. Lithium has been reported as precipitating recurrences. After two weeks of full syndrome resolution a single agent may be reintroduced at a low dose, and slow titration should be continued with regular CPK and vital signs monitoring. The NMS episode gives the opportunity to evaluate what medications are essential and which ones need to be discarded (Rosebush & Mazurek, 2001, p. 6).

Upon suspicion of NMS, all antipsychotics, lithium, and SSRIs should be discontinued. Since most psychiatric settings are not equipped to deal with complex, life-threatening conditions, patients should be immediately transported to a medical center where ICU or other life support measures can be provided.

Anticholinergic Side Effects

Common, Unpredictable, Rarely Serious

Anticholinergic effects result from blockade of cholinergic receptors. Blurred vision, dry mouth, sweating, constipation, tachycardia, delayed micturition, exacerbation of narrow angle glaucoma, impaired memory and learning, and dental disease are common anticholinergic symptoms secondary to neuroleptics, TCAs, and anti-Parkinson medications. More severe anticholinergic toxicity is manifested by seizures, hyperthermia, delirium, central nervous system depression, and coma. Impaired acquisition of new learning is the earliest detectable anticholinergic toxic CNS effect. Dosage increase or cumulative effects of several different anticholinergic medications cause more obvious impairments in attention and cognitive functioning (Ayd, 2000, p. 59). The proposed anticholinergic side effect ranking for SGAs in adults is as follows: Clozapine > quetiapine > olanzapine > risperidone > ziprasidone = aripiprazole.

In the Clinical Antipsychotic Trials of Intervention Effectiveness (CATIE) report, quetiapine was associated with a higher rate of anticholinergic effects than the other medications (olanzapine, risperidone, ziprasidone, perphenazine) (Lieberman, Stroup, et al., 2005, p. 1215).

An anticholinergic side effect that often progresses in silence is constipation; this adverse event may advance to fecal impaction and to paralytic ileus. It is easy to overlook monitoring bowel movements. It is not rare for children with unidentified constipation to require evaluation at the emergency room for abdominal pain or symptoms of abdominal obstruction.

Orthostatic hypotension often causes dizziness and rarely, fainting. Atypicals with higher anticholinergic activity cause this side effect more frequently. In children with a normal heart, this symptom may be inconsequential and simple measures of avoiding rapid standing from a supine or a sitting to a standing position, such as a slow arising to full standing, are sufficient to control this adverse event.

Hematological Side Effects

Uncommon, Unpredictable, Potentially Serious

Agranulocytosis is a well-known and feared clozapine side effect. Changes in blood counts associated with clozapine treatment appear to occur at the same rate in youngsters as in adults. The same hematologic monitoring as in adults is recommended for children on clozapine treatment (Stigler, Potenza, & McDougle, 2001, p. 932).

Less known, are the hematological effects of other atypical medications. For instance, olanzapine may induce a dose related leukopenia (Kodesh, Finkel, Lerner, Kretzner, & Sigal, 2001). Leukopenia has also been reported with risperidone (p. 935). So far, no agranulocytosis has been reported with either quetiapine (Stigler, Potenza, & McDougle, 2001, p. 938), or with ziprasidone (p. 939). To this day, there is no indication that aripripazole has any untoward hematological side effects.

Leukopenia (WBC < 3,500) associated with conventional antipsychotics is usually transitory; it is rather common but not problematic. Agranulocytosis associated with classical antipsychotics occurs most often during the first three months of treatment with an incidence of 1 in 500,000 (Wilkaitis, Mulvihill, & Nasrallah, 2004, p. 438).

Hepatic Side Effects

Rare, Unpredictable, Potentially Serious

Olanzapine produces an increase in the hepatic enzymes and is potentially more toxic than divalproex. It may also be associated with pancreatitis and with steatohepatitis. Fifty-nine percent of patients taking olanzapine alone, had elevations of ALT, AST, or LDH during the treatment period, whereas 26% of the divalproex alone group showed those elevations; 100% of subjects on a combination of olanzapine and divalproex had these elevations. For 42% of the children on combined olanzapine plus divalproex, the elevated peak hepatic enzymes did not return to normal during the observed course of treatment. For these patients, the mean period of time for which the levels of hepatic enzymes were observed after the peak level was 8 ± 6 months (Gonzalez-Heydrich, Raches, Wilens, Leichtner, & Mezzacappa, 2003, p. 1227).

In the case of both peak and mean enzyme levels, the hepatic enzyme elevations were less than three times the upper limit of normal range, and did not meet the threshold for heightened concern. Two patients in olanzapine + divalproex experienced severe complications. One patient developed pancreatitis and was lost to follow-up, and the other developed esteatohepatitis which resolved after the discontinuation of olanzapine. The risk of hepatic failure has been estimated as 1/45,000 for divalproex and 1/12,000 for olanzapine (p. 1231). Olanzapine is, then, more hepatotoxic than divalproex. Olanzapine may cause pancreatitis and steatohepatitis. This risk is further increased when olanzapine is used concomitantly with divalproex (Gonzalez-Heydrich et al., 2003, pp. 1231, 1232; see also Gelenberg, 2002, p. 5).

The conclusion is unavoidable: the combination of olanzapine-divalproex increases the risk of hepatotoxicity and should only be used with caution.

When elucidating liver disease secondary to antipsychotics, the psychiatrist will keep in mind that nonalcoholic fatty liver disease (NAFLD) and nonalcoholic steatohepatitis (NASH), secondary to obesity, need to be ruled out (Tucker, 2004, p. 59). Currently hepatic disease obesity-related surpasses alcohol-related liver disease. Obese persons who drank more than two drinks a day, had close to a sixfold increase of liver damage risk compared to normal weight persons who did not drink alcohol (Zoler, 2004, p. 59).

SEXUAL DYSFUNCTION: UNCOMMON, TROUBLING, PROMOTES NONCOMPLIANCE

Sexual dysfunction, including decreased libido, impaired arousal, and erectile orgasmic dysfunction, is rather common in patients receiving atypicals. These effects may be caused by anticholinergic side effects, alpha-1 inhibition, and hypogonadism secondary to hyperprolactinemia. Erectile dysfunction and anorgasmia are reported with some frequency in patients receiving atypicals (Wirshing et al., 2003, p. 56).

Priapism has been reported with all atypicals except ziprasidone. Alpha-1 blockade can inhibit detumescence via its indirect tendency to increase nitric oxide. Priapism is a urologic emergency. Patients developing abnormally prolonged and painful erections need immediate medical attention (p. 56).

CATARACTS: MOSTLY ASSOCIATED WITH TYPICAL ANTIPSYCHOTICS

Drugs that are most frequently related to the development of lenticular changes include corticosteroids, phenothiazines, miotics, gold, amiodarone, and allopurinol (Ruigomez, Garcia, Dev, et al., 2004, p. 620). Glaucoma and retinal detachment were the strongest predictors of cataracts. Diabetes mellitus increases the risk of cataracts fourfold (p. 623). Overall antipsychotic drug use was not associated with cataracts. Risk is increased with the use of chlorpromazine and prochlorperazine (p. 622).

There is insufficient evidence to associate quetiapine with an increase risk of cataract development. A recent report found 34 cases of lens opacities in 620,000 patient exposures to quetiapine in the United States. Most of these patients had known risk factors (use of medications known to increase the risk for cataracts, ocular trauma, hypertension, or diabetes) or had cataracts at baseline. Some patients could have developed idiopathic cataracts (Marder, Essock, et al., 2004, pp. 1343, 1345). In spite of this, it is recommended that patients older than 40 years should receive an annual ocular evaluation (Marder, Essock, et al., 2004, p. 1345).

In Kasper and Muller-Spahn's (2000) comprehensive overview of quetiapine studies, no mention of cataract as a side effect is mentioned. It is important to remember that there is a high incidence of eye abnormalities in patients with chronic psychosis. A study found that 26% of patients with schizophrenia had cataracts compared to 0.2% of healthy controls with no exposure to psychotropic medications. Many factors predispose a person to cataract development: exposure to typical antipsychotic medications (i.e., thioridazine and chlorpromazine), prior steroid use, increased age, female gender, high blood pressure, diabetes, cigarette smoking, alcohol use, dietary deficiencies, ultraviolet light, and low socioeconomic status (Lieberman, 2004, p. 482).

Reports of lens abnormalities in patients treated with quetiapine are rare, less than 1 in 10,000 cases (p. 482). In the same vein, "So far, no lenticular abnormalities have been found on lit-lamp examinations over a 12 month period" (McConville et al., 2000, p. 257). In spite of this, it is prudent to request yearly ophtalmological evaluations for children on long-term quetiapine treatment. In the CATIE report, there was no difference in cataract rates among the antipsychotic studied (olanzapine, risperidone, quetiapine, ziprasidone, and perphenazine) (Lieberman, Stroup, et al., 2005, p. 1215).

Cognitive Side Effects

Rather Common, Could Become Disabling

Last but not least, antipsychotics produce cognitive side effects. FGAs have an unfavorable impact on the cognitive functions in chronically psychotic patients; this is more so if anticholinergic medications to deal with (or to prevent) EPS are used. Anticholinergic medications disrupt cognitive functions significantly, the memory processes, in particular. Patients on SGAs perform better in neurocognitive testing than patients on conventional antipsychotics. Lowering the dose of conventional antipsychotics yields neurocognitive benefits and decreases the disadvantage of the typical medications; the SGAs are not cognitive enhancers (Velligan & Glahn, 2004, pp. 73–74).

Velligan and Glahn (2004), state that cognitive impairments are central features in schizophrenia and that they are important predictors of community outcomes for schizophrenic patients. Cognitive impairments have a better functional outcome predictive power than clinical symptomatology. Consistently, research has demonstrated that schizophrenic patients perform one to three standard deviations below controls on a wide range of neurocognitive abilities; processing speed, attention, memory, and executive functions, among others, may be relatively more impaired (p. 74).

Other Significant Side Effects

All the atypicals are associated with enuresis; encopresis is less common. Rhinitis, producing "noisy breathing" is a very common side effect. Drooling is not uncommon, particularly in latency children and preschoolers. Antipsychotics interfere with the process of attention, much more if the medication is sedative;

atypicals induce behavioral toxicity in children and adolescents. Atypicals may interfere with temperature regulation. All the atypical medications carry a risk for esophageal dysmotility and photosensitivity. Atypicals are associated with retrograde ejaculation and priapism; see above.

Obsessive–Compulsive Disorder

Atypicals are used to augment the treatment of OCD, but atypicals also worsen OCD symptomatology. Risperidone has been associated with the emergence of obsessive–compulsive disorder (OCD; Diler et al., 2003). The authors presented two cases of rapid-onset OCD associated to risperidone. Case A was an 8-year-old boy with a history of ADHD and chronic tic disorder who developed OCD within two weeks of starting risperidone (0.5 mg TID). Symptoms resolved upon discontinuation of risperidone. Case B, an 11-year-old girl with a history of mental retardation and aggressive behaviors was treated with risperidone 1 mg/day. OCD symptoms started 10 days after risperidone initiation. Symptoms resolved after risperidone discontinuation. The authors conclude that this report adds to several other reports of sudden emergence of OCD and anxiety symptoms in patients treated with atypical antipsychotics.

CHAPTER **14**

Treatment of Atypical Side Effects

Prevention is the best measure to avoid adverse medication events. Prescription of effective medications with minimal likelihood of eliciting adverse events takes precedence over other drugs with increased risks. Systematic monitoring will insure medication effectiveness and prompt detection of and response to emerging side effects. Cardiovascular complications must be kept in mind and avoided at all times. Laryngeal spasm demands immediate emergency treatment. Extrapyramidal side effects (EPS) and galactorrhea demand prompt intervention. Neuroleptic malignant syndrome is a true medical emergency that necessitates intensive and specialized medical care. Weight gain and its related complications (diabetes mellitus, dyslipedemia, and metabolic syndrome) require close monitoring, and a deliberate and coordinated multidisciplinary medical treatment program. Tardive dyskinesia development needs to be anticipated with the use of antipsychotics. The beginning of this complication at its very earliest stages needs timely detection and intervention. For issues related to clozapine side effects see chapter 12 (p. 331).

MEDICAL AND NEUROLOGICAL ISSUES

There are medical and neurological conditions that mimic psychotic disorders; they need a prompt identification. Every child or adolescent with a serious psychotic illness must have a thorough medical and neurological workup, more so if it is the first episode. In these cases, the psychiatrist will make an exhaustive effort to rule out medical or neurological conditions, including the presence of substance abuse. Also, there are complex psychosocial stressors that may not be initially obvious; they require rapid identification and appropriate interventions since they may be a source of medical, behavioral, and emotional destabilization. The psychiatrist needs to insure that the patient's health status is thoroughly reviewed and that the patient is medically cleared of any active medical problem; any ongoing medical problem may contribute to the patient's

419

ongoing behavioral difficulties. Any unresolved medical issues will be attended to by appropriate diagnostic workup or timely referral to appropriate specialists. Any major health problem takes precedence over psychiatric issues, even when patients are agitated and pose a threat to themselves, to others, or to the integrity of the surrounding environment. Agitation should not deter the physician from providing a comprehensive medical evaluation.

The child and adolescent psychiatrist needs to work closely with pediatricians, developmental pediatricians, pediatric neurologists, endocrinologists, and other specialists, and professionals dealing with the specific medical issues or deficits the patient presents. The cooperation and dialogue among treating physicians is essential for dealing with children with complex medical–psychiatric problems (DM, asthma, epilepsy, eating disorders, and others); these patients receive medications from multiple physicians that potentially interact among themselves, and with the psychotropic medications.

ISSUES RELATED TO TORSADES DE POINTES (TDP) AND SUDDEN DEATH: RARE, FEARED, AND POTENTIALLY FATAL, POTENTIALLY PREDICTABLE

Prevention is the most important weapon against TdP, a potentially lethal arrhythmia.

If QTc prolongation is evidenced, a thorough review of the medication the patient is taking, close EKG monitoring, and a prompt cardiovascular consultation will be procured.

TABLE 14.1 Relevant Issues Related to the Prevention of Torsades de Pointes

- A thorough medical history that includes:
  Prior cardiovascular history
  History of fainting and syncope
- A family history that includes:
  History of sudden deaths in the family
  History of drowning, car accidents
  History of Long QTc syndrome
- A review of medications the child is taking that may include QTc prolonging drugs (This review should include OTC drugs, health products, and other herbal products).
- Attention to the impact of psychotropics on the patient's health status and in the cardiovascular system, in particular
- Cardiological consultation requested when the patient has a positive cardiovascular history or is about to receive medications that have the potential for increasing the QTc
- Avoid coprescription of medications that may potentiate QTc prolongation
- Educate the patient about the importance of telling his/her physician(s) about potential risk of adding QTc prolonging medications
- Communicate with primary physician and other specialists on the patient's psychotropic prescriptions and potential risk of adding QTc prolonging coprescriptions

ISSUES RELATED TO OBESITY: COMMON, POTENTIALLY SERIOUS, PREDICTABLE

"Clinicians should focus on preventing initial weight gain and obesity, because subsequent weight loss is very difficult to achieve and existing interventions to promote weight loss are ineffective" (Marder, Essock, et al., 2004, pp. 1336). Clinicians should encourage patients to self-monitor their weight. A gain of one BMI unit in a normal weight or overweight person should lead the clinician to recommend an intervention; for example, nutritional counseling, initiation of an exercise program, use of medications to promote weight loss, or change to a different antipsychotic less likely to be associated with weight gain (p. 1336). The ordering of the described intervention does not represent the sequence of implementation of such interventions. Therefore, change of medications may take precedence over other recommendations.

Currently, issues related to obesity and its consequences are uppermost in physicians' and psychiatrists' minds. Some years back the most relevant adverse concerns were related to EPS, and the dreaded complication of TD. Now, cardio-vascular problems (coronary artery disease, and others) and ketoacidosis associated with diabetes mellitus (secondary to obesity) are the subject of increasing concern. The alarm has been triggered by the progressive realization that the psychotropic medications that are supposed to alleviate mental illness are the cause of significant health complications; mainly, weight increase and diabetes elicitation. Although, antipsychotic medications are the most frequently cited offenders, other psychotropics, including mood stabilizers and antidepressants, contribute to the problem. Why should child and adolescents psychiatrists take an active role in treating obesity?

Recent scientific data have discarded the old idea that obesity reflects a lack of willpower. Obesity is a problem of regulation of energy stores (Wabitsch, 2002, p. 50).

Overweight and obesity are associated with a multiplicity of health risks. Obesity may be considered the worst socioeconomic handicap that women suffer. It is a serious problem in childhood and tends to persist into adulthood, creating major negative, long-term impact on affected subjects (Zwiauer, Caroli, Malecka-Tendera, & Poskitt, 2002, p. 144). Girls overweight at age 16 with a BMI above the 95th percentile when compared with their lean peers seven years later, were found to have completed fewer years of school, earned less, had higher rates of poverty, and were less likely to be married. All of these difficulties were independent of their teenage SES (Hill & Lissau, 2002, pp. 122–123). Primary physicians are not paying the attention that overweight and obese should receive.

Overweight and obesity are associated with significant psychiatric morbidity (depressive disorders, anxiety disorders, eating disorders, suicidal behavior, oppositionality, and others).

Obese patients experience a greater number of lifetime depressive and manic episodes, have more severe and difficult-to-treat index affective episodes, or are more likely to develop an affective depressive recurrence than matched nonobese controls (Strakowski, 2003, p. 58).

Overweight and obesity bring to their sufferers significant social and personal adversity including teasing, rejection, family conflict, and others. When parents become critical of the child's weight the impact is worse.

A school based sample of 4,746 students, 7th to 12th grades at 31 public middle and high schools, was conducted by Eisenberg, Neumark-Sztainer, and Story (2003), to evaluate the association of weight based teasing and body satisfaction, self-esteem, depressive symptoms, and suicidal ideation and suicidal attempts: 81.5% of the students participated; 30.0% of the adolescent girls and 24% of the boys were teased by peers; and 28.7% of adolescent girls and 16.1% of adolescent boys were teased by family members. About 14.6% of adolescent girls and 9.6% of adolescent boys reported teasing from both sources. Teasing about weight was associated with low body satisfaction, low self-esteem, high depressive symptoms, and thinking about suicide and suicidal attempts. The associations held for both adolescent boys and girls, regardless of race, ethnic, or weight groups. Teasing from two sources was associated with a higher prevalence of emotional problems than either teasing from a single source or no teasing.

There is continuity between being overweight at 5 and 10 years of age and overweight in adolescence (and in many cases, into adulthood). About 20% of the children between 12 and 19 years of age are overweight; that is, they are at least in the 85 percentile of weight for their age. The prevalence of overweight and obesity is also increasing in the 2- to 11-year-old range.

The child and adolescent psychiatrist is in a favorable position to promote, implement, and monitor treatment strategies for children and adolescents who have problems with overweight or obesity.

Child and adolescent psychiatrists should not assume this major responsibility by themselves; they should enlist allied specialists' assistance in dealing with these complex issues. The psychiatrist needs to have on his or her team nutritional experts, endocrinologists, cardiologists, physical therapists, and fitness experts to attend to the multiplicity of issues that relate to or complicate the problem of overweight and obesity.

Obesity lowers children's self-esteem; obese children are frequently ostracized and made fun off, and have a negative self-image. Obesity stigmatizes children even before adolescence, and places them outside the social mainstream. When shown drawings of children of different sizes, children rank obese classmates as the least desirable. Parental concern is correlated with children's negative self-image: parental acceptance or lack of concern may be a protective factor for self-esteem (Zametkin, Zoon, Klein, & Munson, 2004, p. 137). See endnote for relevant issues related to obesity and type 2 diabetes.[1]

Even though overweight and obesity are reaching epidemic proportions in childhood, the treatment of severely obese adolescents with comorbid conditions is regarded as investigative at this time, and should be performed as part of closely monitored studies. It is exceedingly difficult for overweight children and adolescents to lose weight, and even more difficult for them to permanently sustain the achieved weight loss. The ultimate goal must be prevention of the development of overweight in children and youth (Yanovski & Yanovski, 2003, p. 1852).

It appears that the amount of weight gained by children and adolescents on atypical antipsychotics is greater than the weight gain reported in adults. Cases of treatment-emergent diabetes have been reported in the absence of weight gain, and this seems to reflect mechanisms other than drug-associated obesity (Carlson, Sowell, & Cavazzoni, 2003, p. 5). Case reports or small case series, associated with treatment emergent hyperglycemia or type 2 diabetes, have been published on patients receiving treatment with clozapine, olanzapine, risperidone, quetiapine, and ziprasidone. To date, the highest frequency of diabetes has been reported in association with clozapine and olanzapine; however, the occurrence and reports of this complication with the other atypicals is on the increase (p. 5). In the CATIE report (Lieberman, Stroup, et al., 2005), olanzapine demonstrated the highest rate of weight increase promotion and the highest prodyslipidemic effect among the agents compared (olanzapine, risperidone, quetiapine, ziprasidone, and perphenazine).

The body mass index (BMI) is a satisfactory measure of the amount of body fat, and is calculated by dividing the weight in kilograms by the square of the height in meters: weight in $kg/height^2$. The measurement of the waist circumference is considered clinically helpful, since the waist circumference is a good marker of abdominal fat content (Amatruda & Linemeyer, 2001, p. 948).[2] Styne and Shoenfeld-Warden (2003, p. 2138) list among others the following medical consequences of childhood and adolescent obesity (see table 14.2).

Is Dieting Counterproductive?

In a large epidemiologic study involving 8,203 girls and 6,769 boys between 9 and 14 years of age, Field et al. (2003) demonstrated that the adolescents who dieted frequently gained more weight than the infrequent dieters or those who did not diet at all. Infrequent dieters were five times more likely to binge eat; frequent dieters were 12 times more likely to report binge eating. Binge eating was a predictor of weight gain in boys. There was also a strong association

TABLE 14.2 Consequences of Childhood and Adolescent Obesity

Insulin resistance (type 2 diabetes mellitus)
Hyperlipidemia
Cardiopulmonary complications
Hypertension
Obstructive sleep apnea
Obesity hypoventilation syndrome (Pickwickian syndrome): CO_2 retention, hypoxia, polycythemia,
    right ventricular hypertrophy
Increased incidence of asthma
Dermatological
        Acanthosis nigricans
        Heat rash
        Intertrigo
        Monilial dermatitis
Orthopedic
        Slipped capital femoral epiphysis
        Blount disease of the tibia
Gastrointestinal
        Hepatic steatosis and fibrosis
        Cholelithiasis
        Gastroesophageal reflux
Other
        Early puberty and menarche, associated with an increase of breast cancer in later life
        Advanced skeletal development: tall child, short adult
        Ovarian hyperandrogenism: hirsutism and irregular menses, polycystic ovarian disease
        Ideopathic intracraneal hypertension
        Lower extremity venous stasis disease
        Urinary stress incontinence
        Increase of mortality from all causes and morbidity from coronary artery disease, and
            atherosclerotic cerebrovascular disease, in both sexes; increase of colorectal cancer in men

Source: Styne & Shoenfeld-Warden (2003, p. 2138).

between frequent dieting and binge eating behavior (pp. 900, 902). Dieting to lose weight is common among preadolescents and adolescent girls, and among adult women. What are the mechanisms to explain the paradoxical weight gain?[3]

Drastic changes in diet are rarely sustainable, so it is not surprising that very few persons maintain the weight loss. For children and adolescents who are overweight, diets carefully supervised by a clinician may be beneficial and appropriate; however, young people and adults who are not severely overweight need to be encouraged to adopt a modest and therefore sustainable weight control strategy that includes physical activity and does not require severe restriction of total calories or components of the diet, such as percentage of calories from fat. Although in the short-term a restrictive diet may be beneficial for weight loss, in the long-term, data suggest that dieting to control weight is not only ineffective but actually may promote weight gain. (pp. 903, 905). For some frustrated dieters the best advice that may be given is for them to stop dieting.

For obese psychotic children, recent atypical antipsychotics offer some promise: aripiprazole and particularly ziprasidone have limited promotion of weight gain. Ziprasidone is the only antipsychotic in current use that improves a number of factors of the metabolic syndrome.

Overweight youth possessing any two of the risk factors for diabetes or metabolic syndrome should be screened every one or two years beginning at age 10 or at the onset of puberty if it occurs at a younger age. The greater the number of risk factors the greater the risk the patient will develop diabetes (pp. 903, 905).

TREATMENT OF OVERWEIGHT AND OBESITY

The fundamental factor in the treatment of overweight conditions and obesity in children and adolescents is patient and family education. The schools have a big role to play in educating children about hygiene and in instilling healthy habits regarding the regular ingestion of balanced meals, and in increasing children's awareness about the importance of quality of nutrition. Contrary to these goals, many schools have gotten in a liaison with the fast food industry and have introduced unbalanced, high caloric meals to their students. This is certainly regrettable. The PTA and other parent organizations should demand appropriate nutritional education and more intense physical education, and advocate for more appropriate nutrition for students. Some schools are beginning to take back "control of the kitchens" and others are taking steps to implement programs to stem the increased epidemic of obesity in children and adolescents.

The psychiatrist should be ready to recommend health-promoting measures, and should be persuasive and determined in challenging lifestyles and dietary habits that put children's health at risk. The psychiatrist's input starts at the time of the diagnostic assessment, when the physician culls medical and family histories, or when he or she carries out the physical examination. Sometimes, the child and adolescent psychiatrist has the advantage of counting on the family to deal with the child's overweight and obesity. Other times, obesity is a family problem, and the treatment of a child's obesity needs to include the coordination of medical and related services for other overweight/obese family members. The focus on educating both child and family with problems of overweight and obesity includes (see table 14.3).

TABLE 14.3 Educational Focus for Overweight and Obese Children and Their Families

- Genetic factors of obesity and diabetes
- Risk factors of overweight and obesity
- Evolution of diabetes mellitus
- Issues related to diet (caloric intake)
- Issues related to energy expenditure (exercise)
- Association of psychiatric disorders with overweight and obesity
- Need to increase active leisure
- Issues related to sedentary life style:
  Excessive time spent in TV viewing, computer involvement
  Lack of exercise
  Snacking ("Munching") on high calorie foods
- Dietary recommendations
- Stress management
- Problem solving techniques
- Danger of drugs and alcohol
- Issues related to hygiene and dental care
- Issues related to sleep hygiene
- Importance of a parental noncritical attitude toward children or adolescents' overweight and obesity

The most effective behavioral treatments for child obesity are outlined in table 14.4.

TABLE 14.4 Effective Behavioral Treatments for Child Obesity

- A group format with individualized behavioral counseling
- Parents participation
- Frequent sessions
- Long-term treatment
- Simple and explicit diets the produce a caloric deficit
- Physical activity programs that emphasizes choice and reward nonsedentary behaviors
- Promotion of changes in the home and family environment to reduce cues and opportunities associated with calorie intake and inactivity
- To increase cues and opportunities for physical activity
- To increase self-monitoring
- To create goal setting and contracting
- To improve parenting skills
- To improve skills for resolving high risk situations
- To improve skills for (habit) maintenance and relapse prevention

Source: Epstein et al. (1994, p. 144).

WEIGHT GAIN ATTENUATION

Pharmacological weight attenuation is a complement to a dietary and exercise program, and it is never a substitute for them. Even with attenuating agents, the expectation for regular exercising and judicious eating should be maintained. A number of medications are showing some promise in slowing the rate of weight increase induced by the atypical antipsychotics and other weight gain promoting medications. The proposed use of the medications to be discussed below, are off label, not FDA approved. Table 14-5 contains a list of the most commonly prescribed weight attenuating agents with potential use in the treatment of children and adolescents, and their suggested doses.[4]

TREATMENT OF OBESITY

A considerable number of patients with chronic psychosis are overweight or downright obese. To complicate matters, most of the mood stabilizers and atypical antipsychotics prescribed to treat these disorders, promote weight gain. Furthermore, child psychiatrists often prescribe combinations of psychotropic medications that cause an undesirable weight increase. Weight reduction and remedial treatment of obesity should take a high priority in the overall comprehensive medico-psychiatric treatment plan because of the social stigmatization and health risks of obesity.

Reducing weight and maintaining a weight reduction expectation demands a sustained effort and enduring determination; it is a very difficult task. If this objective is difficult to achieve for overweight persons without psychiatric problems, it is not hard to imagine that the task will be far more difficult for patients with chronic psychotic disorders whose motivation is unstable. Some pharmaceutical companies have trivialized the seriousness of the obesity problem induced by antipsychotics.

For many families, one of the biggest battles with their children centers on food; most adolescents do not consume regular, balanced, and nutritious meals. Enforcing healthy eating habits can be a losing battle for parents, due to the pernicious influence of TV and the misguided exposure to inappropriate meals in school cafeterias.

The treatment of psychotic obese patients entails, among other things, the following: a comprehensive medical evaluation, an endocrinological evaluation, a cardiological evaluation, and a review of all medications the patients is taking, including over-the-counter medications, herbal supplements, and other health products.

The Expert Committee on Obesity Evaluation and Treatment recommended that the primary goal of child obesity treatment should be to develop healthy eating and activity habits, and not to strive toward an ideal body weight.

The family influence is the most important factor of child obesity treatment; multiple studies have shown that when the family is involved in the treatment, short-term and long-term success rates are higher (Zametkin et al., 2004, p. 144).

Epstein et al. (1994) published a randomized family-based treatment that showed that after 10 years, 34% of the participants (who had entered the study when they were 6 to 12 years old) decreased weight percentage by 20% or more and that 30% were no longer obese. This long-term result demonstrated the importance of family support for modifying eating and activity behaviors, and suggests major differences between early family-based approaches and late adult trials. This study has not been replicated (p. 379–380).

Phases of Medical Treatment of Obesity

There are three principal phases in the treatment of overweight or obesity.

Phase I. Low Calorie Diet; Exercise; Behavioral Therapy

Many pediatricians do not offer treatment to obese children and adolescents in the absence of comorbid conditions. However, the most widespread consequences of childhood obesity may be psychosocial. Obese children and adolescents are at risk for psychosocial maladjustment, including lowered perceived competencies in the social, athletic, and appearance domains, as well as in overall self-worth (Schwimmer, Burwinkle, & Varni, 2003, p. 1813).

The Health-related Quality of Life (QOL) is a comprehensive and multidisciplinary construct that includes physical, emotional, social, and school functioning. Severely obese children score lower in the domains of the QOL inventory than normal children and adolescents, and as low as children who have cancer or who have received chemotherapy (p. 1817).

A significant number of adolescents on depo-medroxyprogesterone (Depoprovera) experience weight gain (2.5 kg after the first year, and 3.7, 6.3, 7.5 kg after two, four, and six years, respectively) (http://www.PharmacyOneSource.comMembers:DrugInformation).

In the treatment of obese patients it is essential to:

- Review eating habits and other behaviors associated with eating.
- Complete a diagnostic inquiry about the patient's perception of his or her body weight and any actions the patient may be taking to reduce it.
- The physician will complete a detailed survey of the patient's eating habits and of the amount and nature of food the child consumes; he or she will encourage the child and family to keep a detailed record of all the food the child ingests.

- Obtain a detailed account of the child's daily levels of activity and exercise. The physician will be cognizant that most patients tend to minimize what they eat, and to exaggerate the amount of exercise they do.
- Diet, exercise and other hygienic measures, such as, good sleep hygiene are important components of the treatment of obesity. Poor sleep decreases insulin, thyroid hormone, growth hormone, and leptin secretion. Of equal, or even more relevance, is the change of behaviors (behavior modification) of habits (rituals) or behavior chains associated with eating; this entails (1) a functional analysis of the association between eating and activity behaviors, and environmental events, and (2) a systematic modification of eating, activity, or other behaviors thought to contribute to or maintain obesity. Cognitive behavioral strategies for weight management should provide concrete skills to children and families to stimulate behavior change and to attain a healthier life style (Styne & Schoenfeld-Warden, 2003, p. 2141).

The greatest success for weight loss is provided by a combination of diet and increased physical activity along with behavioral medication to positively reinforce diet and exercise programs. Exercise lowers blood glucose, helps to promote a healthy lipid profile, and may improve glucose sensitivity. Furthermore, there is evidence that exercise may improve patient's self-esteem and quality-of-life measures in addition to the beneficial effects on weight and metabolism (Carlson, Sowell, & Cavazzoni, 2003, p. 6). A randomized trial of lifestyle modification and pharmacotherapy published by Wadden et al. (2005), in adult obese patients, confirmed that the combination of pharmacotherapy with lifestyle modification has the best outcome. At one year, subjects who received combined therapy lost a mean (± SD) of 12.1 ± 9.8 kg. Patients who received sibutramine alone lost 5.0 ± 7.4 kg; those treated with lifestyle modification alone lost 6.7 kg ± 7.9 kg, and those receiving sibutramine plus brief therapy lost 7.5 kg ± 8.0 kg ($p < 0.001$) (p. 2115). Subjects who received combined therapy lost significantly more weight at all times than subjects in the other three groups (p. 2116).

As has been previously indicated, the inquiry that will best approximate what the patients are or are not doing in pursuing a weight reduction program should be an open, nonleading inquiry. Questions such as are you dieting or are you exercising are useless. The child psychiatrist should rather ask about what the patient is eating, frequency, amount, and the like, as well as, tell me how are you exercising? How long? How often? The weight scales are always the true measure of effective effort, no matter how credible the patients' account may be.

No treatment of obesity is feasible without the help and ongoing consultation of a dietitian. In a parallel fashion, no obese person should embark on exercising or starting a fitness program without expert advice and competent guidance; close medical monitoring is necessary if the patient has hypertension

or cardiological problems. In the latter case, a cardiological consultant is imperative. The role of attenuating agents is described below (also, see table 14.5).

Phase II. Drugs

Pharmacological treatments of obesity help to stabilize weight loss; they are
always supplementary or complementary to diet, exercising, and habit changes.
Most of the obesity and weight reduction studies have been made in adults;
the extension of those results to adolescents and children should be made with
caution. All the medications to be discussed below are off label and do not have
FDA indication for the treatment of obesity in children and adolescents. Please
refer to the section on attenuating agents below.

Pharmacological Treatment of Obesity

Most of the medications used to treat obesity have had a history of failure,
weight regain, drug abuse, and adverse side effects. The most common medications used as adjuvants in the treatment of obesity are listed in tables 14.5a
and table 14.5b.[5]

TABLE 14.5A Medications with Potential Use for Weight Attenuating Effects in Children and Adolescents

Medications	Starting dose	Maximal dose	Remarks
Amantadine	50–100 mg/day	200–300 mg/day	Higher doses produce anticholinergic SE, including memory problems.
Topiramate	12.5–25 mg/day	200 mg/day	Slow upward titration. Language and cognitive side effects are common
Velafaxine	25–50 mg/day	75–300 mg/day or Effexor XR 75–150 mg/day	Concerns with use of antidepressants in children.
Sibutramine	5–10 mg/day	Up to 20 mg/day	May produce hypertension
Nizatidine	50 mg BID	150 mg BID	
Metformine	500 mg/day	500 mg/BID–TID	Contraindicated in patients with renal or hepatic failure, or metabolic acidosis
Zonisamide	50–100 mg/day	200–300 mg/day	Risk of Steven-Johnson syndrome Cognitive side effects are common
Modafanil	25–50 mg/day	100–200 mg/day	
Naltrexone	50 mg/day	100–150 mg/day	

Note: None of the listed medications are FDA approved for weight attenuating purposes for children or adolescents.

TABLE 14.5B Medications with Potential Use for Weight Loss Maintenance in the Treatment of Obesity of Children and Adolescents

Medications	Starting dose	Maximal dose	Remarks
Amphetamines	5–10 mg/day	20–30 mg/day	70%-80% of children using stimulants
Methylphenidate	10–20 mg/day	40–60 mg/day	do not evidence weight loss
Topiramate	12.5–25 mg/day	200 mg/day	Slow upward titration. Language and cognitive side effects are common
Sibutramine	5–10 mg/day	Up to 20 mg/day	May produce hypertension
Nizatidine	50 mg BID	150 mg BID	
Orlistat	120 mg BID	Up to 120 mg TID	Decreases absorption of many vitamins; causes fecal urgency and fecal incontinence
Xenical			
B3 agonists			
Zonisamide	50–100 mg/day	200–300 mg/day	Risk of Steven-Johnson syndrome Cognitive side effects are common
Rimonabant			Not available for medical use yet.

Note: None of the listed medications are FDA approved for weight loss maintenance in children and adolescents.

Phase III. Surgery

In the case of serious heath problems with morbid obesity, when other approaches have failed, surgical treatments need to be considered; 20% of adult obese patients do not respond to medical treatments. Occasionally, morbidly obese adolescents merit a consideration for surgery based on serious health risks, when nonsurgical measures have failed to produced a sustained weight loss or an improvement of a number of cardiovascular or metabolic factors.

For patients with BMIs > 40 who have not responded to behavioral or medication treatments and whose health status is severely compromised by either a metabolic syndrome or cardiovascular problems, surgery should be considered. In adults, there is a 2% operative death rate plus similar perisurgical death rate. Surgery reduces appetite in 70% of cases. However, nutrient assimilation is compromised and many essential mineral and vitamins need to be provided.

The medium and long-term results of gastrointestinal bariatric surgery, published since the mid-1990s, is encouraging, with consistent and persistent losses of 60 to 90% of excess weight and reversal of main metabolic complications in severe and morbid obesity. Fertility also increases after weight loss. Patient selection is very important. Early and late anatomical complications should be considered before recommending bariatric surgery. Deaths and nonfatal serious complications such as sepsis, toxic shock syndrome, thromboembolic disease, fat emboli, and adult respiratory distress syndrome are reported complications. Perioperative complications include cardiorespiratory impairment, infection, gastrointestinal leakage, deep venous thrombosis, and less frequently, wound dehiscence and renal complications. Three categories of long-term surgical complications are likely:

1. Anatomical: incisional hernia, intestinal obstruction, gastroesophageal reflux, gastric ulcer, and staple line disruption;
2. Nutritional: anemia, protein malnutrition, electrolytic imbalance, vitamin deficiency; and
3. Psychological: binge eating and anorexia (Salvatoni, 2002, pp. 356–357).

In summary, treatments for children and adolescent obesity are still investigational, and there are no safe medications to deal with this vexing epidemic problem. Education and prevention are the best tools the profession has available at the present time. The first entails the promotion of balanced and quality diets, and the second stresses the importance of regular exercising; it is important to decrease sedentary behavior stimulated by excessive TV viewing and prolonged computer use, and to instill sanitary habits of adequate sleep hygiene.

Prevention on the part of physicians, relates to the care they need to exercise to avoid writing prescriptions that increase weight and that induce metabolic syndrome, and to redouble their attention to avoiding coprescription of medications whose interactions may result in weight increase or that aggravate metabolic problems that already exist.

NEUROLOGICAL TREATMENTS

The child psychiatrist will be attentive to emerging neurological illnesses. Clinical signs initially thought to be developmental or environment related may turn out to be the result of neurological illness. Even if a child has a bona fide functional disorder, that does not spare him or her from acquiring other neurological or medical illnesses. Complex partial seizure disorders are often difficult to confirm; white matter diseases, infectious disorders, and other genetic and neurodegenerative processes are difficult to diagnose in their beginning stages. There are frequent neurological conditions that may underlie psychiatric symptoms and disorders, and in like manner, there are frequent psychiatric conditions in the neurological population.

"The misdiagnosis of epilepsy is one of the conundrums of modern medicine, one of the legacies of the split between neurology and psychiatry" (Trimble, 2003). There is consensus that as many as 20 to 30% of patients attending chronic seizure clinics in England do not have epilepsy. Pseudoseizures,[6] metabolic and cardiac problems, vasovagal attacks, panic attacks (panic sine panic), dissociative episodes, and others are a source of neurological misidentification. Moreover, up to 20% of the normal population show unspecific EEG abnormalities and 50% of patients with personality disorders, such as borderline personality disorder, show EEG irregularities often temporal (and sometimes focal) and are reported as "epileptiform." Trimble emphasizes the importance of the patient's narrative and the role of a detailed inquiry to clarify the mimicking conditions (p. 288).

TREATMENT OF EXTRAPYRAMIDAL SIDE EFFECTS (EPS)

Children are more susceptible to EPS than adults; preadolescents (latency age and preschoolers) are more prone to EPS reactions than adolescents.

Treatment of Akathisia

Akathisia in children and preadolescents is one of the most common EPS reactions of children exposed to antipsychotic medications, including SGAs. This reaction is characterized by a state of agitation, increased restlessness, driven behavior, dysphoria, insomnia, impulsivity, and involvement in risk related behaviors. The behaviors are more than an intensification of baseline behaviors; for many children akathisia represents a state of agitation that differs qualitatively and quantitatively from the patient's customary demeanors. If the child is not intensely supervised, he might place his own or others' safety at risk, or may get involved in behaviors that endanger the living environment. Aggressive behaviors, self-abusive behaviors, and even suicidal behavior are reported as manifestations of akathisia in preadolescents or adolescents. In counterdistinction to adults, children and even adolescents are seldom able to articulate the subjective distress associated with akathisia.

The most important treatment for akathisia is an accurate diagnosis. Akathisia is frequently misidentified as psychotic agitation, manic behavior, "bad ADHD," anxiety, or others agitated states. If the condition is misidentified, it is likely that the problem remains unresolved and its consequences will intensify. Akathisia is aggravated if the decision to increase antipsychotics is implemented; this is a common mistake because it is assumed that the condition is related to a psychotic agitation.

Any increase of agitation or restlessness in a child who is receiving antipsychotic medication should be construed as a side effect of the antipsychotic; that is, akathisia.

Some preadolescents and adolescents are able to report a relentless dysphoria, an inner state of distress, and a sense of uneasiness that is hard to describe, accompanied by a state of restlessness; patients describe being unable to sit for long, that they need to be moving around, that they need to pace. These patients are unable to focus or to stay on any given task; they may also describe distressing and intruding thoughts of either harming themselves or harming others. It is not unusual to hear from supervising adults that the patients run off, that they run into the streets, that they wander off, or that they ran away.

The examiner will observe a distressed and dysphoric child who is unable to sit still even for a short period of time; if the child sits down, he is unable to keep his feet still; when he stands, he moves and wanders around aimlessly. The child does not respond to redirection; if pressured, he will acquiesce for the shortest time, to continue in his customary restless and pacing behaviors. Since these children do not sleep, they keep the family up; wisely, the parents stay up to supervise them. Because of the driven behavior and impulsivity, these children need supervision all the time.

The first step in the treatment of akathisia is to withhold or discontinue the offending agent. The second step is to select an effective medication. Diphenhydramine or anticholinergic medications have limited impact on this adverse event. Amantadine is not considered effective for the treatment of akathisia. Benzodiazepines have been reported to be beneficial for akathisia; lorazepam has the advantage of having no active metabolites, which eliminates potential side effects and toxicity. Beta-blockers (like propanolol), when not contraindicated, are the medications of choice. Betaxolol is the drug of choice for patients with lung disease because of the beta-1 selectivity at lower doses (Stanilla & Simpson, 2004, p. 529). Once the crisis is resolved, and if the child continues in need of an antipsychotic, a medication with low propensity to produce akathisia/EPS should be selected; quetiapine is a possible alternative.

Suggested Initiating Dosage for akathisia Treatment

Medication	3–6 years	7–12 years	13 and older
Lorazepam	0.25mg TID/QID	0.5mg TID/QID	0.5–1mg TID/QID
Propanolol	5 mg BID	5–10 mg BID	10 mg BID/TID

Treatment of Acute Dystonias

Acute dystonias are common in children and in preadolescents. Hypertonic (spasmodic) reactions of the neck and tongue musculature (with interference of speech and swallowing) are the most common reactions. Oculacephalogeric crises are less common. Opistotonous reactions are very seldom seen. The laryngeal spasm, an extremely serious and potentially lethal complication due to the obstruction of the airway, is fortunately seldom seen. This reaction responds readily to diphenhydramine IV; IM diphenhydramine also works but takes a longer time to produce its effects.

In dystonic reactions, the child complains of a neck discomfort or that he cannot move his neck; frequently, children are alarmed at the progression of the movement disorder; more so, if they experience head deviation, due to neck contraction, or if they feel a progressive inability to move the tongue or to speak. Many children with acute dystonias appear at an emergency room (ER); many parents become alarmed with this reaction and consider it to be a life-threatening event. Parents become so anxious that they forget to implement the measures that were recommended prior to the initiation of the drug. Sometimes, physicians fail to educate parents about an eventual dystonic reaction and what they should do if that AE develops. Seldom, a number of small children between 5 and 9 years of age develop dystonic reactions to the first small dose of antipsychotics and are taken to the ER.

It behooves the physician to alert the caretaker about the potential for acute dystonia and to give instructions as to how to respond if this side effect were to unfold. Since diphenhydramine is commonly effective for acute dystonias, parents should have this medication at hand to dose the child as soon as the first signs of dystonia are identified. The parent should also be told to withhold any further doses of the antipsychotic if the child develops acute dystonia. If the child experiences breathing difficulties, he or she should be rushed to an emergency room. Most of the cases respond to conservative treatment; most of the dystonic reactions do not necessitate emergency room treatment. Not all the dystonias in small children respond to diphenhydramine. This medication is well tolerated, but is very sedating. Diphenhydramine is FDA approved for Parkinsonism and for EPS treatment in adults.

Commonly, diphenhydramine is started at 25 to 50 mg orally; seldom, it needs to be given intramuscularly (IM). The child needs to be assessed periodically to determine medication response; diphenhydramine is repeated every three to four hours; doses of 150 to 200 mg/day are common. Usually, three to four doses a day are necessary for 24 to 36 hours to achieve full resolution of the acute dystonia (Stanilla & Simpson, 2004, p. 526).

If the dystonia does not respond to diphenhydramine, anticholinergic medications are the pharmacologic agents of choice. Benztropine has the advantage of being manufactured in a number of forms (media) allowing for oral or parenteral treatment. For purpose of this discussion, benztropine is selected as the prototypical anticholinergic medication. Benztropine is FDA approved for all forms of Parkinsonism and neuroleptic induced Parkinsonism (p. 525). Alternatives to benztropine are trihexyphenidyl (and its analogue procyclidine), and biperiden. No combination of anticholinergic medications is advised; combination of anticholinergics with amantadine is also discouraged. Amantadine has discordant evidence-based data; in some studies it is equal to or more effective than benztropine; in others, it is no better than placebo. Amantadine could be an alternative option if the dystonia does not respond to anticholinergics (p. 527).

Memory disturbance is the most common side effect of anticholinergic medications because memory is dependent on the cholinergic system; patients with underlying brain pathology are more susceptible to memory disturbances. Patients receiving an antipsychotic and benztropine show increased overall scores in the Wechsler Memory scales when benztropine is withdrawn. Anticholinergic toxicity produces restlessness, disorientation, irritability, hallucinations, and delirium. Toxic doses can produce a clinical situation akin to atropine poisoning, including fixed dilated pupils, flushed face, sinus tachycardia, urinary retention, dry mouth, and fever. This condition can proceed to coma, cardiorespiratory collapse, and death (p. 524). The medication to counteract dystonias and EPS should be continued for two to three days after the adverse event is resolved and then it should be discontinued.

Suggested Initiating Doses for the Treatment of acute Dystonia

Medication	3–6 years	7–12 years	13 and older
Benztropine	0.25 mg BID	0.5 mg BID	0.5 mg TID
	0.25 IM	0.5 IM	1 mg IM
Amantadine	25 mg BID	50 mg BID	100 mg BID

Doses could be adjusted according to tolerance and clinical response. IM medication may be repeated up to two times in 24 hours; it is customary to initiate oral dosing concomitantly with IM medications.

Other Forms of Extrapyramidal Side Effects

Often the observed EPS adverse events are circumscribed to hypertonia/rigidity of limbs and neck. Hypertonia and rigidity is not always bilateral and at the beginning of its manifestation the child may exercise some control over the movements of neck and limbs. The neck is the most revealing area to test for cogwheeling rigidity. Often but not always, when there is neck rigidity, there will also be cogwheel rigidity of the limbs. Findings may be unilateral. The upper arms are the most frequently tested areas at the elbows. By the time there is evidence of muscle rigidity other signs of D2 saturation are reported or detectable: flattening of affect, Parkinsonian tremor, and gait difficulties, including a decrease in involuntary associated movements, shuffling gait, robotic walking, and others. Drooling is another symptom that indicates D2 saturation; this side effect is rather common in preadolescents.

As in the case of dystonias, antipsychotics need to be withheld unless patients are actively psychotic and in need of antipsychotic treatment. If the patient is sensitive to EPS even with the least inducing EPS antipsychotic, a concomitant use of antipsychotics with anti-EPS medications may be indicated. Because amantadine has a less detrimental role in cognitive functions, consideration may be given to its use along the antipsychotic drugs.

Persons on high potency FGAs, in high doses, who are younger (less than 35 years of age), who receive IM medication, who had a prior dystonic reaction, who are male, and those who use cocaine have a higher risk of developing acute dystonic reactions (p. 535). The rabbit syndrome (perioral tremor) was initially considered a form of TD, but is now considered a form of Parkinsonism, and responds well to anticholinergic medications (Mathews et al., 2005, p. 39).

Kafantaris, Hirch, Saito, and Bennet (2005) state that most of the dyskinesias reported in children become evident upon withdrawal of antipsychotics. The authors quote Kumra et al. (1998), who reported an incidence of 28% of withdrawal dyskinesia for a period of 14 to 28 days, after children were taken off antipsychotic medications.

TREATMENT OF TARDIVE DYSKINESIA

The American Psychiatric Association Task Force on TD concluded that there is no consistently effective treatment for TD. If the patient is on anticholinergics medications, they need to be discontinued because they tend to make TD worse (Stanilla & Simpson, 2004, p. 534). Examples of withdrawal dyskinesias and chronic dyskinesia were presented in chapter 13.

Medications that have been used to attempt to deal with the TD condition include clonazepam. This benzodiazepine has been reported to reduce the movements of TD for up to nine months, but tolerance to the benefits of the medication develops. Naltrexone in combination with clonazepam has shown effectiveness in improving TD (Mathews et al, 2005, p. 40). Botulinum toxin has been used in the treatment of drug-induced dystonias. The toxin binds presynaptically to the cholinergic motor nerve terminal preventing release of acetylcholine and producing a denervated muscle. Although the prevention of acetylcholine release starts within a few hours, the clinical effect does not occur for one to three days; the innervation is gradually restored. The FDA has approved the use of botulinum toxin for treatment of strabismus, blepharospasm, and other facial nerve disorders. It also has been used to treat focal neuroleptic-induced dystonias that may occur as part of tardive dyskinesia (TD), such as, laryngeal dystonia and refractory torticollis. For the laryngeal dystonia, the toxin is injected percutaneously through the cricothyroid membrane into the thyroarytenoid muscle bilaterally. The response rate is 80 to 90% and the effects last up to three to four months, and sometimes longer. The toxin has also been effective for the treatment of tardive cervical dystonia (p. 531).

Although initial studies showed some promise for using vitamin E on TD, subsequent studies have failed to demonstrate that alpha-tocopherol is better than placebo (p. 532). However, vitamin E could be considered as prophylaxis against TD among patients who do not yet display TD and who are exposed to D2 antagonists. The chief liability of vitamin E is the development of prolonged bleeding times in vitamin K-deficient patients (Leard-Hansson & Guttmacher, 2004b, p. 31). A double-blind, placebo-controlled, crossover study suggests that melatonin may be effective in the treatment of TD (Mathews et al, 2005, p. 40).

Use of Atypical Antipsychotics for the Treatment of TD

Clozapine decreases the symptoms of severe TD and tardive dystonia. Risperidone and olanzapine have demonstrated antidyskinetic activity in double-blind trials. It appears that olanzapine has less TD risk than risperidone.

Olanzapine

Researchers at Eli Lilly assert that olanzapine reduces the scores of presumptive TD in adult schizophrenics. Kinon, Basson, Stauffer, et al. (1999) reported on a group of 129 adult patients with presumptive TD. The authors concluded that a retrospective analysis of patients with presumptive TD entering olanzapine clinical trials demonstrated a significant reduction of mean AIMS total scores. The marked and persistent effect for up to 30 weeks suggests that olanzapine may contribute to the improvement of TD through a mechanism other than masking of symptoms by the neuroleptic. To address the possibility of olanzapine masking effect on TD symptoms, a second study was conducted by Kinon, Stauffer, Wang, Thi, and Kollack-Walker (2001).[7]

The authors concluded that olanzapine seems to ameliorate rather than mask symptoms of TD; this effect is concurrent with improvement in clinical psychotic status. Olanzapine may offer a potential treatment alternative for patients with schizophrenia and preexisting TD. The two cited studies appear to demonstrate olanzapine's positive antidyskinetic effects in adults; these effects were maintained even with a marked decrease of olanzapine dose (up to 75%), without decrement of the medication antipsychotic properties. There is no literature on the use of olanzapine for the treatment of TD in children.

Risperidone

Risperidone also has beneficial effects on tardive dykinesia. Ya Mei Bali, Shun-Cheih Yu, and Chao-Cheng Lin (2003) reported on a double-blind placebo controlled study on patients with severe tardive dyskinesia treated for a 12-week period with either risperidone or placebo.[8] The authors noted that approximately 70 to 100% of tardive dyskinesia patients show orofacial movements; 20 to 60% limb and truncal movements; and 10 to 50% both orofacial and limb–truncal movements. The study demonstrated that bucco-lingual movements and choreathetoid tardive dyskinesia respond differently to risperidone, supporting the proposition that these are two separate syndromes (pp. 1346–1347).

Aripiprazole

There is a report regarding the beneficial effects of aripiprazole on patients with severe TD.[9] Aripiprazole has not been associated with any significant changes in AIMS scores in adults (Ginsberg, 2004a, p.15), but as has been indicated in chapter 13 in response to aripiprazole, children seem to display significant activation, akathisia, and EPS. Full dystonias have also been observed in both children and adolescents who have been treated with aripiprazole

Use of Anticholinergic Agents

Donazepil

Schopick (2005) using the conceptualization of an imbalance between the dopaminergic and cholinergic systems, used rivastigmine with good results, on a 16-year-old white male with a diagnosis of severe TD, probably secondary to high doses of risperidone, 12 mg/day, for the previous six months. The patient exhibited persistent choreiform movements of upper and lower limbs, torso, head (facio/oral/buccal), and neck. The initial AIMS was 18. Patient had been tapered off risperidone, and was receiving the following medications: quetiapine 50 mg TID; Depakote 1200 mg/day; clonidine 0.075 mg BID + 0.05 mg QHS; benztropine 1 mg BID; clonazepam 0.125 mg BID. He was also taking Claritin D BID. Although the rivastigmine was very helpful, there were breakthrough symptoms during the day (rivastigmine half-life is only 1.5 hours) even with a TID schedule. The change to donazepil brought about significant improvement without breakthrough symptoms. Two months after the initiation of donazepil the AIMS score was 0. At 15 months of follow-up there was no evidence of TD. Final medication regime: clozapine 250 mg/day; atomaxetine 80 q AM; Depakote ER 1000 mg q AM, and 750 mg q HS; clonidine 0.1 mg TID, and donazepil 5 mg/day.

Reserpine and Tetrabenazine

These medications are dopamine depletors and have been shown to be the most effective medications for TD and tardive dystonia (Mathews et al, 2005, p. 40). For the treatment of TD, Jankovic and his group favor the use of tetrabenazine alone or in combination with lithium. In adults, they claim a persistent, excellent response in up to 85% of patients (Menkes, 2006, p. 172).

Use of Branched Chain Aminoacids

The authors reported a decrease in dyskinetic movements with the mixture of branched-chain amino acids (BCAA): L-valine, L-isoleucine, and L-leucine;

this product is food-marketed as Tarvil. The authors quoted a double-blind, placebo-controlled study of the use of BCAAs for adult patients with TD (pp. 1102–1103). The effectiveness and tolerability of this potential treatment for dyskinetic reactions in childhood needs to be validated by controlled research.

TREATMENT OF COGNITIVE SIDE EFFECTS

Even schizophrenic patients who have scored average or above average in cognitive scores have a decrement in cognitive performance compared to their scores before the onset of their illness. The patient level of cognitive functioning might be the most important determinant of real-world outcomes (Keefe & Hawkins, 2005, p. 34).

Evidence for a positive role on cognitive functioning of atypical antipsychotics is accumulating: clozapine appears to improve the domains of attention and verbal fluency, but has limited impact on verbal learning and memory. Risperidone has demonstrated efficacy in improving perceptual and motor processing, reaction time, executive function, working memory, and verbal learning and memory. Olanzapine has overall better results than haloperidol in cognitive functioning. Quetiapine has positive effects on verbal reasoning and fluency, immediate recall, executive function, attention, and verbal memory (Labellarte & Riddle, 2002, pp. 25–27).

Velligan and Glahn (2004) review a number of medications that may hold promise for the treatment of cognitive dysfunction in schizophrenia; these drugs are used as adjunctives. Clinical observations and experiences in the adult field may have implications and applications for the treatment and rehabilitation of chronic and severe psychotic children and adolescents. These medications include:

Guanfacine, an alpha-2 adrenergic agonist, increases spatial working memory and attention when used with SGAs. These effects are consistent with the use of guanfacine in the treatment of ADHD.

Atomaxetine, a selective norepinephrine reuptake inhibitor, increases dopamine and norepinephrine in the frontal cortex. Atomaxetine is currently used for the treatment of ADHD.

Gantamine, which inhibits acetylcholinesterase and modulates nicotinic neurotransmission, is being used for the cognitive improvement of dementia patients.

Glutamine may enhance hypofunction of N-methyl-D-aspartate (NMDA) that appears to be present in schizophrenic patients with cognitive deficits.

Ampakine CX-516 improves attention and memory in patients with schizophrenia. Ampakines may also increase neurotrophin levels that induce neuroprotection (p. 74).

Velligan and Glahn (2004) also review psychosocial interventions, so called, cognitive rehabilitation techniques (CRT), designed to remediate, compensate for, or bypass cognitive deficits, with the goal of improving broad community outcomes for patients with schizophrenia.[10] These techniques may offer some applications for cognitively compromised psychotic children and adolescents. Velligan and Glahn indicate that although the psychosocial techniques have a great deal of appeal, their evaluation has yielded mixed results and learned skills do not generalize to improvements in adaptive functioning (pp. 75–76).

TABLE 14.6 Endogenous Causes of Obesity

Hormonal Causes
    Hypothyroidism
    Hypercortisolism (Cushing's syndrome)
    Primary hyperinsulinism
    Pseudohypoparathyroidism
    Acquired hypothalamic lesions
Genetic Syndromes
    Prader-Willi: Obesity, insatiable appetite, mental retardation, emotional lability, small hands and feet, scoliosis, kyphosis, hypogonadism
    Angelmen (happy puppet syndrome): seizures, developmental delays, and characteristic gait
    Laurence-Moon/Bardet-Biedl: Obesity, mental retardation, pigmentary retinitis, hypogonadism
    Alstrom-Hallingren: Obesity, retinitis pigmentosa, deafness, diabetes mellitus
    Borjeson-Forssman-Lehmann: Obesity, mental retardation, hypogonadism, hypometabolism, epilepsy
    Cohen: Truncal obesity, mental retardation, hypotonia, hypogonadism
    Turner: Short stature, undifferentiated gonads, cardiac abnormalities, obesity, 45X geneotype, female phenotype
    Familial lipodystrophy: Muscular hypertrophy, acromegalic appearance, liver enlargement, acanthosis nigricans, insulin resistance, hypertriglyceridemia
    Beckwith-Wiedemann: exomphalos, macroglosia, and gigantism often associated with visceromegaly, adrenocortical cytomegaly and dysplasia of the renal medulla
    Sotos: cerebral gigantism
    Weaver: large for gestational age, macrosomia, camptodactily, distinctive facies
    Ruvalcaba: Microcephaly, skeletal abnormalities, hypoplastic genitalia, and physical and mental retardation

Source: Modified from Zametkin et al. (2004, p. 140).

APPENDIX A

Drug Interactions

CLOZAPINE DRUG INTERACTIONS

Anticholinergics: Clozapine has potent anticholinergic effects; may potentiate the effects of anticholinergic agents

Antihypertensives: Clozapine may potentiate the effects of antihypertensive agents.

Benzodiazepines: In combination with clozapine may produce respiratory depression and hypotension, especially during the first few weeks of therapy.

Carbamazepine: A case of neuroleptic malignant syndrome has been reported in combination with clozapine. Carbamazepine may alter clozapine levels.

CYP 1A2 enzyme inducers: Metabolism of clozapine may be increased reducing its therapeutic effects. Potential inducers include aminoglutethimide carbamazepine, phenobarbital and rifampin.

CYP 1A2 inhibitors: Serum levels or toxicity of clozapine may be increased; inhibitors include amidiodarone, ciprofloxacin, fluvoxamine, ketoconazole, norfloxacin, ofloxacin, and refecoxib..

CYP 2D6 substrates: Clozapine may increase the levels or effects of CYP2D6 substrates: amphetamines, selected beta-blockers, dextrometorphan, fluoxetine, lidocaine, mirtazapine, nefazodone, paroxetine, risperidone, ritanovir, thioridazine, TCAs, and velafaxine.

CYP 2D6 prodrug substraztes. Clazapine may decrease the level/effects of CYP 2D6 prodrugs: codeine, hydrocodone, oxycodone, and tramadol

Epinephrine: Clozapine may reverse the pressor effect of epinephrine.

Metoclopramide: May increase EPS.

Risperidone: Effects and toxicity may be increased when combined with clozapine.

Valproic acid: May cause reduction in clozapine concentrations (Fuller & Sajatovic, 2005, p. 323).

RISPERIDONE DRUG INTERACTIONS

Antihypertensives: Risperidone may enhance the hypotensive effects of antihypertensives.

Carbamazepine: reduces levels of risperidone and 9-hydroxyrisperidone, up to 50%, with concomitant use.

Clozapine: Decreases the clearance of risperidone and increases its serum concentrations.

CYP 2D6 inhibitors: Metabolism of risperidone may be decreased, increasing blood levels and toxicity. Inhibitors include chlorpromazine, delavirdine, fluoxetine, miconazole, paroxetine, pergolide, quinidine, quinine, ritanovir and ropinirole.

CYP 3A3/4 inhibitors: These effects are minor

Levodopa: At high doses (> 6 mg/day) risperidone may inhibit the antiparkinsonian effect of levodopa.

Metoclopramide: May increase EPS.

Valproic acid: Generalized edema has been reported as a result of concurrent therapy (Fuller & Sajatovic, 2005, p. 1165).

OLANZAPINE DRUG INTERACTIONS

Antihypertensives: Increase the risk of hypotension and orthostatic hypotension.

Carbmazepine: decreases olanzapine levels.

Clomipramine and olanzapine in combination: Have been reported to be associated with seizures (case report).

CNS depressants: Sedative effects may be additive with CNS depressants (i.e., ethanol, barbiturates, narcotic analgesics, and other sedative agents). Caution should be exercised in the use of parenteral olanzapine in patients that are receiving benzodiazepines.

Fluvoxamine: increases olanzapine levels.

Haloperidol: a case of severe Parkinsonism wasa reported.

CYP1A2 and 2D6 are minor substrates; CYP 1A2, 2D; 2C8/9, 2C19, 3A4, are inhibitors but the effects are weak.

Metoclopromide: May incrrese EPS risk

Levodopa: Antipsychotics may inhibit the antiparkinsonian effects of levodopa (Fuller & Sajatovic, 2005, 954).

QUETIAPINE DRUG INTERACTIONS

Antihypertensives: These may increase quetiapine hypotensive effects, particularly orthostasis.

Azole antifungals (fluconazole, itraconazole, ketoconazole): May increase quetiapine considerably (up to 300%).

Cimetidine: May increase quetiapine serum concentration by decreasing its clearance by up to 20%.

CNS depressants: Quetiapine may enhance the sedative effects of other CNS depressants, including antidepressants, benzodiazepines, barbiturates, ethanol, narcotics, and other sedative agents.

CYP 3A3/4 inhibitors: Increase the serum level or toxicity of quetiapine; examples include azole antifungals, ciprofloxacin, clarithromycin, diclofenac, doxycycline, erythromycin, imatinib, isoniazid, nefazodone, nicardipine, propofol, protease inhibitors, quinidine and verapamil.

CYP 3A3/4 Inducers: May decrease the level or effects of quetiapine. Examples include aminoglutethimide, carbamazepine, nafcillin, nevirapine, phenobarbital, phenytoin and rafamycins.

Levodopa: Quetiapine may reduce the antiparkinsonian effects of levodopa.

Lorazepam: Quetiapine may reduce the metabolism of lorazepam; clearance may be reduced by up to 20%.

Metoclopramide: Increases the risks of EPS.

Phenytoin: May increase the clearance/metabolism of quetiapine; up to fivefold changes have been reported.

Thioridazine: May increase the clearance of quetiapine by 65%, decreasing its serum concentration and effects (Fuller & Sajatovic, 2005, 1132).

ZIPRASIDONE DRUG INTERACTIONS

Amphetamine: Efficacy may be decreased by antipsychotics; amphetamines may increase psychotic symptoms.

Antihypertensives: May increase ziprasidone hypotensive side effects, particularly orthostasis.

Carbamazepine: May decrease ziprasidone serum concentration (AUC is decreased by 35%). Other enzyme inducing agents may produce the same effect. Smoking may decrease the levels of ziprasidone.

CNS depressant effects: May be additive to the ziprasidone sedative effects; this includes barbiturates, benzodiazepines, narcotics, ethanol, and other sedative agents.

CYP 3A3/4 inhibitors: Produce a weak effect

Ketoconazole: May increase serum concentration of ziprasidone (AUC is increased by 35% to 40%).

Metoclopramide: May increase the EPS risk.

Levodopa effects: May be inhibited by ziprasidone.

Potassium- and magnesium-depleting agents: May increase the risk of serious arrythmias with ziprasidone; agents include diuretics, aminoglycosides, cyclosporine, and amphotericin.

QTc prolongation agents: May result in additive effects on cardiac conduction, resulting in potentially malignant or lethal arrythmias; concurrent use is contraindicated (Fuller & Sajatovic, 2005, 1387).

Medications that Should Not Be Used Concurrently with Ziprasidone

Amidiodarone, bretylium, cisapride, dofetilide, sotalol, quinidine, other class I and III anti-arrhythmics, dolasetron, ibutilide, mesoridazine, thioridazine, chlorpromazine, droperidol, pimozide, quinolone antibiotics (moxifloxacin, spartfloxacin, gatifloxacin), halofantrine, mefloquine, pentamidine, arsenic trioxide, levomethadyl acetate, probucol or tacrolimus. Ziprasidone is also contraindicated with drugs that have demonstrated pharmacodynamic QT prolongation described in the full prescribing information as a contraindication or a boxed or bonded warning (Geodon, Package Insert). Finally the manufacturer does not rule out that Geodon may increase the TdP risk for susceptible individuals.

ARIPIPRAZOLE DRUG INTERACTIONS

Major drug interactions substrate at CYP2D6 and 3A4

Carbamazepine: May decrease aripiprazole levels.

CYP2D6 Inhibitors: May increase Aripiprazole levels. Examples include chlorpromazine, delavirdine, fluoxetine, miconazole, paroxetine, pergolide, quinidine, quinine, ritonavir, and ropinirole.

CYP3A4 Inducers: May decrease the levels of aripiprazole. Examples include aminoglutethimide, carbamazepine, nafcillin, nevirapine, phenobarbital, phenytoin, and rifamycins.

CYP3A4 Inhibitors: May increase aripiprazole levels. Examples include azole antifungals, ciprofloxacin, clarithromycin, diclofenac, doxycycline, erythromycin, imatinib, isoniazid, nefazodone, nicardipine, propofol, protease inhibitors, quinidine and verapamil.

Ketaconozole: May increase aripiprazole levels. Manufacturer recommends a 50% dose reduction with ketaconazol concomitant therapy (Fuller & Sajatovic, 124).

APPENDIX B

Conventional or Classic Antipsychotics

The modern era of antipsychotic treatment began with the synthesis of chlorpromazine (Largactil) by Paul Charpantier in 1950, and the American psychiatrist William Long, at McLean Hospital, Boston, was the first physician to use chlorpromazine in the United States. Following the success of chlorpromazine many other phenothiazines were synthesized and tested, including haloperidol and thiothixene. The last classical antipsychotic approved by the FDA in 1975 was molindone. The ability of chlorpromazine and other classic antipsychotics to improve psychotic symptoms (hallucinations, delusions, and bizarre behaviors) had a profound impact on chronically hospitalized patients worldwide. In the United States, in only three decades, 80% of hospitalized patients were deinstitutionalized (there were 559,000 hospitalized patients in 1955 and only 107,000 by 1988). Shortly after the spread of chlorpromazine, the phenomenon of extrapyramidal side effects (EPS), including Parkinsonism, dystonia, and akathisia was described. The first report of oral-buccal dyskinesia came from France in 1959. By the beginning of the 1960s the incidence of antipsychotic-related EPS was estimated to be at 40%. Some psychiatrists believed that the antipsychotic action and EPS were inseparable; this belief was dispelled in 1959, when clozapine, which produces antipsychotic action without EPS, was synthesized (Wilkaitis, Mulvihill, & Nasrallah, 2004, pp. 425–426).

Substitutions in the basic phenothiazines' ring at the 10-carbon, divides these drugs into aliphatic, piperidine, and piperazine phenothiazines. Conventional antipsychotic classes with its most representative examples are listed below:

Phenothiazines	Aliphatics	chlorpromazine
	Piperidines	thioridazine, mesoridazine
	Piperazines	fluphenazine, trifluoperazine, perphenazine
Thioxanthenes		thiothixene, chlorprothixene
Dibenzoxapines		loxapine

447

Dihydroindoles	molindone
Butyrophenones	haloperidol
Diphenylbutylpiperidines	pimozide

In general the classical or conventional antipsychotics are effective for the positive symptoms of schizophrenia but have limited or no effect on negative or cognitive symptoms. On the contrary, because of their indiscriminate high binding to the D2 receptor and the consequent high prevalence of EPS, they tend to aggravate negative and cognitive symptoms and to cause hormonal and neurological side effects, which include EPS, tardive dyskinesia (TD), and neuroleptic malignant syndrome (NMS). At least this was the prevailing view prior to the publication of the Clinical Antipsychotic Trial of Intervention Effectiveness results (CATIE; Lieberman, Stroup, et al., 2005). In that study, perphenazine showed effectiveness and tolerability comparable to risperidone, quetiapine, and ziprasidone. It is also remarkable that the average dose used was 20.8 mg/day, that is, about 200 mg of chlorpromazine equivalents per day. Since perphenazine is inexpensive, in comparison to atypical antipsychotics, considerations of cost effectiveness may signal a revival of some FGAs.

Conventional antipsychotics have been used in schizophrenia and schizoaffective disorders; these medications have also been used in affective disorders (depression, bipolar disorders), transient psychotic features associated with personality disorders, psychosis, and movement disorder associated with Huntington's disease, and for the amelioration of nausea, emesis, and hiccups. Haloperidol was for a long time the recommended medication for the treatment of Tourette's disorder.

Conventional antipsychotics are lipophilic and large amounts of these medications are stored in bodily tissues (fat, lung, liver, kidneys, spleen, and others) preventing their removal via dialysis in cases of overdose. Most of the typical antipsychotics are metabolized by the cytochrome 450 subfamilies of 2D6 and 3A4. The major excretion rout is through urine and feces, but they are also excreted in sweat, saliva, tears, and breast milk (pp. 431–433).

The lower potency conventionals (i.e., chlorpromazine, thioridazine) have a broad affinity for antidopaminergic, antihistaminergic, anticholinergic, and antiadrenergic receptors that render them less prone to D2 side effects at a cost of a high anticholinergic activity. The high potency ones (i.e., fluphenazine, haloperidol) have a predominant D2 blocking activity, with limited antihistaminic, anticholinergic, and antiadrenergic properties (pp. 431–433).

IM medications have been very useful pharmacotherapeutic vehicles for patients who have regular problems with medication compliance; these forms are still widely used in Europe and in Japan. The decanoate depot compounds became the most popular forms. SGA depot presentations are beginning to emerge (risperidone), which add new therapeutic options for patients who stray from therapeutic adherence.

BLACK BOXES, WARNINGS, CONTRAINDICATIONS, PRECAUTIONS, AND ADVERSE EVENTS FOR PROTOTYPICAL CONVENTIONAL ANTIPSYCHOTICS

Black Boxes are prominent warnings of serious health risks for a given drug. These warnings are capitalized at the beginning of the PDR product description. At the time of this writing, only thioridazine and mesoridazine have Black Box warnings.

The prototypical side effect profiles of thioridazine, perphenazine, and haloperidol will be described. Brief peculiarities of the other conventionals will be mentioned when pertinent. Physicians are advised to read the PDR or the package insert for the specifics of each classical antipsychotic description, indications, warnings, precautions, and side effect profiles.

THIORIDAZINE

The Black Box warning is listed in the 2004 PDR; Melleril is not a medication listed in the 2006 PDR. In the 2004 listing, there is a capitalized Black Box Warning for Thioridazine Hydrochloride Tablets

Thioridazine has been shown to prolong the QTc interval in a dose related manner, and drugs with this potential, including thioridazine, have been associated with torsade de points-type arrythmias and sudden death. Due to its potential for significant, possibly life-threatening, proarrythmic effects, thioridazine should be reserved for use in the treatment of schizophrenic patients who fail to show an acceptable response to adequate courses of treatment with other antipsychotic drugs, either because of insufficient effectiveness or the inability to achieve an effective dose due to intolerable adverse effects from those drugs (see warnings, contraindications and indications) (p. 2205).

Contraindications

- Thioridazine should be avoided in combination with other drugs that are known to increase the QTc (see p. 446) and in patients with congenital long QTc syndrome.
- Increased QTc prolongation risk may result from using thioridazine in combination with drugs than inhibit the cytochrome P450 2D6 enzyme (e.g., fluoxetine, paroxetine), and with other drugs such as fluvoxamine and pindolol.
- Thioridazine is contraindicated in patients with decreased genetic 2D6 metabolism; this comprises up to 7% of normal American population.
- Thioridazine should not be used in persons with severe central nervous system depression or those in comatose states (p. 2205).

Warnings

- Potential for proarrythmic effects
- Potential for tardive dyskinesia
- Potential for neuroleptic malignant syndrome
- Risk of potentiation of other CNS depressants (e.g., alcohol, anesthetics, barbiturates, narcotics, opiates, and other psychoactive drugs) (pp. 2205–2206).

Precautions

- Impairs mental alertness
- May cause orthostatic hypotension
- Elevates prolactin levels
- May cause leukopenia and agranulocytosis
- May elicit seizure disorders
- May cause pigmentary retinopathy. (p. 2206)

Serentil (mesoridazine besylate), an active metabolic derivative of thioridazine, has a Black Box, exactly like thioridazine, and has parallel listings of contraindications, warnings, precautions, and adverse events similar to those for the parent compound listed above (2004 PDR, pp. 1020–1022).

PERPHENAZINE

Perphenazine has a high affinity for D2, H1, and 5-HT2 receptors; a high affinity for D1, α1 receptors; a moderate affinity for α2, and a low affinity for M1 and 5HT1 receptors. The affinity for D3 and D4 receptors is unknown (Wilkaitis et al., 2004, p. 434).

Side Effects

Perphenazine is moderately sedating, induces EPS and orthostasis, and has a moderate cardiovascular impact. It produces significant sexual dysfunction and anticholinergic side effects; its potential for weight gain and galactorrhea is high (p. 435), and at therapeutic levels (32 to 64 mg/day), has a low risk for skin reactions (photosensitivity, rash, or pigmentation), low risk for ocular complications (lenticular pigmentation or pigmentary retinopathy), and a low propensity for blood dyscrasias, hepatic disorders, or seizures. Perphenazine side effect profile is akin to the one of mesoridazine, fluflenazine, trifluoperazine, haloperidol, loxapine, and thiothixine. Among FGAs, only molindone and pimozide have a better side effect profile (p. 436). However, pimozide prolongs the QTc. In the CATIE trial (2005), perphenazine displayed the highest EPS rate, even though its mean modal dosage was considered moderate (20.8 mg/day). Discontinuation due to EPS was highest with perphenazine and lowest with quetiapine (Nasrallah, 2006, p. 56). Perphenazine was the best antipsychotic medication regarding weight increase (p. 61).

HALOPERIDOL

Haloperidol has double-blind, placebo controlled, randomized studies in children and adolescents for the treatment of schizophrenia (Campbell, Rapoport, & Simpson, 1999, p. 538). No Black Boxes for haloperidol are represented in the 2004 PDR (pp. 2443–2445). The IM product information is applicable to oral forms.

Haloperidol teratogenic risks are classified in the Pregnancy Category C which indicates that teratogenic risks cannot be ruled out.

Warnings

- Tardive dyskinesia
- Neuroleptic malignant syndrome
- General: bronchopneumonia

Precautions

Use of haloperidol poses added risks in patients with

- Cardiovascular disorders
- Seizure disorders
- Known allergies, history of allergic reactions to drugs
- Patients receiving anticoagulants

An encephalopathic syndrome has been described when haloperidol has been combined with lithium.

Adverse Side Effects

- EPS
- Tardive dyskinesia
- Tardive dystonia

- Other CNS effects: insomnia, restlessness, anxiety, agitation, depression, confusion, seizures, catatonialike behaviors, and others.
- Cardiovascular
- Hematological
- Endocrinological: hyperprolactinemia
- Gastrointestinal: hypersalivation, constipation, liver damage.
- Autonomic (anticholinergic): dry mouth, blurred vision, urinary retention, diaphoresis, and priapism.
- Special senses: cataracts, retinopathy, and visual disturbances
- Other: Sudden death

MOLINDONE

No Black Boxes for Moban (molindone hydrochloride) are represented in the 2006 PDR (pp. 1108-1109). Contraindications, warnings, precautions, and adverse events are similar to haloperidol described above.

Persons allergic to sulfides may be at risk when taking molindone because this product contains metabisulfite. Among the conventional antipsychotics, molidone is the least likely to promote weight gain. In this regard, molindone is at least equal to or better than ziprasidone or aripiprazole.

PIMOZIDE

No Black Boxes are presented in the 2006 PDR product information pertaining to Orap (pimozide) (pp. 120–1222). Pimozide does increase the QTc. All the precautions related to drugs that increase the QTc are applicable to pimozide. Other contraindications, warnings, precautions, and adverse effects are as described for haloperidol above. Concomitant use of macrolide antibiotics and other cytochrome P450 3A4 blockers with pimozide is contraindicated.

OVERVIEW OF CONVENTIONAL
ANTIPSYCHOTICS SIDE EFFECTS

Central Nervous System

Ataraxia

This side effect relates to a relative environmental indifference, behavioral inhibition, and diminished emotional responsiveness (Wilkaitis et al., 2004,

p. 429). This is akin to an amotivational syndrome and may be confused with negative symptoms. Promotion or aggravation of negative symptoms is a frequent FGAs side effect..

Neuroleptic Induced Deficit Syndrome

This adverse event is caused by D2 mesocortical receptor antagonism that leads to a blunting of cognitive functioning, frequently difficult to differentiate from the primary negative schizophrenic illness (p. 430).

Extrapyramidal Side Effects (EPS)

Acute onset EPS includes Parkinsonism, dystonia, hypokinesia, rigidity, and akathisia. These adverse events are secondary to the D2 blockade within the nigrostriatal system. EPS symptoms are more frequent with high potency conventionals. It is estimated that up to 10% of patients on conventionals develop acute dystonia within a few hours to a few days of treatment initiation. It is more common in men under 30 and in women under 25 years of age, in recent cocaine abusers, and when intramuscular high-potency medication is used. Among the dystonias, the laryngeal may become a lethal side effect because of respiratory obstruction and arrest (p. 437).

Tardive syndromes include tardive dyskinesia, tardive dystonia, and tardive akathisia, tardive (nongenital) pain, as well as tardive Tourette's.

The most common early manifestations of tardive dyskinesia are the perioral buccolingual masticatory involuntary movements. Risk of TD increases with age and is more common in certain ethnic groups, in women and girls, in patients with mood disorders, and in persons with early onset of EPS (Wilkaitis et al., 2004, p. 437).

Neuroleptic Malignant Syndrome

The incidence of this syndrome has been estimated to be 0.02 to 2% in patients exposed to antipsychotics; the syndrome carries a mortality rate of 20 to 30%. Death occurs secondary to arrythmias, renal failure caused by rhabdomyolysis, aspiration pneumonia, or respiratory failure (p. 437; see NMS section, chapter 9).

Cardiovascular Side Effects

Some conventional antipsychotics such as thioridazine (Melleril) and its metabolite mesoridazine (Serentil), and others such as pimozide have a potential for causing heart arrythmias and sudden death. Prior to the emergence of the second-generation antipsychotics (SGA), child psychiatrists used thioridazine extensively, unaware of its potentially lethal risks. The recognition of this risk, as well as the broader SGA spectrum of therapeutic effectiveness, had rendered conventional use in the United States obsolete. The performance of perphenazine in the CATIE I report (Lieberman et al., 2005) may signal a revival or reconsideration of some FGAs. Classical antipsychotics are still widely prescribed in many countries for children and adolescents.

Other Cardiovascular Side Effects

Alpha-adrenergic blockade causes orthostatic hypotension and reflex tachycardia. This may increase the frequency of falls and related complications. Lower potency antipsychotics have a high risk of producing cardiac arrythmias. Rapid titration, intramuscular administration (and, especially intravenous administration), could cause an increase of the QTc resulting in serious arrythmias such as torsade de pointes (TdP), a polymorphic ventricular tachycardia, terminating in heart arrest.

ENDOCRINOLOGICAL SIDE EFFECTS

Endocrinological side effects include hyperprolactinemia, obesity, diabetes, and dyslipidemias.

Hyperprolactinemia

This adverse event is due to the blockade of the dopaminergic tuberoinfundibular tract. See chapter 13.

Obesity, Diabetes, and Dyslipidemias

Whereas the high potency typical antipsychotic (e.g., haloperidol, fluphenazine, and others) carries a limited risk for obesity and for induction of diabetes and dyslipidemias, the low potency classical antipsychotics (such as chlorpromazine, thioridazine, and others) carry a high risk for obesity and for promoting diabetes and dyslipidemias, as much as the SGAs. Very close monitoring for the unfolding or worsening of the cited disorders is required when patients suffer from these disorders or are at risk of developing them and receive treatment with classical antipsychotics.

COGNITIVE SIDE EFFECTS

Conventional antipsychotics (mostly, lower potency antipsychotics) are prone to cause cognitive side effects (sedation, confusion, memory impairment, delirium) due to the anticholinergic and antihistaminic side effects. Anticholinergic induced delirium, caused by low potency conventional antipsychotics, is the most common cause of medication-related delirium (see delirium section, chapter 4).

GASTROINTESTINAL SIDE EFFECTS

Xerostomia, nausea, and vomiting are fairly common GI side effects of classical antipsychotics; constipation progressing to impaction and paralytic ileus is a serious untoward GI consequence of conventional antipsychotics. Weight gain is more common with lower potency antipsychotics carrying the risk of diabetes development.

Homeostatic jaundice is a hypersensitivity reaction described most commonly with aliphatic antipsychotics. This complication appears early in treatment (first 1–2 months), and usually subsides with discontinuation of the drug (Wilkaitis et al., 2004, p. 438).

GENITOURINARY SIDE EFFECTS

Urinary hesitancy and urinary retention are caused by M1 receptor blockade; urinary retention increases the frequency of tract infection in both genders. Sexual side effects secondary to increased prolactin levels includes diminished libido, gynecomastia, galactorrhea, erectile dysfunction, retrograde ejaculation (and occasionally, priapism), menstrual irregularities, anorgasmia, and infertility (Idem.).

HEMATOLOGIC SIDE EFFECTS

Transient leukopenia (WBC < 3500/mm3) is common but not problematic; agranulocytosis is more commonly caused by aliphatic and piperidine conventionals during the first three months of treatment. This complication has an incidence of 1 in 500,000. This adverse event is more common in adult women and carries a lethality risk of 20 to 30%. Thrombocytopenic or nontrombocytopenic purpura, or pancytopenia, rarely occurs (Idem, p. 438).

OPHTALMOLOGICAL SIDE EFFECTS

Common anticholinergic ocular side effects include blurred vision (mydriasis and cycloplegia) and aggravation of open angle glaucoma. Moreover, there are direct toxic side effects:

1. Lenticular opacities (cataracts) have been reported with chlorpromazine, thioridazine, and perphenazine treatments. Cataracts seem to be more frequent in young schizophrenic patients, with rates or opacities ranging from 22 to 26%. The overall ocular pathology for young schizophrenic patients is 82%.

   Although conventional antipsychotic treatment may be involved, other factors such as diabetes, smoking, exposure to ultraviolet radiation, stress, and facial trauma may be contributory. It has also been suggested that schizophrenia is a risk factor in itself.
2. Irreversible retinal pigmentation with high thioridazine doses (> 800 mg/day). This pigmentation causes reduction in visual acuity and even blindness (Wilkaitis et al., 2004, p. 439).

DERMATOLOGICAL SIDE EFFECTS

Hypersensitivity rashes, mostly, maculo-papular rashes of trunk, face, and limbs, and photosensitivity reaction are most frequently described as dermatological reactions to conventional antipsychotics. A blue-gray discoloration in body areas exposed to sunlight has been described with chlorpromazine (Wilkaitis et al., 2004).

Notes

Preface

1. The SMHC is one of the few remaining nonprofit mental health organizations in the Southwest USA. This organization started out as an orphanage in the last quarter of the 19th century and evolved into a mental health, university affiliated system in the early 1970s. SMHC offers outpatient, partial hospital, acute, and residential psychiatric services to children and adolescents. The SMHC is also a training site for the University of Texas Health Science Center, Department of Psychiatry at San Antonio for medical students, general psychiatric residents, and fellows in child and adolescent psychiatry.

Chapter 3

1. The relationship of command hallucinations and violence is not clear, but delusions are often implicated as mediators of violence. In one study the presence of delusions increased the risk of violence by a factor of 2:6, and the simultaneous presence of hallucinations and delusions increased such a risk by a factor of 4:1; of particular relevance is the assignment of an identity to the voice, which in turn seems to be associated with compliance with the command (Junginger & McGuire, 2001, p. 385).
2. Associations between psychosis and violence have been described in several studies. Scott and Resnick (2002) report that in adult paranoid psychotic patients, violence is usually well planned and in line with their false beliefs. The violence is directed toward a specific person who is perceived as a persecutor. Of particular clinical concern are delusions characterized by threat or override symptoms: beliefs that the person is dominated by forces that are beyond the person's control, that thoughts are being put into the person's head, that people are wishing the person harm, or that the person is being followed (these symptoms are more likely in adolescents, and frightened, anxious, or angry children); these persons are prone to act aggressively. Schizophrenic patients are more likely to be violent if the hallucinations generate negative emotions (anger, anxiety, or sadness) and if the patient has not developed successful strategies to deal with the voices. There is a relationship between command hallucinations to commit violence and actual violence when a delusion is related to the content of the hallucination (Scott & Resnick, 2002, p. 41). Junginger and McGuire (2001) argue that

the presence of command hallucinations is a paradox. Although there is convincing empirical evidence to support the notion that compliance with command hallucinations is not uncommon, no study so far has found a higher rate of actual violence for persons experiencing command hallucinations..When the subject gives an identity to the voice, there is increased risk of compliance with the command hallucination (p. 385).

Chapter 5

1. The Hamilton Rating Scale for Depression (HRSD or HAM-D) is a 17- to 31-item observer rated scale for the assessment of depressive symptoms. It is one of the most widely used instruments for the assessment of depression. The HRSD emphasizes somatic aspects of depression and is best for patients with the most severe depressive syndromes. This protocol relies heavily on the clinical interviewing skills and expertise of the rater. The 17-item version is the more commonly used of the scales, and the questions concentrate on the patient's condition during the previous few days or weeks, on a 5-point scale (absent, doubtful or trivial, mild, moderate, and severe) (Mullen, 2004, p. 7).

The Montgomery Asberg Depression Rating scale (MDRAS) is a 10-item protocol used in the evaluation of symptoms of depression in adults, and the assessment of changes in depressive symptoms. The MDRAS is an obsever rating scale that has a number of advantages including economy and sensitivity to change, and can be used by different professionals. Nine of the items are based on the patient's report, and one on the rater's observation. The MDRAS does not cover somatic or psychomotor symptoms as does the HRSD, but does evaluate core symptoms of depression (sadness, inner tension, lassitude, pessimistic thoughts, and suicidal thoughts; Mullen, 2004, p. 8).

The Beck Depression Inventory (BDI) is a 21-item scale, developed in 1961, designed to measure the behavioral manifestations of depression. It was modified and renamed the BDI-II reflecting DSM-IV criteria. The Beck protocol addresses mood, pessimism, sense of self-punishment, self-dislike, self-accusation, suicidal wishes, crying, irritability, social withdrawal, indecisiveness, distortion of body image, work inhibition, and loss of libido. Symptoms are rated according to intensity from 0 (mild) to 3 (severe). The sum of all the scores determines the severity of the depression: 0–9, minimal; 10–16, mild; 17–29, moderate; 30–60, severe (Mullen, 2004, p. 12).

The Young Mania Rating Scale (YMRS) is an 11-item protocol used to assess the severity of manic symptoms. Depressive symptoms are not assessed. The YMRS needs to be administered by a trained clinician. The severity rating is based on the patient's subjective report regarding the previous 48 hours and on the rater's observations during the interview (Mullen, 2004, p. 13).

The Beck Hopelessness scale (BHS) is a 20-item, self-report scale designed to measure a patient's negative attitude toward the future. Although, not intended for normal populations or adolescents, it is being used with these groups. It has demonstrated usefulness in inpatient, outpatient, and in emergency services. Scores of 10 or greater indicate a high suicidal risk. The Beck Scale for Suicidal Ideation (BSS) is a 21-item, self-report scale designed to measure the intensity, pervasiveness, and characteristics of suicidal ideation in adults and adolescents. The BSS may provide an assessment of risk but does not actually predict eventual suicide (p. 22).

2. No other subcortical structures that were examined (hippocampus, thalamus, and caudate) were different in volume between BP subjects and normal controls. This is the third report of decreased amygdalar volume from studies using high resolution MRI data (Chang et al., 2005, pp. 568–569). The findings reported in adults have been inconsistent: some studies have reported decreased amygdalar size whereas others have reported an increase when compared to healthy controls. The enlargement could be secondary to stress or to illness duration (Chang et al., 2005, p. 570). In this regard, Altshuler et al. (2005) reported functional MRI evidence of increased left amygdala activation during mania. Healthy subjects showed bilateral activation of the lateral orbitofrontal areas, Brodmann's area 47. These findings are interpreted as an indication that there is a lack of inhibitory/modulatory effect on the amygdala as a result of the lateral orbitofrontal hypofunction (pp. 1212–1213).

3. Other findings in bipolar disorder youth include loss of normal frontal lobe asymmetry, reduced intracranial volumes, increased frontal and temporal sulci size, reduced thalamic area, larger putamen volume, and smaller amygdala and hippocampal volumes relative to healthy controls. These findings differ from parallel studies in adults (Altschuler et al., 2005, pp. 1212–1213). If early- and adult-onset bipolar disorders are the same illness, then age at onset may differentially affect the brain structure. On the other hand, pediatric bipolar illness may be a distinct disorder with a different set of neuroanatomical correlates (Frazier et al., 2005, p. 1262). The decrease of size in the right hippocampus may be a finding reflective of the disease (p. 1262). Female subjects with bipolar disorder showed a more significant decrease in volumes than males. Also, the total volume decrement (mean 5.4%, SD = 6.4%) is supportive of the neurodevelopmental and probably the neurodegenerative hypotheses reflecting brains that have developed differently or that have suffered from early apoptotic pruning of neuronal circuits (p. 1262). Alternatively, the neuroanatomical differences between children and adults with bipolar disorder may be responsible for the difference in clinical presentation (Hirschfeld, 2005, p. 1242).

4. The V2 and V3 regions project to the orbitomesial cortex, anterior cingulate gyrus, amygdala, hippocampal, dentate regions, and hypothalalmus, all of which are believed to modulate mood. One confounding factor in previous studies is the exposure to antidepressants because there have several reports of antidepressaqnt-induced cerebellar toxicity (Mills et al., 2005, p. 1532).

5. The posterior section of the hippocampus is most consistently involved in the volume reduction. It is speculated that the volume reduction represents cellular alterations in 5-HT1A and neurotropin mechanisms, possibly related to elevated cortisol levels. These changes may underlie the alterations in learning and memory associated with major depressive disorder (Neumeister, Charney, & Drevets, 2005, p. 1057).

6. ERPs may be used to track the progression of brain abnormalities. The mismatch of negativity ERP is normal at the onset of a first schizophrenic break but becomes abnormal in the course of the illness; such a development is associated with gray matter loss in the auditory cortex (Gur et al., 2005, p. 95).

Chapter 6

1. Visual hallucinations were reported in an elderly woman who had no medical or cerebral degenerative disease and had been receiving sertraline. It is postulated that the

hallucinations were associated predominantly with three neurotransmitters: serotonin, dopamine, and acetylcoline. SSRIs may potentially induce psychotic symptoms by a 5-HT2- and 5-HT3-mediated dopamine in the ventral striate. Sertraline's high affinity to dopamine receptors makes this association more plausible (Ginsberg, 2004b, p.13).

2. Medications associated with psychosis include anabolic steroids, angiotensin-converting enzyme (ACE) inhibitors, anticholinergics and atropine, calcium channel blockers, cephalosporins, dopamine receptor agonists, fluoroquinolone antibiotics, histamine H1 receptor blockers, histamine H2 receptor blockers, HMG-CoA reductase inhibitors, nonsteroidal anti-inflammatory drugs, procaine derivatives (procainamide, procaine penicillin G), salicylates, sulfonamides (Fohrman & Stein, 2006, p. 38).

3. The patient, a 32-year-old male, developed paranoid and grandiose symptoms six months after treatment initiation with topiramate, shortly after the dose was increased from 150 mg BID to 200 mg BID. The patient became paranoid and believed he was "the messiah," and intended to sacrifice himself as directed by God. He also developed disorganized and illogical thinking and flat affect. Patient did not respond to risperidone treatment, up to 6 mg BID, but the psychosis cleared within 24 hours of topiramate discontinuation (Kober & Gabbard, 2005, p. 1542).

4. In opioid use, the Mu1 receptor stimulation produces cortical level analgesia and physical dependence; the Mu2 causes respiratory depression, decrease of gastrointestinal motility, and bradycardia. The Kappa receptor is associated with spinal analgesia, sedation, and inhibition of the antidiuretic hormone release. The Delta receptor produces analgesia, euphoria, and physical dependence. The Sigma receptor induces dysphoria and hallucinations. It is the pattern of receptor activation that characterizes the clinical effects produced by the various opioid drugs. Besides the well-known respiratory depressive effects, these drugs may also depress the cardiovascular, gastrointestinal, genitourinary, and endocrine systems (Schwengel, 2003, pp. 341, 343).

5. Necessary criteria for the diagnosis of Rett's disorders are:
   (a) Normal prenatal, and perinatal development for the first five months (in some cases development appears normal until 18 months).
   (b) Normal head circumference at birth.
   (c) Deceleration of head growth between 5 and 30 months.
   (d) Development of stereotyped hand movements (wringing or squeezing, clapping or tapping, mouthing, washing or rubbing automatisms after purposeful hand movements are lost.
   (e) Development of severe expressive and receptive language deficits.
   (f) Presence of severe psychomotor retardation.
   (g) Evidence of gait and truncal apraxia between 1 and 4 years of age. The diagnosis is tentative until ages 2 to 5 years (Tsai, 2004, p. 325).

   Children with Rett's syndrome develop lower motor neuron difficulties and basal ganglial dysfunction, forcing them to a wheelchair-bound life (p. 328). In addition, 80% of the patients develop seizures, including partial complex seizures, atypical absence, and generalized tonic-clonic and myoclonic seizures (p. 333). The diagnosis of Rett's syndrome is very difficult before 3 years of age but molecular analysis of mutation in the gene encoding for X-linked methyl-CpG-binding protein 2 (MECP2) assists in the diagnosis. Mutation of MECP2 seems to be the main cause of Rett's disorder and is present in approximately 80% of the patients with Rett's syndrome. Rett's children have a prolonged QTc interval, a serious and potentially lethal cardiac abnormality.

Other serious complications include orthopedic problems, oropharyngeal dysfunction, and gastroesophageal dysmotility (pp. 326–327). Some patients develop self-abusive behaviors, such as chewing their fingers and slapping their face (p. 333).

Chapter 7

1. In 49 patients with childhood onset schizophrenia, Nicolson, Lenane, Singaracharlu, et al. (20000 found that: 28 (57%) had premorbid motor development (delays in the development of the milestones); 27 (55%) had deviant social development; 27 (51%) had premorbid speech and language abnormalities; 10 (about 50% of patients) had premorbid speech impairment; 25 (about 50%) patients had very early language abnormalities; Only 2 (about 4%) patients had speech abnormalities without language impairments; 24 (49%) had delayed school entry or repeated grades; 15 (31%) had needed special education; 40% showed transient autistic symptoms such as hand flapping, echolalia, and unusual interests (see Louis case above). If these statistics are turned around, the difficulties of the diagnosis of COS become even more apparent; thus, in a cohort of children diagnosed with COS: 43% of children showed normal milestone development; 45% showed normal social development; 45% had normal premorbid speech/language development; about 80% of children show unremarkable premorbid speech development; about 50% of children did not show any early language abnormalities; about 50% of children did not have delays in school entrance or did not repeat any grades; about 70% of cases have been schooled in regular education; 60% of the cases show no history of autistic features. In regard to schizophrenia aggregation in families, of 132 relatives evaluated, 29 (22%) had schizophrenia spectrum disorders (78% did not). Of 89 relatives who completed the smooth-pursuit eye movement task, 35 (39.3%) had abnormal eye tracking (this is not a specific finding of COS) but 62.7% of those relatives showed no such abnormality.

2. Criterion A (for schizophrenia). Characteristic symptoms: Two (or more) of the following, each present for a significant portion of time during a one-month period (or less if successfully treated): (a) delusions; (b) hallucinations; (c) disorganized speech (e.g., frequent derailment or incoherence); (d) grossly disorganized or catatonic behavior; (e) negative symptoms (i.e., affective flattening, alogia, or avolition).

   Only one criterion A symptom is required if delusions are bizarre or hallucinations consist of a voice keeping a running commentary on the person's behavior or thoughts, or two or more voices converse with each other (DSM-IV-TR (APA, 2000), p. 312).

3. Criteria for inclusion in the Australian Prodromal Study
   (a) Vulnerability:

       i. Presence of a first degree relative with a psychotic disorder, or with schizotypal personality disorder.

       ii. Decrease in mental state (deterioration in mental status) or level of functioning for at least a month and no longer than five years.

       iii. Decrease of functioning that occurred during the last year.

   (b) Attenuated Psychosis:

       i. Presence of at least one of the following symptoms: ideas of reference, odd beliefs or magical thinking, perceptual disturbances, paranoid ideation, odd thinking or speech, odd behavior or appearance.

ii. Delusions are held with a reasonable degree of conviction.

iii. Symptoms are present several times a week.

iv. Change of mental state (deterioration in mental status) for more than a month and no longer than five years.

(c) Brief Limited Intermittent Psychotic Symptoms (BLIPS):

i. Transient psychotic features: presence of at least one of the following: ideas of reference, magical thinking, perceptual disturbance, paranoid ideation, or odd thinking or speech.

ii. Symptoms are held with strong conviction

iii. Episode lasts less than a week

iv. Symptoms resolve spontaneously

The BLIPS must have occurred during the previous year.

By the end of a 12 month follow-up, 41% of patients in the cohort developed an acute psychosis and were started on antipsychotic medications (Phillips et al., 2002, p. 259).

The Australian project supports the proposition that a population at high risk for the development of psychotic disorders could be identified and that early intervention could be implemented. However, early interventions raise many ethical questions (p. 264).

4. Leonhard considered that hebephrenias were caused by a failure of distinct psychic functional "systems," and as such, they represented nosologically "systematic schizophrenias." He even considered some hebephrenia subforms: silly hebephrenia, eccentric hebephrenia, shallow or apathetic hebephrenia, and autistic hebephrenia. Leonhard thought that contrary to the unsystematic schizophrenias where genetics play a role, in systematic schizophrenias, and in hebephrenia in particular, the etiology was environmental, not genetic.

5. Strahl and Lewis provided a classical review of this disorder in 1972. They state that etymologically hebephrenia relates to an adolescent impairment. Reports dealt with adolescents in the midteens, usually between 15 and 18 years of age, who developed a psychosis, sometimes insidiously, but most often in a more acute onset. Hebephrenia does occur in persons older than adolescence, but rarely occurs after the age of 25. Deteriorated hebephrenic schizophrenics have a striking resemblance to organic brain disease. Two salient clinical features are considered characteristic of hebephrenia:

A rapid downward path. It is the most pernicious form of schizophrenia in that it shows the greatest tendency to deterioration. A number of adolescents are "mentally finished" in two to three years of illness progression.

Outstanding gross disorganization of the intellectual and emotional life. Hebephrenia is the schizophrenic form that shows the most massive personality disorganization.

Patients often display incoherence, even word salad, and a marked impairment of the associative function. They are unable to concentrate or to express ideas coherently. There is also severe disorganization of emotional life. The emotional life (the affect) usually becomes inappropriate. Some patients are markedly withdrawn, but the withdrawal is punctuated with hyperactivity and overexcitement. Irritability and asocial behavior are also common. Massive mood changes are also characteristic. Sometimes these patients run the gamut of emotions in a short time, and there is a marked silliness. The subjective experience is that many hebephrenic patients feel "forced" to behave in a silly manner (which they are unable to stop). Silly and unusually bizarre behavior is expressed in their speech patterns. Silly laughter and completely inappropriate affect are frequently the rule. Grimacing, posturing, and stereotypes are common. Marked regressive behavior is common: many hebephrenic patients show very childish, playful, and mischievous behavior. Other hebephrenic patients display infantile and inappropriate sexual behavior while others display unprovoked temper tantrums. Some even evince baby talk. Frequently patients are narcissistic or self-centered, and even hypochondriacal, with bodily centered delusions. Occasionally hebephrenic patients show manic features, and sometimes their silliness is overlaid with elation; at those times, it is difficult to differentiate between flight of ideas and incoherence, and clinicians are likely to confuse the clinical picture with a bipolar disorder. Delusions and hallucinations may be present; delusions are poorly elaborated, and mostly relate to sex and performance (pp. 654–668).

Chapter 8

1. Genes under active investigative scrutiny:
   (a) Catechol-O-methyltransferase (COMT) gene. The COMT gene, involved in the breakdown of catecholamines, plays a role in the pathogenesis of schizophrenia and maps also to chromosome 22q11 (Roper & Voeller, 1998, p. 1061). The polymorphism of Met158Val has received particular attention because it appears to influence CMPT activity in vivo. Two metanalyses have not found support for an association of schizophrenia with this polymorphism (Shirts & Nimgaonkar, 2004, pp. 58, 63). COMT genotype is a predictor of prefrontal cognitive functioning after IQ scores were controlled. Met-hemizygous patients performed better than Val-hemizygous patients (Bearden et al., 2004, p. 1701; Malhotra, 2005, p. 21).
   (b) NOTCH 4 gene. The NOTCH 4 gene codes for ubiquitin that has been reported to be associated with neurodegeneration. A chromosome 6-11 translocation adjacent to the Beta-1,3 gluconyltransferase, and the overexpression of mRNA for NOGO, a myelin associated protein that inhibits the outgrowth of nerve terminals, has been found in postmortem schizophrenic brains (Buckley, Mahadik et al., 2003, p. 42).
   (c) Neuroregulin 1 gene. Neuroregulin 1, a promising genetic factor involved in the development of schizophrenia, is located on the short arm of chromosome 8. This haplotype is present in 15% of schizophrenics, but only in 7.5% of the general population. Neuroregulin 1 is considered a risk factor that can be determined with a high level of reliability. The neuroregulin (NRG-1) system participates in the regulation of cell survival, proliferation, migration, and differentiation of both neurons and glia. NRG-1 and its receptor, ErbB4, are localized at the synapse; the specific functions of these proteins has not been clarified (Law, 2003, p. 1392).
   (d) Dysbindin or Dystrobrevin-Binding Protein 1 (DTNBP1) gene. Dysbindin binds to B-dystrobrevin and it is a likely component of the dystrophin protein complex. This complex plays a role in synapse formation and maintenance and may also be involved in N-methyl-D-aspartate (NMDA) or gamma-aminobutiric acid (GABA) receptor signaling. DTNBP1 is located in chromosome 6q22. There is consistent evidence for association of this factor with schizophrenia in family based analyses. The results from based control analyses are less convincing (Shirts & Nimgaonkar, 2004, pp. 63–64). The size effect of the susceptibility for schizophrenia associated with dysbindin is small to moderate, and it is likely that this effect accounts for a

modest proportion of the total genetic risk (Kendler, 2004, p. 1535). However, two postmortem studies of schizophenic brains with match controls using inmuno-hystochemical methods found a significant reduction of presynaptic dysbindin-1 in the hipppocampal formation in schizophrenic subjects, in particular in the terminal fields of intrinsic glutaminergic afferents to the subiculum, the hippocampus proper, and the inner molecular layer of the dentate gyrus. Equally, dysbindin mRNA was significantly reduced in multiple layers of the dorsolateral prefrontal complex in schizophrenic subjects. This reduction appears to be specific and has not been seen with other markers of synaptic integrity. Dysbindin levels were also correlated with 4 of 11 markers of the dysbindin gene (Kendler, 2004, p. 1535).

(e) Regulator of G-protein signaling 4 (RGS4) gene. The RGS4 gene belongs to a family of GTP-ase activating proteins that modulate many G-protein coupled receptors and could potentially impact on the functions of neurotransmitters. It maps to chromosome 1q21-22, and has been implicated in schizophrenia in some linkage studies; it appears that this gene is downregulated in schizophrenia (Shirts & Nimgaonkar, 2004, p. 64).

(f) G72 and D-amino-acid Oxidase (DAAO) genes. G72 interacts with DAAO, a potent activator of the NMDA receptor. This gene maps to chromosome 13q34. It is believed that polymorphism in G72 and DAAO are associated with schizophrenia. The initial evidence for RGS4, G72, and DAAO is promising, but more replication studies are needed (Idem).

(g) CHRNA7 gene. A weak linkage signal has been found in several genome scans at the 15q gene, a region containing the genes for alpha-7 nicotine receptor (CHRNA7), associated with an intermediate schizophrenia endophenotype: abnormal P50 evoked response. Variants of CHRNA7 are also associated with schizophrenia (Gur et al., 2005, p. 105).

(h) DISC-1 gene. DISC-1 is a gene in 1q43; a chromosomal translocation originating in this gene has been found to be strongly associated with psychosis in Scottish families (p. 105). Malhotra (2005), also reports that his group had completed a comprehensive analysis of DISC1 gene in a controlled cohort of 586 participants (p. 19).

2. Exposure to maternal psychotic features is associated with higher than expected risk of natal and perinatal mortality. There is a twofold relative risk for fetal death/stillbirth among offspring of affected mothers; this risk is comparable to the one associated with smoking during pregnancy (Webb, Abel, Pickles, & Appleby, 2005, p. 1952).

3. In a study exploring a new high temporal resolution measure of functional connectivity,

(a) *Gamma phase synchronicity.* Gamma phase synchronicity revealed marked deficits in functional connectivity in subjects with both acute and chronic schizophrenia. As a group both chronic and first-episode schizophrenia patients exhibited marked disturbance in both early and late gamma phase synchrony (Selewa-Younan, Gordon, Harris, et al., 2004, p. 1599). Findings are consistent with studies demonstrating deficits in cognitive coordination of both early stimulus integration and later processes of selective attention and context, consistent with executive deficits functioning (p. 1601).

(b) *Gamma band.* The term *gamma band* refers to an endogenous brain oscillation near the frequency of 40 Hertz (Hz, 40 times per second). The oscillation reflects synchronization in several columns of cortical neurons, or between cortex and thalamus cells; this synchronization facilitates interneuronal communication. In schizophrenia there is a failure of gamma band synchronization, especially in the 40 Hz range (Gur et al., 2005, p. 89). Schizophrenic patients are unable to modulate the startle response when forewarned that a probe is coming, in contrast to controls. Schizophrenic patients showed a failure in gating.

(c) *Mismatch negativity.* Mismatch negativity (MMN) is a negative ERP that occurs about 0.2 sec after infrequent sounds (deviants) are presented in the sequence of repetitive sounds (standards). MMN is evoked automatically, without conscious attention. The source of this event seems to be in or near the primary auditory cortex (Heschl gyrus), and it is thought to reflect the operation of sensory memory, a memory of past stimuli used by auditory cortex in analysis of temporary patterns (Gur et al., 2005, p. 90). fMRIs have demonstrated the presence of a deficiency in activation (BOLD) in schizophrenic patients to the mismatch stimulus within the Heschl gyrus and the nearby posterior superior temporal gyrus (p. 90). The MMN abnormalities present in schizophrenic psychosis are not present in manic psychosis (p.90).

(d) *P300 and the failure to process unusual events.* The P300 is an ERP that occurs when a low-probability event is detected and consciously processed. The subjects are asked to count a low probability tone that is interspersed with a more frequent occurring stimulus. The P300 response is consciously processed and is thought to reflect an updating of the conscious information–processing stream and expectancy; this event is larger when the stimulus is rare.

(e) *Contingent negative variation (CNV).* Contingent negative variation (CNV), hemispheric asymmetry in the amplitude of the P1/N1 component complex, processing negativity (Pn), and a late positive component of P300 has been studied at UCLA in schizophrenic children. The CNV measures orienting, preparation, and readiness to respond to an expected stimulus. Normal individuals usually have larger visual P1/N1 components over the right hemisphere. CNV differences between normal subjects and schizophrenics were not consistent across studies, but Nps were found to be smaller in schizophrenic children and adults with both the span and the CPT. Reductions in the Np amplitude in schizophrenia result from impairment in executive functions responsible for the deployment and maintenance of attentional functions. Individuals with frontal lobe lesions resemble schizophrenic subjects in this regard: both groups do not show increased Np to attend stimuli in auditory selection tasks. It is considered that the MMN reflects, in part, NMDA-mediated activity; it is speculated that the reason for schizophrenia progression is due to the NMDA-related exotoxicity that causes both a reduction of the neuropil (dendritic regression) and a simultaneous reduction on MMN in the months following the first hospitalization (Gur et al., 2005, p. 91).

4. Children with an early onset of puberty have a high concentration of adrenal androgens, estradiol, thyrotropin, and cortisol; they also manifest more emotional disorders (anxiety disorders, depression, and parent-reported behavioral problems). The relationship between testosterone levels and aggression is more pronounced in adolescence, particularly if the parent–child relationship is conflictive. It is believed that hormones trigger gene expression related to vulnerability to behavioral disorders. On the other hand, estrogens may have an ameliorating effect by reducing dopaminergic activity (p. 91).

5. PANDAS children show antineuronal antibodies with a reactivity similar to the one shown by children with Sydenham's chorea. Obsessive–compulsive disorder onset or

reactivation, and tic disorders have been documented following a streptococcal infection. The elevation of antistreptococcal antibody titers suggests an immunological response in the pathogenesis of these disorders. The MRI of children with Sydenham's chorea shows an increase in the caudate, putamen, and globus pallidus size. The MRIs of children with PANDAS also show bilateral enlargement of the caudate nuclei. Plasma exchanges produced reduction in the basal ganglia size. Basal ganglia abnormalities have been demonstrated in patients with bipolar disorders: magnetic resonance spectroscopy (MRS) indicated increased glutamate/glutamine neuronal activity in 10 bipolar children but not in the controls. PET studies showed increased activity in the left dorsal anterior cingulate and in the left caudate head in five patients with mania. These neuroimaging studies suggest a common anatomical relationship of bipolar disorders with PANDAS, OCD, Sydenham's chorea, and tic disorders (Soto & Murphy, 2003, pp. 194–205).

6. Kapur wonders how a drug that acts on receptors on a cell surface reverses this complex neurochemical and phenomenological experience called psychosis. Antipsychotics are efficacious in psychosis because all of them share a common property of "dampening salience." Two important aspects of this idea are highlighted. First, while antipsychotics may differ in chemical structure or receptor affinity, they share the psychological effect of dampening salience, which is the final pathway of improvement. Second, antipsychotics only provide a platform (of attenuated salience); the process of symptomatic improvement of delusions requires further psychological and cognitive resolution.

   The resolution of symptoms is a dynamic process: antipsychotics lessen the salience of the concerns, and the patient "works through" her symptoms toward a psychological resolution. Symptom resolution may have much in common with the mechanisms whereby all humans give up on cherished beliefs or frightening dread, and it may involve processes of extinction, encapsulation, and belief transformation—which are fundamentally, psychological concepts. Thus, antipsychotics do not excise symptoms; rather, they attenuate the salience of the distressing ideas and percepts, allowing patients to reach their own private resolution of these matters. Certainly, Kapur makes the case for a multidimensional approach for the treatment of chronic psychosis.

7. Anticholinergic treatment may even have an effect on mortality: the lack of treatment with anticholinergics has been associated with reduced survival in elderly patients with schizophrenia. Findings of reduced muscarinic receptor availability are compatible with the results of neuropathological studies that have examined the muscarinic systems in schizophrenia.

8. The Glu receptor family is comprised of two subfamilies: ionotropic and metabotropic; within these subfamilies there are multiple subdivisions. There are three major categories in the ionotropic receptors: NMDA, amino-3-hydroxy-5-methyl-isoxazole-4-propionic acid (AMPA), and the kainic acid (KA) receptors. Within these, multiple subunits and splice variants have been identified (Farber & Newcomer, 2003, p. 130).

9. G proteins modulate noradrenergic, serotonergic, dopaminergic, cholinergic, and histaminergic receptor systems. G proteins have either stimulatory (Gs) or inhibitory (Gi) effects on effector proteins. Receptor activated G proteins modulate ion flows, regulating the activity of the ion channels, and by controlling the activity of several effector enzymes (Frey et al., 2004, p. 181).

10. PKC (an important enzyme in the PIP2 pathway) acts on the regulation of neuronal excitability, neurotransmitter release, genetic expression, and synaptic plasticity (p. 181). Interestingly, tamoxifen has antimanic effects via PKC mechanisms (p. 184).

Chapter 9

1. The book by Kingdon and Turkington (2005) has useful chapters on specific approaches and techniques to deal with a variety of positive and negative symptoms from a cognitive behavioral therapy perspective.

2. During the last couple of years, this writer has noticed a significant deterioration in the quality (adequacy) of the special education programs in the Southwest, and believes that these negative trends may be happening in other parts of the nation. Due to the "No child left behind" ideals, many special education students are being left behind all together. It is likely that special education appropriations are being shifted to the regular education programming to meet federal standards for regular education. Parents are being deceived, and deceive themselves, when their children who are receiving special education, receive the school recommendation for mainstream education; parents falsely believe that the recommended change in educational status to a regular classroom is an indication that the child's educational condition is improving. In this author's experience mainstreaming is being abused. For instance, children who need a highly structured, self-contained classroom are being offered mainstreaming. Furthermore, schools procrastinate in the identification (comprehensive testing) and implementation of "real" special education programs.

Chapter 10

1. In this writer's opinion, the lessons from the CATIE trial are:

   Antipsychotics in general, and second generation antipsychotics (SGAs) in particular, leave much to be desired in terms of effectiveness, tolerability, and staying power.

   First generation antipsychotics (FGAs) are not dead; it is likely that as a result of the performance of perphenazine, this medication and probably other FGAs may be reconsidered as viable alternatives for the treatment of chronic psychosis and related symptoms.

   Olanzapine showed some gradient of superiority in therapeutic effectiveness and staying power over the comparators: perphenazine, quetiapine, risperidone, and ziprasidone. However, (i) this medication was prescribed at higher doses than recommended in the 2006-PDR, and (ii) olanzapine' adiposogenic and prodyslipidemic side effects were the highest among the antipsychotics tried (risperidone, quetiapine, ziprasidone and perphenazine).

   The cardiotoxicity of ziprasidone has been overstated. Another way of saying this is to assert that ziprasidone cardiotoxicity is comparable in risk to one of olanzapine, perphenazine, risperidone, or quetiapine.

   Ziprasidone was the only antipsychotic among the agents tried that had beneficial effects in weight and other metabolic parameters.

2. The CAFE trial, Comparison of Atypicals in First-Episode Psychosis: A Randomized, 52-week Comparison of olanzapine, quetiapine, and risperidone, conducted by Lieberman, McEvoy, et al. (2005), reflected parallel results to CATIE's: 75.9% of patients were drug naïve, and 57.8% received the diagnosis of schizophrenia. Mean daily modal doses were: olanzapine (N = 133), 11.7 mg; quetiapine (N = 134), 506 mg; risperidone (N = 133), 2.4 mg. At 52 weeks, the treatment discontinuation rates were, 68, 70.9, and 71.4%, respectively. There were no significant differences between treatments,

except that fewer quetiapine patients received fewer concomitant medications for Parkinsonism or akathisia compared to olanzapine (3.7% vs. 11.3%). At week 52, 80% of olanzapine treated patients had gained more than 7% of baseline weight, compared to 57.6% (risperidone), and 50% in quetiapine–treated patients ($P = 0.01$) (p. 526). In the CATIE trial, the mean modal doses and rates for all cause discontinuation were, for olanzapine: 20.1 mg and 64%; for perphenazine: 20.8 mg and 75%; for quetiapine: 543.4 mg and 82%; for risperidone: 3.9 mg and 74%; and for ziprasidone: 112.8 mg and 79%, respectively (Nasrallah, 2006, p. 55).

3. Interesting research findings show that the long-term effect of different atypicals on rats' basal ganglia is different for different drugs: There is an increase in volume in animals that received haloperidol or clozapine compared to control animals; the volume is significantly decreased in animals receiving olanzapine compared with controls; and no significant difference was seen in the risperidone-treated animals compared with controls. These drugs "are very different from each other, not only in what receptors they interact within the brain, but also in differences between low and high doses of the same drug affecting different receptor targets" (Rosack, 2002, p. 23; see, http://www.acnp.org/citations/Npp011402225).

4. Kapur, Arenovich, et al. (2005) demonstrated that onset of actions by antipsychotics (olanzapine and haloperidol) may start by the first day of treatment initiation. Their study supports previous reports of significant antipsychotic effects by the third day of treatment, and even a meta-analysis indicating that rate of improvement during the first week was superior to any other ensuing week. The authors proposed an "early-onset hypothesis." This proposition is in line with a well-recognized, substantial blockade of the dopamine system by antipsychotic medications within the first few hours of treatment (p. 944).

5. The atypical clinical effects are broad and powerful. Atypicals are prescribed for major depression without psychotic features, dysthymia, mania without psychotic features, bipolar II disorder, obsessive–compulsive disorder, generalized anxiety disorder, post-traumatic stress disorder, intermittent explosive disorder, insomnia, delirium, Tourette's disorder, anorexia nervosa, personality changes due to neurological or developmental conditions, borderline personality disorder, catatonia, and probably others. Symptoms for which atypicals are prescribed include aggressive behavior, worrying, agitation, reactivity to environmental stimuli, social stress, insomnia, and mood disturbances (Swartz, 2003, pp. 12–13). This parallels antipsychotic pediatric use.

6. Steiner, Saxena, and Chang (2005) consider primary and secondary disorders of aggression. Primary disorders include: oppositional defiant disorder (ODD), conduct disorder (CD), intermittent explosive disorder (IED), paraphilias, kleptomania, antisocial personality disorder (APD), borderline personality disorder (BPD), and pyromania. To the secondary group belong: ADHD, pervasive developmental disorder (PDD), autism, mental retardation (MR), anxiety disorders (PTSD, dissociative disorder, separation anxiety disorder, social phobia), mood disorders, especially bipolar disorder, substance abuse and dependency (SUD), schizophrenia and other psychotic illnesses, and bulimia (p. 4). The authors also subdivide the primary disorders into reactive, affective, defensive, impulsive (RADI or "hot"), and planned, instrumental, proactive (PIP or "cold"). Different neuronal architectures support these processes. For secondary disorders of aggression, treatment of the dysfunctional module (syndrome) reduces aggressive behavior (p. 4).

7. At the SMHC, where this author practices child and adolescent inpatient, partial hospitalization, and residential treatments, ziprasidone injectable has been used about 400 times, in doses ranging from 5 to 20 mg; most of the medication has been used with adolescents, and to a less extent with preadolescents. Most adolescents received 20 mg IM for agitation or behavior dyscontrol; preadolescents usually received 10 mg IM for related reasons. So far, we have not had the first untoward reaction. Of interest, and a great advantage of this medication vehicle, patients calm down without falling sleep. Most of the children resume therapeutic programming in less than 60 to 90 minutes after the injection. Seldom has the dose been repeated, and no patient has received more than 40 mg IM/day. It is important to indicate that 20 mg of ziprasidone IM is equivalent to approximately 120 mg or probably more of oral dose.
8. A number of scales have been developed for the study of prodromal schizophrenia:
   Comprehensive Assessment of At Risk Mental State (CAARMS)
   Melbourne Criteria for Ultra-High Mental State Based on CAARMS
   Scale of Prodromal Symptoms (SOPS)
   Structured Interview of Prodromal Symptoms (SIPS)
   Criteria of Prodromal Symptoms (COPS)
   Schizophrenia Prediction Instrument for Adults (SPI-A)
   (Addington, 2004, pp. 589–593).
9. The high dose range of olanzapine in the CATIE trial (up to 30 mg/day, 50% higher than the approved upper range of 20 mg/day) is undoubtedly the Achilles heel of the argument that olanzapine demonstrated better effectiveness as measured by the "all-cause discontinuation" parameter.... So the debate boils down to which [antipsychotic medication] is better in the decades-long management of schizophrenia: discontinuation after 3 to 5 months for efficacy/tolerability reasons or discontinuation after 6 to 8 months due to metabolic tolerability/safety reasons. (Nasrallah, 2005, p. 17)
10. Only 22% of the subjects (N = 11 of 50) went one year without an exacerbation or relapse following medication discontinuation. By two years, 96% (N = 48) of the subjects had experienced an exacerbation (N = 28) or relapse (N = 20). The mean time to exacerbation or relapse, for the 48 subjects whose psychotic symptoms returned within the time frame of the study, was 235 days, or just under 8 months. The median time to exacerbation or relapse was 245 days. The two subjects who did not experience exacerbation or relapse within the time frame of the study were followed clinically and ultimately developed psychotic symptoms after drug withdrawal: one at 28 months and the other at 93 months (i.e., 7 years, 9 months). Only three (13%) were hospitalized within three months of exacerbation. The rest were successfully managed in outpatient therapy (Gitlin et al., 2001, pp. 1838–1839). "[W]e still do not automatically recommend long-term maintenance treatment after the first episode for every patient" (p. 1840).

Chapter 11

1. Leverich, Altshuler, Frye, et al. (2006) reported on a continuum of manic to hypomanic manifestations during antidepressant augmentation of mood stabilizers in patients with bipolar depression. The continuum ranged from subthreshold (brief and recurrent brief) hypomania to threshold switches, including full-duration hypomania and mania. If only switches into mania are considered, the switch rate is of 7.9% in the acute treatment trials, and of 14.9% in continuation trials. If full duration hypomania lasting a week or

more were to be considered, the threshold switch would be 19.3% during acute trials, and 36.7% during continuation treatment. Bipolar I depressed patients are more likely to switch than bipolar II depressed patients (p. 235). Venlafaxine had a higher switch rate than sertraline or bupropion. The switch rate of venlafaxine is twofold greater than the switch rate of sertraline (p. 235). Bupropion causes low switch rates even when given to rapid cyclers (p. 236).

2. It is proposed that valproate exerts its antiepileptic effects by direct neuronal mechanisms (i.e., reducing sodium influx and increasing potassium efflux). Other effects may include, decrease of dopamine turnover, decrease of NMDA-mediate currents, decreased release of aspartate, and decrease of somatostatin concentrations in the CSF (Bowden, 2004, p. 570).

3. Among CBZ neurochemical mechanisms, the following have been described :
(a) CBZ decreases glutamate and aspartate release by blocking sodium channels; (b) decreases somatostatinlike inmunoreactivity; (c) increases potassium efflux and serum l-tryptophan; (d) decreases serum levothyroxine, cAMP and cGMP; (e) increases serotonin and substance P neurotransmission; (f) has effects at peripheral-type benzodiazepine receptors; (g) blocks adenosine A1 receptors; (h) increases G protein stimulating alpha subunits (Gs-alpha) and inositol monophosphate (IMPase); (i) decreases G protein-inhibitory alpha subunits (Gi-alpha); (j) increases expression of cytoprotective protein bcl-2 and transcription factor AP-1 binding; (k) decreases glycogene synthase kinase-3beta (GSK-3beta), protein kinase C (CPK), and myristoylated alanine–rich C kinase substrate (MARCKS); (l) decreases sodium influx and glutamate release; (m) increases potassium conductance; (n) acts on peripheral benzodiazepine and alpha 2 adrenergic receptors. The actions vary according to the time and length of use of the drug:
(a) Acute actions: CBZ has similar effects over GABA-B receptors as biclofen.
(b) Acute and subchronic actions:
    i. Increases striatal cholinergic neurotransmission. Decreases adenylate cyclase activity stimulated by dopamine, norepinephrine, and serotonin.
    ii. Decreases turnover of dopamine, norepinephrine, and GABA.
    iii. Chronic actions: antidepressant effects; they include:
        A. Increases serum and urinary free cortisol, free tryptophan, substance P sensitivity, and adenosine A1 receptors.
        B. Decreases CSF somatostatinlike inmunoreactivity (Ketter et al., 2004, p. 585).

4. Carbamazepine decreases the serum levels of the following medications:
Antidepressants: bupropion, citalopram, mirtazapine(?), TCAs *Antipsychotics*: aripiprazole, clozapine, fluphenazine(?), haloperidol, olanzapine, risperidone, thiothixene(?), ziprasidone *Anxiolytics/sedatives*: alprazolam,* buspirone, clonazepam,* midazolam, zoplicone(?). Stimulants: methylphenidate, modafinil *Anticonvulsants*: carbamazepine, ethosuximide, felbamate, lamotrigine,* Oxcarbazepine, phenytoin, primidone, tiagabine, topiramate, valproate, zonisamide *Analgesics*: alfentanil, buprenorphine,* fentanyl (?), levobupivacaine, methadone, tramadol *Anticoagulants*: dicumarol (?), phenprocoumon, warfarin *Antimicrobials*: caspofungin, doxycycline *Antivirals*: delavirdine, protease inhibitors *Immunosuppressants*: cyclosporine (?), sirolimus, tacrolimus *Muscle relaxants*: doxacurium, pancuronium, rapacuronium, rocuronium, vecuronium *Steroids*: Hormonal contraceptives,* dexamethasone, mifepristone, prednisone. *Others*:

bepridil, dihydropyridine calcium channel blockers,* oxiracetam(?), paclitaxel,* quinidine, remacemide(?), repaglinide,* theophylline (?), thyroid hormones
*Low medication level renders it ineffective.
5. See note 1.

Chapter 12

1. *Receptor activity*: clozapine demonstrates moderate to high affinity for 5-HT2A, 5-HT2C, alpha-1, alpha-2, M1, and H1 receptors. Clozapine has moderate affinity for D1 and D4 receptors, low to moderate affinity for D2 and D3 receptors, and, like many other atypicals, it has a low affinity for 5-HT1A receptors (Tauscher, Hussain, Agid et al, 2004, p. 1620).
   Cytochrome activity: clozapine is a substrate for CYP 1A2, 2E1, and 3A3/4; it is also a minor substrate for 2C and 2D6.
   Drug interactions: see appendix A.
2. Approximately one in 10 adult patients with schizophrenia will commit suicide each year. Fifty percent of schizophrenics will make a suicide attempt in their lifetime. Suicide is the leading cause of death in patients with schizophrenia under the age of 35. The suicide rate for the U.S. population is 11.4 per 100,000 whereas the rate for schizophrenics is 90 per 100,000. It appears that the suicide risk for patients with schizophrenia continues throughout their lives. Suicide risk factors that have been identified include: (a) prior family history of suicide attempts; (b) depressed mood; (c) hopelessness; (d) life events; (e) male gender; (f) substance abuse; (g) being unmarried, socially isolated, or unemployed; (h) higher level of premorbid functioning; (i) poor response to treatment and fear of further deterioration; and, (j) insight into the effects of illness (Meltzer, 2002, pp. 279–280).
   Clozapine reduces the rate of suicidality (frequency and intensity) and the lethality of the suicidal attempts. The International Suicide Prevention Trial (InterSePT), a prospective, controlled, randomized, parallel-group study, demonstrated clozapine superiority over olanzapine in reducing suicidality (pp. 281–282).

Chapter 13

1. *Lithium–drug interactions.* NSAIDs, Cox-2 inhibitors, metronidazole, and angiotensine-converting enzyme (ACE) inhibitors may increase lithium concentration to toxic levels. Concomitant use of calcium channel blockers may increase neurotoxicity. The same may happen with the concomitant use of SSRIs (PDR, 2006, p. 1407). On the other hand, acetazolamide, urea, xantine derivatives, and alkalinizing agents such as sodium bicarbonate, lower lithium concentrations (p. 1407).
2. *Valproate drug interactions.* Aspirin increases free valproate fourfold when coadministered with valproate (PDR, 2006, pp. 430). *Depakote*
3. Carbamazepine and to a less extent OXC, are enzyme inducing anticonvulsants, which increase the complexity of the treatment of psychotic bipolar disorders. CBZ drug interactions are explained by three factors:
   (a) CBZ is a robust inducer of catabolic enzymes (including CP450 A3/4, and others) and decreases the serum concentration of many medications. CBZ produces

autoinduction and heteroinduction. These effects may render many medications ineffective, and on the contrary, when CBZ is discontinued, other medication concentrations may increase to toxic levels.

(b) CBZ metabolism may be inhibited by a number of enzyme inhibitors, producing CBZ increased levels and CBZ toxicity.

(c) Carbamazepine epoxide (CBZ-E) is an active metabolite. VPA inhibits the epoxide hydrolase, which results in the increased serum level CBZ-E (but not CBZ) and intoxication. VPA also increases free CBZ level displacing CBZ from its protein binding (Ketter, Wang, & Post, 2004, p. 594).

The following is a list of medications whose metabolism is affected by CBZ:

Fluoxetine, fluvoxamine, and nefazodone increase CBZ concentrations. CBZ combination with mirtazapine is of concern because of mirtazapine's association with agranulocytosis (p. 596). Loxapine, chlorpromazine, and amoxapine increase the level of CBZ-E. Clozapine and CBZ combination is not recommended due the possible synergistic bone marrow suppression. Verapamil, diltiazem, and nimodipine increase CBZ concentrations to toxic levels. The "N" rule establishes that N=no: N means no for nifedipine and no for nimopidine (p. 596). CBZ attenuates alcohol withdrawal, but the attenuation affects cocaine cravings, cocaine effects, and seizures have not been substantiated (Ketter et al., 2004, p. 598).

Carbamazepine decreases the serum levels of the following medications:

Antidepressants: bupropion, citalopram, mirtazapine (?), TCAs. *Antipsychotics*: aripiprazole, clozapine, fluphenazine (?), haloperidol, olanzapine, risperidone, thiothixene (?), ziprasidone. *Anxiolytics/sedatives*: alprazolam,* buspirone, clonazepam,* midazolam, zopiclone (?) *Stimulants*: methylphenidate, modafinil. *Anticonvulsants*: carbamazepine, ethosuximide, felbamate, lamotrigine,*Oxcarbazepine, phenytoin, primidone, tiagabine, topiramate, valproate, zonisamide. *Analgesics*: alfentanil, buprenorphine,* fentanyl (?), levobupivacaine, methadone, tramadol. *Anticoagulants*: dicumarol (?), phenprocoumon, warfarin. *Antimicrobials*: caspofungin, doxycycline. Antivirals: delavirdine, protease inhibitors. *Immunosuppressants*: cyclosporine (?), sirolimus, tacrolimus. *Muscle relaxants*: doxacurium, pancuronium, rapacuronium, rocuronium, vecuronium. *Steroids*: Hormonal contraceptives,* dexamethasone, mifepristone, prednisone. *Others*: bepridil, dihydropyridine calcium channel blockers,* oxiracetam (?), paclitaxel,* quinidine, remacemide (?), repaglinide,* Theophylline (?), thyroid hormones

* Low medication level renders it ineffective.

The following medications are increased by CBZ but not by OXC

Antidepressants: fluoxetine, fluvoxamine, nefazodone. *Antimicrobials*: isoniazid, quinupristin/ dalfopristin. *Macrolide antibiotics*: clarithromycin, erythromycin, flurithromycin, josamycin, ponsinomycin. *Calcium channel blockers*: diltiazem, verapamil. *Hypolipidemics*: gemfibrozil, nicotinamide. *Others*: acetazolamide, cimetidine, danazol, omeprazole, D-propoxyphene, ritonavir (?), ticlopidine (?), valproate (increases VPA-E) (Ketter et al., 2004, pp. 595–596).

4. The QT interval varies primarily with the heart rate. The heart rate corrected QT (QTc) interval is calculated by dividing the QT measured by the square root or the RR interval. According to the Bazett's formula, the QTc interval should not exceed 0.44 second, except in infants. A QTc of 0.49 second may be normal in the first 6 months of life. Lead II (usually with a visible q wave) is the best lead to measure the QT interval.

Long QT interval may be seen in hypocalcemia, myocarditis, and diffuse myocardial diseases, including hypertrophic and dilated cardiomyopathies, long QT syndrome (e.g., Jervell and Lange-Nielsen syndrome, Romano-Ward syndrome (see Note 5), head injury, severe malnutrition, and others. A number of drugs are also known to prolong the QT interval, see Note 6. Other conditions that also may prolong the QT interval are: ischemic heart disease, and sinus bradycardia; coadministration of other medications that alter the sensitivity to catecholamines; hypomagnesemia, hypokalemia, or hypothermia, and autonomic instability caused by stress, extremes of emotion, physical exertion, or sudden shock (Pfizer, Inc.). There is caveat regarding the QTc readings. A benign U wave may be mistaken for QTc prolongation. The QTc of children and adolescents must be calculated by hand in the presence of tachycardia, bradycardia, unusual T- or U-wave morphology, arrhythmias (including bundle branch block), or the presence of U waves. The child psychiatrist should consult with a cardiologist familiar with QTc measurements when uncertain about the significance of QTc prolongation at baseline (Labellarte, Walkup, & Riddle, 2003, p. 621).

5. Jervell and Lange-Nielsen (1957) first described families in Norway in whom a long QT interval on the EKG was associated with deafness, syncopal spells, and a family history of sudden death. Syncopal attacks are due to ventricular arrhythmias. This syndrome is transmitted in an autosomal recessive manner. The Romano-Ward syndrome, reported independently (by Romano et al., in Italy) and by Ward (in Ireland), has all the features of the Jervell and Lange-Nielsen syndrome but without the deafness. This syndrome is transmitted in a dominant autosomal mode and is more common than the Jervell and Lange-Nielsen syndrome (Park, 2002, p. 455). "[I]t is prudent to ask apparently healthy patients if they have had syncope, if they have relatives with long QT syndrome or if they have relatives who died suddenly at a young age" (Glassman & Bigger, 2001, p. 1780). Hypertrophic cardiomyopathy (HC) is usually a familiar disorder of the heart muscle and in 30 to 60% of the cases appears to be genetically transmitted as an autosomal dominant trait. It may be seen in children with LEOPARD syndrome (Lentiginous skin lesions, EKG abnormalities, Ocular hypertelorism, Pulmonary stenosis, Abnormal genitalia, Retarded growth, Deafness). Patients with severe hypertrophy and obstruction may experience anginal chest pain, lightheadedness, or syncope. These patients are prone to develop arrhythmias leading to sudden death (presumably for ventricular tachycardia or fibrillation). These patients may be more prone to sudden death (Park, 2002, pp. 268–270).

6. Drugs that prolong the QT interval:

    Antihistaminics: astemizole, terfenadine. *Antiinfectives*: amantadine, clarithromycin, chloroquine, erythromycin, grepafloxacin, moxifloxacin, pentamidine, sparfloxacin, trimethoprim-sulfamethoxazole. *Antineoplastics*: tamoxifen. *Antiarrythmics*: quinidine, sotalol, procainamide, amiodarone, bretylium, disopyramide, flecainide, ibutilide, moricizine, tocainide, dofetilide. *Antilipemic agents*: probucol. *Calcium channel blockers*: bepridil. *Diuretics*: indapamide. *Gastrointestinal agents*: cisapride. *Hormones*: fludrocortisone, vasopressin. *Antidepressants*: amitriptyline, amoxapine, clomipramine, doxepin, imipramine, nortriptyline, protriptyline. *Antipsychotics*: chlorpromazine, haloperidol, perphenazine, quetiapine, risperidone, sertindole, thioridazine, ziprasidone (Zareba & Lin, 2003, p. 292)

7. See note 5.

8. See note 4.

9. See note 4.

10. A pharmacy database of patients who receive antipsychotic medications was analyzed for 3 to 12 months. The patients were divided into two groups. One group of patients received antipsychotics that prolong the QTc, and the other, received antipsychotics that did not prolong the QTc. Attention was drawn to the frequency of coprescriptions of medications that have the potential for prolonging the QTc. Results showed that 51% of the QT antipsychotics received other QT prolonging drugs for at least one day during the follow-up period. Logistic regression indicated that there was no significant difference between the QTc antipsychotic and the non-QTc antipsychotic groups in reference to the concomitant use of other QTc prolonging drugs. Even though women are at a higher risk for torsades de pointes, women were more likely than men to be prescribed other QTc prolonging medications (56.2 vs. 43.2%; $p < 0.001$) and non-QTc drugs (53.1 vs. 43.0%; $p < 0.001$ (Roe, Odell, & Herderson, 2003).

11. See note 10 for medications that increase QTc interval.

12. When a cohort of 90,000 patients treated for schizophrenia with four antipsychotic drugs (clozapine, 9%; haloperidol, 43%; risperidone, 23%; and thioridazine, 25%) was compared with a control cohort of 7,000 patients with psoriasis and 21,000 patients with glaucoma, patients treated with neuroleptics had a two- to threefold higher risk increase of all cardiac arrest and ventricular arrhythmias, and two to five times higher risk for all cause mortality increase than the control patients (Zareba & Lin, 2003, p. 299).

13. Stubbe and Scahill (2002) recommend further cardiological workup or consultation referral, or alternative therapy if:

    There is history of palpitations, syncope, or dizzy spells.
    Sustained resting heart rate is above 130 bpm.
    PR interval > 200 ms.
    QRS > 120 ms.
    QTc > 460 ms

14. Other drugs that are associated with pancreatitis are azathioprine, estrogens, thiazides, furosemide, sulfonamides, and pentamidine (Koller, Cross, Doraiswamy et al., 2003, p. 1124).

15. The risk of diabetes was greatest among olanzapine users (odds ratio 4.4, 1.8 to 11.0); use of conventional antipsychotics slightly increased the risk (1.3, 1.1, to 1.6). Use of risperidone was also associated with a slightly increased risk of diabetes, but this was not significant (Idem). Described findings were corroborated by Canadian investigators (Caro, Ward, Levinton, & Robinson, 2002) in a large cohort of 33,946 patients in a study supported by Janssen Ortho, Inc. The authors noted that after discontinuation of olanzapine there had been an apparent remission of diabetes in nine published cases (p. 1135). When age, gender, and haloperidol use were controlled for, using a proportional hazard analysis, the relative risk of diabetes was increased 20% (95% CI = 0%-43%, $p = .05$) for olanzapine compared to risperidone (p. 1137). The risk for women was higher: 30% (95% CI = 5% to 65%, $p = 0.02$) comparing olanzapine and risperidone, after adjusting for age, schizophrenia diagnosis, and haloperidol use. During the first three months of olanzapine treatment, there was a 90% increase (95% CI = 40–157%, $p < .001$) in the risk of developing diabetes compared to risperidone (Idem). Atypicals may increase the risk for diabetes in a number of ways:

An increase in the adipose tissue can lead to insulin resistance, glucose intolerance, and ultimately, diabetes.

Serotonin receptor antagonism may lead to hyperglycemia by decreasing pancreatic beta cell response to signals that advance insulin production.

Increase in free fatty acids associated with atypicals can alter glucose metabolism. Clozapine and olanzapine, the atypicals with highest potential for hyperlipedemia have the strongest association with new-onset diabetes (Wirshing et al, 2003, p, 51).

16. Eleven of 21 patients who agreed to participate in the Weight Watchers program completed the study. Of the other 10 patients, seven withdrew before starting the program. Patients who completed the WW program lost more weight than participants in the comparison group. Although participants in the WW program lost more weight than participants in the comparison group, no significant differences were noted in weight changes or in changes in body mass between the two groups. Only the male participants lost weight. No correlation was found between weight loss and exercise or change in psychiatric symptoms (Ball, Coons, & Buchanan, 2001, pp. 968).

17. See note 14.

18. Clozapine and haloperidol were associated with significant elevation of mean glucose levels after eight weeks of treatment; olanzapine was associated with significant elevation of glucose levels after 14 weeks of treatment. Risperidone was not associated with glucose level changes. Fourteen percent of patients (six given clozapine, four given olanzapine, three given risperidone, and one given haloperidol), developed abnormally high levels of glucose (> 125 mg/dl) during the course of treatment. Changes in glucose levels were independent of weight increase: the highest association was present in olanzapine treated patients followed by clozapine and risperidone. In a small number of patients (7) with preexisting diabetes, antipsychotic treatment did not have a deleterious effect on glucose metabolism. There was a rate of 14% of diabetes in this study. This corresponds to double the rate of the U.S. population (Lindenmayer et al., 2003, p. 294).

19. In a communiqué, supported by Lilly, Dagogo-Jack (2003) asserted that,

Together, these clamp studies strongly suggest that antipsychotics, particularly the atypical antipsychotics olanzapine and risperidone, do not directly alter insulin production or sensitivity. These agents are, therefore, unlikely to induce hyperglycemia through the primary mechanisms of action in the central nervous system. A more plausible explanation is that antipsychotics, through either weight gain or other metabolic effects, uncover latent diabetes tendencies in predisposed subjects. The effect of weight gain should not be underestimated, since obesity significantly alters glucose homeostasis and may serve as a risk factor for the development of diabetes in predisposed patients. Fortunately, weight gain is manageable. (p. 4)

The CATIE report findings (2005) regarding olanzapine contradicts Dagogo-Jack's propositions, and clinical experience demonstrates that managing weight gain is a very difficult enterprise.

Euglycemic and hyperglycemic clamp techniques have been used to study the effects of antipsychotics on insulin and glucose response. In the euglycemic clamp technique, a steady level of hyperinsulinemia is produced via continuous insulin infusion. Glucose is also infused, and the amount of glucose needed to maintain a basal plasma glucose level provides an estimate of insulin resistance. This is considered the gold standard for the measurement of insulin sensitivity. The hyperglycemia clamp technique uses a continuous infusion of glucose to assess the sensitivity of the B-cell function. This technique is used to assess insulin release (Dagogo-Jack, 2003, pp. 3, 4).

20. Sharma (2003) reported a series of six patients with mood disorders who developed tardive dyskinesia (TD) following treatment with quetiapine. Three patients had a prior history of TD, but none of those had dyskinetic movements at baseline for at least two years.

Chapter 14

1. Adolescent obesity is rapidly becoming a national health problem; the prevalence of obesity increased from 5 to 11% from 1980 to 1994, and to 15.5% by 2000. This increase has been accompanied by a dramatic increase in type 2 diabetes and a host of related health complications (Berkowitz, Wadden, Tershakovec, & Cronquist, 2003, p. 1805). Obesity related diseases (diabetes, dyslipidemias, and their complications, heart and renal diseases) are the leading cause of death in the United States. Obesity, particularly excessive abdominal adipose tissue, is a leading risk factor in the development of type 2 diabetes in adults and in child and adolescent populations (Carlson, Sowell, & Cavaz-zoni, 2003, p. 5).

Obesity is associated with increased hepatic cholesterol synthesis, increased biliary cholesterol secretion, and gallbladder bile supersaturation with cholesterol. Curiously, risk of gallstone formation rises during weight loss in an exponential fashion (Amatruda & Linemeyer, 2001, pp. 955–956). Only 5 to 10% of obesity has an identifiable endogenous cause; 90% of the cases have an idiopathic etiology (see table 14.6, p. 441).

Guillaume and Lissau (2002) indicate that genetic factors explain 50 to 90% of the variation in BMI. Family studies generally report estimates of parent–offspring and sibling–sibling correlations in agreement with heritability of 20 to 80%. Adoption studies suggest genetic factors account for 20 to 60% of the variation in BMI (p. 39).

Obesity rises between 9 and 10 years, dips between 10 and 11 years, flats out between 11 and 13 years, and then rises steadily to 16 years at which point 20% of the children are obese (Mustillo et al., 2003, pp. 853–854). Obesity in adolescents is also associated with an increased risk of mortality and morbidity and, with the exception of diabetes the risk is independent of adult weight. (Amatruda & Linemeyer, 2001, p. 950)

The vicissitudes of obesity in children were studied in the Great Smoky Mountains Study (Mustillo et al., 2003). In this study, a cohort of 991 children, 9 to 16 years old, were followed for eight years. Four trajectories of adolescent obesity were described: 72.8% were never obese; 7.5 %, not obese at baseline, became obese at adolescence; 14.6% were chronically obese; 5.8% who were obese during late childhood lost weight during adolescence. Childhood and chronic obesity were associated with uneducated parents and lower income. Childhood and chronically obese children were more likely to suffer from depression and oppositional defiant disorder (mostly in boys). Between 16 and 24% of the children sampled were obese in at least one of the eight measurements, at any time during the study (p. 854). Boys had a higher prevalence of obesity among whites and Asians, but girls had a higher prevalence among Hispanics and Blacks (p. 856).

Leptin, a hormone produced by adipocytes, interacts with its hypothalamic receptor to regulate feeding through a leptin-melanocortin pathway in the hypothalamus. The average obese person has increased leptin secretion because of an increase of body mass, but the appetite is not reduced, suggesting a degree of resistance to leptin (Styne & Schoenfeld-Warren, 2003, pp. 2138–2139).

Insulin can act at the hypothalamus to enhance leptin-induced phosphorilation of the transcription factor STAT3. This finding seems to indicate that insulin and leptin join effects to decrease body weight, suggesting that these hormones act on common target neurons in the hypothalamus (Figlewicz, 2003, p. 84). Insulin given directly into the CNS can decrease the expression of neuropeptide Y—which stimulates a robust food intake when administered directly to the CNS (NPY)—which occurs in association with fasting or diabetes (p. 84).

In Westernized populations the endogenous adiposity signals are rendered ineffective by high fat diets (p. 85). Given the role of striatal DA (dopamine) in motivation and reward, it is hypothesized that one of insulin's actions in the CNS is to decrease the rewarding aspect of food (p. 86). As a matter of fact, insulin could blunt the ability of opiod peptides to enhance the intake of palatable food (p. 88).

Although type 2 diabetes has been relatively rare in children, current data suggest an epidemic increase of this disease in children and adolescents (Carlson et al., 2003, p. 6).

2. The BMI mortality rate is a U-shaped curve with increased mortality at a BMI < 23 and > 28 (Amatruda & Linemeyer, 2001, p. 949). For obese persons the mortality risks seem to be related to increased health risks associated with obesity: hypercholesterolemia, hypertension, left ventricular hypertrophy, and hyperglycemia. In the Framingham study, only 8% of males and 18% of females, in the highest weight percentile were free of health risks (p. 949).

Those with a BMI between the 85th and 95th percentile are considered a high risk for obesity. Obesity is defined as a BMI greater than the 95th percentile. Hispanics and African Americans have a higher BMI, and are more prone to obesity, and are at a higher risk for type 2 diabetes mellitus, than whites and Asian Americans. Adolescents with a BMI greater than the 95th percentile have a 50% risk of being obese in adulthood. Children with a BMI greater than the 85th percentile are considered worrisome, much more so if the patients have a personal or family history of hypertension or dyslipedimias (Styne & Schoenfeld-Warren, 2003, p. 2137).

There is a clear association between high BMIs and cancer. For persons with extreme obesity, with BMI of 40 or above, the death rates for cancer are higher than for persons of normal weight (for men 52% higher; for women 62% higher). For men and women, extreme obesity is associated with cancer of esophagus, colon and rectum, liver, gallbladder, pancreas, and kidney; the same is true for deaths due to non-Hodgkin lymphoma and multiple myeloma. There are trends of increased death risk for cancer of stomach and prostate in men, and for cancer of breast, uterus, cervix, and ovary in women. It is calculated that obesity accounts for 14% of all deaths from cancer in men and 20% of those in women (Calles, Rodriguez, Walker-Thurmond, & Thun, 2003). However, obesity is protective for osteoporosis.

The ratio of waist circumference to hip circumference is positively associated to all mortality causes in white women 55 to 69 years old. Obesity definitively decreases the life-span: if a person is obese at 40, this person has six years less of life; if the person is obese and a smoker, there will be 13 years less of life for males, and 14 years less for females.

3. Dieting increases metabolic efficiency, and over time, dieters need fewer calories to maintain weight. Metabolic efficiency would result in dieters gaining weight when consuming diets that previously were effective for maintaining weight. Furthermore,
   (a) Restrictive diets are seldom sustained for a long time. Restrictive dieting is frequently followed by bouts of overeating or binge eating.
   (b) Dieters consume diets with a high percentage of carbohydrates. There is a possible connection of glycemic index to weight gain. The authors gave more explanatory weight to the first two mechanisms.
4. What follows is a brief overview of the most common medications used as weight attenuating agents:

   Amantadine: This dopamine agonist may be useful in decreasing weight and BMI with continued use. Although this medication may not prevent the weight increase stimulated by the atypicals, it attenuates its increase. It is believed that amantadine improves the balance between fats and carbohydrates metabolized for energy production. Amantadine may also have a central component effect at the level of the appetite regulatory centers in the hypothalamus (Gracious, Krysiak, & Youngstrom, 2002, p. 255). A double-blind, placebo-controlled study of amantadine in adult patients receiving olanzapine demonstrated that amantadine was able to halt weight gain in some adults with olanzapine-induced weight gain That effect occurred early and reached a plateau at eight weeks. Amantadine has beneficial effects in weight stabilization, even after subjects have gaines substantial weight following months of olanzapine treatment (Graham, Gu, Lieberman, Harp, & Perkins, 2005, p. 1745). Amantadine does not improve insulin or lipid levels, however.

   Amantadine is reasonably safe, has relatively few interactions with other drugs—central nervous system stimulants, antihistamines—does not require laboratory monitoring, appears to have low abuse potential, has a slow onset of action, and is inexpensive. No deterioration of psychiatric symptoms occurred with the use of amantadine, and no worsening of psychosis or other major side effects has been documented (p. 1745). Of further interest is amantadine potential for reversing the neuroleptic induced hyperprolactinemia (Gracious, Krysiak, & Youngstrom, 2002, p. 250). It needs to be remembered that amantadine may increase the QTc interval. At doses above 200 mg/day, amantadine impairs memory and other neurocognitive functions. With some frequency, amantadine is very irritating to the upper GI.

   Dose: 100 mg BID for preadolescents and up to 200 mg BID for older preadolescents and adolescents may be effective; there is a liquid preparation dosed at 10 mg/ml for smaller children. For these, 50 mg BID may be tried. In the author's clinical experience, if the patient has not demonstrated weight attenuation or weight loss with amantadine in the 200 to 300 mg/day range it is unlikely that higher doses would be beneficial.

   Topiramate: This antiepileptic medication is thought to stimulate 5-HT2C receptors, suppressing the increased appetite induced by 5-HT2C antagonism (Nguyen, Yu, & Maguire, 2003, p. 62). Topiramate is thought to act through voltage-specific sodium channel activity or by antagonizing glutamate/kainite/AMPA (alpha-amino-3-hydroxy-5-methyl-4-isoxazolepropionic acid) receptors. It also increases the activation of GABA A (gamma aminobutyric acid-type A) receptors, enhancing chloride ion flow into the neuron (Pavulari, Janicak, & Carbray, 2002, p. 272).

   Topiramate may have an additional positive effect: it may be a useful adjunctive treatment in diabetic patients and its effects may not be solely related to weight loss. This effect may be the result of alteration of regulation of insulin sensitivity (Ryback, Brodsky, & Littman, 2005, p. 57). Eight patients (seven with type 2, one with type 1 diabetes) received treatment with topiramate for weight attenuating effects. Seven patients had been identified as diabetic prior to treatment. For all the eight patients the blood glucose either normalized or decreased near normal levels within a few months of initiating topiramate treatment, and for all the type 2 patients there was a gradual weight loss; the type 1 patient, who was not overweight prior to topiramate treatment, underwent a normalization of the glucose level at the five months of treatment even though his weight remained stable (p. 60). See Note 4. In one study, topiramate enhanced phosphatidylinositol 3(p1-3)-kinase and its downstream effector Akt/PKB kinase, a signal transduction pathway involved in the regulation of insulin sensitivity (Ryback et al., 2005, p. 60).

Topiramate mood stabilizing effects are in question; however, this medication is sometimes effective in promoting weight reduction. Induction of this medication must be slow due to the risk of language disturbances and other neuropsychological impairments. The physician needs to alert the patient and family of the risk of nephrolithiasis, acute glaucoma, and hyperchloremic acidosis, a very serious, potentially fatal side effect.

The most recent warnings about this medication relate to oligohydrosis (decreased sweating) and hyperthermia, particularly in children. These reactions are more common in hot weather. Caution is advised when topiramate is coprescribed with other drugs that predispose patients to heat related disorders, such as, carbonic anhydrase inhibitors and drugs with anticholinergic activity. Topiramate may be associated with more cognitive impairment than some of the new antiepileptic drugs, gabapentin and lamotrigene (McElroy & Keck, 2004, p. 633).

Topiramate is also helpful in the treatment of binge eating disorder associated with obesity. Patients on topiramate showed greater rate of reduction of binge frequency, binge day frequency, BMI, weight, CGI severity scale, and YBOCS, compared with placebo (McElroy, Arnold, et al., 2003, p. 258).

Dose: Slow induction, 12.5 to 25 mg BID; dose may be increased on a weekly basis by 12.5 to 25 mg with close monitoring of the cognitive and language functions. In the author's clinical experience, if the patient does not show weight attenuation or weight decrease at doses of 100 mg BID, it is unlikely that higher doses will produce a positive weight decrease.

Interactions between topiramate and metformin have been observed in normal volunteers. Plasma clearance of topiramate may be decreased with the concomitant use of metformin. Closer monitoring of glucose control is recommended if topiramate is added or withdrawn (Gracious & Meyer, 2005, p. 40). There is limited research data regarding Topiramate use for weight reduction in children and adolescents.

Venlafaxine: This antidepressant boosts serotonin and norepinephrine at the receptor sites; up to 43% of adult patients on venlafaxine showed 5% or more of weight reduction, and up to 88% of adult patients reported 50% or better reduction of bingeing. Venlafaxine was well tolerated; dry mouth, sexual dysfunction, insomnia, and nausea were the most frequently reported side effects. In six adult patients (17%) there was a sustained increase in blood pressure that was considered of no clinical significance. No patients discontinued the medication because of side effects. Mean velafaxine dose was 222 ± 63 mg with a range between 75 to 300 mg (Malhotra, King, Welge, Brusman-Lovins, & McElroy, 2002, p. 802). Of course, psychiatrists prescribing antidepressants in children will remember the Black Box warning regarding increase of suicide ideation, as well as of an eventual provocation of mania by medications of this class.

   Initial dose: 25 to 50 mg BID; if the child is an early adolescent, Effexor XR 75 mg/ could be a safe starting dose. Effective dose range, between 150 and 200 mg/day or Effexor XR, 75 to 150 mg/day.

Phentermine and Sibutramine: These appetite suppressant agents possess a potent inhibitory effect at the presynaptic norepinephrine transporter. This is the ascribed mechanism for appetite suppression. Sibutramine suppresses appetite by a combined norepinephrine and 5-HT reuptake inhibition, increasing both monoamines in the hypothalamus (p. 300).

   Sibutramine has been approved for chronic use since 1998. It is particularly indicated in patients who have lost weight through diet and exercise and need weight maintenance. Sibutramine can be used in patients with a BMI equal or greater that 30 or a BMI equal or greater than 27 in the presence of other heath risks (hypertension, dyslipidemia, diabetes, etc.). In some patients sibutramine raises blood pressure, but there does not seem to be any increase in valvular disease (Amatruda & Linemeyer, 2001, p. 977).

   Note: patients on neuroleptics, antidepressants, and lithium have an increased risk of serotonin syndrome if they take sibutramine (Gelenberg, 2004, p. 3; see "Serotonin Syndrome," chapter 13.

   Starting dose: 5 mg q/day to 5 mg BID. Doses above 20 mg/day are not recommended.

Nizatidine: This medication, a selective histamine (H2) receptor antagonist, is effective in reducing olanzapine-related weight gain at a dose of 300 mg BID (Nguyen, Yu, & Maguire, 2003, p. 62).

   Atmaca, Kuloglu, Tescan, and Gecici (2003) reported on the use of nizatidine for weight gain induced by olanzapine in 59 adult schizophrenics. Out of 59 schizophrenic patients receiving open label olanzapine (5 to 25 mg/day) for three months, 35 gained 2 to 5 kg (5.6 lb). These patients were randomized to a double-blind trial of nizatidine (150 mg BID) and placebo for eight weeks. Patients on nizatidine lost $4.5 \pm$ kg (10 ± 4.9 lb, $p < 0.05$). Patients taking placebo gained $2.3 \pm .9$ kg (5.1 ± 2.0 lb). Serum leptin levels climbed in all patients who gained weight; the nizatidine group showed a decrease in the leptin levels, while the patients on placebo displayed leptin increase. Extrapyramidal symptoms associated with nizatidine use have been reported (see below).

   Dosing: Starting dose 50 mg/day; maximal recommended dose: 150 mg BID.

   Lam (2004) described the case of a 16-year-old female adolescent with a history of paranoid schizophrenia, which had been treated with quetiapine (300 mg/day) and paroxetine (dose unknown). This patient's BMI had increased from 21.7 at baseline to 30 in nine months, necessitating a weight-attenuating agent (nizatidine). The patient developed akathisia and Parkinsonism (with no dystonia or tardive dyskinesia) when the dose of nizatidine was increased from 150 mg/day to 300 mg/day. These symptoms remitted when the nizatidine dose was reduced to the previous 150 mg/day. Lam speculates that the higher doses of nizatidine probably induced a metabolic inhibition of CYP3A4 and CYP2D6 cytochromes. However, nizatidine by itself does not cause involuntary movements and at doses of 150 mg BID is not expected to have a significant inhibition of the cited cytochromes (pp. 2–3).

Ginsberg (2005a) reported on a case of extrapyramidal symptoms associated with nizatidine. A 16-year-old female with a one-year history of paranoid schizophrenia, had an initial weight 141.9 lb and a BMI of 21.7. The physical examination had been unremarkable, and there was no baseline EPS. She received progressive doses of quetiapine up to 300 mg BID. Nine months later, her weight had increased to 196.5 lb and the BMI to 30. The patient appeared depressed and had an increase in appetite. Paroxetine 20 mg was added and three months later, she looked better, although her weight had not changed. Nizatidine 150 mg BID was initiated. Four weeks later, there had been a substantial decrease of weight: 174.9 lb, and the BMI was 26.7. Nizatidine was further increased to 300 mg BID. Four days later, akathisia, bradykinesia, tremor, and rigidity were evident, consistent with EPS. When the nizatidine was decreased to 150 mg BID the EPS resolved. Three months later, the patient's weight was 158.4 lb and the BMI was 24.2, and there was no evidence of EPS. The temporal sequence of clinical events is consistent with nizatidine EPS induced (pp. 19–20).

Metformin: This biguanide agent has become the first-line medication for the management of type 2 diabetes. Its primary function is to decrease the hepatic production of glucose; it also lowers insulin resistance in muscle and fat. Metformine lowers hyperlipedemia and induces a modest weight reduction. Metformine use is contraindicated in patients with renal or hepatic failure, and in patients with metabolic acidosis. Metformine must be discontinued in any acute disorder in which renal clearance may be compromised (including major surgery, severe infection, or use of intravenous iodinated contrast media). Therapy should be started at a low dose and titrated slowly to therapeutic levels (Gitelman, 2003, p. 2136). Doses of 1000 to 1500 mg/day are common, that is, 500 mg BID or 500 mg TID, or alternative dose schedules.

Metformin may cause elevation of liver functions, lactic acidosis, and diarrhea (Gracious & Meyer, 2005, p. 40).

Morrison, Cottingham, and Barton (2002), reported on the use of metformin (500 mg TID) in 19 pediatric patients (age 10 to 18) who had gained more than 10% weight (children had gained from 6 to 59 kg) from baseline after being treated with atypicals (olanzapine, risperidone, quetiapine) or valproate. Subjects were instructed not to alter their diet or level of activity; 15 patients lost weight (mean ± 2.93 kg, and also experienced a decrease in BMI (mean – 2.2 kg/m2).

Zonisamide: This sulfonamide antiepileptic medication is not related to other agents of its kind. Zonisamide is indicated as an adjunctive therapy in partial seizure in adults with epilepsy. Zonisamide has been reported to decrease appetite and to induce some weight loss. Anorexia is reported in 13% of patients vs. 6% of those on placebo.

Zonisamide is being proposed as an alternative medication for the treatment of binge eating disorder. Zonisamide is a synthetic 1, 2 benzisoxazole derivative anticonvulsant, FDA approved for the treatment of partial seizures in adults. Structurally it is similar to serotonin; its complex mechanism of action includes,

blockade of voltage-sensitive sodium and T-type calcium channels, accelerated release of gama-aminobutyric acid, inhibition of lipid peroxidation, and increased free
radical scavenging. It also has biphasic effects on dopamine with therapeutic doses
enhancing and subtherapeutic doses inhibiting dopamine function. Zonisamide is
also a weak anhydrase inhibitor (Ginsberg, 2004a, p. 14).

Ginsberg (2004a) reported on an open-label, prospective, 12-week trial of
zonisamide in 14 patients with DSM-IV-TR diagnosis of binge eating disorder.
After a week of medication-free evaluation, zonisamide was initiated at a dose of 100
mg/day, and medication was increased weekly to a maximum dose of 600 mg/day.
Dose could be adjusted and decreased as low as 100 mg/day if necessary due to
side effects. Binge eating behavior was the primary outcome measure; secondary
measures included, binge day frequency, BMI, weight, CGI-S, YBOCS-BE, Three
Factor Eating Questionnaire (TFEQ), and the Hamilton Rating Scale for Depression
(p. 15).

Eight subjects (53.3%) completed the 12-week study. Of the eight completers,
seven achieved total remission; the other subject achieved a marked reduction (75
to 99%) of binge-eating frequency. The completers lost 8.2 kg (18.1 lb) by the end
of the 12 weeks. There was also significant reduction in BMI, CGI-S, YBOCS-BE,
and TFEQ scores. At endpoint, the mean daily dose of zonisamide was 513 mg/day
and the mean plasma level was 32 mcg/ml (N = 10–40 mcg/ml). The most common
side effects were fatigue (47%), altered taste (47%), dry mouth (47%), cognitive impairment (40%), insomnia (33%), nausea (33%), drowsiness (33%), and dyspepsia
(33%). Seven patients discontinued the trial (Idem).

The 2006 PDR has the following warning for this medication: "Potentially Fatal
Reactions to Sulfonamides: Fatalities have occurred, although rarely, as a result
of severe reactions to sulfonamides (zonisamide is a sulfonamide) including Steven-Johnson syndrome, toxic epidermal necrolysis, fulminating hepatic necrosis,
agranulocytocis, aplastic anemia, and other blood dyscrasias. Such reactions may
occur when a sulfonamide is readministered irrespective of the route of administration. If signs of hypersensitivity or other serious reactions occur, discontinue
zonisamide immediately" (p. 1090).

The 2006 PDR describes the following side effect reactions for zonisamide:

Serious skin reactions. Deaths associated with Steven-Johnson syndrome and
toxic epidermal necrolysis have occurred.

Serious hematological events. Isolated cases of aplastic anemia and agranulocytocis have been reported. Oligohidrosis and hyperthermia in pediatric patients
may occur. Seizures on withdrawal of zonisamide may occur. Teratogenicity with
zonisamide may occur.

Cognitive and neuropsychiatric adverse events. A variety of cognitive and neuropsychiatric side effects are listed (see p. 1090).

Ziprasidone and Aripiprazole: For obese children and adolescents with psychosis there
are promising psychopharmacological options: ziprasidone and maybe aripiprazole,
for the limited effect on weight; a number of psychotic preadolescents have complained of severe loss of appetite when they have been treated with aripiprazole.

Modafanil: Modafanil is an FDA approved wakefulness-promoting agent; it promotes
wakefulness in patients with excessive sleepiness (ES) associated with narcolepsy,
obstructive sleep apnea-hypopnea syndrome (OSAHS), and shift work sleep dis-

order (SWSD). Modafinil does not affect quality or quantity of sleep (e.g., sleep architecture, sleep duration) as measured by polysomnography.

In recent phase III trials, modafinil demonstrated efficacy for ADHD. The average dose range was between 340 mg and 425 mg/day. It is believed that this medication stimulates the anterior cingulated cortex (Kelly, 2005, p. 20).

During clinical trials, the most common adverse events were headache, nausea, nervousness, rhinitis, diarrhea, back pain, anxiety, insomnia, dizziness, and dyspepsia. In six double-blind, parallel group, placebo-controlled studies, there was no clinically significant difference in body weight change in patients treated with modafanil. However, there was an incidence of "anorexia" of 4% in patients treated with modafanil against 1% in placebo-treated patients. Weight gain was reported in 1% of patients treated with modafanil. The manufacturer states that modafanil is not indicated as an anorectic agent (Cephalon, Provigil Product Summary). Various aspects of subjects' eating behaviors were evaluated in a three-way crossover design for five hours after receiving modafanil, d-amphetamine, or placebo. The result of the study demonstrated decreases in total caloric intake in subjects receiving moderate doses of modafanil and a high dose of d-amphetamine, compared with placebo. Frequency of eating was not altered. All subjects remained within ± 2 kg of their baseline weight.

Although this product has a broad range of potentially beneficial effects (narcolepsy, antidepressant adjuvant, cognitive enhancer, ADHD, social phobia, to decrease the sense of anergy, and others) there are incipient reports of the abusive use of this medication (Kutcher, 2004, p. 10). Physicians should be on the alert.

Naltrexone: Eight women who had gained more than 6 kg on TCAs and lithium treatment received naltrexone 50 mg/day. Weight gain was reversed in five women, stopped in two, and was attenuated in one patient. All patients reported dramatic decrease of food craving; transient side effects included nausea, fatigue, and an altered state (Gracious & Meyer, 2005, pp. 40–41).

Lamotrigene: The 2006 PDR has a Black Box for this medication. The black box relates to potentially fatal skin rashes (Steven Johnson's Syndrome and Toxic Epidermal Necrolysis) (p. 1449). Lamotrigene may cause anorexia (Idem, p. 1454).

5. The following medications are frequently use as coadjuvant medications for the treatment of obesity.

Amphetamines: These drugs have consistently been demonstrated to be better than placebo in promoting weight loss; amphetaminelike drugs lead to a weight loss of at least 1 lb/week in 44% of patients on active drug vs. 26% on placebo (Amatruda & Linemeyer, 2001, pp. 976–977). In the long run, the weight reducing effect of these medications decreases, tolerance develops, and the risk of dependency is increased.

Phentermine: This medication is an amphetaminelike drug with a low addictive potential; it is effective in inducing weight loss: 10 kg at the end of 24 weeks vs. 4.4 kg loss for those in placebo.

Fenfluramine: This drug stimulates serotonin release and prevents its reuptake, induced a 7.5 kg loss at the end of 24 weeks. Combination of phentermine (half a regular dose in the mornings), and fenfluramine at night (to take advantage of its sedative effects) produced a loss of 8.5 kg at the end of the study. Side effects were better on the combination of medications than either with phentermine or fenfluramine alone (p. 977).

Dexfenfluramine: This drug's effects at the end of one year (9.82 kg loss) were not considerably superior to placebo (7.15 kg). In spite of the weight reducing effects, dexfenfluramine and fenfluramine were withdrawn from the market in 1997 due to the occurrence of pulmonary hypertension and heart valve abnormalities similar to those seen in patients with carcinoid syndrome (Amatruda & Linemeyer, 2001, p. 977).

Sibutramine: It is postulated that sibutramine, an H2 blocker, decreases weight by an increasing cholecystokinin, a peptide associated with appetite regulation (Gracious & Meyer, 2005, p. 40). Sibutramine was approved for chronic use and has been available since 1998. This drug is a norepinephrine and a serotonin reuptake inhibitor. Patients on placebo, 5 mg and 10 mg of sibutramine, lost at the end of one year: 3.5, 9.8, and 14 lb respectively. For patients who completed the year of study, the weight loss was somewhat higher. Patients who lost at least 6 kg of weight over four weeks, on a very low caloric diet (VLCD), were treated for a year with 10 mg of sibutramine or placebo; these patients lost 28.4 and 15.2 lb, respectively. For patients who completed the study, the weight loss was of 29.7 lb for sibutramine and 16.7 lb for placebo.

Sibutramine may be especially helpful for patients who have lost weight to maintain the weight loss. This drug may be used in the presence dyslipidemia and diabetes. In studies with mean duration of 7.6 months, there have not been excess occurrences of cardiac valvular disease; however, since this drug tends to increase blood pressure in certain patients, blood pressure needs to be monitored regularly. Sibutramine should not be use in cases of uncontrolled hypertension (Amatruda & Linemeyer, 2001, p. 977). Eighty-two adolescents were randomized to receive behavioral therapy and placebo, and behavioral therapy and sibutramine for six months (phase 1); adolescents had a BMI range between 32 and 44. Both groups received the same standardized family based behavioral weight loss program for the first six months. In the open phase (phase 2, from the 7th to the 12th month) of the program, the sessions were held biweekly during first three months; sessions were monthly during the last three months. Adolescents were instructed to consume 1200 to 1500 K/cal diet of conventional foods with approximately 30% from fat, 15% from protein, and the rest from carbohydrates. Patients were expected to engage in exercise activities for up to 120 minutes per week—walking or similar aerobic activities. The participants kept a daily eating and activity log. All the patients received placebo during the first week. Patients on sibutramine received 5 mg at the second week; dose was increased to 10 mg at the third week, and to 15 mg at the seventh week (Berkowitz et al., 2003, p. 1806). Adolescents receiving behavioral therapy and sibutramine lost a mean (SD) of 7.8 Kg (6.3 kg) equal to 8.5% (6.8%) reduction of the initial BMI. In contrast, adolescents receiving BT and placebo lost 3.2 kg (6.1 lb) equal to a significantly smaller 4.0% (5.4%) reduction in the initial BMI (effect size 0.73; 95% confidence interval (CI), 0.28–1.18; $P = .001$). More than twice as many adolescents treated with sibutramine plus BT reduced their initial BMI by 10% ($P = .02$) and 15% ($P = .02$) compared with those treated with BT and placebo (pp. 1807–1808).

In phase 2 (open label sibutramine treatment), participants who had been on placebo before lost an additional 1.3 kg when they started receiving sibutramine; this represented an additional 2.4% reduction in the initial BMI; in contrast, adolescents who had been on sibutramine and continued on it, gained 0.8 kg (10.5 kg) representing a 0.2% (5.4%) of the baseline BMI (p. 1808). In summary, from baseline to month 12, participants receiving BT and sibutramine throughout lost a total of 9.3 kg equal to an 8.6% (9.9%) reduction in the initial BMI; those initially on BT and placebo but switched to BT plus sibutramine from months 7 to 12, lost 4.5 kg (8.8 kg) equal to 6.4% (8.3%) reduction in the initial BMI. There was no significant difference between the groups at month 12 (p. 1808).

During the 12 months of the study, sibutramine was reduced to 10 mg in 16 adolescents, to 5 mg in seven additional ones, and was discontinued in 10 participants (six for increase of BP and/or pulse, two for echymoses, one for premature ventricular contractions [PVCs], and one because of an unspecific rash) (p. 1810). The authors state that weight-loss medications should be used only on an experimental basis in adolescents. Sibutramine is contraindicated for concomitant use with SSRIs because of the risk of serotonin syndrome (Gracious & Meyer, 2005, p. 39). Sibutramine also may inhibit betacarotene and vitamin E absorption (Idem).

Orlistat is an inhibitor of gastric and pancreatic lipases with antiobesity and antilipemic activities. Its pharmachological effect is the reduction of dietary fat. It is primarily used as an adjunct agent to dietary restriction in the management of obesity. Up to a 30% fat reduction has been reported with the use 120 mg TID of this medication. There is minimal change in plasma concentration of several psychotropic agents including clozapine, haloperidol, desipramine, clomipramine, and carbamazepine (Lam, 2003, p. 2). Orlistat (Xenical) decreases the absorption of vitamins A, D, K, acetretin, calcifediol, calcitriol, dihydrotachysterol, doxercalciferol, ergocalciferol, isotretinoin, tretinoin, and betacarotene. These vitamins need to be supplemented.

The difference of weight loss between 1-year treatment of Orlistat 120 mg TID and placebo was 8.6 lb. After two years the difference was 5.3 lb. GI side effects are very common: fatty or oily stools, increased defecation (fecal urgency), oily spotting, flatus with discharge, oily evacuations, and even fecal incontinence (11.8%). In another study, 35.2% of the patients on 120 mg TID regained the loss weight during the second year whereas 51.3% of those on 60 mg TID regained the loss weight during the same period of time. To deal with the embarrassing steatorrhea related to Orlistat, a low fat intake is recommended (Amatruda & Linemeyer, 2001, pp. 977–978). Xenical is indicated in patients with a BMI of 28 and medical complications or a BMI of 30 without medical complications (Gracious & Meyer, 2005, p. 39).

Lam (2003) suggests that orlistat interferes with the INR. This is due to the medication creating a reduction of the level of fat soluble vitamins such as vitamin K. This interferes with the pharmacological effect of warfarin, resulting in a loss of its efficacy. The patients on Orlistat and warfarin require a very close monitoring of the INR and a supplementation of fat soluble vitamins is advised (p. 3).

B3 Agonists: These drugs stimulate thermogenesis in brown adipose tissue and in muscle. A product labeled BRL 26830A reduces weight without any significant systemic side effects, except for tremor. This product also increased energy expenditure two hours after ingestion without altering the resting metabolic rate (Amatruda & Linemeyer, 2001, p. 977).

Rimonabant: Phase III human trials of rimonabant, a selective cannabinoid-1 receptor

(CB1) blocker, are ongoing for obesity and for smoking cessation. In uncontrolled studies, rimonabant has been shown to help people avoid weight gain while quitting smoking. It is expected that this product will reach the market by mid-2006 (Higgins, 2004, p. 74). A publication by Despres, Golay, Sjostrom, et al. (2005) of a randomized trial of rimonabant in adults, demonstrated that the proportion of patients who had a weight loss equal or greater than 5% was 19.5% in the placebo group and 58.4% in the group receiving 20 mg of rimonabant ($p < 0.001$); the proportion of those who had a weight loss equal to or greater than 10% was 7.2% for those in the placebo group, and 32.6% for the rimonabant group ($p < 0.001$) (p. 2126). Patients on rimonabant had also the greatest reduction in waist circumference in relation to the other groups. Rimonabant 20 mg/day produced a more significant improvement of a number of metabolic factors: a greater reduction of triglycerides than the other groups, had the highest increase in HDL cholesterol levels and greatest reduction of total cholesterol; furthermore, patients on rimonabant 20 mg showed favorable changes in LDL particle size, adiponectin levels, glucose tolerance, fasting and postchallenge insulin levels, and plasma C-reactive protein (p. 2132). Whereas at baseline 54% of the patients met criteria for metabolic syndrome, this number dropped to 25.5%, compared to 40.0% and 41% of patients receiving rimonabant 5 mg and placebo, respectively ($p < 0.001$) (p. 2118).

Zonisamide: See Note 4.

6. Psychogenic nonepileptic seizures (PNES) could be differentiated from true seizures in the clinical presentation. PNES have a variable duration, pattern, and frequency; the cause is emotional, and commonly occurs in the presence of others; it rarely elicits incontinence, and rarely occurs during sleep. The convulsion promotes bizarre, trashing pelvic thrust, sexual movements, and rarely causes injuries. The biting involves the tip of the tongue or the lips. Pupillary reflexes are normal and plantar reflex is normal. Patients are oriented after the episode, there is no postictal stupor, and the serum prolactin and EEG are normal.

   The true epileptic seizures have a short duration (20–70 seconds), the pattern is stereotyped, paroxysmal, and may occur in clusters. The cause is organic and may occur in the absence of other people. Seizures occur during sleep and cause incontinence, and biting of the sides of tongue and cheek; the convulsion is tonic-clonic and the injuries may be serious. Pupillary reflexes may be slow or nonreactive, and after the convulsion Babinski is present; there is postictal confusion as well as postictal stupor. Serum prolactin is elevated, and the EEG is abnormal or variable (Adetunji, Mattews, Williams, & Verna, 2004, p. 28).

7. These patients were identified from three controlled multicenter clinical trials that investigated the efficacy and safety of olanzapine (2.5–20 mg/day, double-blind) trial of schizophrenia for up to 52 weeks. Presumptive TD was defined as a severity rating of moderate (≥ 3) in at least one of seven body regions assessed with the Abnormal Involuntary Movement scale (AIMS) at two consecutive drug-free baseline visits (2–9 days apart). Patients were rated weekly for the initial six weeks of olanzapine treatment and then every two to eight weeks thereafter, depending on the study. Analysis included patients treated up to 30 weeks. Mean change from baseline AIMS Total scores (items 1–7) was determined in each visit. Results: The baseline (week 0) mean AIMS Total was 10.55. The mean change from baseline AIMS Total was significantly reduced by week 1 and

remained significantly lower at all subsequent assessments ($p < 0.05$ for all weeks, signed rank test). Mean reduction of 55 and 71% were noted at weeks 6 and 30, respectively.

8. Forty-nine DSM-IV schizophrenic patients were enrolled in the study. After a four-week washout period subjects were randomly assigned to either risperidone or placebo. Risperidone dose was initiated at 2 mg/day and was increased gradually to 6 mg/day over six weeks. The 6 mg/day risperidone dose was maintained for the rest of the study. Subjects were evaluated every two weeks with the AIMS and Extrapyramidal Symptom Rating scale. The final mental status was assessed with the BPRS.

   Results: 22 patients in the risperidone group and 20 patients in the placebo group completed the study. The baseline AIMS for all the patients was 15.9 =/– 4.6. At the end of study, AIMS scores had decreased 1.1 ± 4.8 for the placebo group and 5.5 ± 3.8 for the risperidone group ($p < .05$). Fifteen subjects (68%) in the risperidone group and six subjects (30%) in the placebo group were responders ($p < .05$). The risperidone responders had a mean AIMS scored decrease of 7.5 ± 2.1. Among the risperidone group, tardive dyskinesia improvement was noted from the eighth week and was mostly demonstrated in the bucco-lingual-masticatory (BLM) area rather than in the choreathetoid movement in the extremities (pp. 1343–1345).

9. The patient was a 41-year-old female with the diagnosis of schizoaffective disorder who had a severe TD syndrome and who had not responded to other atypicals. The TD had been diagnosed two years before while she was being treated with haloperidol. She received a sequential treatment with risperidone (discontinued for hyperprolactinemia), olanzapine (discontinued for weight increase), ziprasidone (discontinued for EKG changes), and had also received quetiapine. Of interest, quetiapine aggravated the TD.

   The patient had an AIMS score of 12. She received an initial dose of 15 mg of aripiprazole that was increased to 30 mg after two weeks. After 48 hours of initiating aripiprazole there was a dramatic improvement of the TD; the psychotic symptoms had shown only moderate change. After 1 month of treatment with aripiprazole the AIMS score was 2, in spite that the antipsychotic treatment had been augmented with chlorpromazine 100 mg TID.

10. The following psychosocial interventions are being used for rehabilitation of cognitively compromised schizophrenics:

    Neuropsychological educational approach to rehabilitation (NEAR) teaches techniques to promote intrinsic motivation and task engagement; NEAR uses group therapy and computer technology.

    Integrated psychological therapy (ITP) addresses cognitive deficits and social skills.

    Cognitive remediation therapy (CRT) focuses on the development of problem solving strategies.

    Neurocognitive enhancement therapy (NET) aims at improving cognitive and vocational outcomes by a repeated practice of increasingly complex computerized cognitive tasks.

    Other approaches like *Errorless learning* to improve performance at an entry-level job training task, relative to conventional training, and *adaptive strategies*, used in the rehabilitation of persons with head injuries or mental retardation, are aimed to bypass cognitive deficits by establishing support or prostheses in the living environment to improve functioning, were also reviewed.

References

Addington, J. (2004, August). The diagnosis and assessment of individuals prodromal for schizophrenic psychosis. *CNS Spectrums, 9*, 588–594.

Adetunji, B., Mathews, M., Williams, A., & Verma, S. (2004, November). Psychogenic or epileptic seizures? How to clinch the diagnosis. *Current Psychiatry, 3*, 25–35.

Adler, C. M., & Strakowski, S. M. (2003). Boundaries of schizophrenia. *Psychiatric Clinics of North America, 26*, 1–23.

Adler, C. M., Adams, J., DelBello, M. P., Holland, S. K., Schmithorst, V., Levine, A., et al. (2006, February). Evidence of white matter pathology in bipolar disorder adolescents experiencing their first episode of mania: A diffusion tensor imaging study. *American Journal of Psychiatry, 163*, 322–324.

Aina, Y., Nandagopol, J., & Nasrallah, H. A. (2004). Endocrine disorders in schizophrenia: Relationship to antipsychotic therapy. *Current Psychosis & Therapeutic Reports 2*, 78–83.

Akiskal, H. S. (2005, December). (Commentary). The nature of preschool mania. *The Journal of Bipolar Disorders, 4*, 17.

Akiskal, H. S., & Puzantian, V. R. (1979). Psychotic forms of depression and mania. *Psychiatric Clinics of North America, 2*, 419–439.

Alfaro, C. L., Wudarsky, M., Nicolson, R., Gochman, P., Sporn, A., Lenane, M., et al. (2002). Correlation of antipsychotic and prolactin concentrations in children and adolescents acutely treated with haloperidol, clozapine or olanzapine. *Journal of Child and Adolescent Psychopharmacology, 12*, 83–91.

Allen, M. H., Currier, G. W., Hughes, D. H., Docherty, J. P., Carpenter, D., & Ross, R. (2003). Treatment of behavioral emergencies: A summary of the expert consensus guidelines. *Journal of Psychiatric Practice, 9*, 16–38.

Allen, M. H., Hirschfeld, R. M., Wozniak, P. J., Baker, J. D., & Bowden, C. L. (2006, February). Linear relationship of valproate serum concentration to response and optimal serum levels for acute mania. *American Journal of Psychiatry, 163*, 272–275.

Altman H., Collins, M., & Mundy, P. (1997). Subclinical hallucinations and delusions in nonpsychotic adolescents. *Journal of Child Psychology and Psychiatry 38*, 413–420.

Altshuler, L., Bookheimer, S., Proenza, M. A. Townsend, J., Sabb, F., Firestine, A., et al. (2005). Increased amygdala activation during mania: A functional magnetic resonance imaging study. *American Journal of Psychiatry, 162*, 1211–1213.

Altshuler, L. L., Suppes, T., Black, D. O., Nolen, W. A., Leverich, G., Keck, P. E., et al. (2006, February). Lower switch rate in depressed patients with bipolar II than bipolar I disorder treated adjunctively with second-generation antidepressants. *American Journal of Psychiatry, 163,* 313–315.

Aman, M. G., De Smedt, G., Derivan, A., Lyons, B., Findling, R. L., & The Risperidone Disruptive Behavior Study Group. (2002). Double-blind placebo controlled study of risperidone for the treatment of disruptive disorders in children with subaverage intelligence. *American Journal of Psychiatry, 159,* 1337–1346.

Amatruda, J. M., & Linemeyer, D. L. (2001). Obesity. In P. Felig & L. A. Frohman (Eds.), *Endocrinology and metabolism* (4th ed., pp. 945–991). New York: McGraw-Hill.

American Journal of Psychiatry. (2004, February). Practice guidelines for the treatment of patients with schizophrenia (2nd ed.). *American Journal of Psychiatry, 161*(Suppl.), 1–56.

American Psychiatric Association. (2000). *The diagnostic and statistical manual of mental disorders* (4th ed, text rev.) Washington, DC: Author.

Amminger, G. P., McGorry, P. D., & Leicester, S. (2002). Treatment of adolescents and young adults experiencing attenuated psychotic symptoms. *Child and Adolescent Psychopharmacology News, 7,* 1–5.

Arvanitis, L. A., & Rak, I. W. (1997). (Abstract). Long-term efficacy and safety of Seroquel (quetiapine). *Schizophrenia Research, 24,* 196–197.

Asarnow, J. R., & Tompson, M. C. (1999). Childhood-onset schizophrenia: A follow up study. *European Child & Adolescent Psychiatry, 8*(Suppl. 1), 9–12.

Asarnow, J. R., Tompson, M. C., & Goldstein, M. J. (1994). Outcome of childhood-onset schizophrenia-spectrum disorders. *Schizophrenia Bulletin, 20,* 599–617.

Asarnow, J. R., & Asarnow, R. F. (2003). Childhood onset schizophrenia, In E. N. Mash & R. A. Barkley (Eds.), *Child psychopathology* (2nd ed.). New York: Guildford.

Asarnow, J. R., Tompson, M. C., & McGrath, E. P. (2004). Annotation: Childhood-onset schizophrenia: Clinical and treatment issues. *Journal of Child Psychology and Psychiatry, 45,* 180–194.

Asghar-Ali, A. A., Taber, K. H., Hurley, R. A., & Hayman, L. A. (2004). Pure neuropsychiatric presentation of multiple sclerosis. *American Journal of Psychiatry 161,* 226–231.

Atmaca, M., Kuloglu, M., Tescan, E., & Gecici, O. (2002). Quetiapine augmentation in patients with treatment resistant obsessive-compulsive disorder: A single-blind, placebo controlled study. *International Clinical Psychopharmacology, 17,* 115–119.

Ayd, F. J. (2000). *Lexicon of psychiatry, neurology and the neurosciences* (2nd ed.). Philadelphia: Lippincott Williams & Wilkins.

Bachmann, R. F., Schloesser, R. J., Gould, T. D., & Manji, H. K. (2005, November). Molecular and cellular neurobiologic studies identify novel targets for the long-term actions of mood stabilizers. *Clinical Approaches in Bipolar Disorders, 4,* 46–55.

Bachmann, S., Bottmer, C., & Schröder, J. (2005, December). Neurological soft signs in first-episode schizophrenia: A follow-up study. *American Journal of Psychiatry, 162,* 2337–2343.

Badner, J. A. (2003). The genetics of bipolar disorder. In M. P. DelBello & B. Geller (Eds.), *Bipolar disorder in childhood and early adolescence* (pp. 247–254). New York: Guilford.

Ball, M. P., Coons, V. B., & Buchanan, R. W. (2001, July). A program for treating olanzapine-related weight gain. *Psychiatric Services, 52,* 967–969.

Basil, B., Mathews, M., Sudak, D., & Adetunji, B. (2005, September). The concept of insight in mental illness. *Primary Psychiatry, 12,* 58–61.

Bassett, A. S., Chow, E. W. C., Abdel Malik, P., Gheorghiu, M., Husted, J., & Weksberg, R.

(2003). The schizophrenia phenotype in 22q11 deletion syndrome. *American Journal of Psychiatry, 160,* 1580–1586.

Bearden, C. E., Jawad, A. F., Lynch, D. R., Sokol, S., Kanes, S. J., McDonald-McGinn, D. M., et al. (2004). Effects of a functional COMT polymorphism on prefrontal cognitive function in patients with 22q11.2 deletion syndrome. *American Journal of Psychiatry, 161,* 1700–1702.

Bebadis, S. R., & Wilner, A. N. (2005, December). Pediatric epilepsy: Diagnostic and treatment considerations. *CNS News* (Special ed.), *7,* 85–89.

Bender, K. J. (2005, March). PORT updates schizophrenia treatment recommendations. *Psychiatric Times,* XXII, 36.

Beng-Choon, H., Alicata, D., Mola, C., & Andreasen, N. C. (2005). Hippocampus volume and treatment delays in first-episode schizophrenia. *American Journal of Psychiatry, 162,* 1527–1529.

Benjamin, E., & Salek, S. (2005). Stimulant-atypical antipsychotic interaction and acute dystonia. *Journal of the American Academy of Child and Adolescent Psychiatry, 44,* 510–511.

Berkowitz, R. I., Wadden, T. A., Tershakovec, A. M., & Cronquist, J. L. (2003). Behavior therapy and sibutramine for the treatment of adolescent obesity. *Journal of the American Medical Association, 289,* 1805–1812.

Berrettini, W. H. (2005, August). Editorial. *Psychiatry, 2,* 5.

Bess, A. L., & Cunningham, S. R. (2005, December). (Letter). Important drug warning and new information [regarding Clozaril]. East Hanover, NJ: Novartis Pharmaceutical.

Bhangoo, R. K., Dell, M. L., Towbin, K. Myers, F. S., Lowe, C. H., Pine, D., et al. (2003). Clinical correlates of episodicity in juvenile mania. *Journal of Child and Adolescent Psychopharmacology, 13,* 507–514.

Bhangoo, R. K., Deveney, C. M., & Leibenluft, E. (2003). Affective neuroscience and the pathophysiology of bipolar disorder. In M. DelBello & B. Geller (Eds.), *Bipolar disorder in childhood and early adolescence* (pp. 175–192). New York: Guilford.

Bhat, S. K., & Galang, R. (2002). (letter). Narcolepsy presenting as schizophrenia. *American Journal of Psychiatry, 159,* 1245.

Biederman, J., Mick, E., Faraone, S. V., & Wozniak, J. (2004, September). Pediatric bipolar disorder or disruptive behavior disorder? *Primary Psychiatry,* 36–41.

Biederman, J., Spencer, T., & Wilens, T. (2004). Psychopharmacology. In J. M Wiener & M. K. Dulcan (Eds.), *Textbook of child and adolescent psychiatry* (pp. 931–973). Arlington, VA: American Psychiatric Publishing.

Birmaher, B., Arbelaez, C., & Brent, D. (2002). Course and outcome of child and adolescent major depressive disorder. *Child and Adolescent Psychiatric Clinics of North America, 11,* 619–637.

Birmaher, B. (2003). Treatment of psychosis in children and adolescents. *Psychiatric Annals, 33,* 257–264.

Blair, J., Scahill, L., State, M., & Martin, A. (2005). Electrocardiography changes in children and adolescents treated with ziprasidone: A prospective study. *American Journal of Child and Adolescent Psychiatry, 44,* 73–79.

Bogetto, F., Bellino, S., Vaschetto, P., & Ziero, S. (2000, October). Augmentation of fluvoxamine-refractory obsessive compulsive disorder (OCD): A 12 week open trial. *Psychiatric Research, 96,* 91–98,

Boreman, C. D., & Arnold, L. E. (2003). (letter). Hallucinations associated with initiation of guanfacine. *Journal of the American Academy of Child and Adolescent Psychiatry, 42*, 1387.

Bowden, C. L. (2003). Long-term outcome of treatment with the new atypical antipsychotics. In The role of atypical antipsychotics in the treatment of bipolar disorders, Advancing Mental Heath Expert Opinions, convened at the American College of Neuropsycho-pharmacology, December 8, 2003, San Juan Puerto Rico, 1, 35–48.

Bowden, C. L. (2004). Valproate. In A. L. Schatzberg & C. B. Nemeroff (Eds.). *Textbook of psychopharmacology*. Arlington, VA: American Psychiatric Publishing.

Bowes, M. (2002, July). Maximazing the utility of atypical antipsychotics. *Psychiatric Times*, 57–60.

Boyer, E. W., & Shannon, M. (2005, March 17). The serotonin syndrome. *New England Journal of Medicine, 352*, 1112–1120.

Boza, R. A. Hallucinations and illusions of non-psychiatric etiologies. http://www.priory.com/halluc.htm

Brecher, M., Rak, I. W., Melvin, K., & Jones, A. M. (2000). The long-term effect of quetia-pine (Seroquel™) monotherapy on weight in patients with schizophrenia. *International Journal of Psychiatry in Clinical Practice, 4*, 287–291.

Bremmer, J. D. (2005). *Brain imaging handbook*. New York: W. W. Norton.

Brown, W. A., Kennedy, J. C., & Pollack, W. S. (2005, June). Adolescent violence. What school shooters feel, and how psychiatrists can help. *Current Psychiatry, 4*, 12–16, 22.

The Brown University Child and Adolescent Psychopharmacology Update. (2001, November). Is treatment-emergent weight gain linked to diabetes? *3*, 1, 5–7.

The Brown University Child and Adolescent Psychopharmacology Update. (2003, February). Case Reports. Orofacial dyskinesia reported in child taking methylphenidate, *5*, 8.

Brunnette, M. F., Noordsy, D. L., & Green, A. I. (2005, March). A Challenging mix: Co-oc-curring schizophrenia and substance abuse disorders. *Psychiatric Times*, 29–33.

Bryden, K. E., Carrey, N. J., & Kutcher, S. P. (2001). Update and recommendations for the use of antipsychotic medications in early-onset psychosis. Review. *Journal of Child and Adolescent Psychopharmacology, 11*, 113–130.

Buchanan, R. W., & Heinrichs, D. W. (1989). The Neurological Evaluation scale (NES): A structured instrument for the assessment of neurological signs in schizophrenia. *Psychiatric Research* (Elsevier), *27*, 335–350.

Buckley, N. A., & Sanders, P. (2000). Cardiovascular adverse effects of antipsychotic drugs. *Drug Safety, 23*, 215–228.

Buckley, P. F., Gowans, A., Sebastian, S., Pathiraja, A., Brimeyer, A., & Stirewalt, E. (2004, June). The boundaries of schizophrenia: Overlap with bipolar disorders. In R. O. Friedel & D. L. Evans (Eds.), *Current Psychosis and Therapeutic Reports, 2*, 49–56. Philadelphia: Bristol-Myers Squibb Company, Current Science.

Buckley, P. F., Mahadik, S., Evans, D., & Stirewalt, E. (2003). Schizophrenia: Causes, course and neurodevelopment. *Current Psychosis and Therapeutic Reports, 1*, 41–49.

Buckley, P. F., Sebastian, S., Sinha, D., & Stirewalt, E. M. (2003). Out of the pipeline: Aripip-razole. *Current Psychiatry, 2*, 71–73.

Bukstein, O. G., & Tarter, R. E. (1998). Substance use disorders. In C. E. Coffey & R. A. Brumback (Eds.), *Textbook of pediatric neuropsychiatry* (pp. 595–616). Washington, DC: American Psychiatric Press.

Burniat, W., Cole, T., Lissau, I., & Poskitt, E. (2002). *Child and adolescent obesity*. Cambridge, UK: Cambridge University Press.

Butzlaff, R. L., & Hooley, J. M. (1998). Expressed emotion and psychiatric relapse: a meta-analysis. *Archives of General Psychiatry, 55,* 547–552.

Biutelaar J. K., Van der Gaag R. J., Cohen-Kettenis P., & Melman, C. T. M. (2001). A randomized controlled trial of risperidone in the treatment of aggression in hospitalized adolescents with subaverage intelligence. *Journal of Clinical Psychiatry, 62,* 239–248.

Calabrese, J. R., Keck, P. E., MacFadden, W., Minkwitz, M., Ketter, T. A., et al., & The Bolder Study Group. (2005). A randomized, double-blind, placebo-controlled trial of quetiapine in the treatment of bipolar I or II depression. *American Journal of Psychiatry, 162,* 1351–1360.

Calles, E. E., Rodriguez, C., Walker-Thurmond, K., & Thun, M. J. (2003). Overweight, obesity, and mortality from cancer in a prospectively studied cohort of U.S. adults. *The New England Journal of Medicine, 348,* 1625–1638.

Camacho, A. (2004, September). Are some forms of substance abuse related to the bipolar-spectrum? Hypothetical considerations and therapeutic implications. *Primary Psychiatry, 11,* 42–46.

Campbell, M., Rapoport, J., & Simpson, G. M. (1999). Antipsychotics in children and adolescents. *Journal of the American Academy of Child and Adolescent Psychiatry, 38,* 537–545.

Cannon, M., Jones, P. B., & Murray, R. M. (2002). Obstetric complications and schizophrenia: Historical and meta-analytic review. *American Journal of Psychiatry, 159,* 1080–1092.

Caplan, R. (1994a). Thought disorder in childhood. *Journal of the American Academy of Child and Adolescent Psychiatry, 33,* 605–615.

Caplan, R. (1994b, January). Childhood schizophrenia. Assessment and treatment. *Child and Adolescent Psychiatric Clinics of North America, 3,* 15–30.

Caplan, R., Arbelle, S., Guthrie, D., Komo, S., Shields, W. D., Hansen, R., et al. (1997). Formal thought disorder and psychopathology in pediatric primary generalized and complex partial epilepsy. *Journal of American Academy of Child and Adolescent Psychiatry, 36,* 1286–1294.

Carey, J. C. (2003). Chromosome disorders. In C. D. Rudolph, A. M. Rudolph, M. K. Hostetter, G. Lister, & N. J. Siegel (Eds.), *Rudolph's pediatrics* (21st ed., pp. 731–742). New York: McGraw-Hill.

Carlson, C., Sowell, M. O. & Cavazzoni, P. (2003, May). Atypical antipsychotic treatment of children and adolescents and treatment-emergent diabetes. S. P. Kutcher (Ed.). *Child and Adolescent Psychopharmacology News, 8,* 4–7.

Carlson, G. A. (2005). Diagnosing bipolar disorders in children and adolescents. S. P. Kutcher (Ed.). *Child and Adolescent Psychopharmacology News, 10,* 1–6.

Carlson, G. A., & Kashani, J. H. (2002). What is new in bipolar disorder and major depressive disorder in children and adolescents? *Child and Adolescent Psychiatric Clinics of North America, 11,* xv–xxii.

Caro, J. J., Ward, A., Levinton, C., & Robinson, K. (2002). The risk of diabetes during olanzapine use compared with risperidone use: A retrospective database analysis. *Journal of Clinical Psychiatry 63,* 1135–1139.

Caroff, S. N. (2003). Neuroleptic malignant syndrome. Still a risk, but which may be in danger? *Current Psychiatry, 2,* 36–42.

Carpenter, W. T. (2001). (editorial). Evidence-based treatment for first-episode schizophrenia? *American Journal of Psychiatry 158,* 1771–1773.

Carpenter, W. T., Appelbaum, P. S., & Levine, R. J. (2003). The Declaration of Helsinki and clinical trials: A focus on placebo-controlled trials in schizophrenia. *American Journal of Psychiatry, 160,* 356–362.

Casey, D. E., Daniel, D. G., Wassef, A. A., Tracy, K. A., Wozniak, P., & Sommerville, K. W. (2003). Effects of divalproex combined with olanzapine or risperidone in patients with acute exacerbation of schizophrenia. *Neuropsychopharmacology, 28,* 182–192.

Centorrino, F., Price, B. H., Tuttle, M., Bahk, W. M., Hennen, J., Albert, M. J., & Baldessarini, R. J. (2002). EEG abnormalities during treatment with typical and atypical antipsychotics. *American Journal of Psychiatry, 159,* 109–115.

Cepeda, C. (2000). Evaluation of psychotic symptoms. In *Concise guide to the psychiatric interview of children and adolescents* (pp. 149-161). Washington, DC: American Psychiatric Press.

Chakos, M., Lieberman, J., Hoffman, E., Bradford, D., & Sheitman, B. (2001). Effectiveness of second-generation antipsychotics in patients with treatment-resistant schizophrenia: A review and meta-analysis of randomized trials. *American Journal of Psychiatry, 158,* 518–526.

Chang, K., Karchemskiy, A., Barnea-Goraly, M., Garret, A., Iorgova Simeonova, D., & Reiss, A. (2005). Reduced amygdalar gray matter volume in familial pediatric bipolar disorder. *Journal of the American Academy of Child and Adolescent Psychiatry, 44,* 565–573.

Chang, K., Saxena, K., & Howe, M. (2006, March). An open-label study of lamotrigine adjunct or monotherapy for the treatment of adolescents with bipolar depression. *Journal of the American Academy of Child and Adolescent Psychiatry, 45,* 298–304.

Chaudron, L. (2003, July). Is postpartum psychosis a bipolar variant? A phenomenological question. *Psychiatric Times, XX,* 54–61.

Cheng,-Shannon, J., McGough, J. J., Pataki, C., & McCracken, J. T. (2004). Second-generation antipsychotic medications in children and adolescents. *Journal of Child and Adolescent Psychopharmacology, 14,* 372–394.

Christensen, R. C. (2004, February). Recognition and management of the neuromalignant syndrome. *Primary Psychiatry, 11,* 20–22.

Christensen, R. C. (2006, February). Get serotonin syndrome down cold with SHIVERS. *Current Psychiatry, 5,* 114.

Citrome, L., Bilder, R. M., & Volakva, J. (2002). Managing treatment-resistant schizophrenia: Evidence from randomized clinical trials. *Journal of Psychiatric Practice, 8,* 205–215.

Connor, D. F. (1998, March). (letter). Stimulants and neuroleptic withdrawal dyskinesia. *Journal of the American Academy of Child and Adolescent Psychiatry, 37,* 247–248.

Consensus Development Conference on Antipsychotic Drugs and Obesity and Diabetes. (2004, February). *Diabetes Care, 27,* 596–601.

Corcoran, C., McAllister, T. W., & Malaspina, D. (2005). Psychotic disorders. In J. M. Silver, T. W. McAllister, & S. C. Yudofsky (Eds.), *Textbook of traumatic brain injury* (pp. 213–229). New York: American Psychiatric Publishing.

Cornblatt, B. (2003). (CME program). Studying the prodromal stages of schizophrenia: Interrupting the progression to psychosis. In *Advancing the treatment of pediatric psychotic and behavioral disorders* (pp. 15–18). Littleton, CO: A Jenssen Pharmaceutical supported publication. Medical Educational Resources & Clinical Connexion.

Correll, C. U., Leutch, S., & Kane, J. M. (2004). Lower risk for tardive dyskinesia associated with second-generation antipsychotics: A systematic review of 1-year studies. *American Journal of Psychiatry, 161,* 414–425.

Correll, C. U., & Mendelowitz, A. J. (2003, April). First psychotic episode—A window of opportunity. Seize the moment to build a therapeutic alliance. *Current Psychiatry, 2,* 51–67.

Critical Breakthroughs in Psychiatry. (2001, September). *Antipsychotic use in children.* Optima Educational Solutions.

Croog, D., Naccari, C., & Wong, S. (2005, September). Patients at risk for psychosis have emotional deficits in addition to cognitive deficiencies. *Primary Psychiatry, 12,* 13–14.

Csernansky, J. G., Mahmoud, R., & Brenner, R. (2002). A comparison of risperidone and haloperidol for the prevention of relapse in patients with schizophrenia. *The New England Journal of Medicine, 346,* 16–22.

Cummings, J. L., & Mega, M. S. (2003). *Neuropsychiatry and behavioral neuroscience.* Oxford: Oxford University Press.

Currier, G. W. (2003). The controversy over "chemical restraint" in acute care psychiatry. *Journal of Psychiatric Practice, 9,* 59–70.

Dagogo-Jack, S. (2003). *Mechanistic studies demonstrate no effect of antipsychotics on insulin response.* Carmel, IN: Devorah Wood & Associates (a Lilly sponsored publication).

Daniel, D. G., Copeland, L. F., & Tamminga, C. (2004). Ziprasidone. In A. F. Schatzberg & C. B. Nemeroff (Eds.), *Textbook of psychopharmacology.* Arlington, VA: American Psychiatric Publishing.

Daniel, D. G., Zimbroff, D. L., Potkin, S. G., et al. (1999). Ziprasidone 80 mg/day and 160 mg/day in the acute exacerbation of schizophrenia and schizoaffective disorders: A 6-week placebo controlled trial in the ziprasidone study group. *Neuropsychopharmacology, 20,* 491–505.

Daskalakis, Z. J., Christensen, B. K., Fitzgerald, P. B., Fountain, S. I., & Chen, R. (2005). Reduced cerebellar inhibition in schizophrenia: A preliminary study. *American Journal of Psychiatry, 162,* 1203–1205.

Davis, J. M., Chen, N., & Glick, I. D. (2003). A meta-analysis of the efficacy of second-generation antipsychotics. *Archives of General Psychiatry, 60,* 553–564.

Del Beccaro, M. A., Burke, P., & McCauley, E. (1988). Hallucinations in children: A follow-up study. *Journal of the American Academy of Child and Adolescent Psychiatry, 27,* 462–465.

DelBello, M. P., Schwiers, M. L., Rosenberg, H. L., & Strakowski, S. M. (2002). A double-blind, randomized, placebo-controlled study of quetiapine as adjunctive treatment for adolescent mania. *Journal of the American Academy of Child and Adolescent Psychiatry, 41,* 1216–1223.

DelBello, M. P., Axelson, D., & Geller, B. (2003). Introduction. In M. P. DelBello & B. Geller (Eds.), *Bipolar disorder in childhood and early adolescence.* New York: Guilford.

DelBello, M., & Grcevich, S. (2004). Phenomenology and epidemiology of childhood psychiatric disorders that may necessitate treatment with atypical antipsychotics. *Journal of Clinical Psychiatry, 65*(Suppl. 6), 12–19.

DelBello, M., Ice, K., Fisher, D. O., Versavel, M & Micelli, J. J. (2005). (Poster). Ziprasidone in the treatment of children and adolescents with bipolar mania or schizophrenia: an open label, dose-ranging safety and tolerability study. New Clinical Drug Evaluation Unit, 45th Annual Meeting, Boca Raton, Fl, June 6–9.

DelBello, M. P., Kowatch, R. A., Caleb, A., Sanford, K. E., Welge, J. A., Barzman, D. H., Nelson, E., & Strakowski, S. M. (2006, March). A double-blind randomized pilot study comparing quetiapine and divalproex for adolescent mania. *Journal of the American Academy of Child and Adolescent Psychiatry, 45,* 305–313.

DePaulo, J. R. (2006, February). (Editorial). Bipolar disorder treatment: An evidence-based reality check. *American Journal of Psychiatry, 163*, 175–176.

Després, J. P., Golay, A., Sjöström, L., & the Rimonabant in Obesity–Lipids Study Group. (2005, November 17). Effects of rimonabant on metabolic risk factors in overweight patients with dyslipidemia. *The New England Journal of Medicine, 353*, 2121–2134.

Dhossche, D., Ferdinand, R., Van Der Ende, J., Hofstra, M. B., & Verhulst, F. (2002). Diagnostic outcome of self-reported hallucinations in a community sample of adolescents. *Psychological Medicine, 32*, 619–627.

Diler, R. S., Yolga, A., & Avci, A. (202). Fluoxetine-induced extrapyramidal symptoms in an adolescent: A case report. *Swiss Medical Weekly, 132*, 125–126.

Diler, R. S, Yolga, A., Avci, A. & Scahill, L. (2003). Risperidone-induced obsessive-compulsive symptoms in two children. *Journal of Child and Adolescent Psychopharmacology, 13*(Suppl. 1), S89–S92.

Dilsaver, S. C. (2005, December). Preschool mania does not exist. *The Journal of Bipolar Disorders*, Reviews and Commentaries, *IV*, 15–16.

Dimaio, V., & Dimaio, D. (2001). Sudden death during or immediately after a violent struggle In V. Dimaio & D. Dimaio (Eds.), *Forensic pathology* (2nd ed.). Boca Raton, FL: CRC Press.

Diwadkar, V., & Keshavan, M. S. (2003). Emerging insights on the neuroanatomy of schizophrenia. *Current Psychosis and Therapeutics Reports. 1*, 28–34.

Dolder, C. R., Lacro, J. P., Dunn, L. B., & Jeste, D. V. (2002). Antipsychotic medication adherence: Is there a difference between typical and atypical agents? *American Journal of Psychiatry, 159*, 103–108.

Domon, S. E., & Webber, J. C. (2001). Hyperglycemia and hypertriglyceridemia secondary to olanzapine. Case Report. *Journal of Child and Adolescent Psychopharmacology, 11*, 285–288.

Dorland's Illustrated Medical Dictionary, 28th Ed. (1994). W. B. Saunders.

Doval, O., Gaviria, M., & Kanner, A. M. (2001). Frontal lobe dysfunction in epilepsy. In A. B. Ettinger & A. M. Kanner (Eds.), *Psychiatric issues in epilepsy, a practical guide to diagnosis and treatment* (pp. 261–271). Philadelphia: Lippincott Williams & Wilkins.

Dreikurs, R., & Grey, L. (1968). *The new approach to discipline: logical concequences* (pp. 37–40). New York: Plume.

Duffy, A. (2003, November). The use of family history in selecting long-term treatment for patients with bipolar disorders. *Child and Adolescent Psychopharmacology News.* S. P. Kutcher (Ed.), *8*, 1–3.

Egeland, J. A., Shaw, J. A., Endicott, J., Pauls, D. L., Allen, C. R., Hostetter, A. M., & Sussex, J. N. (2003). Prospective study of prodromal features for bipolarity in well Amish children. *Journal of the American Academy of Child and Adolescent Psychiatry, 42*, 786–796.

Eggers, C. (1989). Schizo-affective psychosis in childhood: A follow-up study. *Journal of Autism and Developmental Disorders, 19*, 327–342.

Eggers, C., Bunk, D., & Burns, B. (2002). Childhood and adolescent schizophrenia: Results from two long-term follow-up studies. *Neurology, Psychiatry and Brain Research, 9*, 183–190.

Ehrmann, D.A. (2005, March 24). Polycystic ovary syndrome. *New England Journal of Medicine, 352*, 1223–1236.

Eisenberg, M. E., Neumark-Sztainer, D., & Story, M. (2003, August). Association of weight-based teasing and emotional well-being among adolescents. *Archives of Pediatrics and Adolescent Medicine, 157,* 733–738.

Epstein, L. H., Valoski, A., Wing, R. R., & McCurley, J. (1994). Ten-year outcome of behavioral family-based treatment of childhood obesity. *Health Psychology, 13,* 373–383.

Farber, N. B., & Newcomer, J. W. (2003). The role of NMDA receptor hypofunction in idiopathic psychotic disorders. In M. P. DelBello & B.Geller (Eds.), *Bipolar disorder in childhood and early adolescence.* New York: Guilford.

Farmer, E. M. Z., Dorsey, S., & Mustillo, S. A. (2004). Intense home and community interventions. *Child and Adolescent Psychiatric Clinics of North America, 13,* 857–884.

Fegert, J. (2003, June). Ethical and legal problems in treating schizophrenic patients with neuroleptics during childhood and adolescence. *Child and Adolescent Psychopharmacology News, 8,* 5–9.

Fenichel, G. M. (2005) *Clinical pediatric neurology. A signs and symptoms approach* (5th ed.). Philadelphia: Elsevier Saunders.

Fennig, S., Susser, E. S., Pilowsky, D. J., Fennig, S., & Bromet, E. J. (1997). Childhood hallucinations preceding the nfirst psychotic episode. *Journal of Nervous and Mental Diseases, 185,* 115–117.

Field, A. E., Austin, S. B., Taylor, C. B., Malspeis, S., Rosner, B., Rockett, H. R. et al. (2003). A. relation between dieting and weight change among preadolescents and adolescents. *Pediatrics, 112,* 900–906.

Figlewicz, D. P. (2003). Insulin, food intake, and reward. *Seminars in Clinical Neuropsychiatry, 8,* 82–93.

Filley, C. M. (2003). White matter disorders. In R. B. Schiffer, S. M. Rao, & B. S. Fogel (Eds.), *Neuropsychiatry* (2nd ed.). Philadelphia: Lippincott Williams & Wilkins.

Findling, R. L., Kusumakar, V., Daneman, D., Moshang, T., De Smedt, G., & Binder, C. (2003). Prolactin levels during long-term risperidone treatment of children and adolescents. *Journal of Clinical Psychiatry, 64,* 1362–1369.

Findling, R. L., McNamara, N. K., & Gracious, B. L. (2003). Antipsychotic agents: Traditional and atypical. In A. Martin, L. Scahill, D. Charney, S. Leckman, & J. F. Leckman (Eds.), *Pediatric psychopharmacology principles and practice.* Oxford University Press.

Findling, R. L., McNamara, N. K., Stansbrey, R., Gracious, B. L., Resaca, E. W., Demeter, C. A., et al. (2006, February). Combination lithium and divalproex sodium in pediatric bipolar symptom restabilization. *Journal of the American Academy of Child & Adolescent Psychiatry, 45,* 142–148.

Fink, M. (2002, September). Catatonia in adolescents and children. *Psychiatric Times,* 28–29.

Fohrman, D. A., & Stein, M. T. (2006, February). Psychosis: 6 steps to rule out medical causes in kids. Time saving algorithm combines efficiency with a thorough evaluation. *Current Psychiatry, 5,* 35–47.

Frazier, J. A., Chiu, S., Breeze, J. L., Makris, N., Lange, N., Kennedy, D. N., et al. (2005). Structural brain magnetic resonance imaging of limbic and thalamic volumes in pediatric bipolar disorder. *American Journal of Psychiatry, 162,* 1256–1265.

Freedman, R. (2005, Sept. 22). (editorial). The choice of antipsychotic drugs for schizophrenia. *The New England Journal of Medicine, 353,* 1286–1288.

Freeman, M. P., Wiegand, C. & Gelenberg, A. J. (2004). Lithium. In A. F. Schatzberg & C. B. Nemeroff (Eds.), *Textbook of psychopharmacology.* Arlington, VA: American Psychiatric Publishing.

Frey, B. N., Rodrigues da Fonseca, M. M., Machado-Vieira, R., Soarese, J. C., & Kapczinski,

F. (2004). Neuropathological and neurochemical abnormalities in bipolar disorder. *Revista Brasileira de Psiquiatria, 26*, 180–188.

Friedman, M., Mull, C., Sharieff, G. & Tsarouhas, N. (2003). Prolonged QT syndrome in children: An uncommon but potentially fatal entity. *Journal of Emergency Medicine 24*,173–179.

Fuller, A. K., & Fuller, J. E. (2005, December). Cases that test your skills. A "bad" boy's behavior problems. *Current Psychiatry, 4*, 77–78, 87–90.

Fuller, M. A., & Sajatovic, M. (2005). *Drug Information Handbook for Psychiatry* (5th ed.). Lexi-Comp Inc.

Gabbard, G. O., & Kay, J. (2001). The fate of integrated treatment: Whatever happened to the biopsychosocial psychiatrist? *American Journal of Psychiatry, 158*, 1956–1963.

Gabbay, V., Silva, R. R., Castellanos, F. X., Rabinovitz, B., & Gonen, O. (2005, September). Structural and functional neuroimaging of pediatric depression. *Primary Psychiatry, 12*, 51–57.

Gaffney, G. R., Perry, P. J., Lund B. C., Bever-Stille, K. A., Arndt, S., & Kuperman, S. (2002). Risperidone versus clonidine in the treatment of children and adolescents with Tourette syndrome. *Journal of the American Academy of Child and Adolescent Psychiatry, 41*, 330–336.

Galanter, C. A., Bilich, C., & Walsh, B. T. (2002). Side effects of desipramine and age. *Journal of Child and Adolescent Psychopharmacology, 12*, 137–145.

Galderisi, S., Maj, M., Mucci, A., Casano, G. B., Invernizzi, G., Rossi, A., et al. (2002). Historical, psychopathological, neurological, and neuropsychological aspects of deficit schizophrenia: A multicenter study. *American Journal of Psychiatry, 159*, 983–990.

Gallagher, R. (2005, September). Evidence-based psychotherapies for depressed adolescents: A review and clinical guidelines. *Primary Psychiatry, 12*, 33–39.

Garralda, M. E. (1984a). Hallucinations in children with conduct and emotional disorders: I. The clinical phenomena. *Psychological Medicine, 14*, 589–596.

Garralda M. E. (1984b). Hallucinations in children with conduct and emotional disorders: II. The follow-up study. *Psychological Medicine, 14*, 597–604.

Gelenberg, A. J. (2002, May. Newer antipsychotics may increase the risk of pregnancy. *Biological Therapies in Psychiatry, 25*, 17.

Gelenberg, A. J. (2003a, March). Venous thromboembolism and antipsychotic drugs. *Biological Therapies in Psychiatry, 26*, 9.

Gelenberg, A. J. (2003b, July). Hazards of clozapine. *Biological Therapies in Psychiatry, 26*, 26–27.

Gelenberg, A. J. (2003c, July). TMS for bipolar patients. *Biological Therapies in Psychiatry, 26*, 25.

Gelenberg, A. J. (2004, January). Coping with antipsychotic induced weight. *Biological Therapies in Psychiatry, 27*, 2–3.

Geller, B., Warner, K., Williams, M., et al. (1998). Prepubertal and young adolescent bipolarity versus ADHD: Assessment, and validity using the WASH-U-KSADS, CBCL and TRF. *Journal of Affective Disorders, 51*, 93–100.

Geodon [Ziprasidone], Package Insert (Revision, May 2005). Roerig, Distributor, Pfizer Inc, New York, New York.

Ghaemi, S. N. (2002). "All the worse for fishes": Conceptual and historical background of polypharmacy in psychiatry. In S. N. Ghaemi (Ed.), *Polypharmacy in psychiatry*. New York: Marcel Dekker.

Gheorghe, M. D., Baloescu, A., & Grigorescu, G. (2004, August). Premorbid cognitive and behavioral functioning in military recruits experiencing the first episode of psychosis. *CNS Spectrums, 9*, 604–606.

Giedd, J. N., Jeffries, N. O., Blumenthal, J., Castellanos, F. X., Vaituzis, A. C., Fernandez, T., et al. (1999). Childhood-onset schizophrenia: Progressive brain changes during adolescence. *Biological Psychiatry, 46*, 892–898.

Gilmer, T. P., Dolder, C. R., Lacro, J. P., Folsom, D. P., Lindamer, L., Garcia, P., et al. (2004). Adherence to treatment with antipsychotic medication and health care costs among medicaid beneficiaries with schizophrenia. *American Journal of Psychiatry, 161*, 692–699.

Ginsberg, D. L. (2004a, March). Psychopharmacology reviews. *Primary Psychiatry, 11*, 14–19.

Ginsberg, D. L. (2004b, June). Psychopharmacology reviews. *Primary Psychiatry, 11*, 13–17.

Ginsberg, D. L. (2005a, January). Psychopharmacology reviews. *Primary Psychiatry, 12*, 17–20.

Ginsberg, D. L. (2005b, March). Psychopharmacology reviews. *Primary Psychiatry, 12*, 21–22.

Ginsberg, D. L. (2005c, September). Psychopharmacology Reviews. *Primary Psychiatry, 12*, 25–29.

Ginsberg, D. L. (2005d, November). Psychopharmacology reviews. Valproate treatment for catatonia *Primary Psychiatry, 12*, 29–30.

Ginsberg, D. L. (2005e, December). Psychopharmacology reviews. Aripiprazole induced psychosis.*Primary Psychiatry, 12*, 30.

Gitelman, S. (2003). Diabetes mellitus. In C. D. Rudolph, A. M. Rudolph, M. K. Hostetter, G. Lister, & N. J. (Eds.), *Rudolph's pediatrics* (21st ed.). New York; MacGraw Hill.

Gitlin, M., Nuechterlein, K., Subotnik, K. L., Ventura, J., Mintz, J., Fogelson, D. L., et al. (2001). Clinical outcome following neuroleptic discontinuation in patients with remitted recent-onset schizophrenia. *American Journal of Psychiatry, 158*, 1835–1842.

Glassman, A. H., & Bigger, J. T. (2001). Antipsychotic drugs: Prolong QT interval, torsade des pointes and sudden death. *American Journal of Psychiatry 158*, 1774–1782.

Goff, D. C. (2004). Risperidone (495-505). In A. F. Schatzberg & C. B. Nemeroff (Eds.), *Textbook of psychopharmacology*. Arlington, VA: American Psychiatric Publishing.

Gogtay, N., Sporn, A., Clasen, L. S., Nuget III, T. F., Greenstein, D., Nicolson, R., et al. (2004). Comparison of progressive cortical gray matter loss in childhood-onset schizophrenia with that in childhood-onset atypical psychosis. American *Journal of Psychiatry, 162*, 1637–1643.

Goldfarb, W. (1974). Distinguishing and classifying the individual schizophrenic child. In S. Arieti & G. Caplan (Eds.), *American handbook of psychiatry* (2nd ed., vol. 2, pp. 85–106). New York: Basic Books.

Gonzalez-Heydrich, J., Raches, D., Wilens, T. E., Leichtner, A., & Mezzacappa, E. (2003). Retrospective study of hepatic enzyme elevations in children treated with olanzapine, divalproex and their combination. *Journal of The American Academy of Child and Adolescent Psychiatry, 42*, 1227–1233.

Goodman, R. (2002). Brain disorders. In M. Rutter, E, Taylor, & L. Hersov (Eds.), *Child and adolescent psychiatry modern approaches* (4th ed., pp. 241–260). Oxford, UK: Blackwell Science.

Goodwin, F. K., & Ghaemi, S. N. (2003, December). (Editorial). The course of bipolar disorder and the nature of agitated depression. *American Journal of Psychiatry, 160*, 2077–2079.

Gracious B. L., & Finding R. L. (2001, March). Antipsychotic medications for children and adolescents. *Pediatric Annals, 30*, 138–145.

Gracious, B. L., Krysiak, T. E., & Youngstrom, E. A. (2002). Amantadine treatment of psychotropic-induced weight gain in children and adolescents: Case series. Case report. *Journal of Child and Adolescent Psychopharmacology, 12*, 249–257.

Gracious, B. L., & Meyer, A. E. (2005, January). Psychotropic-induced weight gain and potential pharmacologic treatment strategies. *Psychiatry, 2*, 36–42.

Graham, K. A., Gu, H., Lieberman, J. A., Harp, J. B., & Perkins, D. O. (2005). Double-blind, placebo-controlled investigation of amantadine for weight loss in subjects who gained weight with olanzapine. *American Journal of Psychiatry, 162*, 1744–1746.

Green, L., Joy, S. P., Robins, D. L., Booklier, K. M., Waterhouse, L. H., & Fein, D. (2003). Autism and pervasive developmental disorders. In R. B. Schiffer, S. M. Rao, & B. S. Fogel (Eds.), *Neuropsychiatry* (pp. 503–551). Philadelphia: Lippincott Williams Wilkins.

Greenhill, L. (2002). Stimulant medication. Treatment of children with attention deficit hyperactivity disorder. In P. S. Jensen & J. R. Cooper (Eds.), *Attention deficit hyperactivity disorder* (pp. 9-1–9-27). State of the Science-Best Practices. Kingston, NJ: Civic Research Institute.

Greenhill, L. L., Vitiello, B., Riddle, M. A., Fisher, P., Shockey, E., March, J. S., et al. (2003, June). Review of safety assessment methods used in pediatric psychopharmacology. *Journal of the American Academy of Child and Adolescent Psychiatry, 42*, 627–633.

Greenspan, S. I., & Glovinsky, I. (2005, May). Bipolar patterns in children: New perspectives on developmental pathways and a comprehensive approach to prevention and treatment. *The Brown University Child and Adolescent Behavioral Letter, 1*, 5–6.

Guillaume, M., & Lissau, I. (2002). Epidemiology. In W. Burniat, T. Cole, I. Lissau, & E. Poskitt (Eds.), *Child and adolescent obesity* Cambridge University Press.

Guilleminault, C. (1996). Sleep and its disorders. In B. O. Berg (Ed.), *Principles of child neurology*. New York: McGraw-Hill.

Gupta, S. (2003). Epidemiological studies demonstrate no differences in diabetes risk between atypical antipsychotics. A Eli Lilly and Company supported publication. Deborah Wood & Associates, Carmel Indiana.

Gur, R. E., Andreasen, N., Asarnow, R., Gur, R., Jones, P., Kendler, K., et al. (2005). Schizophrenia/defining schizophrenia. In D. L. Evans, E. B. Foa, R. E. Gur, H. Hendin, C. P. O'Brien, M. M. P. Seligman, & B. T. Walsh (Eds.), *Treating and preventing adolescent mental health disorders. What we know and what we don't know*. Oxford University Press.

Halbreich, U., & Kahn, L. S. (2003). Hyperprolactinemia and schizophrenia: Mechanisms and clinical aspects. *Journal of Psychiatric Practice, 9*, 344–353.

Harvey, P. D. (2003). (CME). Recognizing the link between cognitive, affective, and social impairment, and long term outcomes. In *Improving outcomes in schizophrenia: Recent advances in the treatment of cognitive and affective domains* (pp. 1–3). PsychCME, Duke University Medical Center, Jontly sponsored by CME Outfitters,

Harvey, P. D., Meltzer, H., Simpson, G. M., Potkin, S. G., Loebel, A., Siu, C. et al. (2004). Improvement in cognitive function following a switch to ziprasidone from conventional antipsychotics, olanzapine or risperidone in outpatients with schizophrenia. *Schizophrenia Research, 66*, 101–113.

Hendren, R. L. (2003). (CME program). Neurodevelopmental findings—The future of identification and treatment of mental disorders. In *Advancing the treatment of pediatric psychotic and behavioral disorders.* Medical Educational Resources, Inc. & Clinical Connexion, LLC.

Heres, S., Davis, J., Maino, K., Jetzinger, E., Kissling, W., & Leucht, S. (2006, February). Why olanzapine beats risperidone, risperidone beats quetiapine, and quetiapine beats olanzapine: An exploratory analysis of head-to-head comparison studies of second-generation antipsychotics. *American Journal of Psychiatry, 163,* 185–194.

Hill, A. J., & Lissau, I. (2002). Psychosocial factors. In W. Burniat, T. Cole, I. Lissau & E. Poskitt (Eds.), *Child and adolescent obesity* Cambridge University Press.

Hirschfeld, R. M. A. (2005). (editorial). Are depression and bipolar disorder the same illness? *American Journal of Psychiatry, 162,* 1241–1242.

Hirshfeld-Becker, D. R., Biederman, J., Henin, A., Faraone, S. V., Cayton, G. A., & Rosenbaum, J. F. (2006, February). Laboratory observed behavioral disinhibition in the offspring of parents with bipolar disorder: A high risk pilot study. *American Journal of Psychiatry, 163,* 265–271.

Ho, B. C., Alicata, D., Mola, C., & Andreasen, N. C. (2005). Hippocampus volume and treatment delays in first-episode schizophrenia. *American Journal of Psychiatry, 162,* 1527–1529.

Ho, B. C., Alicata, D., Ward, J., Mose, D. J., O'Leary, D. S., Arndt, S., et al. (2003). Untreated initial psychosis: Relation to cognitive deficits and brain morphology in first-episode schizophrenia. *American Journal of Psychiatry, 160,* 142–148.

Ho, B. C., Mola, C., & Andreasen, N. C. (2004). Cerebellar dysfunction in neuroleptic naïve schizophrenic patients: Clinical, cognitive, and neuroanatomic correlates of cerebellar neurological signs. *Biological Psychiatry, 55,* 1146–1153.

Hockaday, J. M. (1996). Migraine in childhood. In B. O. Berg (Ed.), *Principles of child neurology* (pp. 693–706). New York: McGraw-Hill.

Hollis, C. (2000). Adult outcomes of child- and adolescent-onset schizophrenia: Diagnostic stability and predictive validity. *American Journal of Psychiatry, 157,* 1652–1659.

Hollis, C. (2001). Diagnosis and differential diagnosis. In H. Remschmidt (Ed.), *Schizophrenia in children and adolescents* (pp. 82–118). Cambridge, UK: Cambridge University Press.

Holmes, G. L. (1996). Epilepsy and other seizure disorders. In B. O. Berg (Ed.), *Principles of child neurology* (pp. 223–284). New York: McGraw Hill.

Honea, R., Crow, T. J., Passingham, D., & Mackay, C. E. (2005, December). Regional deficits in brain volume in schizophrenia: A meta-analysis of voxel-basel morphometry studies. *American Journal of Psychiatry, 162,* 2233–2245.

Hummer, M., Malik, P., Gasser, R. W., Hofer, A., Kemmler, G., Moncayo Naveda, R. C., et al. (2005). Osteoporosis in patients with schizophrenia. *American Journal of Psychiatry, 162,* 162–167.

Hunter, M. D., & Woodruff, P. W. R. (2004). (letter). Characteristics of functional hallucinations. *American Journal of Psychiatry, 161,* 923.

Hussain, M. Z., Waheed, W., & Hussain, S. (2005). (letter). Intravenous quetiapine abuse. *American Journal of Psychiatry, 162,* 1755–1756.

Hwang, J., Lyoo, I. K., Dager, S. R., Friedman, S. D., Oh, J., S., Lee, J. Y., et al. (2006, February). Basal ganglia shape alterations in bipolar disorder. *American Journal of Psychiatry, 163,* 276–285.

Israeli, D., & Zohar, J. (2004). (letter). Is multiple cavernoma a developmental defect in schizophrenia? *American Journal of Psychiatry, 161*, 924.

Ito, H. (2005, January). Effect of gender differences on the cardiovascular system in patients with mental disorders. *Psychiatric Times*, 42-43, 86.

Jabs, B. E., Verdaguer, M. F., Pfuhimann, B., Bartsch, A. J., & Beckmann, H. (2002). The concept of hebephrenia over the course of time with particular reference to the Wernicke-Kleist-Leonhard school. *World Journal of Biological Psychiatry 3*, 200–206.

Jacobsen, L., & Bertolino, A. (2000). Functional imaging in childhood schizophrenia. In M. Ernst & J. M. Rumsey (Eds.), *Functional neuroimaging in child psychiatry* (pp. 189–204). Cambridge University Press.

Jarbin, H., Ott, Y., & von Knorring, A. L. (2003). Adult outcome of social function in adolescent-onset schizophrenia and affective psychosis. *Journal of the American Academy of Child and Adolescent Psychiatry, 42*, 176–183.

Jensen, J. B. (2004, September). Conduct disorder and other disruptive behaviors: Pediatric psychopharmacology. In R. O. Friedel & D. L. Evans (Eds.), *Current Psychosis and Therapeutic Reports, 2*, 104–108.

Jibson, M. D. (2003). First-line atypicals are not equal in efficacy. CON (point of view in response to PRO point of viewed expressed by I. D. Glick & J. M. Davis. *The Journal of Psychotic Disorders: Reviews and Commentaries, 8*(3), 14.

Jibson, M. D., & Tandon, R. (1998). New atypical antipsychotic medications. *Journal of Psychiatric Research, 32*, 215–228.

Jibson, M. D., & Tandon, R. (2003). An overview of antischizophrenic medications. *Pharmacy News* (Special ed.), 59–63; also (2004, December). *CNS News* (Special ed.), 109–115.

Jobson, K. O., & Potter, W. Z. (1995, March). *Psychopharmacology Bulletin, 31*, 457–507.

Joshi, K. G., & Faubion, M. D. (2005, September). Mania and psychosis associated with St. John's Wort and ginseng. *Psychiatry, 2*, 56–61.

Junginger, J., & McGuire, L. (2001). (letter). The paradox of command hallucinations. *Psychiatric Services, 52*, 385.

Kafantaris, V., Coletti, D. J., Dicker, R., Padula, G., & Kane, J. M. (2001). Adjunctive antipsychotic treatment of adolescents with bipolar disorder. *Journal of the American Academy of Child and Adolescent Psychiatry, 40*, 1448–1456.

Kafantaris, V., Hirch, J., Saito, E., & Bennet, N. (2005, November). (letter). Treatment of withdrawal dyskinesia. *Journal of the American Academy of Child & Adolescent Psychaitry, 44*, 1102–1103.

Kane, J. M. (2004, May 5). Improving long-term treatment outcomes and adherence. impact of atypical antipsychotics on functional recovery and long-term outcomes. *APA. Advancing Mental Health* (Expert Opinion Series), *1*, 29–42.

Kane, J. M., Carson, W. H., Saha, A. R., McQuade, R. D., Ingenito, G. G., Zimbroff, D. L., et al. (2002). Efficacy and safety of aripiprazole and haloperidol versus placebo in patients with schizophrenia and schizoaffective disorder. *Journal of Clinical Psychiatry, 63*, 763–771.

Kane, J. M., Leucht, S., Carpenter, D., & Docherty, J. P. (2003). The expert consensus series. Optimizing pharmacologic treatment of psychotic disorders. *The Journal of Clinical Psychiatry, 64*(Suppl.12).

Kane, J. M., & Turner, M. (2003). (CME program). Raising the bar for treatment expectations in schizophrenia. In P. S. Masand (Ed.), *PsycCME Reports* (pp. 2–6). Bethesda, MD: Duke University Medical Center, CME Outfitters.

Kapur, S. (2003). Psychosis as a state of aberrant salience: A framework linking biology, phenomenology, and pharmacology of schizophrenia. *American Journal of Psychiatry, 160,* 13–23.

Kapur, S., Arenovich, T., Agid, O., Zipursky, R., Linborg, S., & Jones, B. (2005). Evidence for onset of antipsychotic effects within the first 24 hours of treatment. *American Journal of Psychiatry, 162,* 939–946.

Kapur, S. & Remington, G. (2001). Atypical antipsychotics: New directions and new challenges in treatment of schizophrenia. *Annual Reviews of Medicine, 52,* 503–517.

Kasper, S., & Muller-Spahn, F. (2000). Review of quetiapine and its clinical applications in schizophrenia. *Drug Evaluation. Expert Opinion of Pharmacotherapy, 1,* 783–801.

Kasper, S., Brecher, M., Fitton, L., & Jones, A. M. (2004). Maintenance of long-term efficacy and safety of quetiapine in open-label treatment of schizophrenia. *International Clinical Psychopharmacology, 19,* 281–289.

Kaur, S., Sassi, R. B., Axelson, D., Nicoletti, M., Brambilla, P., Monkul, E. S., et al. (2005). Cingulate cortical anatomical abnormalities in children and adolescents with bipolar disorder. *American Journal of Psychiatry, 162,* 1637–1643.

Keck, P. E., Marcus, R., Tourkodimitris, S., Ali, M., Liebeskind, A., et al., & Aripiprazole Study Group. (2003). A placebo-controlled, double-blind study of the efficacy and safety of aripiprazole in patients with acute bipolar mania. *American Journal of Psychiatry, 160,* 1651–1658.

Keck, P. E., Versiani, M., Potkin, S., West, S. A., Giller, E., Ice, K., et al. (2003). Ziprasidone in the treatment of acute bipolar mania: A three week, placebo-controlled, double-blind, randomized trial. *American Journal of Psychiatry, 160,* 741–748.

Keefe, R., & Hawkins, K. (2005, March). Assessing and treating cognitive deficits. *Psychiatric Times, XXII,* 33–34.

Keller, A., Castellanos, F. X., Vaituzis, A. C., Jeffries, N. O., Giedd, J. N., & Rapoport, J. L. (2003). Progressive loss of cerebellar volume in childhood-onset schizophrenia. *American Journal of Psychiatry, 160,* 128–133.

Kelly, J. (2005, August). Phase III trials demonstrate modafinil efficacy in ADHD. *Neuropsychiatry, 6*(1), 17–20.

Kendall, R., & Jablensky, A. (2003). Distinguishing between the validity and utility of psychiatric diagnoses. *American Journal of Psychiatry, 160,* 4–12.

Kendler, K. S. (2003, September).(editorial). The genetics of schizophrenia: chromosomal deletions, attentional disturbances, and spectrum boundaries. *American Journal of Psychiatry, 160,* 1549–1553.

Kendler, K. S. (2004). (editorial). Schizophrenia genetics and dysbindin: A corner turned? *American Journal of Psychiatry, 161,* 1533–1537.

Kendler, K. S. (2005). "A gene for...": The nature of gene action in psychiatric disorders. *American Journal of Psychiatry, 162,* 11243–12152.

Kennedy, N., Boydell, J., Kalidindi, S., Fearon, P., Jones, P. B., van Os, J., et al. (2005, February). Gender differences in incidence and age at onset of mania and bipolar disorder over a 35-year period in Camberwell, England. *American Journal of Psychiatry, 162,* 257–262.

Keshavan, M. S. (2005, March). First-episode schizophrenia: Research perspectives and clinical implications. *Psychiatric Times,* 22–28.

Keshavan, M. S., Sanders, R. D. Sweeney, J. A., Diwaldkar, V. A., Goldstein, G., Pettegrew, J. W., et al. (2003). Diagnostic specificity and neuroanatomical validity of neurological abnormalities in first-episode psychosis. *American Journal of Psychiatry 160*, 1298–1304.

Ketter, T. A., Wang, P. W., & Post, R. M. (2004). Carbamazepine and oxcarbazepine. In A. F. Schatzberg & C. B. Nemeroff (Eds.), *Textbook of psychopharmacology*. Arlington, VA: American Psychiatric Publishing.

King, D. J., Burke, M., & Lucas, R. A. (1995). Antipsychotic drug-induced dysphoria. *British Journal of Psychiatry, 167*, 480–482.

King, R. A. (1994). Childhood-onset schizophrenia. Development and pathogenesis. *Child and Adolescent Psychiatric Clinics of North America, 3*, 1–13.

Kingdon, D. G., & Turkington, D. (2005). *Cognitive therapy of schizophrenia*. New York: Guilford.

Kinon, B. J., Basson, B. R., Stauffer, V. L., & Tollefson, G. D. (1999). (abstract). Effects of chronic olanzapine treatment on the course of presumptive tardive dyskinesia. [Abstract]. *Schizophrenia Research, 36*, 363.

Kinon, B. J., Stauffer, V. L., Wang, L., Thi, K. T., & Kollack-Walker, S. (2001). *Olanzapine improves tardive dyskinesia in patients with schizophrenia—Results of a controlled prospective study*. Presented at the American Psychiatric Association 53rd Annual Institute on Psychiatric Services, Orlando, Florida, October 12.

Klin, A., & Volkmar, F. R. (2003). Asperger's syndrome: Diagnosis, and external validity. *Child and Adolescent Psychiatric Clinics of North America, 12*, 1–13.

Knowles, L., & Sharma, T. (2004, August). Identifying vulnerability markers in prodromal patients: A step in the right direction for schizophrenia prevention. *CNS Spectrums, 9*, 595–602.

Kober, D., & Gabbard, G. O. (2005). (letter). Topiramate induced psychosis. *American Journal of Psychiatry, 162*, 1542.

Kodesh, A., Finkel, B., Lerner, A. G., Kretzner, G., & Sigal, M. (2001). Dose-dependent olanzapine-associated leukopenia: Three case reports. *International Clinical Psychopharmacology, 16*, 117–119.

Koller, E. A., Cross, J. T., Doraiswamy, P. M., & P. M., Malozowski, S. N. (2003). Pancreatitis associated with atypical antipsychotics: from the Food and Drug Administration MedWatch Surveillance System and published report. *Pharmacotherapy, 23*, 1123–1130.

Koro, C. E., Fedder, D. O., L'Italien , G. J., Weiss, S. S., Magder, L. S., Kreyenbuhl, J., et al. (2002). Assessment of independent effects of olanzapine and risperidone on risk of diabetes among patients with schizophrenia: population based nested case-control study. *British Medical Journal, 325*, 243–247.

Kowatch, R. A., Davanzo, P. A., & Emslie, G. J. (2000). Pediatric mood disorders and neuroimaging. In M. Ernst & J. M. Rumsey (Eds.), *Functional neuroimaging in child psychiatry* (pp. 205–223). Cambridge University Press. Cambridge, UK.

Kowatch, R. A., Fristad, M., Birmaher, B., Wagner, K. D., Findling, R. L., et al. (2005, March). Treatment guidelines for children and adolescents with bipolar disorder. *Journal of the American Academy of Child and Adolescent Psychiatry, 44*, 213–235.

Kratochwill, T. R., Albers, C. A., & Shernoff, E. S. (2004, October). School-based interventions. *Child and Adolescent Psychiatric Clinics of North America, 13*, 885–904.

Krüger, S., Alda, M., Young, L. T., Goldapple, K., Parikh, S., & Maybereg, H. S. (2006, February). Risk and resilience markers in bipolar disorder: Brain responses to emotional challenge in bipolar patients and their healthy siblings. *American Journal of Psychiatry, 163*, 257–264.

Kumra, S. (2000, January). The diagnosis and treatment of children and adolescents with schizophrenia. *Child and Adolescent Psychiatric Clinics of North America, 9,* 183–199.

Kumra, S., Jacobsen, L. K., Lenane, M., Zahn, T.P., Wiggs, E., Alaghband-Rad, J., et al. (1998, January). "Multidimensionally impaired disorder": Is it a variant of very early-onset schizophrenia? *Journal of the American Academy of Child and Adolescent Psychiatry, 37,* 91–99.

Kuperberg, G. R., & Caplan, D. (2003). Language dysfunction in schizophrenia. In R. B. Schiffer, S. M. Rao & B. S. Fogel (Eds.), *Neuropsychiatry* (2nd ed., pp. 444–466). Philadelphia: Lippincott Williams & Wilkins.

Kupka, R. W., Luckenbaugh, D. A., Post , R. M., Suppes, T., Altshuler, L. L., Keck, P. E., et al. (2005). Comparison of rapid-cycling and non-rapid-cycling bipolar disorder based on prospective mood ratings in 539 outpatients. *American Journal of Psychiatry, 162,* 1273–1280.

Kutcher, S. P. (2004). New research. Quetiapine in the long-term treatment of schizophrenia. *Child and Adolescent Psychopharmacology News, 9,* 10.

Labellarte, M. J., Crosson, J. E., & Riddle, M. A. (2003). The relevance of prolonged QTc measurement to pediatric psychopharmacology. *Journal of the American Academy of Child and Adolescent Psychiatry, 42,* 642–650.

Labellarte, M. J., & Riddle, M. A. (2002). (CME program). Growing up whole: A focus on the use of atypical antipsychotic medications in children and adolescents. The Johns Hopkins University School of Medicine and Quintiles Medical Communications.

Labellarte, M. J., Walkup, J. T., & Riddle, M. A. (2003). (letter). Benign U-wave mistaken for QTc prolongation. *Journal of the American Academy of Child and Adolescent Psychiatry, 42,* 621.

Lacro, J. P., Dunn, L. B., Dolder, C. R., Leckland, S. G., & Jeste, D. V. (2002, October). Prevalence of and risk factors for medication nonadherance in patients with schizophrenia: A complete review of recent literature. *Journal of Clinical Psychiatry, 63,* 892–909.

Lader, M., & Lewander, T. (1994). The neuroleptic-induced deficit syndrome. *Acta Psychiatrica Scandinavica, 89*(Suppl.), 5–13.

Lake, J. (2005, November). Integrative management of depressed mood: Evidence and treatment guidelines. *Psychiatric Times, 22,* 91–97.

Lake, C. R., & Hurwitz, N. (2006, March). 2 Names, 1 Disease. Does schizophrenia = psychotic bipolar disorder? *Current Psychiatry, 5,* 42–60.

Lam, F. Y. W. (2003, July). Obesity: Orlistat may affect INR when added to warfarin. *The Brown University Psychopharmacological Update.*

Lam, Y. W. F. (2004, September). Paroxetine and quetiapine plus nizatidine-possible EPS drug-drug interactions. *The Brown University Psychopharmacology Update, 15,* 2–3.

Lambert, M. V., Schmitz, E. B., Ring, H. A., & Trimble, M. (2003). Neuropsychiatric aspects of epilepsy. In R. B. Schiffer, S. M. Rao, & B. S. Fogel (Eds.), *Neuropsychiatry* (2nd ed., pp. 1071–1131). Philadelphia: Lippincott Williams & Wilkins.

Law, A. (2003) Schizophrenia, IV: Neuregulin-1 in the human brain. In C. A. Tamminga (Ed.), Images in neuroscience. *American Journal of Psychiatry, 160,* 1392.

Leard-Hansson, & Guttmacher, L. (2004, March). Bupropion and schizophrenia (Evidence-based psychiatric medicine), *Clinical Psychiatric News,* 32.

Leard-Hansson, J., & Guttmacher, L. (2004, August). Vitamin E for tardive dyskinesia (evidence-based psychiatric medicine). *Clinical Psychiatric News,* 31.

Leard-Hansson, J., & Guttmacher, L. (2006, January). Can exercise treat depression? (evidence-based psychiatric medicine). *Clinical Psychiatric News, 34,* 29.

LeDoux, M., Braslow, K., & Brown, T. M. (2004). (letter). C-reactive protein and serotonin syndrome. *American Journal of Psychiatry, 161,* 1499.

Lee, C., & McGlashan, T. H. (2003). Treating schizophrenia earlier in life and the potential for prevention. *Current Psychosis and Therapeutics Reports, 1,* 35–40.

Lee, P., Moss, S., Friedlander, R., Donnelly, T., & Honer, W. (2003). Early-onset schizophrenia in children with mental retardation: diagnostic reliability and stability of clinical features. *Journal of the American Academy of Child and Adolescent Psychiatry, 42,* 162–169.

Lefley, H. P. (2004, November). Intercultural similarities and differences in family caregiving and family interventions in schizophrenia. *Psychiatric Times,* 70.

Legido, A., Tenembaum, S. N., Katsetos, C. D., & Menkes, J. H. (2006, 7th ed.). Autoinmune and postinfectious diseases. In J. H. Menkes, H. B. & Sarnat, H. B & Bernard Maria (Eds.), *Child neurology* (pp. 557–657). Philadelphia: Lippincott Williams & Wilkins.

Leslie, D. L., & Rosenheck, R. A. (2004). Incidence of newly diagnosed diabetes attributable to atypical antipsychotic medications. *American Journal of Psychiatry, 161,* 1709–1711.

Leucht, S., Barnes, T. R. E., Kissling, W., Engel, R. R., Correll, C., & Kane, J. M. (2003). Relapse prevention in schizophrenia with new-generation antipsychotics: A systematic review and exploratory meta-analysis of randomized controlled trials. *American Journal of Psychiatry, 160,* 1209–1222.

Levenson, J. L. (2005). Psychosis in the medically ill. *Primary Psychiatry, 12,* 12–18.

Lewinsohn, P. M., Seeley. J. R., & Klein, D. N. (2003). Bipolar disorder in adolescents. Epidemiology and suicidal behavior. In B. Geller & M. P. DelBello (Eds.), *Bipolar disorder in children and early adolescence* (pp. 7–24). New York: Guilford.

Lewis, M. (1994). Borderline disorders in children. *Child and Adolescent Psychiatric Clinics of North America, 3,* 31–42.

Lieberman, J. A. (2004a). Aripiprazole. In A. F. Schatzberg & C. B. Nemeroff (Eds.), *Textbook of psychopharmacology* (pp. 487–494). Arlington, VA: American Psychiatric Publishing.

Lieberman, J. A. (2004b). Quetiapine. In A. F. Schatzberg & C. B. Nemeroff (Eds.), *Textbook of psychopharmacology* (pp. 473–486). Arlington, VA: American Psychiatric Publishing.

Lieberman, D. Z. (2005, September). (letter). Bipolar depression and substance abuse. *Current Psychiatry, 4,* 11.

Lieberman, A. J., McEvoy, J. P., Perkins, D., & Hamer, R. H. (2005). Comparison of atypicals in first-episode psychpsis [Café]: a randomized, 52 week comparison of olanzapine, quetiapine, and risperidone. Summary report. 18th ECNP Congress. *European Neuropsychopharmacology, 15,* S526.

Lieberman, A. J., Stroup, T. S., McEvoy, J. P., Swartz, M. S., Rosenheck, R. A., Perkins, D. O. et al., for the Clinical Antipsychotic Trials of Intervention Effectiveness (CATIE) Investigators. (2005, September 22). Effectiveness of antipsychotic drugs in patients with chronic schizophrenia. *New England Journal of Medicine, 353,* 1209–1223.

Lieberman, A. J., Tollefson, G., Tohen, Green, A. I., Gur, R. E., et al., & GDH Study Group. (2003). Comparative: A efficacy and safety of atypical and conventional antipsychotics drugs in first-episode psychosis: Randomized, double-blind trial of olanzapine versus haloperidol. *American Journal of Psychiatry, 160,* 1396–1404.

Lin, P.-I., McInnis, M. G., Potash, J. B., Willour, V., MacKinnon, D. F., DePaulo, J. R., & Zandi, P. P. (2006, February). Clinical correlates and family aggregation of age at onset of bipolar disorder. *American Journal of Psychiatry, 163,* 240–246.

Lindenmayer, J. P., Czobor, P., Volavka, J., Citrome, L., Sheitman, B., McEvoy, J. P., et al. (2003). *American Journal Psychiatry, 160*, 290–296.

Lindsey, R. L., Kaplan, D., Koliatsos, V., Walter, J. K., & Sandson, N. S. (2003). (letter). Aripiprazole and extrapyramidal symptoms. *Journal of the American Academy of Child and Adolescent Psychiatry, 42*, 1269.

Linehan, M. M. (1993). *Skills training manual for treating borderline personality disorder.* New York: Guilford.

Lishman, W. A. (1998). *Organic psychiatry. The psychological consequences of cerebral disorder.* Oxford: Blackwell Science.

Lochman, J. E., Barry, T. D., & Pardini, D. A. (2003). Anger control training for aggressive youth. In A. E. Kazdin & J. R. Weisz (Eds.), *Evidence-based psychotherapies for children and adolescents* (pp. 263–281). New York: Guilford.

Loebel, A., Miceli, J., Chappel, P., & Siu, C. (2006, June). (letter). Eletrocardiographic changes with ziprasidone. *Journal of the American Academy of Child and Adolescent Psychiatry, 45*, 636–637.

Lohr, D., & Birmaher, B. (1995, January). Psychotic disorders. *Child and Adolescent Psychiatric Clinics of North America, 4*, 237–254.

Lou, H. C. (1998). Cerebral palsy and hypoxic-hemodynamic brain lesions in the newborn. In C. E. Coffey & R. A. Brimback (Eds.), *Textbook of pediatric neuropsychiatry.* Washington, DC: American Psychiatric Press.

Mack, A. H., Feldman, J. J., & Tsuang, M. T. (2002). A case of "pfropfschizophrenia": Kraepelin's bridge between neurodegenerative and neurodevelopmental conceptions of schizophrenia. *American Journal of Psychiatry, 159*, 1104–1110.

Malhotra, S., King, K. H., Welge, J. A., Brusman-Lovins, L., & McElroy, S. L. (2002). Venlafaxine treatment of binge-eating disorder associated with obesity: A series of 35 patients. *Journal of Clinical Psychiatry, 63*, 802–806.

Malhotra, A. K. (2005, March). Current limitations and future prospects in genetics. *Psychiatric Times*, 17–21.

Mann, S. C., Caroff, S. N., Campbell, E. C., & Greenstein, R. A. (2003, September). Identification and treatment of malignant catatonia. *Child and Adolescent Psychopharmacological News*, Ed. S. P. Kutcher, *8*(6), 7–9, 12.

Marangell, L. B., Yudofsky, S. C., & Silver, J. M. (1999). Psychopharmacology and electroconvulsive therapy. In R. E. Hales, S. C. Yudofsky, & J. A, Talbott (Eds.), *Textbook of psychiatry* (3rd ed.). Washington, DC: American Psychiatric Press.

Marder, S. R., Essock, S. M., Miller, A. L., Buchanan, R. W., Casey, D. E., Davis, J. M., et al. (2004). Physical health monitoring of patients with schizophrenia. *American Journal of Psychiatry, 161*, 1334–1349.

Marder, S. R., Glynn, S. M., Wirshing, W. C., Wirshing, D. A., Ross, D., Widmark, C., et al. (2003). Maintenance treatment of schizophrenia with risperidone or haloperidol: 2-year outcomes. *American Journal of Psychiatry, 160*, 1405–1412.

Marder, S. R., & Wirshing, D. A. (2004). Clozapine. In A. F. Schartzberg & C. B. Nemeroff (Eds.), *Textbook of psychopharmacology.* Arlington, VA: American Psychiatric Publishing.

Maria, B. L., & Bale. J. F. (2006). Infections of the nervous system. In J. H. Menkes, H. B. Sarnat, & B. L. Maria (Eds.), *Child neurology* (7th ed.). Philadelphia: Lippincott Williams & Wilkins.

Marin, R. S. (2005, August). (Guest editorial). A different take on motivation. *Clinical Psychiatric News, 33*, 15.

Martin, A., Blair, J., State, M., Leckman, J. F., & Scahill, L. (2006, June). (letter). Reply to Loebel, A., Miceli, J., Chappel, P., & Siu, C. (2006, June). (letter). Eletrocardiographic changes with ziprasidone. *Journal of the American Academy of Child and Adolescent Psychiatry, 45,* 638–639.

Matsumoto, A. M. (2001). The testis. In P. Felig & L. A. Frohman (Eds.), *Endocrinology and metabolism* (4th ed., pp. 635–705). New York: McGraw-Hill.

Mathews, M., Gratz, S., Adetunji, B., George, V., Mathews, M., & Basil, B. (2005, March). Antipsychotic-induced movement disorders: Evaluation and treatment. *Psychiatry, 2,* 36–41.

McClellan, J. (2004). Diagnostic interviews. In J. M. Wiener & M. K. Dulcan (Eds.), *Textbook of child and adolescent psychiatry* (pp. 137–148). Arlington, VA: American Psychiatric Publishing.

McClellan, J., Breiger, D., McCurry, C., & Hlastala, S. A. (2003). Premorbid functioning in early-onset psychotic disorders. *Journal of The American Academy of Child and Adolescent Psychiatry, 42,* 666–672.

McClellan, J., McCurry, C., Speltz, M. L., & Jones, K. (2002). Symptom factors in early-onset psychotic disorders. *Journal of the American Academy of Child and Adolescent Psychiatry, 41,* 791–798.

McClellan, J., & Werry, J. (1994). Practice parameters for the assessment and treatment of children and adolescents with schizophrenia. *Journal of the American Academy of Child and Adolescent Psychiatry, 33,* 1616–1635.

McClellan, J., & Werry, J. (1997). Practice parameters for the assessment and treatment of children and adolescents with schizophrenia. *Journal of the American Academy of Child and Adolescent Psychiatry, 36,* S77–S93.

McClure, E. B., Treland, J. E., Snow, et al. (2005). Deficits in social cognition and response flexibility in pediatric bipolar disorder. *American Journal of Psychiatry, 162,* 1644–1651.

McConville, B. J., Arvanitis, L. A., Thyrum, P. T., Foster, K. D., Sorter, M. T., Friedman, L. M., et al. (2000). Pharmacokinetics, tolerability, and clinical effectiveness of quetiapine fumarate: An open label trial in adolescents with psychotic disorders. *Journal of Clinical Psychiatry, 61,* 252–260.

McConville, B. J., & Sorter, M. T. (2004). Treatment challenges and safety considerations for antipsychotic use in children and adolescents. *Journal of Clinical Psychiatry, 65*(Suppl. 6), 20–29.

McCracken J. T., McGough J., Bhavik, S., Cronin, P., Hong, D., Aman, M. G., et al., & the Research Units on Pediatric Psychopharmacology Autism Network. (2002). Risperidone in children with autism and serious behavioral problems. *New England Journal of Medicine, 347,* 314–321.

McDougle, C. J. (2003, May). (CME Program). Introduction. In Advancing the treatment of pediatric psychotic and behavioral disorders (pp. 4–5). Faculty: C. J. McDougle, R. L. Hendren, L. Scahill, J. Biederman, & B. Cornblatt. *Medical Education Resources, 4.*

McDougle, C. J., Scahill, L., Aman, M. G. , McCracken, J. T., Tierney, E., Davies, M., et al. (2005). Risperidone for the core symptom domains of autism: Results from the Study by the Autism Network of the Research Units on Pediatric Psychopharmacology. *American Journal of Psychiatry, 162,* 1142–1148.

McDowell, D. M. (1999). MDMA, ketamine, GHB, and the "club drug" scene. In M. Galanter & H. D Kleber (Eds.), *Textbook of substance abuse treatment* (2nd ed.). Washington, DC: American Psychiatric Press.

McElroy, S. L., Arnold, L. M., Shapira, N A., Keck, P. E., Rosenthal, N. R., Karim, M. R., et al. (2003). Topiramate in the treatment of binge eating disorder associated with obesity: A randomized, placebo-controlled trial. *American Journal of Psychiatry, 160*, 255–261.

McElroy, S. L., & Keck, P. E. (2004). Topiramate. In A. F. Schatzberg & C. B. Nemeroff (Eds.), *Textbook of psychopharmacology* (3rd ed., pp. 627–636). Arlington, VA: American Psychiatric Publishing.

McEvoy, J. P., Lieberman, J. A., Stroup, T. S., Davis, S. M., Meltzer, H. Y., Rosenheck, R. A., Swartz, M. S., Perkins, D. O., Keefe, R. S.E., Davis, C. E., Severe, J., Hsiao, J. K., for the CATIE Investigators. (2006, April). Effectiveness of Clozapine Versus Olanzapine, Quetiapine, and Risperidone in Patients With Chronic Schizophrenia Who Did Not Respond to Prior Atypical Antipsychotic Treatment. *American Journal of Psychiatry, 163*, 600–610.

McNeil, D. E., Eisner, J. P., & Binder, R. L. (2001). (letter). Reply to the letter "The paradox of command hallucinations." *Psychiatric Services, 52*, 385–386.

Meltzer, H. Y. (2002). Suicidality in schizophrenia: A review of the evidence for risk factors and treatment options. *Current Psychiatry Reports, 4*, 279–283.

Menkes, J. H. (2006). Heredodegenerative diseases. In Menkes, J. H., Sarnat, H. B., & Maria, B. L. (Eds.), *Child neurology* (7th ed., pp. 163–226). Philadelphia: Lippincott Williams & Wilkins.

Merry, S. N., & Werry, J. S. (2001). Course and prognosis. In H. Remschnidt (Ed.), *Schizophrenia in children and Adolescents*. Cambridge University Press.

Miller, A. L., Hall, C. S., Buchanan, R. W., Buckley, P. F., Chiles, J. A., et al. (2004, April). The Texas Medication Algorithm Project Antipsychotic Algorithm for Schizophrenia: 2003 Update. *Journal of Clinical Psychiatry, 65*, 500–508.

Miller, F. G., & Lazowski, L. E. (1990, 2001). *The Adolescent SASSI-2 Manual. Identifying substance use disorders*. Springville, IN: The SASSI Institute.

Mills, N. P., DelBello, M. P., Adler, C. M., & Strakowski, S. M. (2005). MRI analysis of cerebellar vermal abnormalities in bipolar disorder. *American Journal of Psychiatry, 162*, 1530–1532.

Moreno, D., Burdalo, M., Reig, S., Parellada, M., Zabala. A., Desco, M., Baca-Baldomero, E., & Arango, C. (2005, November). Structural neuroimaging in adolescents with first psychotic episode. *Journal of the American Academy of Child and Adolescent Psychiatry, 44*, 1151–1157.

Morrison, J. A., Cottingham, E. M., & Barton, B. A. (2002). Metformin for weight loss in pediatric patients taking psychotropic medications. *American Journal of Psychiatry, 159*, 655–657

Mortensen, P. B., Pedersen, C. B., Melbye, M., Mors, O., & Ewald, H. (2003, December). Individual and family risk factors for bipolar affective disorders in Denmark. *Archives of General Psychiatry, 60*, 1209–1215.

Mullen, J. (2004). *Manual of rating scales for the assessment of mood disorders*. Wilmington, DE: AstraZeneca Pharmaceuticals LP.

Murphy, K. C. (2002, February). Schizophrenia and velo-cardio-facial syndrome. *The Lancet, 359*, 426–430.

Mustillo, S., Worthman, C., Erkanli, A., Keeler, G., Angold, A., & Costello, E. J. (2003). Obesity and psychiatric disorder: Developmental trajectories. *Pediatrics, 111*, 851–859.

Nagera, H. (1966). Early childhood disturbances, the infantile neurosis, and the adulthood disturbances. New York: International Universities Press.

Nasrallah, H. A. (2005, December). (Commentary). The CATIE study: Effectiveness is in the eye of the beholder. *Journal of Psychotic Disorders*, Reviews and Commentaries, *9*, 17.

Nasrallah, H. H. (2006, February). CATIE'S surprises. In antipsychotics' square-off, were there any winners or losers? *Current Psychiatry*, *5*, 48–65.

Nasrallah, H. A., & Newcomer, J. W. (2004, October). Atypical antipsychotics and metabolic dysregulation. Evaluating the risk/benefit equation and improving the standard of care. *Journal of Clinical Psychopharmacology*, *24*, S7–S14.

Nasrallah, H. A., & Smeltzer, D. J. (2002). *Contemporary diagnosis and management of patients with schizophrenia*. Newtown, PA: Handbooks in Health Care.

Navarro, V. J., & Senior, J. R. (2006, February 16). Drug-related hepatotoxicity. *The New England Journal of Medicine*, *354*, 731–739.

Neumeister, A., Charney, D. S., & Drevets, W. C. (2005). Hippocampus. C. A. Tamminga (Ed.), Images in Neuroscience. *American Journal of Psychiatry* (Special issue), *162*, 1057.

Newcomer J. W., Haupt, D. W., Fuetola, R., Melson, A. K., Schweiger, J. A., Cooper, B. P., et al. (2002). Abnormalities in glucose regulation during antipsychotic treatment of schizophrenia. *Archives of General Psychiatry*, *59*, 337–345.

Newcomer, J. W., Nasrallah, H. A., & Loebel, A. D. (2004). The atypical antipsychotic therapy and metabolic issues national survey. *Journal of Clinical Psychopharmacology*, *24*, S1–S6.

Nguyen, C. T., Yu, B., & Maguire, G. (2003). Update in atypicals. Preemptive tactics to reduce weight gain. *Current Psychiatry*, *l2*, 58–62.

Nicolson, R., Lenane, M., Brookner, F., Gochman, P., Kumra, S., Spechler, L., et al. (2001, July/August). Children and adolescents with psychotic disorder not otherwise specified: A 2- to 8-year follow-up study. *Comprehensive Psychiatry*, *42*, 319–325.

Nicolson, R., Lenane, M., Singaracharlu, S., Malaspina, D., Giedd, J. N., Hamburger, S. D., et al. (2000). Premorbid speech and language impairments in childhood-onset schizophrenia. Association with risk factors. *American Journal of Psychiatry*, *157*, 794–800.

Nicolson, R., & Rapoport, J. (1999). Childhood-onset schizophrenia: Rare but worth studying. *Biological Psychiatry*, *46*, 1418–1428.

Nierenberg, A. A., Ostacher, M. J., Calabrese, et al. (2006, February). Treatment-resistant bipolar depression: A STEP-BD equipoise randomized effectiveness trial of antidepressant augmentation with lamotrigine, inositol, or risperidone. *American Journal of Psychiatry*, *163*, 210–216.

Nierenberg, J., Salisbury, D. F., Levitt, J. J., David, E. A., McCarley, R. W., & Shenton, M. E. (2005). Reduced left angular gyrus volume in first-episode schizophrenia. *American Journal of Psychiatry*, *162*, 1539–1541.

Nnadi, C. U., Goldberg, J. F., & Malhotra, A. K. (2005). Genetics and psychopharmacology: Prospects for individualized treatment. *Essential Psychopharmacology*, *6*, 193–208.

Noaghiul, S., & Hibbeln, J. R. (2003, December). Cross national comparisons of seafood consumption and rates of bipolar disorders. *American Journal of Psychiatry*, *160*, 2222–2227.

Oepen, G. (2002). Polypharmacy in schizophrenia. In S. N. Ghaemi (Ed.), *Polypharmacy in psychiatry* (pp. 101–132). New York: Marcel Dekker.

Otnow Lewis, D. (1996). Conduct disorder. In M. Lewis (Ed.), *Child and adolescent psychiatry: A comprehensive textbook* Philadelphia: Williams & Wilkins.

Papolos, D. F. (2003). Bipolar disorder and comorbid disorders: The case for a dimensional nosology. In M. P. DelBello & B. Geller (Eds.), *Bipolar disorder in childhood and early adolescence.* New York: Guilford.

Papolos, F. P., & Papolos, J. (2002). *The bipolar child. The definitive and reassuring guide to childhood's most misunderstood disorder.* New York: Books New York.

Pappadopulos, E. A., Guelzow, B. T., Wong, C., Ortega, M., & Jensen, P. S. (2004). A review of the growing evidence base for pediatric psychopharmacology. *Child and Adolescent Psychiatric Clinics of North America, 13,* 817–855.

Pappadopulos, E., Jensen, P. S., Schur , S. B., MacIntyre II, J. C., Ketner, S., Van Order, K. D., et al. (2002). "Real world" atypical antipsychotic prescribing practices in public child and adolescent inpatient settings. *Schizophrenia Bulletin, 28,* 111–121.

Pappadopulos, E., MacIntyre II, J. C., Crismon, M. L., Findling, R. L., Malone, R. P., Derivan, A., et al. (2003). Treatment recommendations for the use of antipsychotics for aggressive youth (TRAAY). Part II. *Journal of the American Academy of Child and Adolescent Psychiatry, 42,* 145–161.

Park, M. K., & Troxler, R. G. (2002). *Pediatric cardiology for practitioners* (4th ed.). St. Louis, MO: Mosby.

Parker G. F. (2002). (letter). Clozapine and borderline personality disorder. *Psychiatric Services, 53,* 348–349.

Patel. N. C., Crismon, M. L., Hoagwood, K., & Jensen, P. (2005). Unanswered questions regarding atypical antipsychotic use in aggressive children and adolescents. *Journal of Child & Adolescent Psychopharmacology, 15,* 270–284.

Patel, N. C., Sanchez, R. J., Johnsrud, M. T., & Crismon, M. L. (2002). Trends in antipsychotic use in a Texas Medicaid population of children and adolescents. *Journal of Child and Adolescent Psychopharmacology, 12,* 221–229.

Patel, N. C., DelBello, M. P., Bryan, H. S, Adler, C. M., Kowatch, R. A., Stanford, K., & Strakowski, S. M. (2006, March). Open-label lithium for the treatment of adolescents with bipolar depression. *Journal of the American Academy of Child and Adolescent Psychiatry, 45,* 289–297.

Pavuluri, M. N., Birmaher, B., & Naylor, M. W. (2005). Pediatric bipolar disorder: A review of the past 10 years. *Journal of the American Academy of Child and Adolescent Psychiatry, 44,* 846–871.

Pavuluri, M. N., Henry, D. B., Devineni, B., Carbray, J. A., Naylor, M. W., & Janicak, P. G. (2004). The pharmacotherapy algorithm for stabilization and maintenance of pediatric bipolar disorder. *Journal of the American Academy of Child and Adolescent Psychiatry, 43,* 859–867.

Pavuluri, M. N., Herbener, E., & Sweeney, J. (2004, May). Psychotic symptoms in pediatric bipolar disorder. *Journal of Affective Disorders, 80,* 19–28.

Pavuluri, M. N., Janicak, P. G., & Carbray, J. (2002). (letter). Topiramate plus risperidone for controlling weight gain and symptoms in preschool mania. *Journal of Child and Adolescent Psychopharmacology, 12,* 271–273.

Pavuluri, M. N., & Naylor, M. W. (2005, May). Multi-modal integrated treatment for youth with bipolar disorder. *Psychiatric Times, 12,* 24–27.

Pavuluri, M. N., Schenkel, L. S., Aryal, S., et al. (2006, February). Neurocognitive function in unmedicated manic and medicated euthymic pediatric bipolar patients. *American Journal of Psychiatry, 163,* 286–293.

Pearlson, G. D. (2004). Neuroimaging findings are different in schizophrenia and bipolar disorders. *CON. The Journal of Psychotic Disorders: Reviews & Commentaries, 8*(3), 15.

Perisse, D., Amoura, Z., Cohen, D., et al.(2003). Case study: Effectiveness of plasma exchange. *The American Academy of Child and Adolescent Psychiatry, 42,* 497–499.

Perlis, R. H., Brown, E., Baker, R. W., & Nierenberg, A. A. (2006, February). Clinical features of bipolar depression versus major depressive disorder in large multicenter trials. *American Journal of Psychiatry, 163,* 225–231.

Perlis, R. H., Ostacher, M. J., Patel, J. K., Marangell, L. B., Zhang, H., Wisniewski, S. R., et al. (2006, February). Predictors of recurrence in bipolar disorders: Primary outcomes from the systematic treatment enhancement program for bipolar disorder (STEP-BD). *American Journal of Psychiatry, 163,* 217–224.

Phillips, L. J., Leicester, S. B., O'Dwyer, L. E., Francey, S. M., Koutsogiannis, J., Abdel-Baki, A., et al. (2002). The PACE clinic: Identification and management of young people at "ultra" high risk of psychosis. *Journal of Psychiatric Practice, 8,* 255–266.

Physicians' Desk Reference (2004) (58th ed.). Montvale NJ: Thompson PDR

Physicians' Desk Reference (2006) (60th ed.). Montvale NJ: Thompson PDR

Pierre, J. M., Shnayder, I., Wirshing, D. A., & Wirshing, W. C. (2004). (letter). Intranasal Quetiapine Abuse. *American Journal of Psychiatry, 161,* 1718.

Pierre, J. M., Wirshing, D. A., & Wirshing, W. C. (2004, August). High-dose antipsychotics. Desperation or data driven? *Current Psychiatry, 3,* 30–37.

Pies, R. (1997). (Editorial). Must we now consider SSRIs neuroleptics? *Journal of Clinical Psychopharmacology, 17,* 443–445.

Pies, R. (2002, August). Seized by psychosis. Clinical puzzles. *Psychiatric Times,* 16–18.

Pies, R. (2003, April). The colorful masquerader. *Psychiatric Times, XX,* 16–17.

Pilowsky, D. (1986). Problems in determining the presence of hallucinations in children. In D. Pilowsky & W. Chambers (Eds.), *Hallucinations in children.* Washington, DC: American Psychiatric Press.

Pilowsky, D. (1998). Problems in determining the presence of hallucinations in children. In D. Pilowsky & W. Chambers (Eds.), *Hallucinations in children.* Washington, DC: American Psychiatric Press.

Pinninti, N. R., & Sosland, M. (2004, July). Delusions: How cognitive therapy helps patients let go. *Current Psychiatry, 3,* 98.

Poulton, R., Caspi, A., Moffitt, T. E., Cannon, M., Murray, R., & Harrington, H. L. (2000). Children's self-reported psychotic symptoms and adult schizophreniform disorder. *Archives of General Psychiatry, 57,* 1053–1057.

Powell, H., Tindall, R., Schultz, P., Paa, D., O'Brien, J., & Lampert, P. (1975). Adrenoleukodystrophy. *Archives of Neurology, 32,* 250–260.

Powers, P. S., Simpson, H., & McCornick, T. (2005a, April). Anorexia nervosa and psychosis. *Primary Psychiatry, 12,* 39–45.

Powers, P. S., Simpson, H., & McCornick, T. (2005b, April). Anorexia nervosa and psychosis. *Primary Psychiatry, 12,* 39–45.

Preskorn, S. H. (2004, August). Why patients may not respond to usual recommended dosages. 3 variables to consider when prescribing antipsychotics. *Current Psychiatry, 3,* 38–43.

Preskorn, S. H., & Flockhart, D. (2004). 2004 guide to psychiatric drug interactions. *Primary Psychiatry, 11,* 39–60.

Procyshyn, R. M., Ihsan, N., & Thompson, D. (2001). A comparison of smoking behaviors between patients treated with clozapine and depot neuroleptics. *International Clinical Psychopharmacology, 16,* 291–294.

Pryse-Phillips, W. (2003). *Companion to clinical neurology* (2nd ed.). Oxford: Oxford University Press.

Purdon S. E., Jones, B. D. W., Stip, E., Labelle, A., Addington, D., David, S. R., et al. (2000). The Canadian Collaborative Group for Research on Cognitive in Schizophrenia. Neuropsychological change in early phase schizophrenia during 12 months of treatment with olanzapine, risperidone, or haloperidol. *Archives of General Psychiatry, 57,* 249–258.

Raedler, T. J., Knable, M. B., Jones, D. . W., Urbina, R. A., Gorey, J. G., et al. (2003). Endocrinological challenge studies in patients with schizophrenia have reported a greater growth hormone response to cholinergic tone. *American Journal of Psychiatry, 160,* 118–127.

Rao, U. (2003). Sleep and other biologic rhythms. In M. P. DelBello & B. Geller (Eds.), *Bipolar disorder in childhood and early adolescence.* New York: Guilford Press.

Ratzoni, G., Gothele, D., Brand-Gothele, A., Reidman, J., Kikinson, L., Gal, G., et al. (2002). Weight gain associated with olanzapine and risperidone in adolescent patients: A comparative prospective study. *Journal of the American Academy of Child and Adolescent Psychiatry, 43,* 337–343.

Ray, W. A., & Meador, K. G. (2002). Antipsychotics and sudden death: Is thioridazine the only bad actor? *British Journal of Psychiatry, 180,* 483–484.

Reddy, R., Smith, M., & Robinson, D. (2005, April). (letter). Non-psychotic hallucinations. *Psychiatry, 2,* 11–12.

Reimherr, J. P., & McClellan, J. M. (2004). Diagnostic challenges in children and adolescents with psychotic disorders. *Journal of Clinical Psychiatry, 65*(Suppl. 6), 5–11.

Reinherz, H. Z., Paradis, A. D., Giaconia, R. M., Stashwick, C. K., & Fitzmaurice, G. (2003, December). Childhood and adolescent predictors of major depression in the transition to adulthood. *American Journal of Psychiatry, 160,* 2141–2147.

Remschmidt, H., Martin, M., Henninghausen, K., & Schulz, E. (2001). Treatment and rehabilitation (pp.192–267). In H. Remschmidt (Ed.), *Schizophrenia in children and adolescents.* Cambridge, UK: Cambridge University Press.

Resnick, P. J., & Knoll, J. (2005, November). Faking it. How to detect malingered psychosis. *Current Psychiatry, 4,* 12–25.

Rey, J. M., Martin, A., & Krabman, P. (2004, October). Is the party over? Cannabis and juvenile psychiatric disorder: The past 10 years. *Journal of the American Academy of Child and Adolescent Psychiatry, 43,* 1194–1205.

Rizzo, M., & Eslinger, P. J. (2004). *Principles and practice of behavioral neurology and neuropathology.* Philadelphia: W.B. Saunders.

Robinson, D. G., Woerner, M. G., McMeniman, M., Medelowitz, A., & Bilder, R. M. (2004). Symptomatic and functional recovery from a first episode of schizophrenia or schizoaffective disorder. *American Journal of Psychiatry, 161,* 473–479.

Robinson, R. G., & Jorge, R. E. (2005). Mood disorders. In J. M. Silver, T. W. McAllister, & S. C. Yudofsky (Eds.), *Textbook of traumatic brain injury* (pp. 201–212). Arlington, VA: American Psychiatric Publishing.

Roe, C. M., Odell, K. W., & Herderson, R. R. (2003). Concomitant use of antipsychotics and drugs that may prolong the QT interval. *Journal of Psychopharmacology, 23,* 197–200.

Rogers, D. (2002, January). Comparing atypical antipsychotics. *Psychiatric Times, XIX*, 40–43.

Rosack, J. (2002, July 19). Atypical antipsychotics affect brain structures differently. *Psychiatric News, 37*, 23.

Rosebush, P., I., & Mazurek, M. F. (2001, June). Identification and treatment of neuroleptic malignant syndrome. *Child and Adolescent Psychopharmacology News, 6*, 1–6.

Rosenbaum-Asarnow, J., & Asarnow, R. F. (2003). Childhood-onset schizophrenia. In E. J. Masch & R. A. Barkley (Eds.), *Child psychopathology* (2nd ed., pp. 455–485). New York: Guildford.

Rosenstock, J. (2006, February). Make tardive dyskinesia passé with PASST principle. *Current Psychiatry, 5*, 101–102.

Ross, R. G. (2006, July). Psychotic and manic-like symtoms during stimulant treatment of attention deficit hyperactivity disorder. *American Journal of Psychiatry, 163*, 1149–1152.

Rosso, I. M., Cannon, T. D., Huttunen, T., Huttunen, M. O., Londqvist, J., & Gasperoni, T. L. (2000). Obstetric risk factors for early-onset schizophrenia in a Finnish birth cohort. *American Journal of Psychiatry, 157*, 801–807.

Rothner, A. D. (1999). Headaches in children and adolescents. *Child and Adolescent Psychiatric Clinics of North America, 8*, 727–745. W B Saunders.

Ruigomez, A., Garcia Rodriguez, L. A., Dev, V. J., Arellano, F., & Raniwala, J. (2000). Are schizophrenia or antipsychotic drugs a risk factor for cataracts? *Epidemiology, 11*, 620–623.

Rund, B. R., Melle, I., Friis, S., Larsen, T. K., Midboe, L. J., Opjordsmoen, S., et al. Neurocognitive dysfunction in first-episode psychosis: Correlates with symptoms, premorbid adjustment and duration of untreated psychosis. *American Journal of Psychiatry, 161*, 466–472.

Ryan, M. C. M., Collins, P., & Thakore, J. H. (2003). Impaired fasting glucose tolerance in first-episode, drug-naïve patients with schizophrenia. *American Journal of Psychiatry, 160*, 284–289.

Ryan, R. (2001, December). Recognizing psychosis in nonverbal patients with developmental disabilities. *Psychiatric Times*, 51–52.

Ryback, R., Brodsky, L., & Littman, R. (2005, January). Topiramate as an adjunctive treatment in psychiatric patients with diabetes. *Primary Psychiatry, 12*, 57–60.

Saha, A. R., McQuade, R. D., Carson, W. H., et al. (2001, July 1–6). *Efficacy and safety of aripiprazole and risperidone vs. placebo in patients with schizophrenia and schizoaffective disorders.* Poster session presented at the 7th World Congress of Biological Psychiatry Meeting, Berlin, Germany.

Saito, E., Correll, C. U., Gallelli, K., McMeniman, M., Parikh, U. H., Malhotra, A. K., & Kafantaris, V. (2004). A prospective study of hyperprolactinemia in children and adolescents with atypical antipsychotic agents. *Journal of Child and Adolescent Psychopharmacology, 14*, 350–358.

Saito, E., Correll, U. C., & Kafantaris, V. (2003). Hyperprolactinemia in children and adolescents treated with atypical antipsychotics [Abstract]. *Journal of Child and Adolescent Psychopharmacology, 13*, 411–424.

Sallee, F. R., Gilbert, D. L., Vinks, A. A., Miceli, J. J., Robarge, L., & Wilner, K. (2003). Pharmacodynamics of ziprasidone in children and adolescents: impact on dopamine transmission. *Journal of The American Academy of Child and Adolescent Psychiatry, 42*, 902–907.

Salvatoni, A. (2002). Surgical treatment In W. Burniat, T. Cole, I. Lissau, & E. Poskitt (Eds.), *Child and adolescent obesity.* Cambridge University Press.

Samuel, R. Z., & Mittenberg, W. (2005, December). Determination of malingering in disability evaluations. *Primary Psychiatry, 12,* 60–68.

Sandson, N. B. (2003). *Drug interaction casebook. The cytochrome P450 system and beyond.* Arlington, VA: American Psychiatric Publishing.

Sassi, R. B., Stanley, J. A., Axelson, D., Brambilla, P., Nicoletti, M. A., & Keshavan, M. S., et al. (2005). Reduced NAA levels in the dorsolateral prefrontal cortex of young bipolar patients. *American Journal of Psychiatry, 162,* 2109–2115.

Sauer, J., & Howard, R. (2002). (letter). The beef with atypical antipsychotics. *American Journal Psychiatry, 159,* 1249.

Schaffer, J. L., & Ross, R. G. (2002). Childhood-onset schizophrenia: premorbid and prodromal diagnostic and treatment histories. *Journal of the American Academy of Child and Adolescent Psychiatry, 41,* 538–545.

Scharko, A. M., Baker, E. H., Kothari, P., Khattak, H., & Lancaster, D. (2006, January). Case study: Delirium in an adolescent girl with human immunodeficiency virus-associated dementia. *Journal of the American Academy of Child & Adolescent Psychiatry, 45,* 104–108.

Schaumburg, H. H., Powers, J. M., Raine, C. S., Suzuki, K., & Richardson, E. P. (1975). Adrenoleukodystrophy. *Archives of Neurology, 32,* 577–591.

Schieveld, J. N. M., & Leentjens, A. F. G. (2005, April). Delirium in severely ill young children in the pediatric intensive care unit. *Journal of the American Academy of Child and Adolescent Psychiatry, 44,* 392–394.

Schopick, D. (2005, February). (letter). Donazepil and tardive dyskinesia. *American Journal of the American Academy of Child and Adolescent Psychiatry, 44,* 112.

Schreier, H. A. (1999). Hallucination in nonpsychotic children: more common than we think? *Journal of the American Academy of Child and Adolescent Psychiatry, 38,* 623–625.

Schubert, E. W., & McNeil, T. F. (2004). Prospective study of neurological abnormalities in offspring of women with psychosis: Birth to adulthood. *American Journal of Psychiatry, 161,* 1030–1037.

Schultz, S. C., Olson, S., & Kotlyar, M. (2004). Olanzapine. In A. F. Schatzberg & C. B. Nemeroff (Eds.), *Textbook of psychopharmacology* (pp. 457–472). Arlington, VA: American Psychiatric Publishing.

Schur, S. B., Sikich, L., Findling, R. L., Malone, R. P., Crismon, M. L., Derivan, A. et al. (2003). Treatment recommendations for the use of antipsychotics for aggressive youth (TRAY), Part I: A review. *Journal of the American Academy of Child and Adolescent Psychiatry, 42,* 132–144.

Schwartz, J. E., Fennig, S., Tanenberg-Karant, M. Carlson, G., Craig, T., Galambos, N., et al. (2000). Congruence of diagnoses 2 years after a first-admission diagnosis of psychosis. *Archives of General Psychiatry, 57,* 593–600.

Schwengel, D. (2003). Pain management. In C. D. Rudolph, A. M. Rudolph, M. K. Hostetter, G. E. Lister, & N. J. Siegel (Eds.), *Rudolph's pediatrics* (21st ed., pp. 341–348). New York: McGraw Hill.

Schwimmer, J. B., Burwinkle, T. M., & Varni, J. W. (2003, April). Health-related quality of life of severely obese children and adolescents. *Journal of The American Medical Association, 289,* 1813–1819.

Scott. C. L., & Resnick, P. J. (2002, April). Assessing risk of violence in psychiatric patients. *Psychiatric Times,* 40–43.

Scott, J., & Pope, M. (2002). Nonadherence with mood stabilizers: Prevalence and predictors. *Journal of Clinical Psychiatry, 63*, 384–390.

Seay, A. R., & De Vivo, D. C. (2003). Viral infections of the central nervous system. In C. D. Rudolph, A. M. Rudolph, M. K. Hostetter, G. Lister, & N. J. Siegel (Eds.), *Rudolph's pediatrics* (21st ed., pp. 2305–2317). New York: McGraw-Hill.

Seeman, M. V. (2004). Gender differences in the prescribing of antipsychotic drugs. *American Journal of Psychiatry, 161*, 1324–1333.

Semper, T. F., & McClellan, J. M. (2003). The psychotic child. *Child and Adolescent Psychiatric Clinics of North America, 12*, 679– 691.

Senecky, Y., Lobel, D., Diamond, G. W., et al. (2002), Isolated orofacial dyskinesia: a methylphenidate-induced movement disorder. *Pediatric Neurology, 27*, 224–226.

Sharma, V. (2003). (letter). Treatment-emergent tardive dyskinesia with quetiapine in mood disorders. *Journal of Clinical Psychopharmacology, 23*, 415–417.

Shaw, J. A., Egeland, J. A., Endicott, J., Allen, C. R., & Hostetter, A. M. (2005, November). A 10-year prospective study of prodromal patterns for bipolar disorder among Amish youth. *Journal of the American Academy of Child and Adolescent Psychiatry, 44*, 1104–1117.

Shelton, M. D., & Calabrese, J. R. (2004). Lamotrigine. In A. F. Schatzberg & C. B. Nemeroff (Eds.), *Textbook of psychopharmacology*. Arlington, VA: American Psychiatric Publishing.

Shelton, R. C., Tollefson, G. D., Tohen, M., Stahl, S., Gannon, K. S., Jacobs, T. G., Buras, W. R., Bymaster, F. P., Zhang, W., Spencer, K. A., Feldman, P. D., & Meltzer, H. Y. (2001, January). A novel augmentation strategy for resistant major depression. *American Journal of Psychiatry, 158*, 131–134.

Shirts, B. H., & Nimgaonkar, V. (2004, June). The genes for schizophrenia: Finally a breakthrough? The boundaries of schizophrenia: Overlap with bipolar disorders. In R. O. Friedel & D. L. Evans (Eds.), *Current Psychosis and Therapeutic Reports* (Vol. *2*, pp. 57–66).

Shores, L. E. (2005, March). Normalization of risperidone-induced hyperprolactinemia with the addition of aripiprazole. *Psychiatry 2005*, 42–45.

Shorter oxford english dictionary on historical principles (5th ed.). (2002). Oxford: Oxford University Press.

Sikich, L., Hamer, R., Malekpour, A. H., Sheitman, B. B., & Lieberman, J. A. (2001, December 9–13). *Double-blind trial comparing risperidone, olanzapine and haloperidol in the treatment of psychotic children and adolescents*. Poster session at the 40th Annual Meeting of the American College of Neuropsychopharmacology (ACNP), Wikoloa, Hawaii.

Silva, R. R. (2005, September). (editorial). Youth depression, treatments, and science. *Primary Psychiatry, 12*, 31–32.

Silva, R. R., Gabbay, V., Minami, H., Munoz-Silva, D., & Alonso, C. (2005, September). When to use antidepressant medication in youths. *Primary Psychiatry, 12*, 42–50.

Silva, R. R., Munoz, D. M., Alpert, M., Perlmutter, I. R., & Diaz, J. (1999). Neuroleptic malignant syndrome in children and adolescents. *Journal of the American Academy of Child and Adolescent Psychiatry, 38*, 187–194.

Siris, S. G., & Bermanzhon, P. C. (2003). Two models of psychiatric rehabilitation: a need for clarity and integration. *Journal of Psychiatric Practice, 19*, 171–175.

Slewa-Younan, S., Gordon, E., Harris, A. W., Haig, A. R., Brown, K. J., Flor-Henry, P., & Williams, L. M. (2004, September). Sex differences in functional connectivity in first-episode and chronic schizophrenia patients. *American Journal of Psychiatry, 161*, 1595–1602.

Snyder, P. J. (2001). Diseases of the anterior pituitary. In P. Felig & L. A. Frohman (Eds.), *Endocrinology and metabolism* (4th ed., pp. 173–216). New York: McGraw-Hill.

Snyder, R., Turgay, A., Aman, M., M., Binder, C., Fisman, S., Carroll, A., et al. (2002). Effects of risperidone on conduct and disruptive behavior disorders in children with subaverage IQs. *Journal of the American Academy of Child and Adolescent Psychiatry, 41,* 1026–1036.

Sobin, C., Kiley-Brabeck, K., & Karayiorgou, M. (2005, June). Lower prepulse inhibition in children with the 22q11 deletion syndrome. *American Journal of Psychiatry, 162,* 1090–1099.

Soto, O., & Murphy, T. K. (2003). The immune system and bipolar affective disorder. In M. P. DelBello & B. Geller (Eds.), *Bipolar disorder in childhood and early adolescence* (pp. 193–214). New York: Guilford.

Souza, O., Moll, J., & Eslinger, P. J. (2004). Neuropsychological assessment. In M. Rizzo & P. J. Eslinger (Eds.), *Principles and Practice of Behavioral Neurology and Neuropsychology.* Saunders.

Sporn, A., & Rapoport, J. L. (2001, April). Childhood onset schizophrenia. Mini-review. *Child and Adolescent Psychopharmacology News,* 1–6.

Sporn, A. L., Greenstein, D. K., Gogtay, N., Jeffries, N. O., Lenane, M., Gochman, P., et al. (2003, December). Progressive brain volume loss during adolescence in childhood-onset schizophrenia. *American Journal of Psychiatry, 160,* 2168–2189.

Staat, M. A. (2003). Syphilis. In C. D. Rudolph, A. M. Rudolph, M. K. Hostetter, G. Lister, & N. J. Siegel (Eds.), *Rudolph's pediatrics* (21st ed., pp. 1002–1005). New York: McGraw-Hill.

Stahl, S. M. (2006, February). A rash proposal for treating bipolar disorder. *Current Psychiatry, 5,* 92–100.

Stanilla, J. K., & Simpson, G. M. (2004). Drugs to treat extrapyramidal side effects. In A. F. Schatzberg & C. B. Nemeroff (Eds.), *Textbook of psychopharmacology* (pp. 519–544). Arlington, VA: American Psychiatric Publishing.

Steinberg, A., Brooks, J., & Remtulla, T. (2003). Youth hate crimes: Identification, prevention, and intervention. *American Journal of Psychiatry, 160,* 979–989.

Steiner, H. (2004). (CME program). Symptoms- and diagnosis-based treatment strategies with antipsychotic against aggression. Recommendations on employing antipsychotics in children and adolescents (REACH). Sponsored by the Dannemiller Memorial Educational Foundation & Medical DecisionPoint, educational grant from Janssen Medical Affairs, LLC. Dannemiller Foundation, San Antonio, TX.

Steiner, H., Carrion, V., Plattner, B., & Koopman, C. (2003). Dissociative symptoms in post-traumatic stress disorder: Diagnosis and treatment. *Child and Adolescent Psychiatric Clinics of North America, 12,* 231–249.

Steiner, H., Saxena, K., & Chang, K. (2004, July). The pharmacological treatment of primary and secondary disorders of aggression. *Child and Adolescent Psychopharmacology News, 9,* 1–5.

Sternbach, H. (2003). Serotonin syndrome. How to identify and treat dangerous interactions. *Current Psychiatry, 2,* 14–24.

Stigler, K. A., Potenza, M. N., & McDougle, C. J. (2001). Tolerability profile of atypical antipsychotics in children and adolescents. *Pediatric Drugs, 3,* 927–942.

Stoll, A. L. (2005, December). In session with Andrew L. Stoll. *Primary Psychiatry, 12,* 24–27.

Strahl, M. O., Lewis, N. D C. (1972). *Differential diagnosis in clinical psychiatry. The lectures of Paul H. Hoch, M. D.* Science House.

Strakowski, S. M. (2003, June). How to avoid ethnic bias when diagnosing schizophrenia. *Current Psychiatry, 2*, 72–82.

Strakowski, S. M. (2003a, December 8,). *Safety and tolerability: Using antipsychotics in bipolar maintenance.* Presentation at The Role of New Antipsychotics in the Treatment of Bipolar Disorder, Convened at the American College of Neuropsychopharmacology, San Juan, Puerto Rico. *Advanced Mental Health Expert Opinion Series, UCLA, Neuropsychiatric Institute, 1*, 49–67.

Strakowski, S. M. (2003b, January). Schizoaffective disorder. Which symptoms should be treated first? *Current Psychiatry*, 22–29.

Strakowski, S. M. (2004). Neuroimaging findings are different in schizophrenia and bipolar disorders. PRO. *The Journal of Psychotic Disorders: Reviews and Commentaries, 8*, 3, 14.

Strakowski, S. M., Adler, C. M., Holland, S. K., Miles, N. P., DelBello, M. P., & Eliassen, J. C. (2005). Abnormal fMRI brain activation in euthymic bipolar disorder patients during a counting stroop interference test. *American Journal of Psychiatry, 162*, 1697–1705.

Straus, S. M. J. M., Bleumink, G. S., Dieleman, J. P., van der Lei, J., 't Jong, G. W., Kingma, H., et al. (2004, June). Antipsychotics and the risk of sudden cardiac death. *Archives of Internal Medicine, 164*, 1293–1297.

Stubbe, D. E., & Scahill, L. (2002, October). Critical issues in the use of psychotropic medication and prolonged QTc. *Child and Adolescent Psychopharmacology News. 7*, 6–7, 10–12.

Styne, D. M., & Schoenfeld-Warden, N. (2003). Obesity. In C. D. Rudolph, A. M. Rudolph, M. K. Hostetter, G. Lister, & N. J. Siegel (Eds.), *Rudolph's pediatrics* (21st ed., pp. 2136–2142). New York: McGraw-Hill.

Sudak, D. M. (2004, September). Cognitive-behavioral therapy for schizophrenia. *Journal of Psychiatric Practice, 10*, 331–333.

Suppes, T., Dennehy, E. B., Hirschfeld, F. M. A., Altshuler, L., Bowden, C. L., et al. (2005, July). The Texas Implementation of Medication Algorithms. Update on Algorithms for Treatment of Bipolar Disorders. *Journal of Clinical Psychiatry, 66*, 870–886.

Sussman, N. (2005, September). (editorial). Why did this happen to me? *Primary Psychiatry, 12*, 11.

Swain, J. E., Leckman, J. F., & Volkmar, F. R. (2005, November). The wolf boy. Reactive attachment disorder in an adolescent boy. *Psychiatry, 2*, 55–61.

Swann, A. C. (2006, February). (Editorial). What is bipolar disorder? *American Journal of Psychiatry, 163*, 177–179.

Swartz, C. M. (2003, January). Antipsychotics as thought simplifiers. *Psychiatric Times, XX*, 12–14.

Swartz, C. M. (2004, October). Antipsychotic psychosis. *Psychiatric Times*, 17–18, 19–20.

Swinton M. (2001). Clozapine and severe borderline personality disorder. *Journal of Forensic Psychiatry, 12*, 580–591.

Tamminga, C. A. (2003). Schizophrenia, V. Images in psychiatry. *American Journal of Psychiatry, 160*, 1578.

Tamminga, C. A. (2005). The cerebellum. *American Journal of Psychiatry, 162*, 1253.

Tandon, R., & Jibson, M. D. (2001). Pharmacologic treatment of schizophrenia: what the future holds. *CNS Spectrums, 6*, 980–986.

Tandon, R., & Jibson, M. D. (2005, December). Applying available evidence to the real life pharmacotherapy of schizophrenia. Parameters of reasonable care. *CNS News*, 7(Special ed.), 91–94.

Tandon, R., Taylor, S. F., DeQuardo, J. R., Eiser, A., Jibson, M. D., & Goldman, M. (1999). The cholinergic system in schizophrenia reconsidered: Anticholinergic modulation of sleep and symptom profiles. *Neuropsychopharmacology, 21*, S189–S202.

Tanguay, P. E. (2000). Pervasive developmental disorders: A 10-year review. *Journal of the American Academy of Child Adolescent Psychiatry, 39*, 1079–1095.

Tantam, D. (2003). The challenge of adolescents and adults with Asperger's syndrome. *Child Adolescent Psychiatric Clinics of North America, 12*, 143–163.

Taylor, M. A., & Fink, M. (2003). Catatonia in psychiatric classification: A home of its own. *American Journal of Psychiatry, 160*, 1233–1241.

Tenenbein, M. Toxic ingestions and exposures. In C. D. Rudolph, A. M. Rudolph, M. K. Hostetter, G. Lister, & N. J. Siegel (Eds.), *Rudolph's pediatrics* (21st ed.). New York: McGraw-Hill..

Tillman, R., & Geller, B. (2005). A brief screening tool for a prepuberal and early adolescent bipolar disorder phenotype. *American Journal of Psychiatry, 162*, 1214–1216.

Todd, R. D., & Botteron, K. N. (2002, July). Etiology and genetics of early-onset mood disorders. *Child and Adolescent Psychiatric Clinics of North America, 11*, 499–518.

Tohen, M., Baker, R. W., Altshuler, L., Zarate, C. A., Suppes, T., Ketter, T. A., et al. (2002). Olanzapine versus divalproex in the treatment of acute mania. *American Journal of Psychiatry, 159*, 1011–1017.

Tohen, M., Calabrese, J. R., Sachs, G. S., Banov, M. D., Detke, H. C., Risser, R., et al. (2006, February). Randomized placebo-controlled trial of olanzapine as maintenance therapy in patients with bipolar I disorder responding to acute treatment with olanzapine. *American Journal of Psychiatry, 163*, 247–256.

Tohen, M., Zarate, C. A., Hennen, J., Kaur Khalsa, H. M., Strakowski, S. M., Gebre-Medhin, P., et al. (2003, December). The McLean-Harvard First-Episode Mania Study: Prediction of recovery and first recurrence. *American Journal of Psychiatry, 160*, 2099–2107.

Took, K. J., Buck, B. L., Paradise, N. F., & El-Dadah, M. (2000, October 25–29). *Quetiapine as an alternative to risperidone in children and adolescents with the side effect of weight gain*. Poster session presented at the 52nd Institute of Psychiatric Services, American Psychiatric Association, Philadelphia, Pennsylvania.

Towbin, K. E. (2003). Strategies for pharmacologic treatment of high functioning autism and Asperger's syndrome. *Child Adolescent Psychiatric Clinics of North America, 12*, 23–45.

Tran, P. V., Hamilton, S. H., Kuntz, et al. (1997). Double-blind comparison of olanzapine versus risperidone in the treatment of schizophrenia and other psychotic disorders. *Journal of Clinical Psychopharmacology, 17*, 407–418.

Trimble, M. R. (2003). Epilepsy in England. *CNS Spectrums, 8*, 288.

Tsai, L. Y. (2004). Other pervasive developmental disorders. In J. M. Wiener & M. K. Dulcan (Eds.), *Textbook of child and adolescent psychiatry* (pp. 317–349). Arlington, VA: American Psychiatric Publishing.

Tsai, L. Y., & Champine, D. J. (2004). Schizophrenia and other psychotic disorders. In J. M. Wiener & M. K. Dulcan (Eds.), *Textbook of child and adolescent psychiatry* (pp. 379–435). Arlington, VA: American Psychiatric Publishing.

Tucker, G. J. (2005). Seizures. In J. M. Silver, T. W. McAllister T. W., & Yudofsky, S. C.

(Eds.), *Textbook of traumatic brain injury.* Arlington, VA: American Psychiatric Publishing.

Tucker, M. E. (2004, August). Rising obesity rates boosting liver disease risk. *Clinical Psychiatric News, 39,* 59.

Twemlow, S. W., Fonagy, P., Sacco, F. C., O'Toole, M. E., & Vernberg, E. (2002). Premeditated mass shootings in school: Threat assessment. *Journal of the American Academy of Child and Adolescent Psychiatry, 41,* 475–477.

Ulloa, R. E., Birmaher, B., Axelson, D., Williamson, D. E., Brent, D. A., Ryan, N. D., Bridge, J., & Baugher, M. (2000). Psychosis in a pediatric mood and anxiety disorders clinic: Phenomenology and correlates. *Journal of the American Academy of Child and Adolescent Psychiatry, 39,* 337–345.

Urraca, N., Arenas-Sordo, MdlL., Ortiz-Dominguez, A., Martinez, A., Molina, B., Galvez, A., Nicolini, H. (2005, November). An 8q21 deletion in a patient with comorbid psychosis and mental retardation. *CNS Spectrums, 10,* 864–867.

Van Bellinghen, M., & De Troch, C. (2001). Risperidone in the treatment of behavioral disturbances in children and adolescents with borderline intellectual functioning: A double-blind, placebo-controlled pilot trial. *Journal of Child and Adolescent Psychopharmacology, 11,* 5–13.

Van Os, J., Hanssen, M., Bijl, R. V., & Volleberg, W. (2001, July). Prevalence of psychotic disorder and community level of psychotic symptoms. *Archives of General Psychiatry, 58,* 663–668.

Velligan, D. I. (2003, June). (CME). Case 1. A disorganized lifestyle and irregular schedule lead to partial medication compliance in a patient with schizophrenia. *The Patient Compliance Challenge. Practice with the Experts. Case Reviews in Clinical Psychiatry.* New York: The Albert Einstein College of Medicine; Stanford, CT: Suasion Group.

Velligan, D. I., & Glahn, D. (2004). Treating the cognitive deficits of schizophrenia. In R. O. Friedel & D. L. Evans (Eds.), *Current Psychosis & Therapeutic Reports, Bristol-Myers Squib Co./Otsuka American Pharmaceuticals, 2,* 73–77.

Velligan, D. I., Newcomer, J., Pultz, J., Csernansky, J., Hoff, A. L., Mahurin, R., & Miller, A. L. (2002). Does cognitive function improve with quetiapine in comparison to haloperidol? *Schizophrenia Research, 53,* 239–248.

Victor, M., & Ropper, A. H. (2001). Epilepsy and other seizure disorders. In M. Victor & A. H. Roper (Eds.), *Adams and Victor's principles of neurology* (7th ed., pp. 331–365). New York: McGraw-Hill.

Vieweg, W. V., & Fernandez, A. (2003). How to prevent hyperprolactinemia in patients taking antipsychotics. *Current Psychiatry, 2,* 57–64.

Vieweg, W. V., & McDaniel, N. L. (2003-I, February). Drug-induced QT interval prolongation and torsade de pointes in children and adolescents. Part I. *Child and Adolescent Psychopharmacology News, 8,* 1–7.

Vieweg, W. V., & McDaniel, N. L. (2003-III, May). Drug-induced QT interval prolongation and torsade de pointes in children and adolescents. Part III. *Child and Adolescent Psychopharmacology News, 8,* 1–4.

Vinks, A. A., & Watson, P. D. (2003). Pharmacokinetics I: Developmental principles. In A Martin, L. Scahill, D. S. Charney, & J. F. Leckman (Eds.), *Pediatric psychopharmacology, principles and practices* (pp. 44–53). New York: Oxford University Press.

Vitiello, B., Riddle, M. A., Greenhill, L. L., March, J. S., Levine, J., Schachar, R. J., et al. (2003). How can we improve the assessment of safety in child and adolescent psychopharmacology? *Journal of the American Academy of Child and Adolescent Psychiatry, 42,* 634–641.

Volkmar, F. R. (1994). Childhood disintegrative disorder. *Child and Adolescent Psychiatric Clinics of North America, 3,* 119–129.

Volkmar, F. R. (1996). Childhood and adolescent psychosis: A review of the past 10 years. *Journal of the American Academy of Child and Adolescent Psychiatry, 35,* 843–851.

Wabitsch, M. (2002). Molecular and biological factors with emphasis on adipose tissue development. In W. Burniat, T. Cole, I. Lissau, & E. Poskitt (Eds.), *Child and adolescent obesity* (pp. 50–63). Cambridge University Press.

Wadden, T. A., Berkowitz, R. I., Womble, L. G., Sarwer, D. B., Phelan, S., Cato, R. K., et al. (2005, November 17). Randomized trial of lifestyle modification and pharmacotherapy for obesity. *The New England Journal of Medicine, 353,* 2111–2120.

Wagner, K. D., Kowatch, R. A., Findling, R. L., et al. (2005, October 18–23.). *Oxcarbazepine in the treatment of children with bipolar disorder: A multicenter, double-blind, placebo-controlled trial.* Poster session at the Joint Annual Meeting of the American Academy of Child and Adolescent Psychiatry and Canadian Academy of Child and Adolescent Psychiatry, Toronto, Canada.

Wahlbeck, K., Tuunainen, A., Ahokas, A., & Leucht, S. (2001). Dropout rates in randomized antipsychotic drug trials. *Psychopharmacology, 155,* 230–233.

Walker, E., Kestler, L., Bollini, A., & Hochman, K. M. (2004). Schizophrenia: etiology and course. *Annual Review of Psychology, 55,* 401–430.

Wang, P. S., Walker, A. M., Tsuang, M. T. et al. (2002). Dopamine antagonists and the development of breast cancer. *Archives of General Psychiatry, 59,* 1147–1154.

Wassef, A. A., Winkler, D. E., Roache, A. L. Boma Abobo, V., Lopez, L. M., Averill, J. P., et al. (2005, February). Lower effectiveness of divalproex versus valproic acid in a prospective, quasi-experimental clinical trial involving 9,260 psychiatric admissions. *American Journal of Psychiatry, 162,* 330–339.

Webb, R., Abel, K., Pickles, A., & Appleby, L. (2005). Mortality in offspring of parents with psychotic disorder: A critical review and meta-analysis. *American Journal of Psychiatry, 162,* 1045–1056.

Weiden, P. J. (2002). Why did John Nash stop his medications. *Journal of Psychiatric Practice, 8,* 386–392.

Weiden, P. J., Simpson, G. M., Potkin, S. G., & O'Sullivan, R. L. (2003, May). Effectiveness of switching to ziprasidone for stable but symptomatic outpatients with schizophrenia. *Journal of Clinical Psychiatry, 64,* 580–588.

Weinberg, W. A., Harper, C. R., & Brumback, R. A. (1998). Examination II: Clinical evaluation of cognitive/behavioral function. In C. E. Coffey & R. A. Brumback (Eds.), *Textbook of Pediatric Neuropsychiatry.* Washington, DC: American Psychiatric Press.

Weisbrot, D., & Ettinger, A. B. (2001). Psychiatric aspects of pediatric epilepsy. In A. B. Ettinger & A. M. Kanner (Eds.), *Psychiatric issues in epilepsy, a practical guide to diagnosis and treatment.* Philadelphia: Lippincott Williams & Wilkins.

Weller, E. B., Kloos, A. L., Hitchcock, S., & Weller, R. A. (2005, August). Are anticonvulsants safe for pediatric bipolar disorder? *Current Psychiatry, 4,* 31–48.

Weller, E. B., Weller, R. A., & Danielyan, A. K. (2004). Mood disorders in prepuberal children. In J. M. Wiener & M. K. Dulcan (Eds.), *Textbook of child and adolescent psychiatry* (pp. 411–435). Arlington, VA: American Psychiatric Publishing.

Werry, J. S., McClellan, J. M., & Chard, L. (1991). Childhood and adolescent schizophrenia, bipolar and schizoaffective disorders. A clinical outcome study. *Journal of The American Academy of Child and Adolescent Psychiatry, 30,* 457–465.

Wicks, S., Hjern, A., Gunnell, D, Lewis, G., & Dalman, C. (2005). Social adversity in childhood and the risk of developing psychosis: A national cohort study. *American Journal of Psychiatry, 162,* 1637–1643.

Wilkaitis, J., Mulvihill, T., & Nasrallah, H. A. (2004). Classic antipsychotic medications. In A. F. Schatzberg & C. B. Nemeroff (Eds.), *Textbook of psychopharmacology* (pp. 425–441). Arlington, VA: American Psychiatric Publishing.

Winans, E. (2003). Switching antipsychotics. A balanced approach to ease the transition. *Current Psychiatry, 2,* 52–64.

Williams, D. T. (1996). Neuropsychiatric signs, symptoms, and syndromes. In M. Lewis (Ed.), *Child and Adolescent Psychiatry. A Comprehensive Textbook* (2nd ed., pp. 344–249). Baltimore, MD: Williams & Wilkins.

Williams, H. J., Glaser, B., Williams, N. M., Norton, N., Zammit, S., Macgregor, S., et al. (2005). No association between schizophrenia and polymorphisms in COMT in two large samples. *American Journal of Psychiatry, 162,* 1736–1738.

Winnas, E. A. (2003, August). Switching antipsychotics. A balanced approach to ease the transition. *Current Psychiatry, 2,* 52–64.

Wirshing, D. A., Danovitch, I., Erhart, S. M., Pierre, J. M., &Wirshing, W. C. (2003). Update on atypicals, Practical tips to manage common side effects. *Current Psychiatry, 2,* 49–57.

Wise, M. G., & Brandt, G. T. (1992). Delirium. In S. C. Yudofsky & R. E. Hales (Eds.), *The American Psychiatric Press textbook of neuropsychiatry* (2nd ed.). Washington, DC: American Psychiatric Press.

Woerner, M. G., Robinson, D. G., Alvir, J. M. J., Sheitman, B. B., Lieberman, J. A., & Kane, J. M. (2003). Clozapine as a first treatment of schizophrenia. *American Journal of Psychiatry, 160,* 1514–1516.

Woods, S. W., Martin, A., Spector, S. G., & McGlashan, T. H. (2002). Effects of development on olanzapine-associated adverse events. *Journal of the American Academy of Child and Adolescent Psychiatry, 41,* 1439–1446.

Wozniak, J., & Biederman, J. (1996). A pharmacological approach to the quagmire of comorbidity in juvenile mania. *Journal of The American Academy of Child and Adolescent Psychiatry, 35,* 926–928.

Yanovski, J. A., & Yanovski, S. Z. (2003). Treatment of pediatric and adolescent obesity. *Journal of the American Medical Association, 289,* 1851–1853.

Yatham, L. N., Grossman, F., Augustyns, I., Vieta, E., & Ravindran, A. (2003). Mood stabilizers plus risperidone or placebo in the treatment of acute mania. *British Journal of Psychiatry, 182,* 141–147.

Yu, V. (2004, September). considering inherited, basal ganglia diseases in the differential diagnosis of first-episode psychosis. *Primary Psychiatry, 11,* 69–72.

Yung, A. R., & McGorry, P. D. (2004). Precursors of schizophrenia. In R. O. Friedel & D. L. Evans (Eds.), *Current Psychosis & Therapeutic Reports, Bristol-Myers Squib Co./ Otsuka America Pharmaceutical,* (Vol. 2, pp. 67–72).

Yurgelun-Todd, D. A., & Renshaw, P. F. (2000). MRS in child psychiatric disorders. In M. Ernst & J M. Rumsey (Eds.), *Functional neuroimaging in child psychiatry* (pp. 59–76). Cambridge, UK: Cambridge University Press.

Zametkin, A. J., Zoon, C. K., Klein, H. W., & Munson, S. (2004). Psychiatric aspects of child and adolescent obesity: A review of the past 10 years. *Journal of the American Academy of Child and Adolescent Psychiatry, 43*, 134–150.

Zarcone, J. R., Hellings, J. A., Crandall, K., Reese, R. M., Marquis, J., Fleming, K., et al. (2001). Effects of risperidone on aberrant behavior of persons with developmental disabilities: I. A double-blind crossover study using multiple measures. *American Journal of Mental Retardation,106*, 525–538.

Zareba, W., & Lin, D. A. (2003). Antipsychotic drugs and qt interval prolongation. *Psychiatric Quarterly, 74*, 291–306.

Zoler, M. (2004, August). Obesity beats alcohol use as risk factor for liver disease. *Clinical Psychiatric News*, 59.

Zonfrillo, M. R., Penn, J. V., & Leonard, H. L. (2005, August). Pediatric polypharmacy. *Psychiatry, 2*, 14–19.

Zwiauer, K. F. M., Caroli, M., Malecka-Tendera, E., & Poskitt, E. M. E. (2002). Clinical features, adverse effects and outcome. In W. Burniat, T. Cole, I. Lissau, & E. Poskitt (Eds.), *Child and adolescent obesity* (pp. 131–153). Cambridge University Press.

Zygmunt, A., Olfson, M., Boyer, C. A., & Mechanic, D. (2002). Interventions to improve adherence in schizophrenia. *American Journal of Psychiatry, 159*, 1653–1664.

Web Sites

Striatal volume changes in the rat following long-term administration of typical and atypical antipsychotic drugs. Retrieved http://www.acnp.org/citations/Npp011402225

http://www.torsades.org/ for information related to QTc prolongation and related issues.

http://www.preskorn.com for psychiatric drug interactions

htpp://www.drug-interactions.com for Cythochrome 450 interactions

http://vm.cfsan.fda.gov/~lrd/fdinter.html FDA food and drug interactions

http://www.personalhealthzone.com/herbsafety.html for herbal–drug interactions

http://www.hiv-druginteractions.org/ for HIV drug interactions

http://www.projinf.org/fs/drugin.html for HIV Interactions

http://www.powermetdesign.com/grapefruit/ for grapefruit juice drug interactions

www.cdc.gov/growthcharts for BMI charts for boys and girls.

www.research.buffalo.edu/quarterly/vol10/num02/f1.shtml. for information about the Stoplight Diet

http://www.PharmacyOneSource.comMembers:DrugInformation

http://www.26.addr.com/~y/mn/ New articles on schizophrenia

http://www.stanleylab.org/ The Stanley Division of Developmental Neurobiology, Johns Hopkins University

http://www.hubin.org/index_en.html Hubin Human Brain Informatics

http://www.abilify.com Caregiver's roadmap for family and friends

http://www.psychiatry.unc.edu/STEP/step.htm Schizophrenia treatment and evaluation program (Department of Psychiatry, University of North Carolina)

http://www.dbsalliance.org/indcex.html Depression and Bipolar Support Alliance

http://intramural.nimh.nih.gov/mood/index.html Mood and Anxiety Disorders Program

http://www.nelh.nhs.uk Center for Evidence-Based Medicine, Oxford, UK

http://www.psych.org/clin_res/bipolar_revisebook_index.cfm American Psychiatric Association Clinical Resources

http://www.bpkids.org/ The Child and Adolescent Bipolar Foundation

http://www.drada.org/ Depression and Related Disorders Association

http://cebmh.warne.ox.ac.uk/cebmh/nelmh/schizophrenia/index.html National Electronic Library for Mental Health

http://www.psychosissupport.com/ Peer Support for Parents of Psychosis Sufferers

http://www.iris-initiative.org.uk/guidelines.htm Initiative to Reduce the Impact of Schizophrenia

http://www.psychosissucks.ca/epi/ Psychosis Intervention Program

http://www.clozarilregistry.com Clozaril Administration Registry Enrollment

http://www.clozapineregistry.com Clozapine Patient Registry

http://www.bpkids.org/learning/6-02.pdf To obtain samples of mood charts

http://www.aacap.org American Academy of Child and Adolescent Psychiatry

http://www.aap.org American Academy of Pediatrics

http://www.autism-society.org Autism Society of America

http://www.bpkids.org Child and Adolescent Bipolar Foundation, provides education about pediatric bipolar disorder.

http://www.dbsalliance.org Depression and Bipolar Disorder Support Alliance (DBSA)

http://www.jbrf.org Juvenile Bipolar Research Foundation

http://www.maapservices.org MAAP Service for Autism and Asperger's syndrome

http://www. nami.org National Alliance for the Mentally Ill (NAMI)

http://www.narsad.org National Alliance for Research on Schizophrenia and Depression

http://www.nimh.nih.org National Institute of Mental Health

http://www.nmha.org National Mental Health Association

http://www.schizophrenia.com provides high quality information and education for patients, caregivers, and families.

Index

Page numbers in italics refer to Tables or Figures.

525

side effects, 369–370
Ventricular size, 108
Very early onset schizophrenia, 171–176, 188,
  222–225
  differential diagnosis, 176–178
  drawings, *98,* 98–100, *99, 100*
  prevalence, 173–176
  risperidone, 342
Victimization, 14–15
Violence
  command hallucinations, 80
  delusions, 78
  risk assessment, 78–82, *79*
Visceral hallucinations, drug related, 130
Visual attention, 107
Visual hallucinations
  drug related, 129, 130
  elements, *29,* 29–38, *30*
Vocational goals, 249–250
Vocational problems, 13–14

Voice identity, auditory hallucinations, 33
Vulnerability markers, *289*

W
WASH-U-KSADS, 103
Weapons, 68
Weight gain
  antipsychotics, 381–383
  mood stabilizers, 12
  second generation antipsychotics, 300, *301*
White matter diseases, 137–139
Wilson's disease, 139
Wraparound, 267–268

Z
Ziprasidone, 352–356, *356*
  clinical acivity, 354–355
  dosing, 354, *356*
  drug interactions, 445–446
    concurrent use contraindicated, 446